RESPIRATORY CARE REGISTRY GUIDE

RESPIRATORY CARE REGISTRY GUIDE

James R. Sills, M.Ed., C.P.F.T., R.R.T.

Director, Respiratory Care Programs
Rock Valley College
Rockford, Illinois

M Mosby

St. Louis   Baltimore   Berlin   Boston   Carlsbad   Chicago   London   Madrid
Naples   New York   Philadelphia   Sydney   Tokyo   Toronto

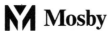

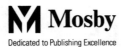
Mosby

Dedicated to Publishing Excellence

Editor: James Shanahan
Developmental Editor: Jennifer Roche
Cover Designer: Sheilah Barrett
Manufacturing Supervisor: Kathy Grone

Printed in the United States of America
Composition by TCSystems, Inc.
Printing/binding by Western Publishing Company

Mosby-Year Book, Inc.
11830 Westline Industrial Drive
St. Louis, MO 63146

International Standard Book Number 0-8016-6201-X

94 95 96 97 98 9 8 7 6 5 4 3 2 1

This book is dedicated to my wife Deborah and our children Rachael and David, who make my life full and complete and will now have me back as a full-time husband and parent; our dog Amber, who still keeps me company when I work at home; my parents; and all of my past, present, and future students.

The journey of 1000 miles begins with a single step.

Hope for the best but plan for the worst.

FOREWORD

The *Respiratory Care Registry Guide* completes the set of two books designed to prepare graduates of respiratory care programs for the Entry Level Examination and the Advanced Practitioner Examinations. In this textbook, the reader is given a clear and precise presentation of the advanced areas of knowledge, skills, and professional attributes that are identified by the National Board for Respiratory Care (NBRC) as essential for **respiratory therapists.** Similar to Jim Sills' first textbook, the *Respiratory Care Certification Guide,* this textbook is based on the NBRC's *most recent* Written Registry Examination Content Outline. Additionally, there is invaluable information *and practice* for the Clinical Simulation Examination. Thus, if your goal is to successfully pass the Written Registry Examination and Clinical Simulation Examinations—and to earn the Registered Respiratory Therapist (RRT) credential—this textbook now serves as your outstanding resource.

The first book in the set, *Respiratory Care Certification Guide* (now in its second edition), provides the reader with the basic knowledge, skills, and professional attributes that are identified by the NBRC for **entry level practitioners.** Thus, if your goal is to successfully pass the NBRC's Entry Level Exam—and to earn the Certified Respiratory Therapy Technician (CRTT) credential—the *Respiratory Care Certification Guide* is the superb resource.

With the completion of this nicely written and straightforward set of textbooks, both the student and the educator can now quickly and easily retrieve what the essential curricular base is, according to the NBRC, for either the technician or the therapist. I am confident that Jim's contributions to the profession of respiratory care will long be appreciated.

Terry Des Jardins, M.Ed., R.R.T.
Parkland College
Department of Respiratory Care
Champaign, Illinois

PREFACE

This textbook, *Respiratory Care Registry Guide*, is designed to complement and supplement *Respiratory Care Certification Guide*, which was written for technician students or anyone preparing for the certification examination. This book is written for therapist students or anyone preparing for the registry examinations. I have attempted to write a standard textbook that covers all the material that the National Board for Respiratory Care (NBRC) has determined therapists, on a national level, must know about or be able to perform. I hope that it proves helpful to those individuals who aspire to become registered respiratory therapists and to advance themselves within our profession.

A close look at the format and content shows that this book is similar in style to *Respiratory Care Certification Guide*. Hopefully, this will make it easier for the user to determine what it is that a *therapist* needs to know in contrast to what it is that a *technician* needs to know. As an educator speaking to other educators, I would suggest that this book is not appropriate for use in technician programs. Educators in 1 + 1 technician and therapist programs will find that *Respiratory Care Certification Guide* is well suited for technician-level students, whereas this book is designed for therapist-level students. Educators in therapist programs should use both books. Corresponding sections can be easily matched when a particular subject is presented (e.g., Pulmonary Function Testing). The overlap in content that is sometimes seen is unavoidable. This is because of the way that the NBRC has differentiated the knowledge, skills, and attitudes required of technicians and therapists on a national level. These different abilities have been incorporated into the two levels of credentialing exams. Although the therapist student needs to "know it all," he or she will only be tested on some of that knowledge and skill on the Entry Level Exam. Other areas will be tested on the Advanced Practitioners Examinations.

James R. Sills, M.Ed., C.P.F.T., R.R.T.

INTRODUCTION FOR STUDENTS AND EDUCATORS

This book is designed to cover in detail all the knowledge areas and skills required and tested of therapists on the registry exams by the National Board for Regulatory Care (NBRC). To offer some guidance on what can be tested, the NBRC has made up two detailed lists. One is the Examination Content Outline for the Entry Level Exam. That list was used in the design of *Respiratory Care Certification Guide*. The second list is the Examination Content Outline for the Written Registry Exam. It was used in the design of this textbook. This second list is also useful in preparing for the Clinical Simulation Exam. These two lists were released to all respiratory care programs in July or August 1993.

It is assumed that the student using this book is already certified. If not, refer to *Respiratory Care Certification Guide,* or other standard textbooks, for guidance on preparing for the Entry Level Examination to earn the Certified Respiratory Therapy Technician (CRTT) credential. This book will build on that important foundation to help the therapist student prepare for the Advanced Practitioner Examinations to earn the Registered Respiratory Therapist (RRT) credential.

The sections in this text are designed to progress logically from patient assessment through the various floor therapies to mechanical ventilation and, finally, special procedures. Patient assessment should be reviewed with each specific therapy and procedure because it is the cornerstone of appropriate care. Each section is followed by a series of self-assessment questions to help the student judge his or her understanding. In addition, two posttests are offered. The first is modeled after the Written Registry Examination and the second offers two problems similar to those seen on the Clinical Simulation Examination. Together they should help the student prepare for the Advanced Practitioner Examinations because both must be passed to become a registered respiratory therapist. See the Introduction for Examinees for more information on how to prepare for these two exams.

Almost every heading that is used in this text is followed by two specially marked codes. The first, (**NBRC tested**), indicates which subjects are specifically listed in the Detailed Content Outline. The user may wish to refer back to the outline for the specific wording used by the NBRC. Occasionally a heading will appear without an NBRC coding after it. Sometimes these headings are added in because they are vital to understanding what the NBRC is testing. This background information will not, in itself, be tested; however, it must be understood to grasp what will be tested. Other non-NBRC coded headings are added because the information has appeared on one or more of the Advanced Practitioner Examinations, but is not specifically listed on the Detailed Content Outline. (It must be understood that at times the NBRC uses rather broad language.)

The second code [**in brackets**] is the NBRC code for the difficulty level of the questions that will be used to test the examinee's understanding of the material. **R** stands for Recall. **Ap** stands for Application. **An** stands for Analysis. See the Introduction for Examinees for a more detailed explanation, if needed.

It is important to understand also what this text does *not* discuss. The learner and educator must look elsewhere for textbooks on human anatomy and physiology, microbiology, mathematics/algebra, chemistry, or any other areas that may be important background information for the therapist student. It is certainly important for the student to have a solid understanding of these areas to which he or she can add understanding of the science of respiratory care. These subjects are not presented in this text because they will not be tested by the NBRC on the Advanced Practitioner Examinations. Although cardiopulmonary pathologic and abnormal conditions are specifically listed on the Detailed Examination Outline, it is beyond the scope of this text to specifically address the various cardiopulmonary pathologic conditions in detail. Some discussion of pathologic processes is included in the general discussion of each section as it relates to the treatment or procedure that the respiratory therapist would perform. It is recommended that the student study the major types of adult and infant disease states and abnormal conditions.

INTRODUCTION FOR EXAMINEES

A graduate of a therapist program who is preparing for the Advanced Practitioner Examinations (Written Registry Exam and Clinical Simulation Exam) can use this text to help focus on what needs to be studied. Just as important, it will help in understanding what will *not* be on the exams. Some of what you learned has already been tested on the Entry Level Examination. In addition, some therapist program graduates may find that part of the information that they studied will not be tested on the Advanced Practitioners Examinations. It is also important to realize that although the National Board for Respiratory Care (NBRC) will not test you on the same information twice, you cannot afford to forget what was studied in preparation for the Entry Level Examination.

Almost every heading that is used in this text is followed by two codes. The first, (**NBRC tested**), indicates that the subject is listed in the Examination Content Outline. The user may wish to refer to the outline for specific wording used by the NBRC. My choice of words is a paraphrasing of theirs. Occasionally a heading will appear without an NBRC coding after it. Sometimes headings are added because they are vital in understanding what the NBRC is testing. This background information will not, in itself, be tested, but the information must be understood to grasp what will be tested. Other non-NBRC coded headings are added because the information has appeared on one or more Advanced Practioner Examinations but is not specifically listed on the Detailed Content Outline. Finally, even though cardiopulmonary pathologic and abnormal conditions are specifically listed on the Examination Content Outline it is beyond the scope of this text to specifically address the various cardiopulmonary pathologic conditions. Some discussion of pathologic processes is included in the general discussion of each section as it relates to the treatment or procedure that the respiratory therapist would perform. It is recommended that the examinee study the major types of adult and infant disease states and abnormal conditions.

The second code, [**in brackets**], is the NBRC code for the difficulty level of the questions asked on the Written Registry Examination. **R** stands for Recall. **Ap** stands for Application. **An** stands for Analysis. More information on this follows.

Written Registry Examination

The Written Registry Examination (WRE) is a 100-question, multiple choice exam that the examinee is given 2 hours to complete. The exam is designed to sample understanding of the full range of knowledge, skills, and professional attitudes that a therapist is expected to display. This textbook is written to cover that entire scope of practice; however, it is impossible to know the content of any given examination. The

NBRC is continuously updating its question bank and creating new exams. Two or three different versions are given at a single time. Therefore your exam may not be the same as someone next to you. Older versions are retired and later offered for sale by Applied Measurement Professionals as self-assessment exams. As mentioned earlier, the examinee will find that the NBRC asks questions at these three different levels of difficulty:

Recall [R]

Recall refers to remembering some factual information that was previously learned. "Identify" would be a commonly used action verb in these types of questions. The examinee may be asked to identify specific facts, terms, methods, procedures, principles, concepts, and so forth.

Prepare for these types of questions by studying the full range of factual information, equations, and so forth seen in respiratory care practice. These types of questions are on the lowest order of difficulty. You either know the answer or you do not; there is little to ponder more deeply. It is very important to have a solid understanding of the factual basis of respiratory care to do well in this and the next two categories of questions. The Written Registry Examination is *less* heavily weighted with Recall questions than the Entry Level Exam.

Application [Ap]

Application refers to being able to use factual type information in real clinical situations that may be new to you. "Apply," "classify," and "calculate" would be commonly used action verbs in these types of questions. The examinee may be asked to apply laws, theories, concepts, and/or principles to new, practical clinical situations. Calculations may have to be performed. Charts and graphs, such as seen in pulmonary function testing, may need to be used.

These types of questions are on a higher order of difficulty than the Recall [R] types. Critical thinking must be applied to the factual information to answer these questions.

Analysis [An]

Analysis refers to being able to separate a patient care problem into its component parts or elements to evaluate the relationship of the parts or elements to the whole problem. "Evaluate," "compare," "contrast," "revise," and/or "select" would be commonly used action verbs in these types of questions. You may be questioned about revising a patient care plan or evaluating therapy.

These types of questions require the highest level of critical thinking. You may have to recall previously learned information, apply it to a patient care situation, and make a judgment as to the best way to care for the patient. The Written Registry

Examination is *more* heavily weighted with Analysis type questions than the Entry Level Exam.

The examinee will find that the Written Registry Examination has these two different types of questions:

One Best Answer (Multiple Choice)

This type of question has a stem (the question) followed by four possible answers coded A, B, C, and D. You must select the *best* answer from among those presented. Only one is clearly best even though other possible answers may be good. Carefully read the stem to make sure that you do not misunderstand the clear intent of the question. Controversial issues may be questioned. The use of "should" in the stem will clue you in to the need to select the answer that would be selected by the majority of practitioners.

Some questions may be worded in a way that you need to exclude a *false* answer. In other words, four answers are correct and one is incorrect. The use of EXCEPT will clue you in to this type of question.

Multiple True-False (Multiple-Multiple Choice)

This type of question has a stem (the question) followed by five possible answers coded with roman numerals I, II, III, IV, and V; then four combinations of the answers coded by letters A, B, C, and D. The stem may ask you to include all true statements or all false statements in the final answer. You must select the letter that represents the correct combination of answers.

There should not be any controversial answers offered. They are all either clearly correct or incorrect. That is the key to selecting the best answer. Read each possible answer as separate from the others. It is suggested that you mark each possible answer as true or false. Next, find the final answer from among those offered. Even if you do not find a final answer that included all the answers that you selected, you will be able to find the best answer through the process of eliminating the final answers offered that you know are incorrect.

Situational Sets

These are only seen on the Entry Level Examination. They have been replaced with the Clinical Simulation Examination for advanced practitioners.

Suggestions for Preparing for the Written Registry Examination

1. Pace yourself so that you have enough time to get through the 100 questions before the 2-hour time limit is reached. That works out to 1.2 minutes or

72 seconds per question. You should be at about question 25 in ½ an hour, question 50 in 1 hour, and so forth. Put a check mark by any difficult questions that you skip. This will help to prevent from marking your answers out of sequence. Come back if there is time at the end. Do not leave any blank questions. You will not be penalized for guessing on the last few questions if you are running out of time.

2. Completely read each question. Determine what it is that you are really being asked. Look for qualifying words such as not, except, most, least desirable, undesirable, and so forth.

3. Separate the important information from that which is not important. Many questions contain patient information and data on blood gases, pulmonary function, hemodynamics, ventilator settings, and so forth. Disregard what does not pertain to the question being asked. Interpret the important data.

4. Do not read beyond the question. Resist the temptation to "psych out" what you think the question writer wants. Use only what is given to you.

5. Carefully read every answer that is offered.

6. In one best answer (multiple choice) questions, pick the best one that is offered. The answer that you might like best may not be offered. Regardless, you must pick from among those that are offered.

7. In multiple true-false (multiple-multiple choice) questions, use the following strategy: a) Find an option that you know to be incorrect. Cross off any of the answers that contain it. b) Find an option that you know to be correct. Cross off any answers that do not contain it. c) Find the remaining question. It must be correct.

8. Again, answer every question. There is no penalty for guessing incorrectly.

9. Take a practice Written Registry Examination under actual testing conditions. Evaluate your strengths and weaknesses and spend more time studying your weak areas. A practice exam is offered at the end of this book in Appendix 1. Others are available, for a fee, from Applied Measurement Professionals.

Relative Weights of the Various Tested Areas on the Written Registry Exam

I have attempted to analyze the content of each of the 100 questions on versions I, II, and III of the Written Registry Self-Assessment Examination. Each question has been placed into one of the following sections. The numbers of questions and percentages are averages and may not be followed exactly on other versions of the examination. However, the relative weights can offer some guidance as to what content is relatively more important or less important. Study time can be spent accordingly.

Sections	*Questions/ Percentage*
1. Patient Assessment	12
2. Blood Gas Analysis and Monitoring	4
3. Pulmonary Function Testing	11
4. Advanced Cardiopulmonary Monitoring	14
5. Oxygen and Helium/Oxygen Therapy	5
6. Hyperinflation Therapy	1
7. Humidity and Aerosol Therapy	3
8. Pharmacology	8
9. Postural Drainage Therapy	1
10. Cardiopulmonary Resuscitation (Emergency Care)	4
11. Airway Management	8
12. Suctioning the Airway	1
13. Intermittent Positive Pressure Breathing (IPPB)	1
14. Mechanical Ventilation of the Adult	16
15. Mechanical Ventilation of the Neonate	2
16. Home Care and Pulmonary Rehabilitation	2
17. Special Procedures	7
TOTAL	100

It is my opinion that the content of Sections 1, 2, 3, and 4 must be thoroughly understood. This information is questioned directly and also incorporated into questions covering all the other sections. The content in Section 14 is the most heavily questioned.

Clinical Simulation Examination

The Clinical Simulation Examination (CSE) is composed of 10 broad-based problems. They are designed to evaluate how well the examinee is able to gather information, evaluate it, and make clinical decisions that relate to simulated real patient situations. This test does *not* look at the recollection of simple facts. Table I-1 lists the types of patient care problems that may be seen.

The examination process is unique for three reasons. First, the answers are printed with invisible ink (so-called latent image). They are only revealed when a special felt tip marker is rubbed over them. There is no way to erase an answer if you should change your mind later. Second, problems are designed in a branching logic format. This means that there is more than one way to solve them. To some extent, you choose your own pathway; however, there is only one that is best. There may be one or two that are acceptable. There may be another one or two that are unacceptable. Third, the pages that make up the 10 problems are scrambled within the examination booklet. You will not start on the first page and work your way through to the last. Rather, you will be flipping back and forth through the booklet as the scenario directs you. It is

Table I-1. A Common Mix of 10 Problems Found on the Clinical Simulation Examination

1. Two problems deal with a chronic obstructive pulmonary disease patient (asthma, emphysema, bronchitis). This may include, but is not limited to, oxygen therapy, pulmonary function testing, home care, rehabilitation, preoperative and postoperative care, mechanical ventilation, and so forth.
2. One problem deals with a trauma patient. This could be a chest, spinal, head, or other injury.
3. One problem deals with a cardiovascular disease patient. This could be a patient with congestive heart failure, myocardial infarct, chest pain, mitral stenosis, preoperative and postoperative open heart surgery, and so forth.
4. One problem deals with a patient with neuromuscular disease. This could include a patient with muscular dystrophy, myasthenia gravis, Guillain-Barré syndrome, and so forth.
5. One problem deals with a neonate or infant. This could involve management in the delivery room, neonatal resuscitation, infant apnea, meconium aspiration, infant respiratory distress syndrome (IRDS), congenital heart defects, and so forth.
6. One problem deals with a child. This could involve epiglottitis, laryngotracheobronchitis (croup), asthma, cystic fibrosis, aspiration of a foreign body, ingestion of a toxic substance, and so forth.
7. Three miscellaneous problems do not fit into the above categories. These may include drug overdose; smoke inhalation; carbon monoxide inhalation; surface burns; cardiopulmonary resuscitation; obesity; hypothermia; thoracic, abdominal, neck, or head surgery; acquired immunodeficiency syndrome (AIDS); near drowning; and so forth.

extremely important that you do not cross over from one scenario to another as you turn through the pages. (More suggestions on how to avoid mistakes with the examination process will be given later.) The examinee is allowed 4 hours to complete the exam. That works out to 20 minutes per problem.

There are three components to the clinical simulation problem: a) the scenario, b) information-gathering sections, and c) decision-making sections. Each is discussed in turn.

Scenario

The scenario establishes the setting for the patient and for you as the respiratory therapist. Typically, it includes the type of hospital, where the patient is within the hospital, and the time of day. General information about the patient is given such as his or her name, age, sex, some general presenting conditions, and a brief history of the illness or event. Your role as a respiratory therapist is described. You may have to gather more information or may need to make a clinical decision. Determine if the situation is an emergency. If it is, you will have to take immediate steps to help the patient. (The examinee should assume that any and all services needed to give optimal care are available in any of the patient scenarios.)

Information-Gathering Sections

Usually the respiratory therapist is directed to gather more information. A list of about 15 to 30 parameters will be available from which to choose; for example, vital signs, blood gases, pulmonary function tests, various laboratory studies, and so forth. You will be instructed to select as many as you feel are important based on what you know at that point in time. Obviously, do not select information that is unnecessarily risky, irrelevant, delays care, and so forth. The latent image marker is now used to reveal the data. Interpret the data that you find to make proper decisions in the next section. When you have finished gathering and interpreting the data, you will be directed to go to a decision-making section.

Decision-Making Sections

It is now required that you make a decision on the best care for the patient based on the information that you have at this point in time. Usually you are instructed to "choose only one" from 4 to 8 options. One of the choices is best, one or two may be acceptable, and the others are not acceptable. The

Table I-2. Scoring of the Clinical Simulation Problem and Examination

All the options selected on each problem are scored on the following scale. The score is based on how appropriate it is to the condition of the patient at the time it was selected.

Score	Rationale
+3	Critically important for good patient care. It is necessary for prompt, proper care. Omitting it would result in the patient being seriously damaged from delays in care, pain, cost, and increased chance of morbidity and/or mortality.
+2	Very important for good patient care.
+1	Helpful for good patient care.
0	Neither helpful nor harmful to patient care.
−1	Somewhat counterproductive to good patient care.
−2	Quite counterproductive to good patient care.
−3	Extremely counterproductive to good patient care. Detrimental to prompt, proper care. Its inclusion will result in the patient being seriously damaged from delays in care, pain, cost, and increased chance of morbidity and/or mortality.

Each problem is individually scored for information-gathering and decision-making based on the judgment of the problem author and the examination committee. The scores in these two areas on all 10 problems are totaled to give two final scores. Both the information-gathering and decision-making areas must be passed to pass the examination. The examination committee determines the two required scores to pass the Clinical Simulation Examination. Because these scores may vary from exam to exam, it is not possible to predict a minimal pass level for any given examination offering.

latent image marker is used to reveal the answer. Usually it will say "Physician agrees. Done," or something to that affect. One or more of the available answers will reveal "Physician disagrees. Make another selection in this section" when it is exposed. This may or may not mean that a bad choice was made. It is possible that the author of the scenario does not want to follow that particular course of action.

Occasionally, you will be directed to "select as many as indicated" for the situation you are dealing with. This would solve a scenario where proper care would involve several procedures being done simultaneously with a patient.

Whether you are directed to make one or several decisions, when finished you will be instructed to go to a new area. This usually takes you to another information-gathering section. You will now need to evaluate how the patient responded to your earlier decision. You will then need to make another decision on care. This pattern will repeat itself until the problem is ended. You will then go on to the next problem until all 10 have been completed. See Table I-2 for how this unique examination is scored.

Suggestions for Preparing for the Clinical Simulation Examination
Things you should do:

1. Carefully follow all directions. If instructed to make only one choice, make only one. Remember, incorrect choices *cannot* be erased. Visually check the section heading for the patient's name and section heading before revealing any choices. This will prevent you from accidentally skipping from one simulation problem to another. This kind of technical error can result in both problems not being scored any further than where the error occurred.
2. Read the scenario to understand the patient's situation and what you are required to do. Is this an emergency? If it is, you will only want to gather the most vital information needed to make a decision on care. Quick action will be required to decide on the best care to give. If it is not an emergency, a more thorough gathering of data is called for. Then, a more well-considered decision for patient care can be made.
3. Thoroughly read all options. With information-gathering sections, lightly mark each desirable option with a pencil before revealing it with the latent image marker. Choose all the options that will give you important information. You will be penalized for skipping over important data and also for making dangerous or wasteful choices. When sure of your selections, reveal them all and then review and interpret them. Avoid the temptation to reveal and interpret one piece of data at a time. You may mistakenly decide not to gather some important

information later. Get the exam supervisor if an answer cannot be read or if the booklet is defective.

4. Try to visualize yourself in the real situation as described. Do what it is that you would do on the job. Make the best choice(s) that you can based on what you know at this point in time. This is true for both information-gathering and decision-making sections. It may be necessary to go back over past information or choices.

5. It is recommended that you make a map of where you have been for each of the 10 problems. This will help you go back to past choices. There are some blank pages included in the test booklet. Notes and calculations can also be written down. It is acceptable to write in the left-hand margin of the test booklet. Do not write in the areas where the latent image answers will appear, on the right-hand margin, or near the bar codes.

6. Completely expose all answers. You will know that the end of an answer has been reached when a double asterisk (**) is revealed. Note: A partially exposed answer (even if accidental) will be counted against you if you are only to make one choice and then make another. In this case, continue with your first choice in that section even if it is not really what you want. If two choices are revealed in a "make one choice" area, the problem will not be scored beyond that point.

7. If a technical error was made, clearly and precisely describe it on the inside of the front cover of your exam booklet. For example, "In Simulation number 7, I was instructed to go to Section C but revealed response number 4 in Section G before I discovered I was in the wrong section." Then, go back to Section C and continue with the simulation. There is no guarantee that your error will be allowed but it will at least be considered.

8. Pace yourself to get through all 10 problems in the 4-hour time limit. That gives you 20 minutes per problem. For example, you should be finishing your third problem after an hour. Unlike the Written Registry Exam, you should *not* rush ahead at the end and pick just anything. You will be penalized for incorrect choices.

9. Take a practice Clinical Simulation Examination. Two are offered at the end of this book in Appendix 2. Others are available, for a fee, from Applied Measurement Professionals.

Things you should avoid:

1. Do not try to jump ahead in the problem or guess what it is that the author is leading to. With the branching logic format, there are several possible

pathways. Work only with what you know now and from the past.

2. Try not to become flustered if you are faced with a scenario you have never experienced at work. Imagine what it is that you would do if faced with this problem and go from there. Also, do not become frustrated if the choice that you prefer is not available. There is more than one way to take care of patient's problems. Make your next best choice and move on.

3. Do not select everything in the information-gathering section. You will lose points by choosing unimportant, time-consuming, unnecessarily expensive, or dangerous procedures.

4. Avoid selecting new or unusual procedures that you are not familiar with, for example, jet ventilation. You will hurt yourself if you do not know how to operate the equipment properly.

5. Do not misinterpret the data you are given. Avoid assumptions about things that are not printed out for you.

Summary—General Suggestions for Either Examination

1. Begin studying about 2 months before the exam. Pace yourself so that everything can be covered in the time that you have. Avoid "cramming" a few days before the examination; these tests will demand more than the simple recall of facts.

2. Study the most important and heavily tested areas first. Work down to the less important ones.

3. Focus on the areas where you are weakest; especially if they are heavily tested.

4. Arrive at the city where the test will be given the evening before the exam. Make a practice drive from your motel to the test site and where you will park. Check the time required and add more for the morning traffic.

5. Get a good dinner. Avoid alcohol, even if nervous, to give you a clear head in the morning.

6. Do not cram for the exam back at the motel. Unfortunately, if you are not prepared by now, a few more hours will not really help. If necessary, brush up on only a few test areas.

7. Set the alarm to get you up in plenty of time to be ready. Get a good night's sleep. Avoid sleeping pills.

8. Eat a good breakfast to get you through to lunch. Minimize caffeine. You will have plenty of adrenaline running through your system to keep you awake while taking the test!

9. Attempt to relax with the self-confidence that comes from knowing that you are well prepared.

BIBLIOGRAPHY

Assmann DC, Hixon SJ, Kacmarek RM: *Clinical simulations for respiratory care practitioners*, Chicago, 1979, Year Book Medical.

Baker MD: Update from the clinical simulation examination committee, *NBRC Newsletter* 12(11):1–4, Nov 1986.

Kacmarek RM, Hixon SJ, Assmann DC: *Clinical simulations for respiratory care practitioners*, vol 2, Chicago, 1985, Year Book Medical.

Study guide for the clinical simulation examination, National Board for Respiratory Care, 8310 Nieman Road, Lenexa, KS 66214.

Study guide for the registry examinations for advanced respiratory therapy practitioners, National Board for Respiratory Care, 8310 Nieman Road, Lenexa, KS 66214.

Van Hooser DT: Do's and don'ts for the clinical simulation exam, *NBRC Horizons* 16(3):1–5, May 1990.

IMPORTANT ADDRESSES AND PHONE NUMBERS

For information on the examination process contact:

National Board for Respiratory Care
8310 Nieman Rd
Lenexa, KS 66214
(913) 599-4200

For information on purchasing self-assessment examinations contact:

Applied Measurement Professionals
11015 W. 75th Terrace, Suite 110
Shawnee Mission, KS 66214
(913) 268-6362

For information on accredited respiratory therapist educational programs contact:

Joint Review Committee for Respiratory Therapy Education
1701 W. Euless Blvd
Suite 200
Euless, TX 76039
(817) 283-2835

For information on state credentialing requirements contact:

American Association for Respiratory Care
11030 Ables Lane
Dallas, TX 75229
(214) 234-AARC

CONTENTS

1 | Patient Assessment

Module A. **Review the patient's chart for the following data; and recommend the following diagnostic procedures based on the current information.**

Note: the following discussion involves noninvasive, bedside procedures and applies primarily to adults. Topics and laboratory values that relate to neonates and children are included as appropriate. Specific areas of neonatal or pediatric assessment are found in Module H.

1. Review the results of the patient's serum electrolyte levels and other blood chemistries (IA1a) [An]; and recommend the tests for additional data (IA2a)[R, Ap, An].

The serum (blood) electrolytes are commonly measured in most patients as they are being admitted to the hospital. This is to determine if they are within the normal ranges listed in Table 1-1. Any abnormality should be promptly corrected so that the patient's nervous system, muscle function, and cellular processes can be optimized. Diet and a number of medications have effects on the various electrolytes. Most abnormalities can be corrected by dietary adjustments or, if necessary, by intravenous supplement.

Potassium (K$^+$)

Potassium is the most important electrolyte to follow because of its effect on general nerve function and cardiac function. Hyperkalemia is a high blood level of potassium and will cause the following electrocardiogram (ECG) changes: high, peaked T waves and depressed S-T segments, widening QRS complex, and bradycardia. Hypokalemia is a low blood level and will cause the following ECG changes: flat or inverted T waves, depression of the S-T segments, premature ventricular contractions (PVC), and ventricular fibrillation if severe enough. (Section 10 offers a more complete discussion of ECG interpretation.) Hypokalemia may be caused by the use of diuretic medications.

Chloride (Cl$^-$)

Hyperchloremia is a high blood level of chloride and will cause a significant prolongation of the S-T segment and the Q-T interval on the ECG. Hypochloremia is a low blood level and will cause the Q-T interval to be shortened and perhaps widen and round off the T waves on the ECG.

Table 1-1. Normal Serum Electrolyte and
Glucose Levels

Normal electrolyte values*	
Chloride (Cl$^-$)	95-106 mEq/L
Potassium (K$^+$)	3.5-5.5 mEq/L
Sodium (Na$^+$)	135-145 mEq/L
Calcium (Ca^{++})	4.5-5.5 mEq/L
Bicarbonate (HCO$_3^-$)	22-25 mEq/L
Normal glucose values*	
Serum or plasma	70-110 mg/100 ml (dl)
Whole blood	60-100 mg/100 ml (dl)

* These values may vary somewhat among references.

Sodium (Na$^+$)

Hypernatremia is a high blood level of sodium and might be seen in a patient who is dehydrated or has been given excessive amounts of sodium by the intravenous route. Hyponatremia is a low blood level and might be seen in a patient who has lost a lot of gastrointestinal secretions because of vomiting, nasogastric tube drainage, or diarrhea.

Bicarbonate (HCO$_3^-$)

Altered bicarbonate levels are commonly seen in patients with pulmonary conditions. Patients with a chronically elevated PaCO$_2$ will typically retain bicarbonate to moderate the respiratory acidosis caused by the elevated carbon dioxide level. Conversely, patients with a chronically decreased PaCO$_2$ level will excrete bicarbonate to moderate the respiratory alkalosis caused by the decreased PaCO$_2$ level.

Calcium (Ca^{++})

Hypercalcemia is an elevated level and may be associated with patients taking diuretics. ECG changes associated with an increased calcium level include a shortened Q-T interval and widened and rounded T waves. Hypocalcemia is a decreased level. ECG changes include a lengthening of the S-T segment and the Q-T interval.

Glucose

The blood glucose level is important to follow because it directly relates to how much sugar is available to the patient for energy for daily activities. The normal values are listed in Table 1-1. Hypoglycemia is a low blood level of glucose; it could mean that the patient is malnourished. Hyperglycemia is a high blood level that could indicate the patient has diabetes mellitus, Cushing's disease, or is being treated with corticosteroids. More specific testing would have to be done to prove the diagnosis.

2.   Review the patient's fluid balance (intake and output). (IA1b) [R]

Intake refers to all the fluids that a patient has taken in a set time period. Usually this includes all oral and intravenous fluids taken in a shift (8 hours) or day (24 hours). Output refers to all of the fluids that a patient has lost in a shift or day. Output includes urine and, if appropriate, emesis or diarrhea.

The additional loss of 500 to 1000 ml of fluid through a normal adult's respiratory system should result in a fairly close matching of intake and output in a day. Dehydration will result if a person should have a significantly lower fluid intake than output for several days. Drying of secretions and hypotension are complications. Overhydration may result if a person is given much more fluid than the kidneys can excrete. This can cause pulmonary edema if the patient has a history of congestive heart failure.

3.   Review the results of the patient's hemoglobin and hematocrit count (IA1a) [R]; and recommend the tests for additional data (IA2b) [R, Ap, An].

The hemoglobin and hematocrit values are important because they directly relate to the patient's oxygen carrying capacity. This, along with the patient's cardiac output, PaO_2, and the affinity of the hemoglobin for oxygen determines the amount of oxygen that will be available to the tissues.

Decreased hemoglobin and hematocrit values indicate that the patient is anemic. An anemic patient has less oxygen carrying capacity and places more stress on the heart when exercising. Hypoxemia from a cardiopulmonary abnormality places this patient at great risk. A transfusion is indicated if the hematocrit is below what the physician considers to be a clinically safe level.

Increased numbers of circulating erythrocytes indicate that the patient is polycythemic. When this is seen as a response to chronic hypoxemia from chronic obstructive pulmonary disease (COPD), cyanotic congenital heart disease, or another disorder, it is labeled as secondary polycythemia. This patient is at added risk because the thickened blood causes an increased afterload for the heart to pump against. These patients are also more prone to blood clots. Supplemental oxygen or other clinical treatment to raise the PaO_2 to at least 55-60 mm Hg will, over a period of time, result in the erythrocyte and hematocrit levels returning to normal. See Table 1-2 for normal values.

Table 1-2. Normal Hemoglobin, Hematocrit, and Erythrocyte Counts for Adults and Children

	Adult*	Infant*	Child*
Hemoglobin (Hb) In gm/100 ml (g/dL)			
Female	12.0-16.0	12.2-20.0	11.2-13.4
Male	13.5-18.0	Same	Same
Hematocrit (Hct) In ml/100 ml (ml/dL)			
Female	38%-47%		
Male	40%-54%		
Erythrocyte (red blood cell [RBC]) count In millions/ml			
Female	4.2-5.4	5.0-5.1	4.6-4.8
Male	4.6-6.2	Same	Same

* These values may vary somewhat among references.

4. Review the results of the patient's leukocyte (white blood cell) count and analysis (IA1a) [R]; and recommend the tests for additional data (IA2b) [R, Ap, An].

A normal leukocyte count and differential count reveals two things about the patient. First, there is no active bacterial infection. Second, the patient has the ability to produce the normal number and variety of white blood cells (WBCs) to combat an infection (see Table 1-3 for the counts).

A mild to moderate increase in the leukocyte count is called leukocytosis. It is seen as a WBC count of 11,000 to 17,000 per cubic millimeter (mm^3). Usually the higher the count is, the more severe the infection. A WBC count of more than 17,000/mm^3 is seen in patients with severe sepsis, miliary tuberculosis, and other overwhelming infections. An extreme shift to the left in the differential count means that there is a significant increase in the number of neutrophils. This is usually seen when a patient has an acute, severe bacterial infection. Exceptions to this are patients who are elderly, have acquired immunodeficiency syndrome (AIDS), or have other immunodeficiencies. They may show only a mildly elevated WBC count while having an infection.

Leukopenia is a low absolute WBC count of 3,000 to 5,000 cells per mm^3 or less. An acute viral infection can cause a mild to moderate decrease in the neutrophil count. The patient who has a low WBC count is at great risk of bacterial or other infections.

5. Review the patient's sputum culture results, antibiotic sensitivity, and Gram's stain results (IA1e) [R]; and recommend the tests for additional data (IA2c) [R, Ap, An].

It is important to get a sputum sample for evaluation whenever bronchitis and/or pneumonia are suspected. A sputum culture is the attempt to grow organisms found in the sputum. Sputum is the mix of mucus from the lungs and saliva from the mouth, therefore, the organisms that are grown may have come from either place. A sample suctioned from the lungs and cultured should only show pulmonary organisms. This is the best thing to do when trying to identify a bronchitis or pneumonia pathogen.

Sensitivity is the act of exposing the cultured organisms to a variety of antimicrobial drugs. The goal is to find which drug(s) will kill the pathogen most effectively. The patient is then treated with that antibiotic.

Table 1-3. Leukocyte Count and Differential Count

Leukocyte count (white blood cell [WBC] per cubic mm (mm^3)*	
Adult	4500-11,000
Infant and child	9000-33,000
Differential count*	
Segmented neutrophils	40%-75%
Lymphocytes	20%-45%
Monocytes	2%-10%
Eosinophils	0%-6%
Bands	0%-6%
Basophils	0%-1%

* These values may vary somewhat among references.

Gram's stain is a special staining process to colorize bacteria into one of two groups. Gram$^+$ (g$^+$) bacteria are stained violet. The most common bacteria that cause bronchitis and pneumonia are Gram$^+$. In general, they are killed by penicillin or related drugs and sulfa-type antibiotics.

Gram$^-$ (g$^-$) bacteria are stained pink. These organisms, unfortunately, are found in many of the sickest and weakest patients. Often these bacteria will only be killed by a specific antibiotic to which they have been proven sensitive. So called "broad spectrum" antibiotics, such as tetracycline, may also be used.

Viruses cannot be identified by this simple staining process. The Ziehl-Neelsen stain is used to identify the *Mycobacterium tuberculosis* (TB) organism. Other pathogens, such as protozoa and fungi, need specialized stains for identification.

6. Review the culture, sensitivity, and Gram's stain results from a patient's blood, urine, or pleural drainage sample. (IA1f) [R]

The same general principles of culture, sensitivity, and Gram's stain apply here as discussed previously. A person without infection would have negative results of testing blood, urine, and/or pleural drainage. If an infection is found, note the organism(s) and antibiotic(s) being used. Positive results from a blood sample (septicemia) would indicate that the patient has a systemic infection; however, further testing will be needed to pinpoint the original site of the infection. Contaminated urine could be the result of an infection in any or several parts of the urinary system. Again, further testing would be needed to determine the origin of the infection.

To evaluate any pleural drainage, fluid must first be removed from the pleural space by a thoracentesis (pleurocenteses) procedure. This procedure is discussed in detail in Section 17. Infected pleural fluid could result from either a lung infection or a blood-born infection that reached the pleural space.

7. Review the results of the patient's ECG. (IA1c2) [R]

A 12-lead diagnostic ECG is indicated in any patient who has heart disease, a suspected myocardial infarction, or who is critically ill with a cardiopulmonary condition. Look for written documentation of the patient's heart condition. See Section 10 for the complete discussion on performing an ECG and interpreting the results.

Module B. X-ray imaging.

1. Make the recommendation for a chest x-ray for additional data (IA2d)[R]; and to evaluate the patient's response to therapy (IIIA1b) [R, Ap].

A chest x-ray should be recommended in the following situations:

a. After an endotracheal or tracheostomy tube has been placed or repositioned
b. When a pneumothorax is suspected
c. After a chest tube has been placed into the pleural space
d. Hemoptysis (bloody sputum)
e. After the jugular/subclavian route has been used to insert a central venous pressure (CVP) or pulmonary artery (Swan-Ganz) catheter

f. If there is a sudden deleterious change in the patient's cardiopulmonary status

g. If there is a sudden, unexplained drop in the patient's oxygenation

h. If the pulmonary artery catheter balloon has been left inflated for a prolonged period and a pulmonary infarct is suspected

2. Review the results of the patient's upper airway x-ray (IA1g) [R]; and recommend one be taken for additional data (IA2e) [R, Ap, An].

An anteroposterior and/or lateral x-ray of the upper airway should be recommended in any patient who presents with a history or symptoms of upper airway obstruction. The normal lateral x-ray of the upper airway will reveal a continuous, unobstructed column of air (dark line) through the mouth, pharynx, larynx, and trachea. Remember that an upper airway obstruction is a medical emergency. A complete obstruction must be quickly cleared or it will result in asphyxiation of the victim.

3. Inspect the patient's chest x-ray to evaluate the patient's response to care. (IIIA1c) [R, Ap, An]

Note: The first part of this presentation is not listed on the Examination Content Outline developed by the National Board for Respiratory Care (NBRC). It is included for the purpose of helping the learner understand the basic principles of radiology and the science of interpreting chest x-rays results.

Fundamentals of Radiology

Images of the internal body structures are recorded on an x-ray film when high frequency and power electromagnetic (x-ray) waves penetrate the body and, to some extent, pierce through it to strike the film. If the thorax is between the x-ray source and the film, a chest x-ray results. The chest x-ray is also known as a chest radiograph, chest roentgenograph, or CXR.

There will be absorption of the x-rays by the body tissues in direct proportion to their densities. In other words, very dense tissues such as bones will absorb more x-rays, allowing fewer to pass through to the film than less dense tissues such as the lungs. What is then seen on the x-ray film is a negative or reverse image of the densities of the structures within the chest. When viewing an x-ray film, a range of shadings will be seen progressing from black to white. Black is seen around the edge of the body because air does not stop the x-rays that then strike and expose the film. Partial absorption is seen as varying degrees of white shadows on the film. The body's tissues absorb the x-rays to a degree proportional to their density. The most dense tissues are the bones and will be clearly seen as solid, white shapes. Water or fluids are the next most dense and will be seen as less solid white shapes or shadows. If there is enough fluid in an area, the x-rays will be completely absorbed and a solid, uniform white shadow will be seen. The heart and any fluid in or around the lungs are clearly seen this way. Lastly, the soft tissues of the skin and lungs are the least dense. Air-filled spaces, such as the lungs, will be seen as almost black. Because the lungs do contain some tissues, they are not seen as entirely black. Metallic objects such as bullets, wire sutures, parts of artificial heart valves, and so forth totally absorb all x-rays and will appear as a sharply outlined white shadow.

It is helpful to the learner to review the normal anatomy of the chest cage, lungs, airways, heart, and so forth before learning the various positions used to obtain chest x-rays or the findings of normal or abnormal chest x-rays. See Fig. 1-1 for the common patient positions for a chest x-ray.

Patient Positioning for a Chest X-ray

The *posterior to anterior view* (P-A, PA, or posteroanterior) is the standard for finding the proper anatomical positions of the thoracic organs. The patient is instructed to take in a maximal inspiration. This lowers the hemidiaphragms of the adult to the level of the ninth to eleventh ribs, and of the infant to the eighth rib posteriorly. The P-A position is preferred to the anterior to posterior position because the heart is less magnified and any fluid level in a pleural space is easier to see. If ordered, a full expiratory x-ray can be taken to compare to the full inspiratory

Radiographic Projection	Explanation	Graphic Demonstration
AP (anteroposterior)	The anterior surface of the body is closest to the x-ray source with the posterior body surface closest to the film. The x-ray beam enters the anterior surface and exits the posterior surface to strike the film forming the radiographic image.	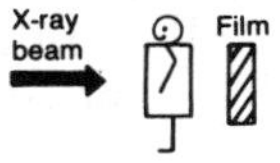
PA (posteroanterior)	The posterior surface of the body is closest to the x-ray source with the anterior body surface closest to the film. The x-ray beam enters the posterior surface and exits the anterior surface to strike the film forming the radiographic image.	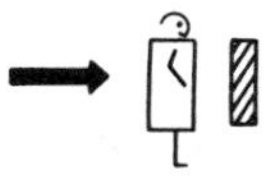
Lateral	So-named for the side of the body closest to the film, that is, a left lateral projection is obtained with the patient's left side closest to the film and the x-ray beam enters the right side to obtain the radiograph.	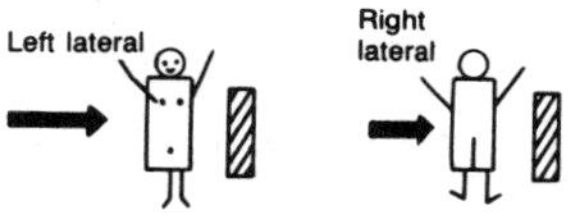
Oblique	A position in which the patient's body part is rotated so that it does not produce either an AP/PA or a lateral projection. RAO (right PA oblique): The patient's right side is rotated toward the film. LAO (left PA oblique): The patient's left side is rotated toward the film. RPO (right AP oblique): The patient's right posterior side is rotated toward the film. LPO (left AP oblique): The patient's left posterior side is rotated toward the film.	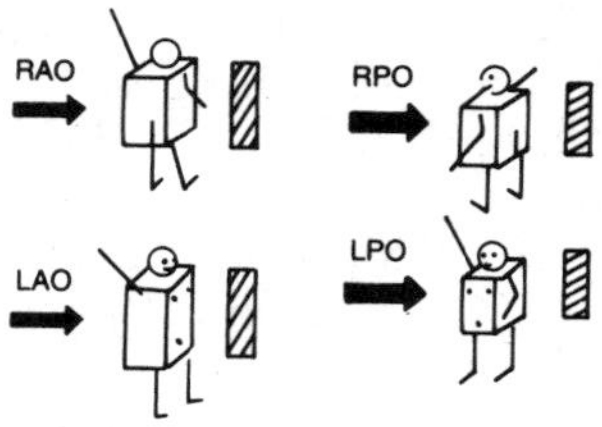
Lateral decubitus	Patient is positioned lying on either the right or the left side; the x-ray beam is directed parallel to the floor and perpendicular to the film. The patient can also be placed in a ventral or dorsal position. (Patient shown is on right side.)	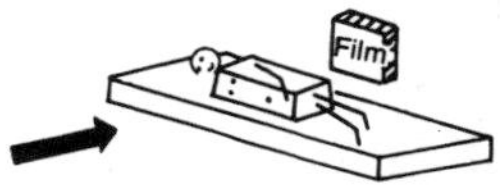
Lordotic	Patient is postured in an AP orientation, tilted back away from the vertical; the x-ray beam is directed with a cephalic angulation, that is, the x-ray beam is directed toward the head.	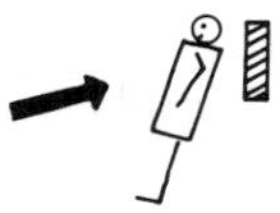

Fig. 1-1 Radiographic projections for the chest and lungs. (From DiPietro JS, Mustard MN: *Clinical guide for respiratory care practitioners*, Norwalk, Conn, 1987, Appleton & Lange. Used by permission.)

film. This is needed to show the excursion of the hemidiaphragms, their symmetry, or to make a small pneumothorax more detectable.

The *anterior to posterior view* (A-P, AP, or anteroposterior) is often used when the patient is too ill to be transported to the radiology department for a standard P-A chest x-ray. It is often referred to as a "portable" chest x-ray because the machine can be moved to the patient's bedside. The patient who is on a mechanical ventilator should be given a sigh breath by the respiratory care practitioner to fill the lungs and lower the diaphragm as much as possible.

The standard *lateral view* is taken with the patient standing upright with both arms raised above the head and the left side against the film cassette. This is because the heart is left of center in the chest. A lateral view is used to see behind the heart and hemidiaphragms and to localize any lesions found on a P-A film.

The *oblique view* provides a third angle to the internal chest structures. This is especially helpful when the physician is checking the heart borders, mediastinal structures, hilar structures, and lung masses.

The *lateral decubitus view* is very helpful in evaluating known or suspected fluid in the pleural space. As little as 25 to 50 ml can be detected in the adult as it flows to a horizontal position. An air-fluid level in a lung cavity can also be evaluated by the shifting of the fluid line by gravity. The dorsal decubitus view is used to help identify a small pneumothorax in an infant.

The *lordotic (apical lordotic) view* is used when it is necessary to look at the upper lung fields without the clavicles and first and second ribs obscuring them. The apices, right middle lobe, and lingula can be clearly seen.

Normal Adult Chest X-ray Findings

Posterior to anterior (P-A, PA, or posteroanterior) view (see Figs. 1-2 and 1-3).

- The chest will be roughly rectangular in shape.
- Faint lung markings should be seen to the edges of the chest wall.
- All lung fields should be clear of infiltrates or any other densities.
- The right hemidiaphragm will be about one intercostal space higher than the left hemidiaphragm.
- The left hilum will be about one intercostal space higher than the right hilum.
- The costophrenic angles should be acute and clear.
- The heart should be predominantly on the left side of the chest.
- The cardiothoracic (C-T) ratio should be less than .5 or 50%.
- The trachea and other mediastinal structures should be midline.
- An air bubble may be seen in the stomach below the left hemidiaphragm.

Lateral view (see Fig. 1-4).

- Faint lung markings should be seen to the edges of the chest wall.
- All lung fields should be clear of infiltrates or any other densities.
- The right hemidiaphragm will be about one intercostal space higher than the left hemidiaphragm.
- The costophrenic angles should be acute and clear.
- The heart should be anterior of midline in the chest.

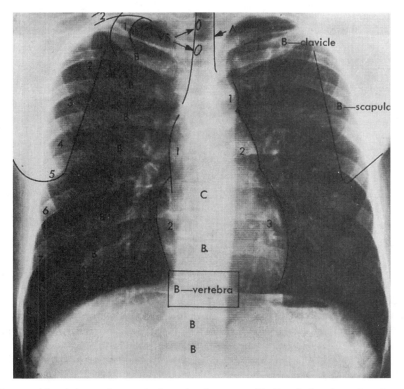

Fig. 1-2 A normal adult posteroanterior chest x-ray with the following structures marked: *A,* trachea. *VS* marks the vertebral spinous processes, which should be seen within the tracheal air column when the patient is properly positioned. *B,* bones, including scapula, vertebra, clavicle, and ribs. Ribs 1 to 8 are marked on the right chest over their anterior surfaces. *C,* Cardiac shadow. Right side marks show: *1,* the superior vena cava; *2,* the right atrium. Left side marks show: *1,* aortic arch; *2,* pulmonary artery segment; *3,* left ventricle. (From Sheldon RL, Dunbar RD: Systematic analysis of the chest radiograph. In Scanlan CL, Spearman CB, Sheldon RL, editors: *Egan's fundamentals of respiratory care,* ed 5, St. Louis, 1990, CV Mosby. Used by permission.)

Normal Neonatal Chest X-ray Findings

Posterior to anterior (P-A, PA, or posteroanterior) view (see Fig. 1-5).

- The chest will be roughly triangular or conical in shape.
- Faint lung markings should be seen to the edges of the chest wall.
- All lung fields should be clear of infiltrates or any other densities.
- The right hemidiaphragm will be about one intercostal space higher than the left hemidiaphragm.
- The left hilum will be about one intercostal space higher than the right hilum.
- The costophrenic angles should be acute and clear.
- The heart will be more midline than in the adult but the left ventricle shifts the overall shadow to the left.

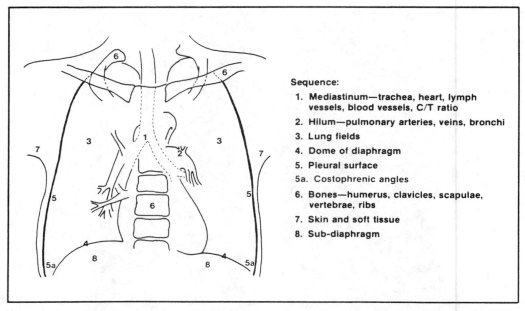

Sequence:

1. Mediastinum—trachea, heart, lymph vessels, blood vessels, C/T ratio
2. Hilum—pulmonary arteries, veins, bronchi
3. Lung fields
4. Dome of diaphragm
5. Pleural surface
5a. Costophrenic angles
6. Bones—humerus, clavicles, scapulae, vertebrae, ribs
7. Skin and soft tissue
8. Sub-diaphragm

Fig. 1-3 A suggested sequence for evaluating the structures seen on a frontal chest x-ray. (From Rau JL, Pearce DJ: *Understanding chest radiographs.* Denver, 1984, Multi-Media Publishing. Used by permission.)

- The cardiothoracic (C-T) ratio should be less than .6 or 60%.
- The trachea and other mediastinal structures should be midline.

Lateral view.

- Faint lung markings should be seen to the edges of the chest wall.
- All lung fields should be clear of infiltrates or any other densities.
- The right hemidiaphragm will be about one intercostal space higher than the left hemidiaphragm.
- The apex of the diaphragm has a more anterior location than in the adult.
- The costophrenic angles should be acute and clear.
- The ribs will be seen sloping down from back to front.
- The heart may appear enlarged from top to bottom because the infant's thymus gland is enlarged compared to the adult's, and its shadow blends in with the cardiac shadow (silhouette sign).

The following three x-ray signs are important to look for because their presence or absence will give important clues to a patient's diagnosis.

Cardiothoracic (C-T) Ratio

The cardiothoracic (C-T) ratio is the ratio of the width of the heart at the diaphragm compared to the widest lateral diameter inside the chest wall (see Fig. 1-6). It should be measured from a posterior to anterior chest x-ray. The normal adult's C-T ratio is less than .5 or 50% and the normal infant's C-T ratio is less than .6 or 60%.

If the patient's chest size is normal, a large C-T ratio shows that the heart is

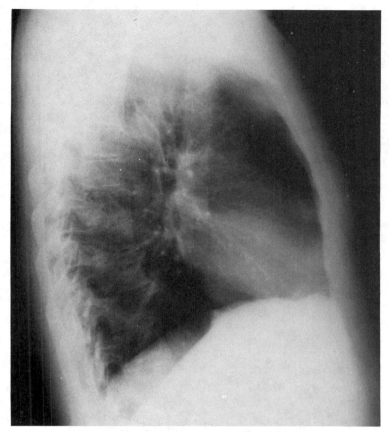

Fig. 1-4 A normal adult lateral chest x-ray. The spinal column can be seen on the left. The cardiac shadow can be seen right of center within the chest cavity and behind the sternum. (From Eubanks DH, Bone RC: *Comprehensive respiratory care,* ed 2, St. Louis, 1990, CV Mosby. Used by permission.)

enlarged. This can be seen in congestive heart failure, cor pulmonale or right ventricular failure, and some congenital heart defects. A small C-T ratio is seen in patients who have severe emphysema because the lung volumes are enlarged and the heart is elongated as the diaphragm is depressed.

Air Bronchogram

Air bronchograms are seen on the chest x-ray as dark, air-filled airways within an area of white, airless lung tissue (see Fig. 1-7). This faint difference in densities is often difficult to see and will not be revealed at all in an underexposed x-ray. Examples of conditions where an air bronchogram can be seen include atelectasis, pneumonia, and infant respiratory distress syndrome (IRDS).

Silhouette Sign

The silhouette sign is seen as a density (white shadow) that is continuous between a pulmonary consolidation, infiltrate, or mass and the heart, aorta, or diaphragm such that the usual border between the two organs is obliterated. Instead,

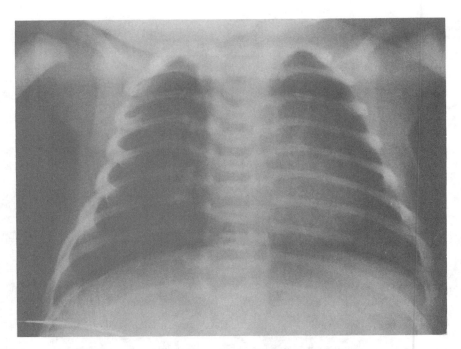

Fig. 1-5 A normal newborn chest film. (From Carlo, Chatburn: *Neonatal respiratory care,* St. Louis, Mosby–Year Book. Used by permission.)

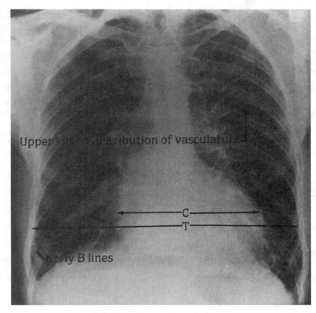

Fig. 1-6 The cardiothoracic (C-T) ratio is measured from a posteroanterior x-ray. It is the ratio of the width of the heart to the width of the thorax at the diaphragm. The normal C-T ratio is less than 50% in an adult and less than 60% in an infant. This patient has congestive heart failure. Note that the C-T ratio is greater than 50%; there is an increase in vascular markings in the upper lobes and horizontal Kerly B lines can be seen in the right lower lobe. (From Sheldon RL, Wilkins RL: Clinical application of the chest radiograph. In Wilkins RL, Sheldon RL, Krider SJ, editors: *Clinical assessment in respiratory care,* ed 2, St. Louis, 1990, CV Mosby. Used by permission.)

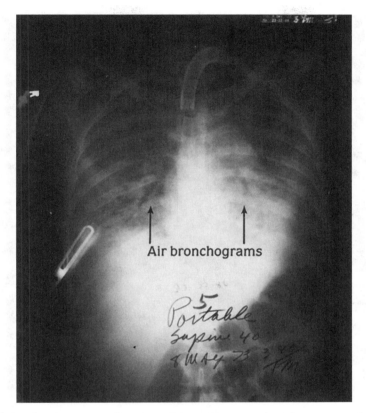

Air bronchograms

Fig. 1-7 Air bronchograms are shown on this anteroposterior chest x-ray of an adult. This patient also has a tracheostomy tube that is properly positioned. (From Sheldon RL, Wilkins RL: Clinical application of the chest radiograph. In Wilkins RL, Sheldon RL, Krider SJ, editors: *Clinical assessment in respiratory care,* ed 2, St. Louis, 1990, CV Mosby. Used by permission.)

the abnormal pulmonary tissue and the other organ appear to be a single density (see Fig. 1-8). A right middle lobe consolidation or infiltrate from pneumonia will result in the loss of the right heart border. Instead, the lobe and right heart border will appear to be continuous. A consolidation or infiltrate in the lingula from pneumonia will result in the loss of the left heart border. The lingula and left heart border will appear to be continous. If either the right or left heart border can be seen as separate from a pulmonary consolidation, infiltrate, or mass that is adjacent to it, the pulmonary problem has to be in the lower lobe.

a. Look for the presence of, or any changes in, pneumothorax, subcutaneous emphysema, or any other extrapulmonary air. (IB6a) [R, Ap]

Free air that leaks into the interstitial spaces of the lung or body cavities is abnormal in any patient. Causes for an air leak include barotrauma (alveolar rupture related to the use of a mechanical ventilator), a ruptured bleb (congenital or acquired blister on the visceral pleura), puncture wound through the chest wall, and needle puncture through the pleural space during the insertion of a central venous pressure

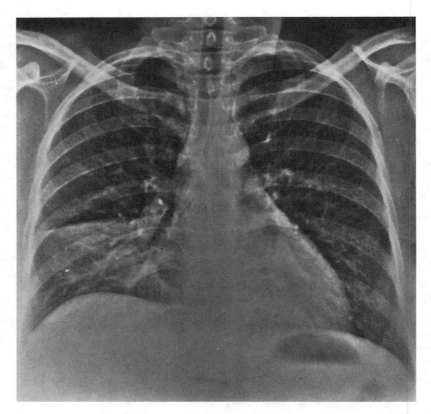

Fig. 1-8 The silhouette sign is demonstrated by the merging of the right cardiac shadow and the consolidation shadow of a right middle lobe pneumonia. This indicates that the two areas are in direct contact. (From Sheldon RL, Wilkins RL: Clinical application of the chest radiograph. In Wilkins RL, Sheldon RL, Krider SJ, editors: *Clinical assessment in respiratory care*, ed 2, St. Louis, 1990, CV Mosby. Used by permission.)

or pulmonary artery catheter via the subclavian or jugular vein. Once air under pressure is forced through a bronchial or alveolar tear into the interstitial tissues, it will tend to follow the path of least resistance. This may result in air being found in any of the following areas singly or in combinations.

Pneumothorax is air in the pleural space. The lung tends to collapse toward the hilum. A pneumothorax is identified on the chest x-ray as an area of black, indicating air that surrounds the collapsed lung. No lung markings will be visible in the air filled space and the edge of the lung can be seen (see Fig. 1-9). A small amount of air does not necessarily need to be evacuated if the patient's breathing, blood gases, and vital signs are stable. A chest tube should be placed to withdraw the air if the lung is more than 10% collapsed or if the patient is experiencing difficulty breathing, hypoxemia, and unstable vital signs. If the air is under sufficient pressure to shift the lung and mediastinal structures to the opposite side it is called a *tension pneumothorax*. These patients will have a great deal of difficulty breathing, will be severely hypoxemic, and show tachycardia and hypotension. This is a most serious condition and can lead to the death of the patient if it is not quickly identified and treated. A pleural chest tube is always placed into the affected side to remove the air so that the lung will reexpand.

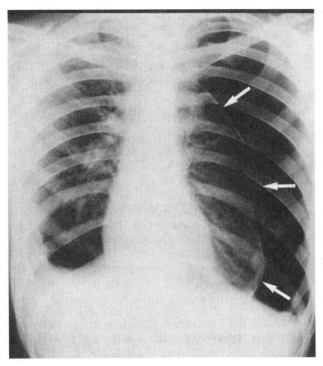

Fig. 1-9 Frontal x-ray of an adult male with a left-sided tension pneumothorax. The edge of the collapsed lung is shown by the arrows. Note how the mediastinum is shifted to the right, the right lung is compressed, and the left hemidiaphragm is depressed. (From Des Jardins TR: *Clinical manifestations of respiratory disease,* ed 2, Chicago, 1990, Year Book Medical. Used by permission.)

Subcutaneous emphysema is air found in the soft tissues such as the skin, axilla, shoulder, neck, or breast of the affected side. In extreme cases, the air will force its way into skin and soft tissues throughout the body. The chest x-ray appearance is one of scattered dark areas (air pockets) in the various soft tissues (see Fig. 1-10). A small leak is gradually reabsorbed into the blood stream. A large air pocket can be removed by a chest tube as shown.

The following are other locations where free air can be pathologically found: *Pneumomediastinum* is air in the mediastinal space. *Pneumopericardium* is air in the pericardial space (see Fig. 1-11). Both of these conditions can be very serious. A cardiac tamponade is created if the pressure around the heart is great enough to interfere with its function. When the heart is compressed the patient will show a drop in blood pressure, rising heart rate, and jugular vein distension. *Pneumoperitonium* is air in the peritoneal space. This condition can be dangerous in an infant if a large enough volume of air is below the diaphragm that its movement is limited. *Pulmonary interstitial emphysema (PIE)* is air that has disseminated throughout the intersitial spaces of the injured lung(s). The lungs appear "bubbly" on the chest x-ray as shown in Fig. 1-11. The air may further leak into any of the above locations. This condition is most commonly seen in infants with IRDS who require mechanical ventilation.

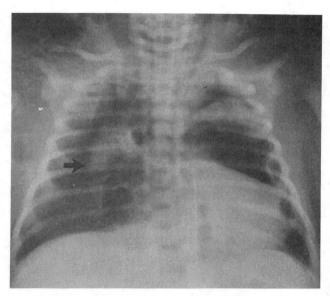

Fig. 1-10 Frontal x-ray of a neonate showing subcutaneous emphysema in the shoulders and neck area. Other abnormal air in the patient's chest includes a pneumomediastinum, which outlines the right lobe of the thymus gland (arrow) and a left anterior pneumothorax. (From Carlo, Chatburn: *Neonatal respiratory care,* St. Louis, Mosby–Year Book. Used by permission.)

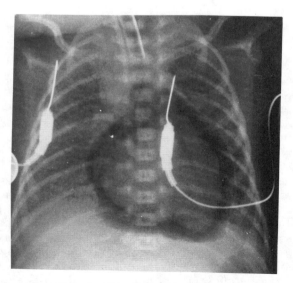

Fig. 1-11 Frontal x-ray of a neonate showing a pneumopericardium that resulted from pulmonary interstitial emphysema. Note the dark outline of air around the heart. Chest tubes have been placed to remove air from around the heart and the right pleural space from an earlier pneumothorax. An endotracheal tube is also seen. (From Koff PB, Eitzman DV, Neu J: *Neonatal and pediatric respiratory care,* St. Louis, 1988, CV Mosby. Used by permission.)

b. Look for the presence of, or any changes in, mediastinal shift. (IB6j) [R, Ap]

The mediastinum is the area between the lungs that contains the heart and great vessels, trachea, hilar structures, and esophagus. In the neonate, the heart and other mediastinal structures should be approximately in the center of the chest with the left ventricle to the left of center. In the adult, the majority of the heart and mediastinal structures should be left of center in the chest. A shift from any cause is abnormal and can be caused by several conditions as shown in Fig. 1-12. Atelectasis, if unilateral and great enough, will result in a shift *toward* the problem area (see Fig. 1-12, A). Pulmonary fibrosis, if unilateral and great enough, will result in a shift *toward* the problem area (see Fig. 1-12, B). Tension pneumothorax will result in a shift *away* from the problem area (see Fig. 1-12, C). Fluid in the pleural space, if great enough, will result in a shift *away* from the problem area (see Fig. 1-12, D).

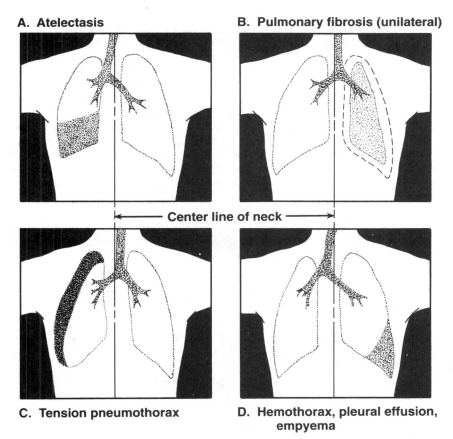

A. Atelectasis

B. Pulmonary fibrosis (unilateral)

← — Center line of neck — →

C. Tension pneumothorax

D. Hemothorax, pleural effusion, empyema

Fig. 1-12 Conditions causing tracheal deviation and mediastinal shift (simulated chest x-ray findings). **A,** Unilateral atelectasis with tracheal deviation toward the affected lung. **B,** Unilateral pulmonary fibrosis with tracheal deviation toward the affected lung. **C,** Tension pneumothorax with tracheal deviation away from the affected lung. **D,** Pleural fluid with tracheal deviation away from the affected lung. (From Sills JR: *Respiratory care certification guide,* St. Louis, 1991, Mosby–Year Book. Used by permission.)

c.   Look for the position of any chest tubes. (IB6c) [R, Ap]

Chest tubes are placed to remove any abnormal collection of air or fluid from the thoracic cavity so that the function of the heart and/or lungs will return to normal. A pleural chest tube is placed to remove air or fluid from the pleural space. The insertion site and depth of insertion of the tube depend on the patient's disorder. See Section 17 for more discussion on the placement of pleural chest tubes.

A mediastinal or pericardial chest tube is placed to remove air or fluid from either of these spaces (see Fig. 1-11). Cardiac tamponade can result from either the pressure of air or fluid compressing the heart. Most postoperative open heart surgery patients will have one or more mediastinal chest tubes in place for several days to remove any blood from around the heart. The insertion site is below the sternum and the tube(s) are placed posterior to the heart in the pericardial and/or mediastinal space.

A chest or chest and abdominal x-ray will be needed to check the position of the various tubes after the initial insertion. They should be located properly in the patient to remove the abnormal collection of air or fluid. Another x-ray will be needed to check the tube's position if there is a sudden change in the patient's condition such as no air or fluid leaking out when it had been earlier.

d.   Look for the presence of, or any changes in, pulmonary infiltrates (IB6m) [R, Ap] or consolidation (IB6b) [R, Ap].

A pulmonary infiltrate occurs when a fluid such as water passes from the pulmonary vascular bed into the lung tissues. Usually this fluid moves into the lung because the alveolar capillary membrane is damaged. On a chest x-ray, an infiltrate often appears as a faint white blurring of the lung and other associated structures.

A consolidation is a filling of the alveoli with fluid such as pulmonary edema; an infiltrate; or aspirated vomitus, blood, or water. It is often segmental or lobar. Consolidation is noticed on the chest x-ray as a dense white shadow because all the air has been replaced by the fluid. The mediastinum and heart will be seen in their normal location. (See Fig. 1-13 for the P-A and lateral chest x-ray appearance of consolidation in each of the segments of both lungs.) Air bronchograms may also be noticed on a x-ray film that reveals consolidation.

e.   Look for the presence of, or any changes in, atelectasis. (IB6b) [R, Ap]

Atelectasis is the collapse of alveoli; no air or fluid will be found in them. This problem is commonly seen postoperatively in the lower lobes of patients who have had abdominal or thoracic surgery and do not breathe deeply because of the pain. The x-ray appearance of atelectasis will be an increase in lung markings and a decrease in the lung volumes. If one sided, the mediastinum may shift toward the affected side. For example, a localized atelectasis of a segment or lobe most commonly is seen after a patient has a bronchial obstruction. The air distal to the obstruction is absorbed into the blood stream resulting in alveolar collapse (see Fig. 1-12, A). If bilateral, the mediastinum will be properly located; for example, this condition would be seen in a premature infant with IRDS. The x-ray will reveal a reticulogranular ("ground glass") appearance of diffuse atelectasis. If severe enough, the lungs will appear a uniform white (see Fig. 1-14).

f. Look for the positions of, or any changes in, the hemidiaphragms. (IB6e) [R, Ap]

The normal infant's and adult's A-P or P-A chest x-ray will reveal a domed shape to the hemidiaphragms with the edges turning down to acute costophrenic angles (see Fig. 1-2). A lateral chest x-ray will reveal the same domed shape with the edges turning down to acute costophrenic angles (see Fig. 1-4). The edges of the hemidiaphragms should be smooth without any unusual dips or peaks. The following conditions will result in one or both hemidiaphragms being positioned abnormally: unilateral atelectasis, fibrosis, and pleural fluid; tension pneumothorax, check-valve bronchial obstruction, and chronic obstructive pulmonary disease (COPD) (see Figs. 1-9, 1-12, 1-15, 1-16, and 1-17 for examples). An improvement in the patient's condition should result in a return of the hemidiaphragm(s) to a closer to normal position.

g. Look for the presence of, or any changes in, hyperinflation. (IB6f) [R, Ap]

Hyperinflation is an excessive amount of air in one or both lungs. The specific chest x-ray findings, to some degree, depend on the underlying condition that causes the hyperinflation. Unilateral hyperinflation is caused by a check-valve obstruction as shown in Fig. 1-15. At first glance, a tension pneumothorax appears as unilateral lung hyperinflation. Remember that with this condition the chest is hyperinflated while the lung is collapsed (see Figs. 1-9 and 1-12, C).

The adult with COPD, such as asthma, bronchitis, and emphysema, will show both lungs to be overinflated and both hemidiaphragms depressed (see Figs. 1-16 and 1-17). Other x-ray findings include widened intercostal spaces; hyperlucent lung fields; small, vertical heart; small cardiothoracic diameter; and decreased vascularity of peripheral areas of the lungs with enlarged hilar vessels. The lateral chest x-ray findings in the COPD patient are the same plus they include anterior bowing of the sternum, increased retrosternal air space, and kyphosis.

The newborn with meconium aspiration will often show signs of bilateral hyperinflation from air trapping. The P-A chest x-ray findings may include hyperlucent lungs, depressed hemidiaphragms, and wide rib spaces. The lateral chest x-ray may reveal that the upper ribs lose their downward slope to become more horizontal, the anterior chest protrudes, and there is an increase in the retrosternal air space.

h. Look for the presence of, or any changes in, pleural fluid. (IB6g) [R, Ap]

Abnormally large amounts of pleural fluid will typically be seen on a P-A or A-P film as obscuring the costophrenic angle. This is because gravity will tend to draw the fluid to the lowest level (see Figs. 1-18 and 1-19). Small amounts of fluid can sometimes be better visualized by taking a lateral decubitus x-ray. If the fluid is able to freely move in the pleural space, it will shift in a few minutes to the side that is down (see Fig. 1-20). An empyema that is loculated (fixed) by adhesions will not move when the patient lies on his or her side. If large amounts of fluid are removed by a thoracentesis procedure, a chest x-ray should be taken to confirm the removal of fluid, the reexpansion of the lung, and that a pneumothorax was not caused.

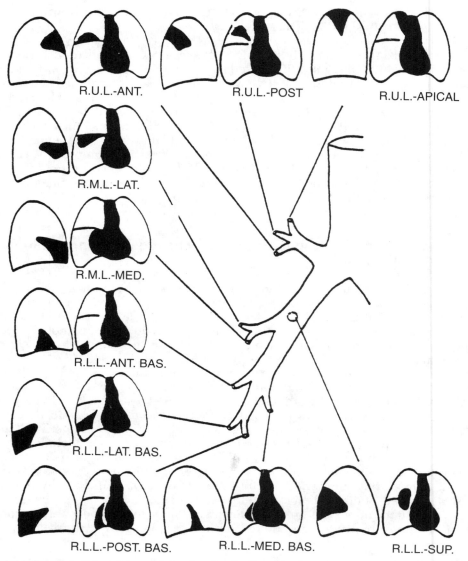

Fig. 1-13 Simulated frontal and lateral x-ray findings for consolidation in the various segments of both lungs. (From Cherniack RM, Cherniack L: *Respiration in health and disease,* ed 3, Philadelphia, 1983, WB Saunders. Used by permission.)

i.   Look for the presence of, or any changes in, pulmonary edema. (IB6h) [R, Ap]

Pulmonary edema is watery fluid that has leaked out of the pulmonary capillary bed into the interstitial spaces and alveoli. It is most commonly caused by left ventricular failure (also known as congestive heart failure), but can also be the result of fluid overload, pulmonary capillary damage, or decreased osmotic pressure in the blood from a low level of protein.

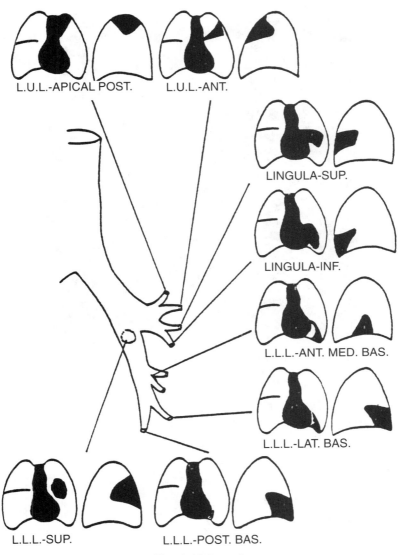

L.U.L.-APICAL POST.   L.U.L.-ANT.

LINGULA-SUP.

LINGULA-INF.

L.L.L.-ANT. MED. BAS.

L.L.L.-LAT. BAS.

L.L.L.-SUP.   L.L.L.-POST. BAS.

Fig. 1-13 *(cont.)*

It is noticed on a P-A or A-P chest x-ray as fluffy, white infiltrates in both lung fields. These tend to be seen more extensively in the lower lobes due to gravity pulling the fluid to the basilar vessels where it leaks out. If the root cause is left ventricular failure, the vessels in the hila will also be engorged and the left ventrical enlarged (see Fig. 1-21). A worsening primary problem will result in more fluid leaking into the lungs and the appearance of more white infiltrates on succeeding chest x-rays. Once the problem is corrected, the lungs will return to normal as the fluid is reabsorbed and removed.

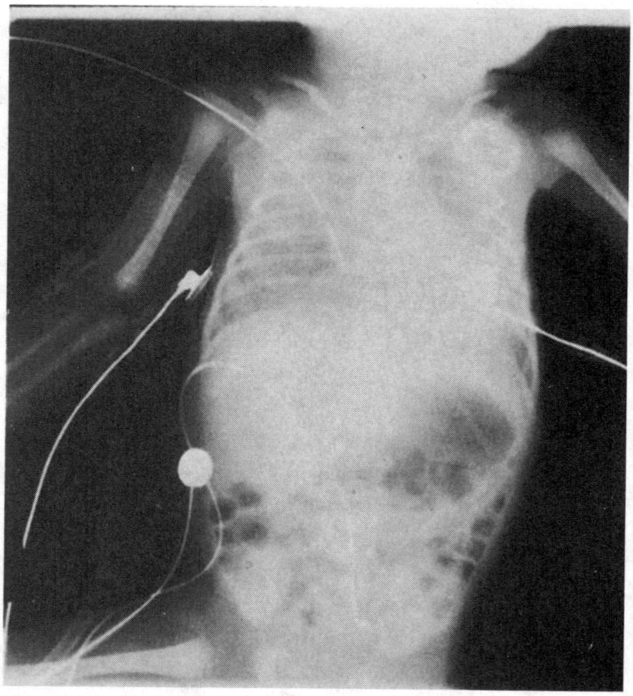

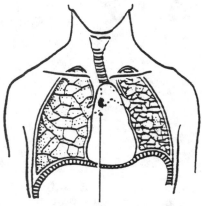

Fig. 1-14 Frontal x-ray of a neonate with severe atelectasis from infant respiratory distress syndrome (IRDS). Also note the right pleural chest tube and wires to various monitoring systems. (From Des Jardins TR: *Clinical manifestations of respiratory disease,* ed 2, Chicago, 1990, Year Book Medical. Used by permission.)

CHECK VALVE OBSTRUCTION
(on exp.)

Fig. 1-15 Simulated frontal x-ray showing a check-valve bronchial obstruction in the right lung in an adult. Note how the mediastinum is shifted away from the overinflated lung and the right hemidiaphragm is depressed. (From Cherniack RM, Cherniack L: *Respiration in health and disease,* ed 3, Philadelphia, 1983, WB Saunders. Used by permission.)

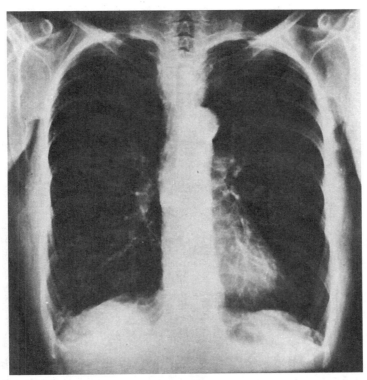

Fig. 1-16 Frontal x-ray of an adult with advanced chronic obstructive pulmonary disease (COPD). Both lungs are overinflated and hyperlucent. The ribs are spread more widely than normal. Often these patients have a cardiothoracic ratio that is smaller than normal because the heart is elongated and the lateral chest diameter is increased. Contrast this film with that of a normal adult as shown in Fig. 1-2. (From Sheldon RL, Wilkins RL: Clinical application of the chest radiograph. In Wilkins RL, Sheldon RL, Krider SJ, editors: *Clinical assessment in respiratory care,* ed 2, St. Louis, 1990, CV Mosby. Used by permission.)

j.   Look for the presence and position of any foreign bodies. (IB6d) [R, Ap]

A foreign body is anything that is not naturally found in the chest. That includes catheters and other medical devices placed there for therapeutic purposes and any nonmedical objects. It is essential that the practitioner know the normal anatomy of the chest to notice when a foreign body is present in it. Metallic objects are easily noticed because they completely block any x-ray penetration through the chest and are clearly outlined on the film as solid, white shadows. Examples include swallowed or aspirated coins or metal buttons, surgical clips or wires, artificial heart valves, internal catheters, and bullets (see Figs. 1-22 to 1-24). Other, nonmetallic foreign objects are much more difficult to identify because they have about the same densities as normal body tissues. This includes plastic pieces from toys and foods such as peanuts. Determining the exact location of a foreign body may require taking P-A, lateral, and oblique chest x-rays.

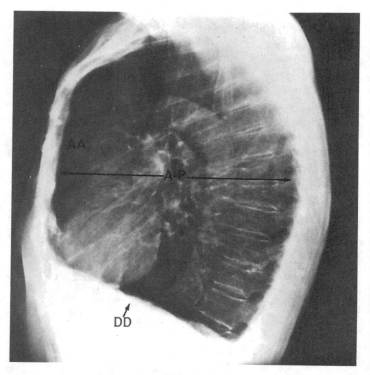

Fig. 1-17 Lateral x-ray of an adult with advanced COPD. Note the characteristic shape of a "barrel chest" from the overinflated lungs. The anteroposterior (A-P) diameter of the chest is increased. *AA* marks an increased anterior airspace between the heart and sternum. The angle of the manubrium and body of the sternum is more obtuse than normal. *DD* marks depressed hemidiaphragms that are flattened. Contrast this film with that of a normal adult as shown in Fig. 1-4. (From Sheldon RL, Wilkins RL: Clinical application of the chest radiograph. In Wilkins RL, Sheldon RL, Krider SJ, editors: *Clinical assessment in respiratory care,* ed 2, St. Louis, 1990, CV Mosby. Used by permission.)

k. Check the chest x-ray for the size and patency of the patient's major airways. (IB6i) [R, Ap]

The trachea and both the right and left mainstem bronchi should be seen on a properly taken chest x-ray film. They will be seen as straight, dark air columns in contrast with the white shadows of the various surrounding tissues (see Figs. 1-2 and 1-3). A white shadow within the airway could be a foreign body or tumor. A lung tumor that is pressing on the airway will cause it to narrow or be occluded.

l. Check the chest x-ray for the position of the patient's endotracheal or tracheostomy tube. (IB6k) [An]

The distal end of all these tubes should be seen within the lumen of the trachea and about midway between the larynx and the tracheal bifurcation to the right and left mainstem bronchi (see Figs. 1-11 and 1-23 for the endotracheal tube placement). The proximal end of the tracheostomy tube (or transtracheal oxygen catheter) will be seen on the film coming out of the surgical insertion site in the suprasternal notch. The distal end should be centered within the trachea above the carina (see Fig. 1-7). Most of these tubes are made of a radio opaque material or have a line

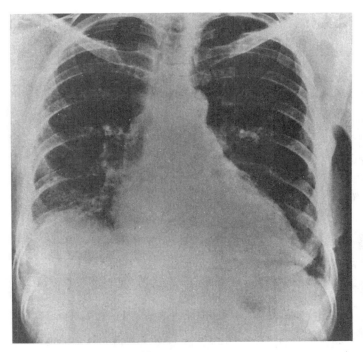

Fig. 1-18 Frontal x-ray of an adult showing a small pleural effusion in the right chest. Note how the costophrenic angle and hemidiaphragm are obscured by the white shadow of fluid. (From Sheldon RL, Wilkins RL; Clinical application of the chest radiograph. In Wilkins RL, Sheldon RL, Krider SJ, editors: *Clinical assessment in respiratory care,* ed 2, St. Louis, 1990, CV Mosby. Used by permission.)

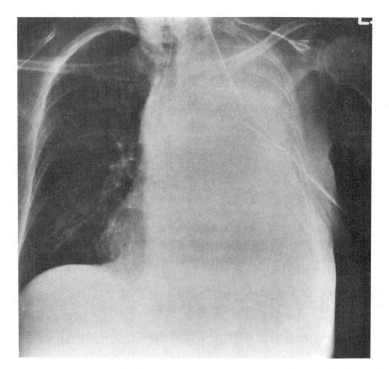

Fig. 1-19 Frontal x-ray of an adult showing a massive pleural effusion in the left chest. Note how the shadow from the fluid causes a "white out" that obscures all left-sided structures. (From Sheldon RL, Wilkins RL: Clinical application of the chest radiograph. In Wilkins RL, Sheldon RL, Krider SJ, editors: *Clinical assessment in respiratory care,* ed 2, St. Louis, 1990, CV Mosby. Used by permission.)

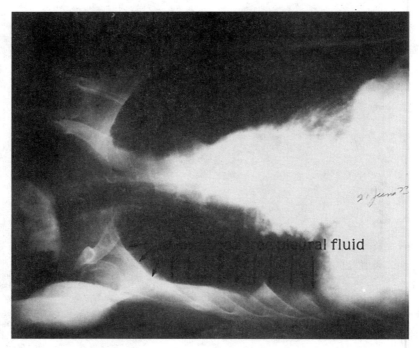

Fig. 1-20 Lateral decubitus x-ray of an adult showing the shift of a small pleural effusion to the now dependent part of the pleural space. The layer of fluid is marked by the arrows. (From Sheldon RL, Wilkins RL: Clinical application of the chest radiograph. In Wilkins RL, Sheldon RL, Krider SJ, editors: *Clinical assessment in respiratory care,* ed 2, St. Louis, 1990, CV Mosby. Used by permission.)

of radio opaque material imbedded into them so that they can be easily seen on the x-ray film.

Care must be taken not to push the endotracheal tube deeper into a bronchus—usually the right—or to pull it out. The tracheostomy tube and transtracheal oxygen catheter are less likely to be displaced if they are properly cared for. Take another x-ray to check the position of any of these tubes if there is clinical evidence that a position may have changed.

m. Check the chest x-ray for a sign that the cuff on the endotracheal or tracheostomy tube is overinflated. (IB61) [R, Ap]

A properly inflated cuff will fill the space between the tube and the patient's trachea; an airtight seal will be made. If the cuff is overinflated it will put excessive pressure on the trachea. This could cause it to dilate and be seen as a wider dark area than the rest of the tracheal air column. If this is noticed, the cuff pressure should be measured. Excessive pressure should be reduced to a safer level (see Section 11, Airway Management, for more discussion on managing cuff pressures.)

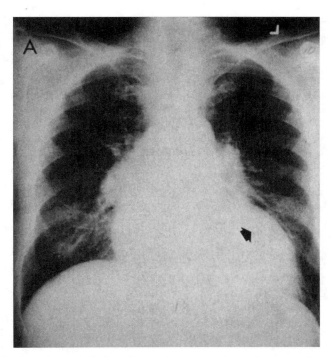

Fig. 1-21 Frontal x-ray of an adult showing pulmonary edema, increased pulmonary vascular markings, and enlarged left ventricle. The cardiothoracic diameter is increased, with the arrow showing where the border of the left ventricle should normally be seen. (From Des Jardins TR: *Clinical manifestations of respiratory disease,* ed 2, Chicago, 1990, Year Book Medical. Used by permission.)

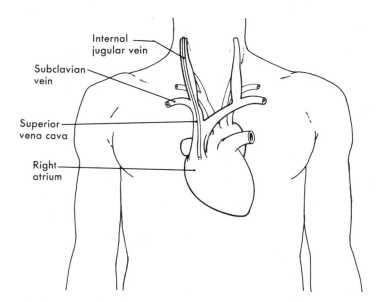

Fig. 1-22 Drawing of an adult with a properly placed central venous pressure (CVP) catheter. (From Daily EK, Schroeder JS: *Techniques in bedside hemodynamic monitoring,* ed 4, St. Louis, 1989, CV Mosby. Used by permission.)

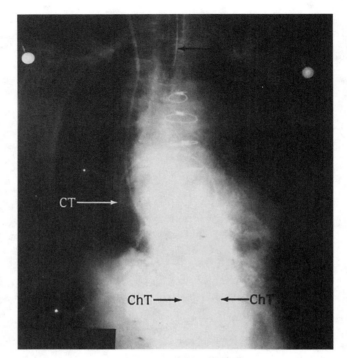

Fig. 1-23 Frontal x-ray of an adult postoperative open heart surgery patient with several medically necessary foreign bodies. A properly placed pulmonary artery (Swan-Ganz) catheter is noted to loop through the right side of the heart and out into the right pulmonary artery. The catheter tip is marked at *CT.* Other foreign bodies include a properly placed endotracheal tube marked at *TT,* sternal wire sutures, ECG chest leads on each shoulder, and pericardial chest tubes marked by *ChT.* (From Sheldon RL, Wilkins RL: Clinical application of the chest radiograph. In Wilkins RL, Sheldon RL, Krider SJ, editors: *Clinical assessment in respiratory care,* ed 2, St. Louis, 1990, CV Mosby. Used by permission.)

Module C. *Interview* the patient in order to find out what his or her sputum production is like. (IB5a) [An]

Time of Maximum and Minimum Expectoration.—Interview the patient to determine the following:

1. Time of maximum expectoration. Ask the patient, "When do you cough up the most? For example, is it in the morning, after eating spicy foods, after a breathing treatment, after smoking, during work, or during exposure to dusts?"
2. Time of minimum expectoration. Ask the patient, "When do you cough up the least? For example, is it during certain nonallergic seasons of the year, after a breathing treatment, or after eating milk or milk products?"

Quantity.—Some practitioners prefer to know of a specific amount such as a teaspoon, tablespoon, 10 ml, and so forth. Others prefer to use subjective measures such "a little" or "a lot." Interview the patient to determine the following:

1. How the quantity of sputum relates to the times of maximum and minimum expectoration and the patient's lifestyle. Ask the patient, "Is

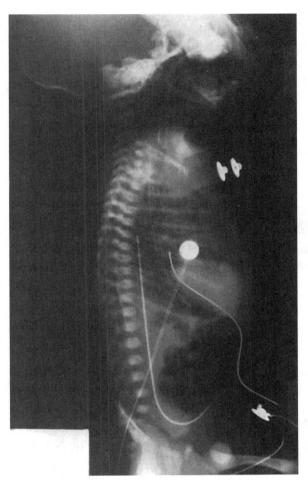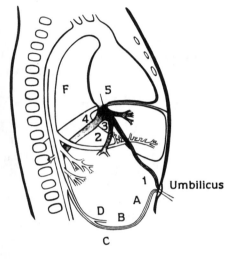

Fig. 1-24 Lateral x-ray and drawing of the internal vascular structures of an infant with an umbilical artery catheter (UAC) and umbilical vein catheter (UVC) in place. The UAC passes through the umbilicus, umbilical artery (*A*), hypogastric artery (*B*), internal iliac artery (*C*), common iliac artery (*D*), abdominal aorta (*E*), to the thoracic aorta (*F*). The umbilical vein catheter passes through the umbilicus, umbilical vein (*1*), portal vein (*2*), ductus venosus (*3*), inferior vena cava (*4*), to the right atrium (*5*). Other foreign bodies include an endotracheal tube and ECG leads. (From Sheldon RL, Wilkins RL: Clinical application of the chest radiograph. In Wilkins RL, Sheldon RL, Krider SJ: *Clinical assessment in respiratory care,* ed 2, St. Louis, 1990, CV Mosby. Used by permission.)

there anything that you do that increases or decreases the amount you cough out?" For example, the patient states that he coughs up 20 cc after his breathing treatments but can cough nothing up after eating a bowl of ice cream.

2. Does the amount coughed up change in a cyclical way? Ask the patient, "Do you cough up the most in the mornings or at night? Is there a work or lifestyle habit that changes how much you cough up? Is there a seasonal allergic condition that influences your asthma and sputum production?"

Adhesiveness of the Sputum.—Interview the patient to determine the following:

1. "Are there times of the day or things that you do in the day that seem to result in your secretions becoming thicker or thinner?"
2. "Do your medications (e.g., Mucomyst) make the secretions easier to cough out?"
3. "Are there foods that make your secretions easier to cough out?"

Module D.   Determine the patient's complete respiratory condition in the following ways by *observation.*

1.   Evaluate the patient's general appearance. (IB1d) [An]

Start by inspecting the patient quickly from head to toe including how he is dressed and found in the room. Ideally, this is done without the patient knowing that he is being observed. The patient who is not suffering from cardiopulmonary disease should be able to lie flat in bed or on either side without any breathing difficulty. He or she should appear to breathe comfortably without any undue effort. The patient with one-sided lung disease may prefer to lie with the good side down. This also might be the case with lobar pneumonia, pleurisy, or broken ribs. The patient with severe airway obstruction, as seen with asthma, bronchitis, or emphysema, will tend to sit up in a chair or on the edge of the bed and lock the arms and shoulders for support. This enables the patient to use the accessory muscles of ventilation. The patient with orthopnea will not want to lie flat because of the resulting shortness of breath. This is commonly seen in patients with congestive heart failure and pulmonary edema.

2.   Determine if the patient is cyanotic. (IB1j) [An]

Cyanosis is an abnormal blue or ashen gray coloration of the skin and mucus membranes. It is most easily seen in Caucasians by looking at the lips and nail beds. It can be seen in darker pigmented people by looking at the inner lip, inner eye lid, or looking at the nail beds.

Commonly, cyanosis is said to be caused by hypoxemia, and that the more bluish a patient's color the more hypoxemic he or she is. This is often the case; however, cyanosis is *not* an accurate measurement of a patient's oxygenation. Cyanosis occurs when more than 5 volumes percent (vol %) of hemoglobin is desaturated. This happens whenever an insufficient amount of oxygen is delivered to the skin and other tissues to meet its metabolic needs (as in a cardiopulmonary arrest). There are three fairly common clinical situations where cyanosis is not a good observational tool to judge the patient's oxygen level. First, the anemic patient may be hypoxic but not cyanotic. This could happen if he or she did not have enough hemoglobin to desaturate 5 volumes percent. Second, the polycythemic patient may appear cyanotic even though he or she is not hypoxic. This would be seen if he had more than 5 volumes percent of desaturated hemoglobin despite having an acceptable PaO_2. Third, the patient in shock may have a normal PaO_2, but be cyanotic because the blood pressure is low and not delivering the oxygen to the tissues. To be safe, the patient with cyanosis should have a blood gas sample drawn for PaO_2 measurement or pulse oximetry performed for SpO_2 measurement to evaluate his oxygenation.

3.   Determine if the patient is diaphoretic. (IB1f) [An]

Diaphoresis is profuse sweating. It is normally seen after vigorous exercise. You would expect to see a patient sweating after a stress test or even an oxygen assisted walk. Diaphoresis in the patient who is resting in bed is a sign of serious trouble. When the body is severely stressed, it releases adrenaline into the blood stream. Diaphoresis is one of a number of bodily effects caused by the release of adrenaline. Similar sweating may be seen if a large enough dose of the drug epinephrine is given.

Diaphoresis is a nonspecific sign of serious cardiopulmonary difficulties. It may be seen any time the patient is in shock and/or hypoxemic. Patients suffering from a myocardial infarct are commonly diaphoretic. The practitioner should promptly evaluate the diaphoretic patient's pulse, respiratory rate, blood pressure, and arterial blood gases.

4.   Determine if the patient has nasal flaring. (IB1q) [An]

Nasal flaring is a dilation of the nares on inspiration. The normal person breathing comfortably should have little or no nasal flaring. The person who is exercising vigorously may have it. It is abnormal to see nasal flaring in a patient who is resting in bed. In this case, it is a sign of increased effort at breathing; the patient is attempting to reduce airway resistance by dilating the nares. Patients of any age will nasal flare when experiencing an increased effort at breathing; however, it is most commonly seen in the premature newborn (see Fig. 1-25).

Nasal flaring is not specific to any disease or condition. Examples of conditions where nasal flaring is seen include IRDS, adult respiratory distress syndrome (ARDS), or any condition where the pulmonary compliance is decreased or the airway resistance is increased.

5.   Determine if the patient has clubbing of the fingers. (IB1i) [An]

Clubbing of the fingers (also known as digital clubbing) is an abnormal thickening of the ends of the fingers. It can also occur in the toes. The key finding is an angle of more than 160° between the top of the finger and the nail when seen from the side. Clinically, you will notice both a lateral and an anteroposterior thickening of the ends of the fingers (see Fig. 1-26 for a comparison of normal to clubbed fingers). The fingernail and toenail beds may be cyanotic.

The underlying cause is not completely understood, but at least in part seems to be chronic hypoxemia. This results in arterio-venous anastomosis with thickening of the tissues. The list of diseases where clubbing is seen includes COPD, bronchogenic carcinoma, bronchiectasis, sarcoidosis, and infective endocarditis.

6.   Determine if the patient has peripheral edema. (IB1c) [An]

Peripheral edema is seen when fluid leaks from the capillary bed into the tissues. It is most commonly seen in the ankles and feet or along the back when the patient is lying supine in bed. You measure the extent of the edema by pressing a finger into the tissues. Normal skin will spring back while edematous skin will be pitted. The pitting edema is graded as plus 1 for 1 mm, plus 2 for 2 mm, and so forth, of indentation. Obviously, the deeper the pitting the more peripheral edema the patient has.

Peripheral edema is most commonly seen in patients with congestive heart failure or who are fluid overloaded. Patients with septicemia will often have periph-

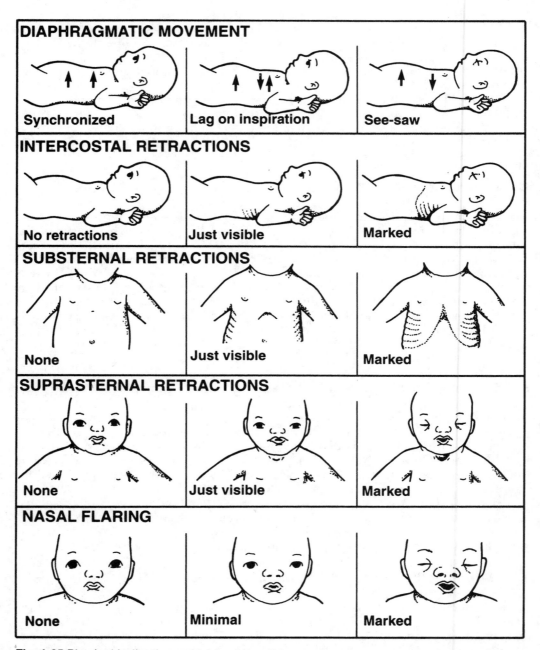

Fig. 1-25 Physical indications of labored breathing. (From Sills JR: *Respiratory care certification guide*, St. Louis, 1991, Mosby–Year Book. Used by permission.)

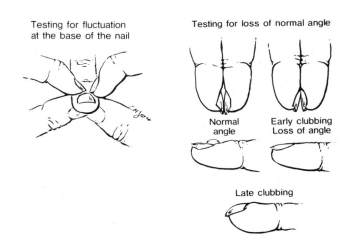

Testing for fluctuation at the base of the nail

Testing for loss of normal angle

Normal angle

Early clubbing Loss of angle

Late clubbing

Fig. 1-26 Signs of and test for clubbing. (From Lehrer S: *Understanding lung sounds*, Philadelphia, 1984, WB Saunders. Used by permission.)

eral edema because the blood-born pathogen (usually *Staphylococci*) will cause abnormal capillary leakage.

7. Determine if the patient has excessive venous distension. (IB1b) [R, Ap]

The internal jugular vein and external/anterior jugular vein are observed in the normal person by having him or her lie supine with the head elevated 30°. The crest of the vein column should be seen just above the border of the midclavicle. A rough measure of the intravascular volume and central venous pressure is made by pressing on the veins at the base of the neck. The returning blood should fill the veins and make them distend (see Fig. 1-27). When the pressure is released the veins should return to their previous level of distension just above the level of the midclavicle. Increased venous distension is noted when the veins stand out at a level above the clavicle. This is seen in patients with right heart failure (cor pulmonale), fluid overload, COPD, and when high airway pressures and positive end-expiratory pressure (PEEP) are needed for mechanical ventilation. The higher the veins are distended, the more the patient is compromised.

It is not normal for the veins to collapse below the clavical when the obstructing finger is removed. If seen, this patient should then have his or her head laid flat. Normally, when flat, the external jugular vein should be seen as partially distended. If the vein collapses on inspiration, low venous pressure is confirmed and the patient is probably hypovolemic. This is commonly seen with dehydration, hemorrhage, or increased urine output following the use of diuretics.

8. Determine the patient's capillary refill. (IB1e) [R, Ap, An]

Capillary refill is the time needed for blood to refill the capillary bed after it has been forced out. The procedure is to pinch the finger or toe nail until it blanches, then release the pressure. The pink color of the nail bed should return in less than 3 seconds. Any delay in the return to pink color would indicate reduced blood flow to the extremities. Cyanotic nail beds would also be seen with reduced blood flow.

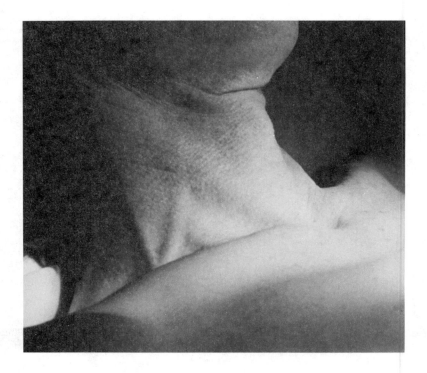

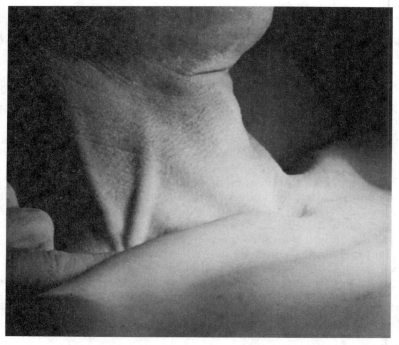

Fig. 1-27 Evaluating distension of the external jugular vein. These photographs show a patient with right-sided heart failure. Note that the top photograph shows the external jugular vein distended above the level of the clavicle. The bottom photograph shows how pressing a finger over the external jugular vein results in its further filling with blood and distending. In a normal person, when the pressure is released the vein should collapse to just above the superior border of the mid-clavicle. See the text for further discussion. (From Daily EK, Schroder JS: *Techniques in bedside hemodynamic monitoring,* ed 4, St. Louis, 1989, Mosby. Used by permission.)

Examples of conditions that would result in a decreased capillary refill include decreased cardiac output, low blood pressure from any cause, and the use of vasopressor medications.

9. Determine if the patient has muscle wasting. (IB1a) [R, Ap]

Muscle wasting is an abnormal condition of decreased muscle mass. The muscle wasting can be generalized or localized depending on the underlying cause. Examples of conditions where muscle wasting is seen include:

a. COPD such as emphysema and bronchitis. This lung disease often results in muscle wasting because the patient is consuming an unusually large number of calories through the act of breathing. In addition, these patients often do not eat well because a full stomach restricts the movement of the diaphragm and worsens their work of breathing and shortness of breath. Because of this, they are frequently malnourished or undernourished. Their arms and legs will be thin; their shoulder, elbow, and knee joints will be prominent; and their ribs will be clearly outlined by deep intercostal spaces.

b. Lung cancer or other cancers usually result in a loss of muscle mass. This is because the growing tumor consumes many calories that are not available to the normal body tissues. These patients usually also have thin arms and legs with prominent joints during advanced disease.

c. Neurological injuries, such as transsection of the spinal cord, result in atrophy of the affected muscles. Atrophy of the muscles is a decrease in their size due to the lack of use. This is an unavoidable consequence of the permanent loss of nerve input to the affected muscles. For example, transsection of the spinal cord at the first lumbar vertebrae (L1) results in loss of nerve input to the legs. The patient is a paraplegic. In time, the muscles of the legs will atrophy; however, if the arms are exercised, they retain their normal muscle mass. If the patient has a spinal transsection that results in the loss of nerve input to both the arms and legs (quadreplegia), all of the limbs will atrophy.

10. Determine the shape of the patient's chest. (IB1k) [An]

The patient should be sitting up straight or standing erect when being examined for chest configuration. Look at the patient from the front, back, and both sides to see the symmetry. See Fig. 1-28 for the appearance of the normal infant's and adult's chest, barrel chest, funnel chest, pigeon chest, and thoracic kyphoscoliosis. The spinal column can be curved in several ways. Kyphosis is an exaggerated A-P curvature of the upper spine. Lordosis is an exaggerated A-P curvature of the lower spine. Scoliosis is either a right or left lateral curvature of the spine. Kyphoscoliosis is either a right or left lateral curvature combined with an A-P curvature of the spine.

11. Determine if the patient has asymmetrical chest movement when breathing. (IB1o) [An]

The normal infant and adult will have symmetrical chest movement when breathing at rest or during exercise. All breathing efforts are best observed when the patient is not wearing a shirt. In females, it may be necessary to observe only the uncovered back to judge chest movement. Any kind of asymmetrical chest movement is abnormal. The asymmetrical movement may be from an abnormality of the chest wall, abdomen, or from a pulmonary disorder.

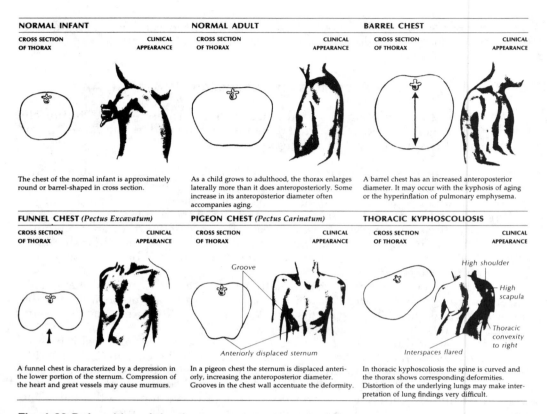

NORMAL INFANT		NORMAL ADULT		BARREL CHEST	
CROSS SECTION OF THORAX	CLINICAL APPEARANCE	CROSS SECTION OF THORAX	CLINICAL APPEARANCE	CROSS SECTION OF THORAX	CLINICAL APPEARANCE

The chest of the normal infant is approximately round or barrel-shaped in cross section.

As a child grows to adulthood, the thorax enlarges laterally more than it does anteroposteriorly. Some increase in its anteroposterior diameter often accompanies aging.

A barrel chest has an increased anteroposterior diameter. It may occur with the kyphosis of aging or the hyperinflation of pulmonary emphysema.

FUNNEL CHEST *(Pectus Excavatum)*		PIGEON CHEST *(Pectus Carinatum)*		THORACIC KYPHOSCOLIOSIS	
CROSS SECTION OF THORAX	CLINICAL APPEARANCE	CROSS SECTION OF THORAX	CLINICAL APPEARANCE	CROSS SECTION OF THORAX	CLINICAL APPEARANCE

A funnel chest is characterized by a depression in the lower portion of the sternum. Compression of the heart and great vessels may cause murmurs.

Groove

Anteriorly displaced sternum

In a pigeon chest the sternum is displaced anteriorly, increasing the anteroposterior diameter. Grooves in the chest wall accentuate the deformity.

High shoulder

High scapula

Thoracic convexity to right

Interspaces flared

In thoracic kyphoscoliosis the spine is curved and the thorax shows corresponding deformities. Distortion of the underlying lungs may make interpretation of lung findings very difficult.

Fig. 1-28 Deformities of the thorax. (From Bates B: *A guide to physical examination and history taking,* ed 4, Philadelphia, 1987, JB Lippincott. Used by permission.)

Thoracic Scoliosis or Kyphoscoliosis.—Patients with either of these problems will have greater chest wall movement on the side to which the spine is curved. The other side of the chest will be compressed and move less with inspiration.

Flail Chest.—The flail segment will move in the opposite direction of the rest of the chest (also known as paradoxical movement). That is, with inspiration, the flail segment will move inward while the rest of the chest moves outward, and during expiration the flail segment will move outward as the rest of the chest moves inward. As the ribs heal, the segment will stabilize and move with the rest of the chest.

Pneumothorax.—The side with the collapsed lung will not move as much as the chest wall over the normal lung (see Fig. 1-12, C).

Atelectasis/Pneumonia.—The side with the atelectasis or pneumonia will not move as much as the chest wall over the normal lung (see Fig. 1-12, B).

12. Determine if the patient has intercostal and/or sternal retractions when breathing. (IB1p) [An]

Intercostal retractions are noticed when the soft tissues between the ribs are drawn inward during inspiration as the chest wall moves outward (see Fig. 1-25). Suprasternal retractions are noticed when the soft tissues *above* the sternum are drawn inward during an inspiration as the chest wall moves outward. Substernal retractions are noticed when the soft tissues *below* the sternum are drawn inward during an inspiration as the chest wall moves outward (see Fig. 1-25 for both).

The typical person who is breathing at rest should not have any retractions. That same person may have some minor retractions during vigorous exercise. Retractions of any kind are abnormal in any patient of any age who is resting in bed. Retractions are commonly seen in conditions where the airway resistance is increased or the lung compliance is decreased. Both of these will increase a patient's work of breathing. The patient must generate a more negative intrathoracic pressure to breathe and as a result the various soft tissues are drawn inward during inspiration. Conditions where this is seen include IRDS, ARDS, pulmonary edema, pneumonia, asthma, bronchitis, and emphysema.

13. Determine if the patient uses accessory muscles when breathing. (IB1n) [An]

Accessory muscles of ventilation should not be needed during passive, resting breathing. They may be used when breathing vigorously during exercise. The dyspneic patient is likely to use them even when resting. The accessory muscles of inspiration are the intercostals, the scalenii, sternocleidomastoids, trapezii, and rhomboids. The abdominal muscles are used during active expiration. The easiest accessory muscles of inspiration to observe in action are the sternocleidomastoids from the front and side of the patient and the trapezii from the back of the patient.

Accessory muscle use in a patient who is resting should make you realize that the work of breathing is greatly increased. The finding is not specific for any one condition, but it is seen commonly in the patient with emphysema.

14. Determine if the patient has diaphragmatic movement when breathing. (IB1l) [An]

Normally the adult's diaphragm moves downward several centimeters toward the abdomen during inspiration as the chest wall moves outward. This is seen as the abdomen protrudes when its contents are forced forward. The chest and abdomen should rise and fall together during quiet and vigorous breathing efforts.

There are two conditions where this normal chest and abdominal movement does not occur. First is a patient with emphysema, severe air trapping, and a barrel chest. This patient's diaphragm is depressed and flat rather than domed because of the air that is trapped in the lungs. On inspiration, the diaphragm still contracts but is unable to displace the abdominal contents down to permit air to be drawn into the lungs. You will notice that this patient does not have the expected abdominal movement during inspiration. This patient will use the accessory muscles of inspiration to assist his breathing.

Second is any condition where the airway resistance is increased or lung compliance is decreased. The greater negative intrathoracic pressure needed to draw the tidal volume into the lungs can cause the chest wall to collapse inward as the abdominal contents are displaced outward. The result is a kind of "see-saw" or paradoxical movement relationship between the chest wall and abdomen. On inspiration, the chest wall may move inward as the abdomen moves outward. This is most commonly seen in IRDS because the premature neonate's rib cage is relatively compliant compared to the stiff lungs (see Fig. 1-25).

15. Determine the patient's breathing pattern. (IB1m) [An]

The various respiratory patterns can be identified by their characteristic respiratory rate, respiratory cycle, and tidal volume as follows.

A. Eupnea (normal breathing)
  1. Normal respiratory rate for the age of the patient.
  2. Normal respiratory cycle. When timing the flow of air into and out of the lungs, the inspiratory : expiratory (I : E) ratio is 1 : 1.5 to 1 : 2. A pause of variable time will follow the exhalation of the tidal volume. This will change the true I : E ratio to 1 : 2 to 1 : 4.
  3. Tidal volume is normal for the size of the patient. Inspiration is achieved without the use of accessory muscles of inspiration; exhalation is passive.
B. Hypopnea (shallow breathing)
  1. Respiratory rate is usually somewhat slower than normal.
  2. Normal respiratory cycle.
  3. Tidal volume is decreased for the size of the patient.
  4. Possible causes: deep sleep, sedation, coma, hypothermia, alkalemia, restrictive lung disease.
  5. May be combined with bradypnea.
C. Hyperpnea (deep breathing)
  1. Respiratory rate may be normal or somewhat faster.
  2. Normal respiratory cycle.
  3. Tidal volume is increased for the size of the patient.
  4. Possible causes: acidemia, fever, pain, fear, anxiety, increased intercranial pressure.
  5. May be combined with tachypnea.
D. Bradypnea (slow breathing)
  1. Slower than normal respiratory rate.
  2. Expiration may be longer than normal due to a longer pause.
  3. Tidal volume will be decreased for the size of the patient.
  4. Possible causes: deep sleep, sedation, coma, hypothermia, alkalemia.
  5. May be combined with hypopnea.
E. Tachypnea (rapid breathing)
  1. Faster than the normal respiratory rate.
  2. Inspiration may be faster than normal with the help of inspiratory accessory muscles. Expiration may be shorter than normal and expiratory accessory muscles may be used to force the air out faster. The pause seen in eupnea will be gone. The inspiratory : expiratory ratio may be 1 : 2 or less.
  3. The tidal volume may be increased for the size of the patient.
  4. Possible causes: acidemia, fever, pain, anxiety, increased intracranial pressure.
  5. May be combined with hyperpnea.
F. Obstructed inspiration
  1. Normal to slower respiratory rate.
  2. Inspiratory time will be equal to or longer than expiratory time. Inspiration will be aided by the use of the inspiratory accessory muscles. Expiration will be passive.
  3. Tidal volume may be normal, larger, or smaller than normal depending on how the patient adapts to the increased work of breathing. It is most common to see a slower rate with a larger tidal volume.
  4. Possible causes: croup, epiglottitis, foreign body aspiration with partial airway obstruction, postextubation laryngeal edema, airway tumor, or airway trauma.
G. Obstructed expiration
  1. Normal to slower respiratory rate.

2. Expiratory time will be longer than normal. Accessory muscles of inspiration and expiration may be used.
3. Tidal volume may be normal or decreased for the size of the patient.
4. Possible causes: asthma, emphysema, bronchitis, cystic fibrosis, bronchiectasis, airway tumor, or airway trauma.

H. Kussmaul respiration (rapid, large breaths)
1. Faster than normal rate.
2. Inspiratory : expiratory ratio will approach 1 : 1. Both inspiratory and expiratory accessory muscles may be used.
3. Tidal volume will be increased for the size of the patient.
4. Probable cause: acidemia (pH 7.2 to 6.95) from diabetic ketoacidosis.

I. Cheyne-Stokes respiration (waxing and waning tidal volumes)
1. The respiratory rate varies from normal or faster and may have short periods of apnea.
2. The respiratory cycle is normal or approximates it except if the patient has periods of apnea.
3. The tidal volumes "wax and wane" over a variable time cycle. A 20-second cycle is fairly common. There may be periods of apnea between the decreased tidal volumes.
4. Possible causes: head injury, stroke, increased intracranial pressure, or congestive heart failure.

J. Biot's respiration (unpredictably variable)
1. The respiratory rate will vary from rapid to short periods of apnea.
2. The respiratory cycle will vary considerably.
3. The tidal volume will vary from shallow to large.
4. Possible causes: head injury, brain tumor, increased intracranial pressure.

K. Apnea (cessation of breathing at the end of exhalation)
1. Apnea that lasts long enough to result in hypoxemia, bradycardia, and hypotension must be treated aggressively. Artificial respiration, with or without supplemental oxygen, must be started immediately.
2. It is important to evaluate the patient's previous breathing pattern to determine the cause of the apnea. Normal breathing followed by apnea might lead you to consider causes of heart attack, stroke, or upper airway obstruction. An abnormal breathing pattern followed by apnea might lead you to consider the cause(s) of the original abnormal breathing.
3. Evaluate the previous tidal volume variation for the same reasons as above.
4. Possible causes: airway obstruction, heart attack, stroke, or head injury.

16. Determine the kind of cough the patient has. (IB1r) [An]

Normal Cough

The normal cough has four parts: 1) a deep inspiration is taken in, 2) the epiglottis and vocal cords close to keep the air trapped in the lungs, 3) the abdominal and other expiratory muscles contract to raise the air pressure in the lungs, and 4) the epiglottis and vocal cords open to allow the compressed air to explosively escape and remove any mucus or foreign matter. All these components must work individually and in a coordinated manner for the patient to have an effective cough. The following are possible variations used by patients who for some reason cannot cough normally.

Serial Cough

All the actions of a normal cough take place in a serial cough except that the patient performs a series of smaller coughs rather than a single large one. This method of coughing may be used by postoperative patients who complain of too much abdominal or thoracic pain to cough normally. As the pain lessens, the patient should be able to cough normally.

Midinspiratory Cough

All the actions of a normal cough take place in a midinspiratory cough except that the patient does not take as deep a breath. This is sometimes used by emphysema and bronchitis patients to help prevent airway collapse when they cough.

Huff Cough

A huff cough is used by patients with artificial airways. They cannot close the epiglottis and vocal cords, so they can only take a large breath and blow out with as much force as possible. It is still an effective way to clear secretions if they are thin enough.

Assisted Cough

With an assisted cough, the patient needs direct help from the practitioner. The patient is given a deep breath by means of an IPPB machine or manual ventilator. Then the practitioner helps the patient blow the air out quickly by pushing on the abdominal area to move the diaphragm up. This procedure is limited to conscious patients with neuromuscular defects who cannot cough effectively on their own.

Module E.   Determine the patient's complete respiratory condition in the following ways by *palpation.*

1.   Determine the patient's pulse rate, rhythm, and force. (IB2c) [An]

The heart rate is most commonly counted by palpating the following locations: carotid, femoral, radial, and brachial arteries, and apical pulse of the heart. Other arterial sites such as the temporal, dorsalis pedis, and posterior tibial can be used but are more difficult to find. The pulse should be counted for a minimum of 30 seconds with 1 minute being the most accurate.

Palpating a pulse at any of the sites mentioned reveals the timing between the heart beats. This rhythm is normally regular in people who are at rest or exercising at a steady level. The rhythm is felt and mentally timed as the pulse rate is counted. The time period between beats should be about the same.

The respiratory effort may have some influence on the rhythm. Fairly common in children and sometimes in adults, the heart rhythm and rate speed up on inspiration and slow down on expiration. This sinus arrhythmia is not really abnormal; it is caused when the negative intrathoracic pressure during inspiration draws blood more quickly into the thorax and heart. The opposite may be true during mechanical ventilation with a high peak pressure or mean airway pressure. Then the heart rhythm and rate may slow during inspiration and speed up during expiration. In any other case, an irregular rhythm would indicate some sort of cardiac problem. An ECG would be needed to help determine the specific cause.

The force of the pulse is an indicator of the strength of the heart's contraction and blood pressure. Normally each heartbeat should be felt with the same amount of force. The clinical experience of feeling the pulse of many patients with normal blood pressure and without heart disease will lead to the development of a sense of touch for a "normal" heart's force of contraction.

A "thready" or variable force felt with each heartbeat is usually a sign of heart disease. Atrial fibrillation is an example of an irregular heart rhythm that results in an irregular force. The irregular rate and rhythm cause variable volumes of blood to be pumped with each contraction. A large volume of blood will be felt as a strong pulse whereas a small volume of blood will be felt as a weak pulse.

A "bounding" or greater than normal force felt with each beat is usually a sign of hypertension. In either case, for safety's sake, blood pressure should be taken. Compare it to the patient's previous blood pressure to see if there has been a change.

2. Determine if the patient has palpable rhonchi indicating secretions in the airway. (IB2d) [An]

Palpable rhonchi (also known as tactile fremitus) are noticed when vibrations from airway secretions can be felt through the chest wall as the patient breathes. They are abnormal because they indicate that the patient has a significant secretion problem. Palpable rhonchi would not be detected in a patient with clear airways. Having the patient cough or suctioning the airway to remove secretions will result in the reduction or complete elimination of palpable rhonchi. Remember that an airway that is completely occluded by a mucus plug or foreign body will *not* reveal palpable rhonchi because there is no airflow. Breath sounds would also be absent in this area.

There are different methods of detecting palpable rhonchi. Some practitioners may prefer to use their fingertips whereas others prefer the edge of the open or closed hand. It is important to assess all areas of the patient's chest for palpable rhonchi to detect their exact location(s), symmetry, and anterior and posterior differences.

3. Determine if the patient has tactile fremitus. (IB2a) [R, Ap]

Tactile fremitus is a vibration felt through the chest wall when the patient speaks. Normally, when a sound is created in the larynx, its vibration is carried throughout the tracheobronchial tree to the lung parenchyma and to the chest wall. The intensity of the vibration or its absence gives the practitioner important information on the patient's condition.

Fig. 1-29 shows different methods of detecting tactile fremitus. Some practitioners may prefer to use their fingertips as in Fig. 1-29, A and B, whereas others prefer the ulnar edge of the open or closed hand as in Fig. 1-29, C and D. It is important to assess all areas of the patient's chest for tactile fremitus to detect any variations. Fig. 1-29, E and F show that this should be done over both lung fields to compare their symmetry as well as anterior and posterior differences. Fig. 1-30 shows the posterior and anterior locations for the evaluation of tactile fremitus. Start with the supraclavicular fossae and proceed to alternate intercostal spaces. An attempt must be made to preserve the adult female patient's modesty when evaluating over the anterior locations. The patient may be asked to lift the breast in order to palpate beneath it.

The procedure for evaluating tactile fremitus is to have the patient say "99" in a normal voice as the practitioner's fingers or hand are moved from location to

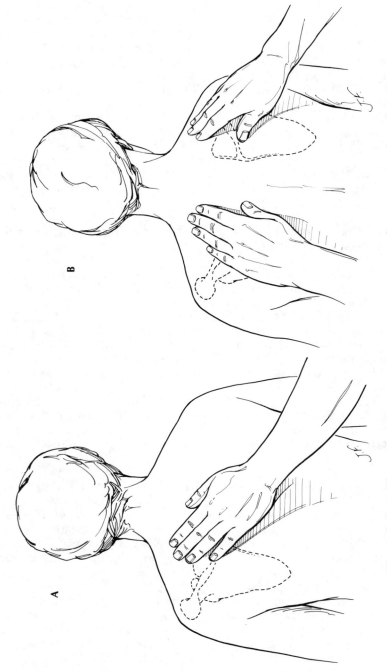

Fig. 1-29 Techniques for feeling tactile fremitus. (See the text for a complete discussion.) (From Eubanks DH, Bone RC: *Comprehensive respiratory care*, ed 2, St. Louis, 1990, CV Mosby. Used by permission.)

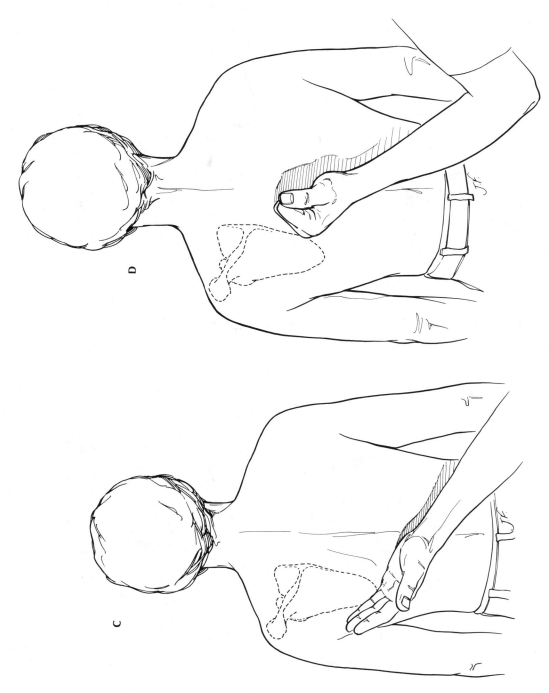

Fig. 1-29 *(cont.)*

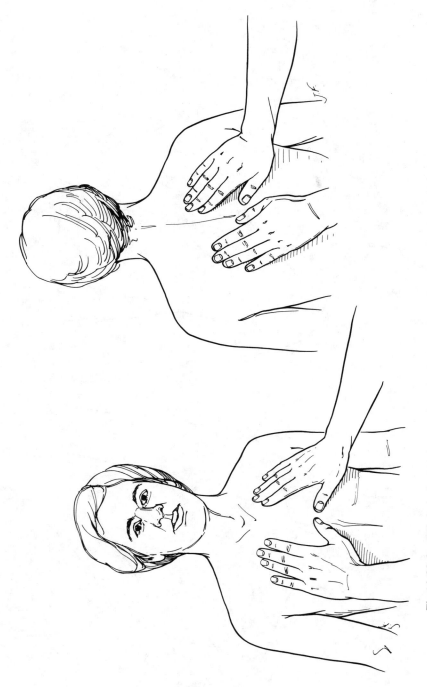

Fig. 1-29 (cont.) Anterior and posterior placement of hands to detect bilateral changes in tactile fremitus. (From Eubanks DH, Bone RC: *Comprehensive respiratory care*, ed 2, St. Louis, 1990, CV Mosby. Used by permission.)

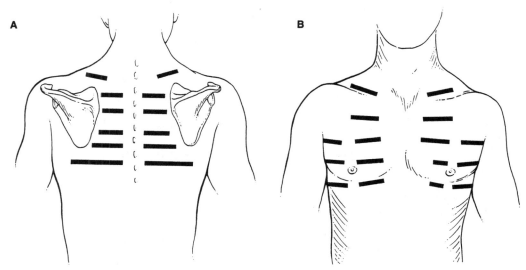

Fig. 1-30 A, Locations on the posterior chest for feeling tactile fremitus and performing percussion. **B,** Locations on the anterior chest for feeling tactile fremitus and performing percussion. (From Swartz MH: *Textbook of physical diagnosis*, Philadelphia, 1989, WB Saunders. Used by permission.)

location. This procedure is also called palpation for bronchophony. The "99" should be spoken at least once for each location to determine any variations. Having the patient speak more loudly or deeply should increase the intensity of the vibrations felt. The intensity of the vibrations directly relates to the density of the underlying lung and chest cavity. Conditions that increase density will result in more intense vibrations. Conversely, conditions that decrease density will result in less intense vibrations. Vibrations are also reduced when they are blocked from penetrating through to the surface. See Table 1-4 for conditions that alter tactile fremitus.

4. Determine if the patient has any tracheal deviation. (IB2e) [R, Ap, An]

Normally the trachea is in a midline position within the neck and thorax. The location of the trachea is found by gently inserting the index finger into the suprasternal notch of an upright or supine patient (see Fig. 1-31). The trachea

Table 1-4. Abnormal Tactile Fremitus

Increased	Decreased
Unilateral	Unilateral
Pneumonia	Pneumothorax
Atelectasis	Pleural effusion
Consolidation	Bronchial obstruction
Bilateral	Bilateral
Pulmonary edema	Thick chest wall (fat or muscle)
Adult respiratory distress syndrome (ARDS)	Chronic obstructive pulmonary disease (COPD)

should be detected in midline with soft tissues on both sides. A trachea that is shifted off to one side is abnormal and can be caused by the following (see Fig. 1-12):

    a. Atelectasis, which causes the trachea to be pulled *toward* the affected side.

    b. Pulmonary fibrosis, which causes the trachea to be pulled *toward* the most affected side.

    c. Tension pneumothorax, which causes the trachea to be pushed *away* from the affected side.

    d. Hemothorax, pleural effusion, and empyema, which push the trachea *away* from the affected side.

Correction of the underlying pulmonary problem will result in the trachea returning to its normal midline position.

5. Determine if the patient has any tenderness. (IB2b) [R, Ap]

Tenderness is an increased local sensation of pain when the chest is gently hit with the ulnar area of the fist. This tapping is done in a symmetrical pattern over the posterior and anterior lung areas and normally should not cause any pain. Intercostal tenderness would be felt at the site of an inflamed pleura. Local tenderness and a history of trauma to an area of the chest would lead to the conclusion of musculoskeletal pain. A chest x-ray might be indicated to determine if any ribs have been fractured. The absence of chest wall tenderness should lead to a further investigation as to the cause of the chest pain. Consider angina pectoris (hypoxic heart pain).

Module F. Determine the patient's complete respiratory condition in the following ways by *auscultation*.

Note: Knowledge of normal and abnormal breath sounds will be tested on the Written Registry Exam. Breath sounds are discussed in detail in *Respiratory Care*

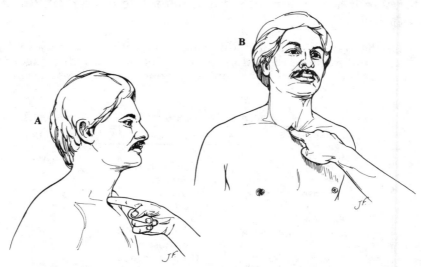

Fig. 1-31 A and **B,** Detecting the position of the trachea by pressing the index finger into the suprasternal notch. (From Eubanks DH, Bone RC: *Comprehensive respiratory care,* ed 2, St. Louis, 1990, CV Mosby. Used by permission.)

Certification Guide (Sills, 1994) and other respiratory care textbooks. They will be presented here again in a shortened form. It must be presumed that the student or examinee has practical experience in the proper use of a stethoscope for listening to breath sounds. Also, it is presumed that he or she has had the clinical opportunity to listen to a number of patients with normal and abnormal breath sounds.

1.   Determine if the patient has bilaterally normal breath sounds. (IB4f) [An]

A Joint Pulmonary Nomenclature Committee of the American College of Chest Physicians and the American Thoracic Society has recommended the following three terms:

1. *Normal.* Normal breath sounds are also called vesicular (Eubanks and Bone, 1985; Wilkins, Hodgkin, & Lopez, 1988), alveolar (Burton, 1988), and normal vesicular (Lehrer, 1984). These normal breath sounds would be heard over all areas of normally ventilated lungs. Normal breath sounds have been variously described as "leaves rustling," "like a gentle breeze," and so forth. These faint sounds are made as air is moved through the small airways of the lungs during the breathing cycle. They should be heard equally in all lung fields. The inspiratory to expiratory phase ratio is about 3 : 1. The inspiratory sound is louder than the expiratory sound and there is no pause between inspiration and expiration. See Table 1-5 for a graphic representation and other information about normal/vesicular breath sounds.

2. *Bronchial.* Bronchial breath sounds are also called tubular (Eubanks and Bone, 1985), tracheal (Burton, 1988), and tracheobronchial (Wilkins et al., 1988). These normal breath sounds would be heard over the trachea and main bronchi. Bronchial breath sounds have been described as being louder, harsher, and higher pitched than normal. They have a fairly uniform pitch on inspiration and expiration with a distinct pause in the transition of flow. The I : E ratio is about 1 : 1.5.

Lehrer (1984) and Wilkins et al (1988) describe a *tracheal* breath sound that is normally heard over the laryngeal area. It is very loud and high pitched. The I : E ratio is about 1 : 1 with a distinct pause between the phases. This normal sound heard in the larynx will be contrasted later with the abnormal sound of stridor. (See Table 1-5 for a graphic representation and other information about bronchial/tubular/tracheal breath sounds.)

Bronchial breath sounds are abnormal if heard in any other areas except those mentioned in this section. When bronchial sounds are heard over areas that should normally be vesicular, it is a sign of consolidation or atelectasis with a patent airway.

3. *Bronchovesicular.* Eubanks and Bone (1985), Burton (1988), Lehrer (1984), and Wilkins et al (1988) describe the third breath sound, bronchovesicular, as normal. Eubanks and Bone (1985) and Burton (1988) say that this sound is heard normally over the right supraclavicular area because large bronchi are relatively close to the surface. Lehrer says that this sound is heard normally anteriorly between the first and second intercostal spaces and posteriorly between the scapula. (Note that Eubanks and Bone call the sound in this location tubular.)

The sound is a cross between bronchial and vesicular. It is more muffled than bronchial but louder than vesicular, and it has the same pitch throughout inspiration and expiration. The I : E ratio is about 1 : 1. (See Table 1-5 for a graphic representation and other information about bronchovesicular breath sounds.)

Bronchovesicular breath sounds are abnormal if heard in any other areas except those mentioned here. When bronchovesicular sounds are heard over areas that should be normal vesicular, it is a sign of partial consolidation or atelectasis with a patent airway.

Table 1-5. Normal Breath Sounds

Breath Sound	Graphic Representation*	Location	Quality	I : E Ratio
Vesicular	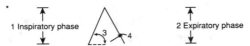	Areas other than trachea and large airways	Lower pitched and less loud than other normal breath sounds, breezy sounding	3 : 1
Tracheal		Over trachea	Loudest and highest pitched of the normal breath sounds, harsh and tubular	5 : 6
Bronchial		Over larger airways	Loud and high pitched but less loud and lower pitched than tracheal sounds, hollow sounding	2 : 3
Bronchovesicular		Near large airways	Moderately loud, lower pitch than bronchial sounds of vesicular and bronchial breath sounds	1 : 1

From DiPietro JS, Mustard MN: *Clinical guide for respiratory care practitioners*, Norwalk, Conn, 1987, Appleton & Lange. Used by permission.

* 1 Inspiratory phase   2 Expiratory phase

1. Graphic representation of inspiration. Line length represents duration. 2. Graphic representation of expiration. Line length represents duration. 3. Graphic representation of the pitch of the breath sound, as demonstrated by the angle. 4. Line thickness, graphically representing the amplitude of the breath sound.

2. Determine if the patient has increased, decreased, absent, or unequal breath sounds. (IB4b) [An]

This discussion is limited to variations in normal vesicular breath sounds. The abnormal appearance of bronchial and bronchovesicular breath sounds was discussed earlier.

a. Increased normal vesicular breath sounds:

• Found most often in children and in debilitated adults because their thinner chest walls transmit the sounds better.

b. Decreased normal vesicular breath sounds:

• Most commonly caused by a pleural effusion, hemothorax, or empyema because of fluid between the lung and the stethoscope (see Fig. 1-12, D).
• Pulmonary fibrosis due to decreased airflow (see Fig. 1-12, B).
• Emphysema due to decreased airflow.
• Pleural thickening due to dampening from the thicker pleural tissues.

c. Absent normal vesicular breath sounds:

- Pneumothorax due to the lung being forced away from the chest wall (see Fig. 1-12, C).
- Atelectasis because no air moves into the collapsed area (see Fig. 1-12, A).
- Endotracheal tube placed into a bronchus instead of the trachea. In this case, the right bronchus is most commonly intubated so that the breath sounds are absent over the left lung.
- Large pleural effusion.
- Very obese patient.

d. Unequal normal vesicular breath sounds:

- Pneumonia, consolidation, or atelectasis that decreases airflow into a segment or lobe.
- Foreign body or tumor in a bronchus that decreases airflow to the distal lung.
- Spinal or thoracic deformity that reduces airflow to the underlying lung.

3. Determine if the patient has rhonchi (wheezing) or rales (crackles). (IB4g and h) [An]

Rhonchi

Rhonchi (also known as wheeze and rhonchus) have the following features or characteristics:

- They are continuous sounds.
- They are more commonly heard on expiration than inspiration.
- Low-pitched, polyphonic expiratory sounds are commonly associated with secretions in the airways. Coughing or tracheal suctioning will often cause these sounds to be modified or eliminated. Common pulmonary conditions include asthma, bronchitis, pneumonia, or any other secretion-causing problem. Common terms for these sounds include rhonchus, sonorous rhonchus, low-pitched wheeze, sonorous wheeze, and polyphonic wheeze.
- High-pitched, monophonic expiratory sounds are commonly associated with closure of the small airways. Coughing or tracheal suctioning is unlikely to eliminate these sounds. Common pulmonary conditions include asthma, emphysema, congestive heart failure, foreign body aspiration, airway tumor, asbestosis, and interstitial fibrosis. Common terms for these sounds include wheeze, high-pitched wheeze, sibilant rhonchus, sibilant rale, and monophonic wheeze.

See Fig. 1-32 and Table 1-6 for more information on interpreting abnormal/adventitious breath sounds.

Rales (Crackles)

Rales have the following features or characteristics:

- They are discontinuous sounds.
- They are more commonly heard on inspiration than expiration.

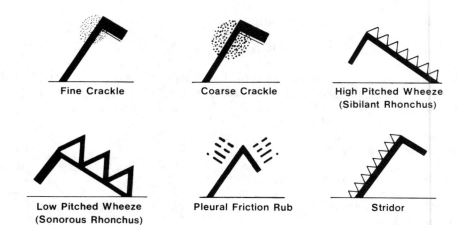

Fine Crackle   Coarse Crackle   High Pitched Wheeze (Sibilant Rhonchus)

Low Pitched Wheeze (Sonorous Rhonchus)   Pleural Friction Rub   Stridor

Fig. 1-32 Graphic representation of abnormal breath sound patterns. (From Lehrer S: *Understanding lung sounds.* Philadelphia, 1984, WB Saunders. Used by permission.)

- They are caused by the sudden opening of collapsed airways.
- They are heard as a repeated sound during the same phase of the respiratory cycle.
- Early inspiratory crackles are heard in patients with obstructive lung diseases such as chronic bronchitis, bronchiectasis, asthma, and emphysema.

Table 1-6. Adventitious Breath Sounds

Crackling	Short, burst of noise, primarily in I*	Popping of bubbles and/or opening of small airways	Local to pathology— mostly at bases	Fibrosis, CHF pulmonary edema, alveolar proteinosis, peripneumonic
Fibrotic	High frequency (like hair rubbing together)			
Peripneumonic and CHF	Medium frequency			
Pulmonary edema	Low frequency (both I and E)*			
Wheeze	Prolonged sound—E more than I but can be both; often musical. The higher pitched are from smaller airways	Air currents at point of airway bifurcation	Local to pathology	Airway constriction
Rub	Low pitched, duration is very specific—often at end inspiration	Pleural surfaces rubbing together	Local to pathology	Pleural inflammation or mass

From Eubanks DH, Bone RC: *Comprehensive respiratory care,* ed 2, St. Louis, 1988, Mosby–Year Book. Used by permission.
* I = inspiration; E = expiration; CHF = congestive heart failure

The bronchitis and bronchiectasis patient may have some clearing of the sounds with coughing or tracheal suctioning. Common terms for these sounds include course crackle, rale, bubbling rale, and course crepitation.

- Late inspiratory crackles are heard in patients with restrictive lung diseases such as interstitial fibrosis and asbestosis. These sounds do not clear with coughing or suctioning. Common terms for these sounds include fine crackle, rale, crackle, and fine crepitations.
- The Joint Pulmonary Nomenclature Committee states that rales and crackles mean the same thing; however, the term *rales* is used by some to describe the sound heard in the lungs of patients with congestive heart failure and pulmonary edema. These sounds will clear with the correction of the pulmonary edema.

4. Determine if the patient has any stridor. (IB4e) [An]

- Stridor is heard as a harsh, monophonic, high-pitched inspiratory sound over the larynx. (It is not the normal tracheal sound.)
- Stridor can often be heard without a stethoscope.
- Common pediatric conditions include acute epiglottitis, laryngotracheobronchitis (croup), and laryngomalacia (congenital stridor).
- Common adult conditions include postextubation laryngeal edema and a laryngeal tumor.
- When stridor is heard on inspiration and expiration it is commonly caused by an aspirated foreign body, tracheal stenosis, or a laryngeal tumor.
- Severe stridor is a respiratory emergency because the airway may rapidly close completely.

5. Determine if the patient has a friction rub. (IB4a) [R, Ap]

A friction rub (also known as a pleural friction rub) is the sound caused by the rubbing together of the inflamed and adherent visceral and parietal pleura as seen in pleurisy. It is heard through a stethoscope and is described as loud and grating, clicking, or the creaking of old leather. The inspiratory sound frequently is reversed from the expiratory sound as the pleural tissues rub against each other in the opposite direction.

A friction rub is heard most commonly over the lower lung areas. Commonly the sound is found at the site where the patient complains of pleural pain on breathing. Coughing and suctioning do not affect it. The causes include pulmonary infarct or any pneumonia that leads to an abscess or empyema. Rarely, a bronchial tumor will block the clearance of secretions leading to pneumonia, abscess, and empyema.

6. Determine if the patient has dysrhythmias. (IB4d) [R, Ap]

By listening at the point of maximal impulse, the patient's heart rhythm can be easily determined. A steady rhythm will have approximately equal amounts of time between ventricular contractions. It is considered normal to have a slight increase in the rate and faster rhythm during an inspiration than during an expiration. This is due to the increase in blood brought into the chest during the inspiration when the intrathoracic pressure is more negative. The opposite pattern might be seen when a patient is being mechanically ventilated with high peak airway pressures. This would indicate that the venous return to the heart is decreased during a mechanically delivered inspiration.

Any sudden variations in rate and rhythm not related to the respiratory cycle are abnormal. It is difficult to determine the origin of most dysrhythmias solely on the basis of their sound patterns; an ECG is indicated. A premature ventricular contraction (PVC) can be noted by the following rhythm characteristics: 1) the heartbeat is premature, and 2) there is a complete compensatory pause between the PVC and the following normal beat. The complete compensatory pause is the time interval of two normal heartbeats. (See the representative rhythm strip in Section 10.)

7.   Determine the patient's blood pressure. (IB4c) [An]

The blood pressure is the result of the pumping ability of the left ventricle (made up of the heart rate and stroke volume), arterial resistance, and blood volume. The normal blood pressure is caused by all three factors being in balance against each other. If one factor is abnormal, the other two have some ability to compensate. For example, if the patient has lost a lot of blood, the body attempts to maintain the blood pressure by increasing the arterial resistance and increasing the heart rate.

> Normal blood pressures:
> Adult: 120/80 mm Hg
> Infant to a child of less than 10 years: 60-100/20-70 mm Hg

As with the other vital signs, there is some variation of blood pressure among individuals. It is important to know what the patient's normal blood pressure is in order to compare it to his or her current value. Carefully measure the blood pressure in any patient who has cardiopulmonary disease or a history of hypotension or hypertension.

Hypotension in the adult is a systolic blood pressure of less than 80 mmHg. Recommend a blood pressure measurement in any patient who has a history of hypotension, appears to be in shock, has lost a lot of blood, has a weak pulse, shows mental confusion, is unconscious, or has low urine output.

Hypertension in the adult is a systolic blood pressure of 140 mmHg or greater and/or a diastolic blood pressure of 90 mmHg or greater. Carefully measure the blood pressure of any patient with a history of hypertension, bounding pulse, or symptoms of a stroke (mental confusion, headache, and sudden weakness or partial paralysis). Fear, anxiety, and pain will also cause the patient's blood pressure to temporarily rise.

The practitioner should have experience taking blood pressures with either a mercury column or anaeroid-type sphygmomanometer. The mercury types are limited in that the mercury column must be kept in a stable, upright position to be accurate. For that reason the anaeroid type is preferred for patient transport or when exercising.

The arm (or leg) cuff must be the right size for the patient. They come in different sizes for adults and pediatrics. Loose connections or disconnections between the air bladder and the hoses that connect the pressure manometer and bulb will result in the inability to inflate the bladder. Tightly reconnect the hoses and other components to create an airtight seal so that blood pressure can be measured.

Module G.   Determine the patient's complete respiratory condition in the following ways by *percussion.*

Percussion of the chest is performed to determine normal and abnormal densities of the lungs and related structures. It must be performed properly to be a reliable diagnostic tool. There are two generally accepted methods of performing percussion. Both must be performed with equal force and speed or the resulting sound will reflect the technique rather than the condition of the lungs. Avoid percussing over a woman's breast tissue.

Immediate percussion involves striking the tip of the middle finger of one hand directly onto the chest wall in a symmetrical pattern. This is useful for finding large general differences in density and for finding landmarks such as the sternum and other bony structures, the liver, and the heart. Mediate percussion involves striking the tip of the middle finger of one hand onto the central section of the middle finger of the other hand (see Fig. 1-33). The finger to be struck is fitted firmly between the ribs in a symmetrical pattern shown in Fig. 1-30. Mediate percussion is better for precisely locating an abnormal area and will be used in the following discussions.

1. Determine the patient's diaphragmatic excursion. (IB3a) [R, Ap]

It is helpful to determine the patient's diaphragmatic excursion during both normal tidal volume breathing and during maximal inspiration and expiration. Both hemidiaphragms should move the same amount during both the normal and maximal efforts. It should be remembered that, because of the liver, the right hemidiaphragm is usually found to be about 1 cm higher than the left.

The following procedure is for determining diaphragmatic excursion during tidal volume breathing:

1. The patient should be sitting up straight.
2. Have the patient exhale passively and hold.
3. Percuss down the posterior chest to find the level of both hemidiaphragms. The air-filled lungs will have a resonant sound whereas the more solid tissues below the lungs will have a dull sound. (See next section for a more detailed discussion of the sounds.)
4. Have the patient inhale a normal tidal volume and hold.
5. Percuss down the posterior chest to find the level of both hemidiaphragms.
6. Note the range of movement on both sides by the intercostal space when the dull sound was heard at the end of expiration and at the end of

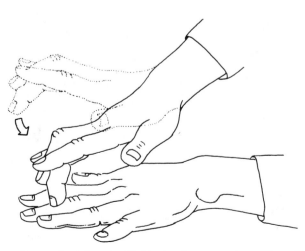

Fig. 1-33 Technique for performing mediate chest percussion. (From Shapiro BA, Kacmarek RM, Cane RD, Peruzzi WT, Hauptman D: *Clinical application of respiratory care,* ed 4, St. Louis, 1991, Mosby–Year Book. Used by permission.)

inspiration. During a quiet tidal volume breath, the adult's hemidiaphragms will move down about 1.5 cm on both sides. For example, the dull sound was heard at the 9th intercostal space at the end of exhalation and the 10th intercostal space at the end of inspiration.

Procedure for determining diaphragmatic excursion during maximal expiratory and inspiratory (vital capacity) breathing:

1. The patient should be sitting up straight.
2. Have the patient exhale as completely as possible and hold.
3. Percuss down the posterior chest to find the level of both hemidiaphragms. The air-filled lungs will have a resonant sound whereas the more solid tissues below the lungs will have a dull sound.
4. Have the patient inhale as completely as possible and hold.
5. Percuss down the posterior chest to find the level of both hemidiaphragms.
6. Note the range of movement on both sides by the intercostal space when the dull sound was heard at the end of expiration and at the end of inspiration. During the vital capacity effort, the adult's hemidiaphragms will move down about 5 cm on both sides. For example, the dull sound was heard at the 7th intercostal space at the end of exhalation and the 11th intercostal space at the end of inspiration (see Fig. 1-34).

Table 1-7 shows conditions that can affect the position of one or both hemidiaphragms.

2.   Determine if the patient has areas of altered resonance. (IB3b) [R, Ap]

Mediate percussion with proper technique should be performed over the posterior and anterior areas of the chest as shown in Fig. 1-30 (avoid breast tissue). The

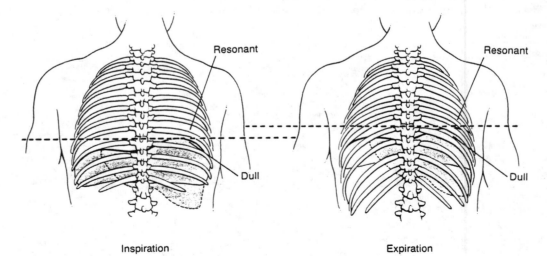

Inspiration   Expiration

Fig. 1-34 The excursion of the hemidiaphragms can be determined by percussing the patient's posterior chest. This should be done at the end of inspiration, as shown on the left, and expiration, as shown on the right. The change from a resonant (lung) sound to a dull (abdominal) sound indicates the border of the hemidiaphragm on each side. (From Swartz MH: *Textbook of physical diagnosis*, Philadelphia, 1989, WB Saunders. Used by permission.)

Table 1-7. Conditions that Affect the
Position of the Hemidiaphragms

Elevated
Unilateral:
   Atelectasis (on the affected side)
   Paralysis of the hemidiaphragm (on the
     affected side)
   Enlarged liver (right side only)
Bilateral:
   Third trimester of pregnancy
   Obesity
   Ascites
   Atelectasis (if bilateral)
Depressed
Unilateral:
   Pneumothorax (on the affected side)
   Check-valve obstruction to exhalation (on the
     affected side)
   Pleural effusion (on the affected side)
Bilateral:
   Emphysema
   Asthma

usual pattern is to proceed from the top down and side to side to compare for symmetrical sounds. The shoulders should be rolled forward when percussing the posterior chest to move the scapulae as much out of the way as possible. Table 1-8 shows the different types of percussion notes, their common characteristics, and example locations. See Fig. 1-35 for the location of the normal percussion sounds over the anterior chest.

Sounds such as hyperresonance are always abnormal when found over lung areas. They indicate that more air than normal is present. Be careful not to confuse it with the normal sound of tympany found over an air-filled stomach. An increase in the density of the underlying lung or related structures will result in a dull sound at an abnormal location. This sound is associated with pneumonia, consolidation, or atelectasis when the alveoli are fluid filled or airless; tumor; and pleural fluid such as effusion, blood, pus, or chyle. It is normal to hear dullness over the heart and liver.

Table 1-8. Percussion Notes and Characteristics

	Relative Intensity	Relative Pitch	Relative Duration	Example Locations
Resonant/resonance	Loud	Low	Long	Normal lung
Flat/flatness	Soft	High	Short	Sternum, spine, scapula
Dull/dullness	Medium	Medium	Medium	Liver, heart
Tympanic/tympany	Loud	High	Longer	Stomach air
Hyperresonant/hyperresonance	Very loud	Lower	Longer	Bilateral: emphysema asthma Unilateral: pneumothorax bleb

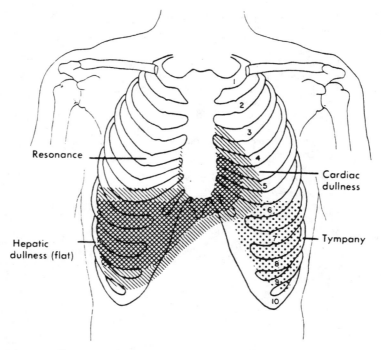

Fig. 1-35 Areas over the normal anterior thorax where resonance, dullness, tympany, and flatness can be heard during percussion. (From Prior JA, Silberstein JS, Stang JM: *Physical diagnosis,* ed 6, St. Louis, 1981, CV Mosby. Used by permission.)

Module H.   Neonatal Assessment.

1.   Review the perinatal/neonatal patient's chart for the following data.
a.   Review the maternal and perinatal history and data (IA1h1 and 2) [R]

Perinatal refers to the time period toward the end of a pregnancy and for up to 4 weeks after the neonate is born. The NBRC has specifically listed assessment of lung maturity, APGAR scores, and gestational age in the Examination Content Outline. The additional discussion is based on information presented in several of the most recent neonatal respiratory care textbooks and journal articles.

Antenatal Assessment (Assessment During the Pregnancy)

Maternal History

The medical and personal history of the mother is obviously important because it directly relates to the health of the fetus she is carrying. The mother's age is important because women younger than 16 and older than 40 years are more likely to have a high-risk pregnancy. This is especially true if a woman older than 40 is having her first child. Gravida is the term that relates to pregnancy; primagravida refers to a woman's first pregnancy. Para is the term that relates to delivering a potentially live infant; primapara/primaparous refer to a woman's first delivery of an infant. Table 1-9 lists a number of maternal and other factors that can result in the anticipation of a high-risk infant being born. It must be noted that about 25% of high-risk infants are born with no indication from the history of there being any problem.

Table 1-9. Some Factors Associated with a High-Risk Newborn Infant

Maternal Factors:
Maternal age of less than 16 or greater than 40 years
Low socioeconomic status
Poor nutrition
Lack of medical care during pregnancy
Smoking, drug, or alcohol abuse
Underweight or overweight
Abnormal fetal growth
Hereditary anomalies
Vaginal bleeding early in pregnancy
Low maternal urinary estriol
Polyhydramnios or oligohydramnios
Toxemia of pregnancy/preeclampsia
Previous history of infant(s) with jaundice, respiratory distress, or previous premature delivery
Chronic disease:
   Hypertension unrelated to pregnancy
   Diabetes mellitus
   Cardiovascular
   Pulmonary
   Anemia
   Renal
Labor and Delivery/Obstetric Factors:
Premature rupture of the membranes
Prolonged rupture of the membranes over 24 hours
Premature labor (less than 38 weeks gestation)
Postmature labor (greater than 42 weeks gestation)
Rapid or prolonged labor
Prolapsed umbilical cord
Previous or primary cesarean section
Breech or other abnormal presentation
Analgesia and anesthesia
Fetal Factors:
Multiple births
Meconium in amniotic fluid
Abnormal fetal heart rate or rhythm
Fetal acidosis
Prematurity or postmaturity
Small or large for gestational age
Rh factor sensitization
Congenital malformation
Immature lecithin/sphingomyelin (L/S) ratio or negative phosphatidylglycerol (PG) test
Birth trauma

b.   Studies indicating lung maturity. (IA1h5) [R]

In order to determine the lung maturity of the fetus, a sample of amniotic fluid must be obtained by an amniocentesis. The maturity of the fetus's lungs can be determined by evaluating three components of surfactant released by the developing alveolar type II cells.

The first test of lung maturity is the lecithin/sphingomyelin (L/S) ratio. The test is a comparison of the relative amounts of these two surfactant components. In general, the more lecithin there is compared to sphingomyelin, the more mature the lungs are. There is usually a significant increase in the lecithin level at about 35 weeks of gestation. (See Table 1-10 for more information on the interpretation of this and the next test.) A weakness of the L/S ratio test is that borderline values are difficult to interpret and false-positive values are sometimes found.

The second test is determining the presence of phosphatidylglycerol (PG) in the amniotic fluid. It appears at about 36 weeks of gestation and increases through the duration of the pregnancy. The laboratory reports PG as either present or absent from the sample of amniotic fluid. Its presence always indicates lung maturity.

Intrapartum Assessment (Assessment During Labor)

Table 1-9 lists a number of intrapartum and other factors that can result in the anticipation of a high-risk infant being born. The following are widely used to evaluate how the fetus is tolerating the stress of labor and delivery.

Fetal Heart Rate

Fetal heart rate is normally between 120 and 160 beats/min. (The fetal heart rate is also known as fetal heart tones [FHT].) It is normally variable with the fetus's waking and sleeping periods. The fetal heart rate can be measured externally through the mother's abdominal wall. During a contraction of the uterus, the heart rate commonly slows to near or less than 120 beats/min. This is because of the vagal nerve stimulation during the compression of the head into the birth canal (see Fig. 1-36, A). The heart rate returns to normal when the contraction is over.

Table 1-10. Lecithin/Sphingomyelin (L/S) Ratio and Phosphatidylglycerol (PG) as Markers of Fetal Lung Maturity

Clinical Finding	Interpretation
L/S ratio 2 : 1 (2.0) or greater	Mature lungs; less than 5% chance of IRDS
L/S ratio 1.5 : 1 (1.5)	Transitional lungs; about a 50% chance of IRDS
L/S ratio 1 : 1 (1.0) or less	Immature lungs; about a 90% chance of IRDS
Phosphatidylglycerol present	Mature lungs
Phosphatidylglycerol absent	Immature lungs

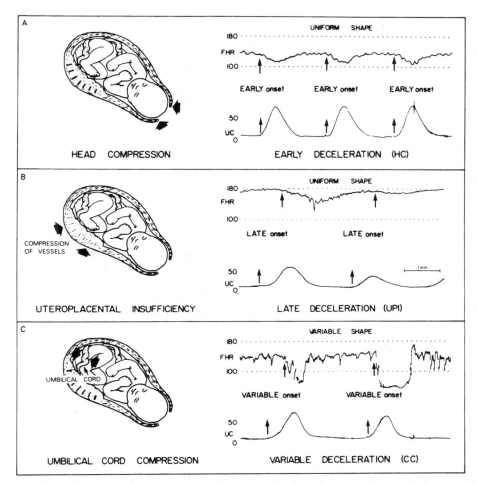

Fig. 1-36 Fetal heart rate patterns showing normal early deceleration and abnormal late deceleration and variable deceleration. (From Avery GB: *Neonatology: pathophysiology and management of the newborn,* ed 2, Philadelphia, 1981, JB Lippincott. Used by permission.)

This normal decrease and increase in FHT that is related to uterine contractions is called early deceleration or type I dips.

Late deceleration or type II dips are seen when the fetal heart rate slows sometime after the contraction begins and does not return to normal until sometime after the contraction is over (see Fig. 1-36, B. This is often caused by uteroplacental insufficiency from compression of the vessels in the placenta. It is frequently associated with low Apgar scores and fetal asphyxia and acidosis.

Variable deceleration is seen when the fetal heart rate slows and increases in an unpredictable pattern in comparison to the contractions (see Fig. 1-36, C). This pattern is more commonly seen than late deceleration and is believed to be caused by compression of the umbilical cord by a body part. During the compression, little or no blood reaches the fetus. It is also often associated with low Apgar scores and fetal asphyxia and acidosis.

With late and variable deceleration, the mother's heart rate and blood pressure should be monitored. Treatment includes giving the mother supplemental oxygen and placing her in a head-down, left lateral position. If the fetus is felt to be at risk of asphyxia, a cesarean section will need to be performed.

Other heartbeat irregularities are not related to labor and delivery. Tachycardia of greater than 160 beats/min can be associated with infection, fetal immaturity, congenital heart malformations, and the effects of maternal drugs. Bradycardia of less than 120 beats/min and decreased beat-to-beat variability (fixed heart rate) are seen with fetal asphyxia and distress.

Fetal Scalp pH

Fetal scalp pH is only indicated when the fetus is known to be distressed. This would be shown by a heart rate of more than 160 or less than 120/min, when variable or late decelerations are seen, or when meconium (fetal stool) is seen in the amniotic fluid.

When the head (or buttocks) are seen in the birth canal, a blood sample is taken. This must be done between contractions so that there is a normal amount of blood flow to the sampling site. The site is disinfected, lanced, and the blood sample drawn into a capillary tube that is then sealed and sent to the lab for pH analysis. A pH value of 7.25 or greater is considered normal. A pH value between 7.25 and 7.20 is considered to be preacidotic. A pH value of less than 7.20 shows fetal acidosis indicating that the fetus is hypoxemic. Between 40% and 80% of infants born with a fetal scalp pH of less than 7.20 have a low Apgar score.

Postpartum/Neonatal Assessment

Table 1-9 lists a number of postpartum and other factors that can result in the anticipation of a high-risk infant being born.

Resuscitation and Vital Signs

All newborns require some level of resuscitation. This is usually limited to suctioning amniotic fluid out of the nose and mouth, drying the skin, providing warmth, and the newborn receiving tactile stimulation that comes from these procedures. Newborns with moderate Apgar scores may need to breathe in some supplemental oxygen until they are more vigorous and ventilating better. The newborn with a low Apgar score requires cardiopulmonary resuscitation. Table 1-11 lists the vital signs seen in a normal newborn.

Table 1-11. Normal Newborn Vital Signs

Heart rate	Greater than 120/min		
	Less than 160/min		
Blood pressure	*Birth weight in grams*	*Systolic*	*Diastolic*
	1000-2000	55 mmHg	30 mmHg
	More than 3000	65 mmHg	40 mmHg
Respiratory rate	30-60/min		
	Periodic breathing with apneic spells of less than 10 seconds are common; there should be no bradycardia or cyanosis associated with them		
Temperature	Keep abdominal skin temperature at 36.5°C		
	Keep rectal (core) temperature between 35.5° and 37.5°C		

Weight

The relationship between birth weight and gestational age is important to evaluate. Fig. 1-37 shows this relationship for preterm (less than 38 weeks gestation), term (38-42 weeks gestation), and postterm (more than 42 weeks gestation) infants. In general, if an infant is between the 10th and 90th percentile of normal weight for gestational age, the infant is within normal limits. Any infant who is either large or small for gestational age is at increased risk of complications during and after delivery. Large postterm infants and small preterm infants are especially at risk.

Silverman Score

The Silverman score (sometimes called the Silverman-Anderson score) is an evaluation system for the newborn's respiratory difficulty and work of breathing. The following parameters are evaluated: upper chest movement, lower chest movement, xiphoid retraction, chin movement, and expiratory grunt (see Fig. 1-38 for the grading of the five parameters). A grade of 0 indicates no increase in the work of breathing; a grade of 1 indicates some increase in the work of breathing; and a grade of 2 indicates greatly increased work of breathing. The five parameters are

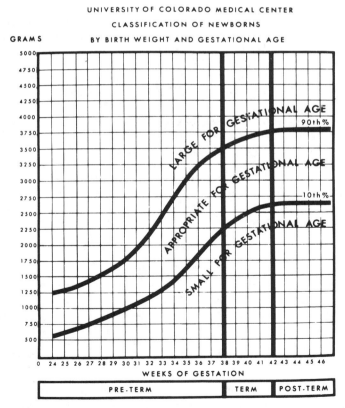

Fig. 1-37 The Colorado intrauterine growth chart for determining the appropriateness of a newborn's birth weight for its gestational age. (From Avery GB: *Neonatology: pathophysiology and management of the newborn,* ed 2, Philadelphia, 1981, JB Lippincott. Used by permission.)

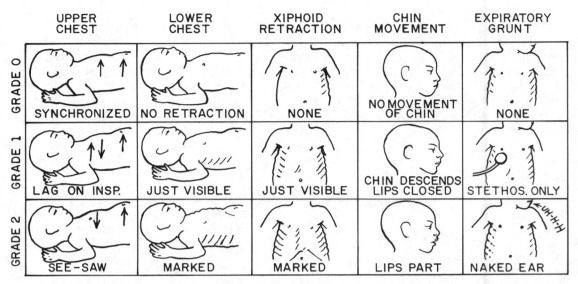

	UPPER CHEST	LOWER CHEST	XIPHOID RETRACTION	CHIN MOVEMENT	EXPIRATORY GRUNT
GRADE 0	SYNCHRONIZED	NO RETRACTION	NONE	NO MOVEMENT OF CHIN	NONE
GRADE 1	LAG ON INSP.	JUST VISIBLE	JUST VISIBLE	CHIN DESCENDS LIPS CLOSED	STETHOS. ONLY
GRADE 2	SEE-SAW	MARKED	MARKED	LIPS PART	NAKED EAR

Fig. 1-38 The Silverman score for determining the severity of a newborn's lung disease and work of breathing. (From Silverman WA, Anderson DH: *Pediatrics* 17:1, 1956. Used by permission.)

then scored on a scale of 0 to 10. A score of 0 indicates that the newborn is normal with no respiratory difficulties. The more the infant is laboring to breath, the higher the score will be. A score of 10 indicates that the newborn is having major respiratory difficulties. Medical intervention will definitely be needed.

c. Determine the patient's APGAR scores. (IA1h3) [R]

The Apgar scoring system is used in the delivery room to give a general evaluation of how a newborn infant is responding. The following five parameters are judged: heart rate, respiratory effort, muscle tone, reflex response, and color. Table 1-12 shows how the five parameters are scored on a scale of 0, 1, and 2. The newborn is evaluated soon after birth to calculate a 1-minute Apgar score. A 5-minute evaluation and Apgar score are also calculated. The infant is rated as good if the score is 7 to 10, fair if the score is 4 to 6, and poor if the score is 0 to 3. If the 5-minute score is less than 7, the newborn is rescored every 5 minutes up to 20 minutes after the delivery.

Table 1-12. Apgar Scoring Chart

Sign	0	1	2
Heart rate	Absent	Slow (below 100)	Over 100
Respiratory effort	Absent	Weak cry, hypoventilation	Good strong cry
Muscle tone	Limp	Some flexion of extremities	Well flexed

Reflex response
  Response to catheter in
    nostril or to other
    cutaneous stimulation
	No response	Grimace	Cough, sneeze, or cry

Color	Blue, pale	Body pink, extremities blue	Completely pink

From Lough MD, Doershuk CF, Stern RC: *Pediatric respiratory therapy,* ed 3, Chicago, 1985, Year Book Medical. Used by permission.

d. Determine the patient's gestational age (Dubowitz score). (IA1h4) [R]

The Dubowitz score is made up of 11 physical and 10 neurological criteria that develop at a set rate during gestation. Ballard and co-workers modified the scoring system by simplifying it to six physical and six neurological criteria. Fig. 1-39 shows the criteria, scoring system, and scale for rating the maturity of the newborn. A score of between 35 and 45 would indicate that the infant was born between 38 and 42 weeks of gestation; this would be a normal score for a term infant. A premature infant would have a score of less than 35 and a postterm infant would have a score of greater than 45. The maturity rating scale can be used to give an estimation of gestational age accurate within 2 weeks.

Neuromuscular Maturity

	-1	0	1	2	3	4	5
Posture							
Square Window (wrist)	>90°	90°	60°	45°	30°	0°	
Arm Recoil		180°	140°-180°	110°-140°	90-110°	<90°	
Popliteal Angle	180°	160°	140°	120°	100°	90°	<90°
Scarf Sign							
Heel to Ear							

Physical Maturity

Skin	sticky friable transparent	gelatinous red, translucent	smooth pink, visible veins	superficial peeling &/or rash. few veins	cracking pale areas rare veins	parchment deep cracking no vessels	leathery cracked wrinkled
Lanugo	none	sparse	abundant	thinning	bald areas	mostly bald	
Plantar Surface	heel-toe 40-50mm:-1 <40mm:-2	>50mm no crease	faint red marks	anterior transverse crease only	creases ant. 2/3	creases over entire sole	
Breast	imperceptible	barely perceptible	flat areola no bud	stippled areola 1-2mm bud	raised areola 3-4mm bud	full areola 5-10mm bud	
Eye/Ear	lids fused loosely:-1 tightly:-2	lids open pinna flat stays folded	sl. curved pinna; soft; slow recoil	well-curved pinna; soft but ready recoil	formed &firm instant recoil	thick cartilage ear stiff	
Genitals male	scrotum flat, smooth	scrotum empty faint rugae	testes in upper canal rare rugae	testes descending few rugae	testes down good rugae	testes pendulous deep rugae	
Genitals female	clitoris prominent labia flat	prominent clitoris small labia minora	prominent clitoris enlarging minora	majora & minora equally prominent	majora large minora small	majora cover clitoris & minora	

Maturity Rating

score	weeks
-10	20
-5	22
0	24
5	26
10	28
15	30
20	32
25	34
30	36
35	38
40	40
45	42
50	44

Fig. 1-39 The Ballard modification of Dubowitz Gestational Age Assessment. (From Ballard JL, Novak KZ, Driver M: *Journal of Pediatrics* 119:417, 1991.)

2. Determine the perinatal/neonatal patient's complete respiratory condition in the following ways by *observation*.
a. Determine the patient's APGAR scores. (IB1g) [R, Ap]

The newborn is evaluated soon after birth to calculate a 1-minute Apgar score. A 5-minute evaluation and Apgar score are also calculated. The infant is rated as good if the score is 7 to 10, fair if the score is 4 to 6, and poor if the score is 0 to 3. A good score indicates that the infant is adjusting normally; no further resuscitation efforts are needed. The newborn with a fair score is given supplemental oxygen directed to the face. If the heart rate is less than 100, the infant is bag-mask ventilated with 100% oxygen at a rate of 40/min. A newborn with a poor score requires major resuscitative efforts. Bag-mask ventilation with 100% oxygen will be needed. If the heart rate is less than 60/min, chest compressions at a rate of 120/min will be needed for perfusion. If the 5-minute score is less than 7, the newborn is rescored every 5 minutes up to 20 minutes after the delivery.

The 1-minute Apgar score is a good index of how the newborn tolerated the delivery process. The 5-minute Apgar score is a good index of how the newborn's cardiopulmonary system is adjusting from fetal to adult conditions. A low 5-minute Apgar score is associated with increased mortality in the first month of life. Survivors have a high risk of mental impairment and cerebral palsy.

b. Determine the patient's gestational age (Dubowitz score). (IB1h) [R, Ap]

The descriptions of gestational development for the criteria of physical maturity are listed in Fig. 1-39. As can be seen, more points are earned for each step of gestational development. A term infant will score 3–4 points for each of the 12 criteria. The illustrations of gestational development for the criteria of neurological/neuromuscular maturity can be seen in the figure; however, because the infant must be manipulated to perform the rating, the following descriptions will be helpful.

Posture.—The infant should be supine and quiet. Simply observe how the infant positions its arms and legs. The more mature infant will fully flex its elbows and hips and knees.

Square Window.—Flex the hand at the wrist. Exert gentle pressure to have the wrist flex as much as possible. The more mature infant will have full flexibility of the hand against the forearm.

Arm Recoil.—With the infant supine, fully flex the forearms for 5 seconds. Then, fully extend the forearms by pulling on the hands. When released, the more mature infant will quickly return its forearms to full flexion.

Popliteal Angle.—The infant must lie supine with the pelvis flat on the examining surface. The lower leg is flexed onto the thigh and the thigh fully flexed to the abdomen. One hand is used to hold the thigh in the flexed position while the other hand is used to extend the lower leg. The angle between the thigh and lower leg is then measured. The more mature infant will have less joint flexion and a smaller angle.

Scarf Sign.—With the infant supine, take one of the infant's hands and extend it as far as possible across the neck toward the opposite shoulder. The infant is scored as follows:

0 = The elbow reaches the opposite anterior axillary line.
1 = The elbow reaches closer to the opposite anterior axillary line than the
    midline of the chest.
2 = The elbow reaches midway between the opposite anterior axillary line
    and the midline of the chest.
3 = The elbow reaches the midline of the chest.
4 = The elbow does not reach the midline of the chest.

Heal-to-Ear Maneuver.—The infant should be supine on the examining table with the pelvis flat. Take the infant's foot in one hand and move it as near to the head as possible. Do not force it! The more mature infant will have less joint flexibility and will not be as able to move the foot as near the head as a less mature infant.

3. *Inspect* a lateral neck x-ray to evaluate the following:

Note: The following discussion usually applies to a child but could also apply to an adult.

a. Look for the presence of epiglottitis. (IB7a) [R, Ap]

Epiglottitis is an inflammation of the epiglottis and surrounding supraglottic structures. It is a medical emergency and is usually diagnosed on the basis of the history and physical examination resulting in the child being intubated. If a lateral neck x-ray is taken, it will show a white haziness in the supraglottic area. This is the swollen epiglottis and is sometimes obvious enough to be called the "thumb sign." This is seen when the usually thin and grassile epiglottis is swollen and looks like the end of the thumb. It must be emphasized that under no circumstances should the child be laid supine for the neck x-ray. This could result in the swollen epiglottis fatally closing over the opening to the trachea. Allow the child to sit upright in the most comfortable position. (See Fig. 1-40 for a drawing of the epiglottis and Fig. 1-41 for a lateral neck x-ray of the epiglottis. Table 1-13 lists the general history and physical findings for distinguishing between epiglottitis and laryngotracheobronchitis.)

b. Look for the presence of subglottic edema. (IB7b) [R, Ap]

Subglottic edema is an inflammation of the subglottic mucus membranes of the larynx, trachea, and bronchi. This condition is also known as laryngotracheobronchitis (LTB) and croup. Subglottic edema is usually treated by the inhalation of a cool aerosol in a mist tent and racemic epinephrine for mucosal vasoconstriction. If a lateral neck x-ray is taken, it will show a white haziness in the subglottic area. This is the swollen laryngeal and tracheal tissue and is sometimes obvious enough to be called the "pencil sign" or "steeple sign." This is seen when the usually blunt end of the trachea at the vocal cords is thinned to a narrow point by the swollen mucus membrane. (See Fig. 1-40 for a drawing of subglottic edema and Fig. 1-41 for a lateral neck x-ray of this problem.)

c. Look for the presence and position of any foreign bodies. (IB7c) [R, Ap]

The history of sudden breathing difficulty, cough, and inspiratory stridor combined with a physical examination of the patient will usually point to the suspicion of aspiration. A lateral neck x-ray and/or P-A or A-P chest and neck x-ray will often

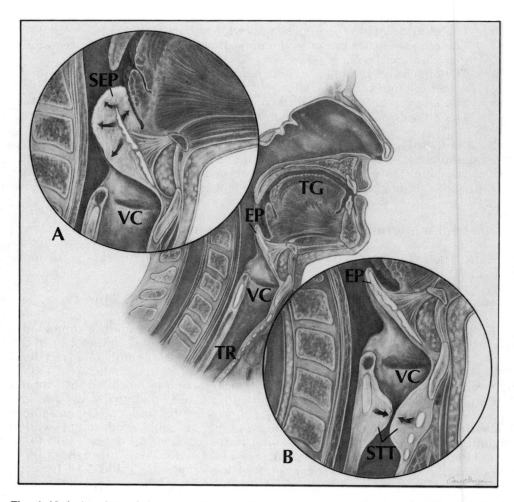

Fig. 1-40 A drawing of the normal upper airway is shown in the middle. Contrast it with: **A,** epiglottitis; and **B,** laryngotracheobronchitis (croup). *TG,* tongue; *EP,* epiglottis; *VC,* vocal chords; *TR,* trachea; *SEP,* swollen epiglottis; *STT,* swollen trachea tissue. (From Des Jardins TR: *Clinical manifestations of respiratory disease,* ed 2, Chicago, 1990, Year Book Medical. Used by permission.)

help to confirm the presence and position of a foreign body. Fig. 1-42 shows an A-P chest and neck x-ray. Note the clearly-seen solid white shape of the foreign body. This indicates that the object is metallic. Plastic toy pieces and foods such as peanuts are much harder to see because their densities are closer to those found in the body. Look for distortion of the dark air column of the upper airway and trachea to indicate the location of a foreign body.

Note: This ends the discussion on specific aspects of physical assessment of the neonate or child. The following modules would apply to adults or children.

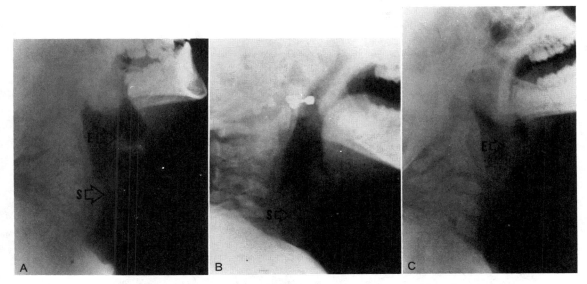

Fig. 1-41 Lateral neck x-rays on children showing: **A,** normal upper airway during an inspiration; **B,** laryngotracheobronchitis (croup) showing haziness of the subglottic trachea from mucosal edema; **C,** epiglottitis with a swollen, rounded epiglottis. Areas marked *E* show the epiglottis; areas marked *S* show the subglottic trachea. (From Williams JL: Radiographic evaluations. In Koff PB, Eitzman DV, Neu J, editors: *Neonatal and pediatric respiratory care.* St. Louis, 1988, CV Mosby. Used by permission.)

Module I.   Determine and continue to monitor how the patient responds to the treatment or procedure.

1.   Make a recommendation to measure the patient's hemoglobin, hematocrit, serum electrolytes and other blood chemistries, and leukocyte count and analysis. (IIIA1g) [R, Ap, An]

The normal values for these items were listed previously. Make a recommendation to measure the hemoglobin and hematocrit in any patient who has hemorrhaged. A transfusion may be needed to enable the patient to carry more oxygen.

Table 1-13. General History/Physical Findings of Laryngotracheobronchitis and Epiglottitis

Clinical Finding	LTB	Epiglottitis
Age	3 mo–3 yr	2–4 yr
Onset	Slow (24–48 hr)	Abrupt (2–4 hr)
Fever	Absent	Present
Drooling	Absent	Present
Lateral neck x-ray	Haziness in subglottic area	Haziness in supraglottic area
Inspiratory stridor	High pitched and loud	Low pitched and muffled
Hoarseness	Present	Absent
Swallowing difficulty	Absent	Present
White blood count	Normal (viral)	Elevated (bacterial)

From Des Jardins TR: *Clinical manifestations of respiratory disease,* ed 2, Chicago, 1990, Year Book Medical. Used by permission.

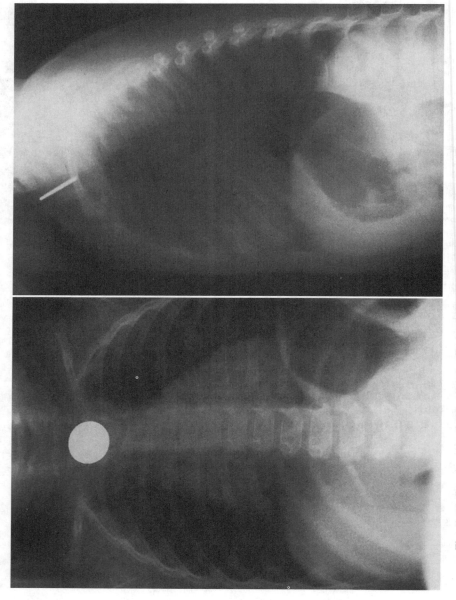

Fig. 1-42 Foreign body obstruction in an 18-month-old girl. **A** shows a frontal x-ray with the solid white disk of a coin clearly seen in the hypopharynx. **B** shows a lateral view of the chest with the edge of the coin seen as a solid white line. (From Hunter TB, Bragg DG: *Radiologic guide to medical devices and foreign bodies*, St. Louis, 1994, Mosby–Year Book. Used by permission.)

Make a recommendation to measure the hemoglobin and hematocrit in any patient who has chronic hypoxemia. Secondary polycythemia would be confirmed by an elevated level of RBCs.

Make a recommendation to measure the patient's serum electrolytes and other blood chemistries in any patient who shows a cardiac dysrhythmia, displays mental confusion, has had severe vomiting or diarrhea, has sweated profusely and shows signs of heat stroke, or has been given diuretic medications to increase urine output. Electrolyte or nutritional deficiencies can cause these problems or worsen an existing condition.

Make the recommendation to perform a leukocyte count and analysis in any patient who has a high fever and signs of bacterial infection. A person with a normal immune response will show an increase in the leukocyte count and an increase in immature forms in response to an acute, severe bacterial infection.

2. Evaluate the patient's fluid balance (intake and output). (IB9n, IC2f, and IIIA1h) [R, Ap, An]

Intake and output (I and O) should be approximately equal in the normal person with a properly functioning heart and kidneys. Insensible water loss through perspiration and breathing are usually ignored in adults because the amount lost is relatively small and can only be estimated as about 500–1000 ml per day. Insensible water loss is a risk in the low birth weight infant. Prevent this by keeping the infant's environmental temperature within one degree of its body temperature (neutral thermal environment or NTE). Oxygen should be humidified. This normal person would have expected vital signs and urine specific gravity.

The dehydrated patient will likely show some or all of the following signs and symptoms: tachycardia, hypotension, high urine specific gravity, oliguria (low urine output), low central venous and pulmonary wedge pressure readings, tenting of the skin when pinched, and mental confusion. This patient will have the need for a fluid intake that far exceeds the output.

The fluid overloaded patient will likely show some or all of the following signs and symptoms: tachycardia, hypertension, low urine specific gravity, increased urine output, increased CVP and PWP readings, peripheral edema in the dependent parts of the body, and pulmonary edema with crackles/rales. This patient will need to be fluid and sodium restricted. In addition, diuretics will help to rapidly increase the urine output.

Any patient who has a history of heart or kidney problems or who has a current serious cardiopulmonary disorder should have his or her intake and output monitored closely. This is done by adding all the patient's intake (oral, intravenous, etc.) and output (urine, blood work, etc.) for each 8-hour shift. See Table 1-14 for the normal adult's values for fluid intake, urine output, and urine specific gravity.

3. Make the recommendation for a chest x-ray, as needed, to help determine the patient's condition. (IIIA1b) [R, Ap]

Indications for a chest x-ray include the need to evaluate any patient with a suspected or known cardiopulmonary condition or after an invasive treatment for the condition. This may include, but is not limited to: COPD, pneumonia, IRDS, ARDS, near drowning, aspiration, thoracic trauma, congestive heart failure with pulmonary edema, thoracic surgery, pneumothorax, postinsertion of a pleural or pericardial chest tube, and postinsertion of an endotracheal tube.

Table 1-14. Normal Adult's Fluid Intake, Urine Output, and Urine Specific Gravity

---

The normal, minimal daily water requirement for an adult patient is about 1500–2000 ml.

The average urine output is 0.5–1 ml/kg/hr.

Polyuria is a urine output of more than 1500 ml/hr.

Oliguria is a urine output of less than 400 ml in 24 hr.

Anuria is a urine output of less than 100 ml in 24 hr.

The normal range for specific gravity of urine is 1.002–1.030. The adult with a normal fluid intake should have a specific gravity of 1.016–1.022.

---

4. Inspect the patient's chest x-ray as necessary. (IIIA1c) [R, Ap, An]

It is appropriate to inspect any previous or new chest x-ray to determine the patient's condition or to detect a change in the patient's condition.

Module J. Evaluate the physician's orders and the patient's respiratory care plan; make any recommendations or changes as needed.

1. Examine all of the data to determine the patient's pathophysiological condition. (IC3a) [R, Ap, An]

It is beyond the scope of this text to discuss in detail all the various cardiopulmonary conditions and disorders that can befall the patients that respiratory therapists help to care for; however, because the NBRC is known to ask questions on cardiopulmonary pathologies, it is recommended that the student and examinee study at least the most commonly seen. Table 1-15 is included as a summary of some common adult conditions. Table 1-16 is included as a guide to the differential diagnosis of neonatal respiratory distress.

2. Take part in the development of the respiratory care plan. (IC3c) [An]

This relates to the respiratory therapist being involved with the patient care team of the physician, nurse, and others in deciding how to best care for the patient. Be prepared to use the information contained in this section and the rest of the text to help you make decisions on how to care for your patients. The NBRC will ask questions that relate to what would be the best recommendations for care. Minimally, the following steps are needed in the respiratory care plan for any patient:

1. Determine an expected outcome or goal(s).
2. Develop a plan to achieve success.
3. Decide how to measure the patient's achievement of the goal.

Table 1-15. Physical Signs of Abnormal Pulmonary Pathology

Abnormality	Initial Impression	Inspection	Palpation	Percussion	Auscultation	Possible Causes
Acute airway obstruction	Appears acutely ill	Use of accessory muscles	Reduced expansion	Increased resonance	Expiratory wheezing	Asthma, bronchitis
Chronic airway obstruction	Appears chronically ill	Increased anteroposterior diameter, use of accessory muscles	Reduced expansion	Increased resonance	Diffuse reduction in breath sounds; early inspiratory crackles	Chronic bronchitis, emphysema
Consolidation	May appear acutely ill	Inspiratory lag	Increased fremitus	Dull note	Bronchial breath sounds; crackles	Pneumonia, tumor
Pneumothorax	May appear acutely ill	Unilateral expansion	Decreased fremitus	Increased resonance	Absent breath sounds	Rib fracture, open wound
Pleural effusion	May appear acutely ill	Unilateral expansion	Absent fremitus	Dull note	Absent breath sounds	Congestive heart failure
Local bronchial obstruction	Appears acutely ill	Unilateral expansion	Absent fremitus	Dull note	Absent breath sounds	Mucous plug
Diffuse interstitial fibrosis	Often normal	Rapid shallow breathing	Often normal; increased fremitus	Slight decrease in resonance	Late inspiratory crackles	Chronic exposure to inorganic dust
Acute upper air obstruction	Appears acutely ill	Labored breathing	Often normal	Often normal	Inspiratory and/ or expiratory stridor	Epiglottitis, croup, foreign body aspiration

From Wilkins RL, Sheldon RL, Krider SJ: *Clinical assessment in respiratory care*, ed 2, St. Louis, 1990, Mosby–Year Book. Used by permission.

Table 1-16. Differential Diagnosis of Neonatal Respiratory Distress

| | Respiratory Disorders | |
Common	Less Common	Mechanical
Respiratory distress syndrome	Pulmonary hemorrhage	Upper airway obstruction
Transient tachypnea	Pulmonary hypoplasia/ agenesis	Tracheal lesions
Meconium aspiration	Congenital lung cysts, tumors	Rib cage anomalies
Pneumonia	Congenital lobar emphysema	Extrinsic masses
Pneumothorax/air leaks	Tracheoesophageal fistula	Diaphragmatic hernia
		Abdominal distension
		Pleural effusion/ chylothorax

| | Extrapulmonary Disorders | |
Cardiac/Vascular	Metabolic	Neurologic/Muscular
Hypovolemia	Acidosis	Cerebral edema
Anemia	Hypoglycemia	Cerebral hemorrhage
Polycythemia	Hypothermia	Drugs
Persistent fetal circulation	Hyperthermia	Muscle disorders
Cyanotic heart disease		Spinal cord problems
Congestive heart failure		Phrenic nerve damage

From Lough MD, Doershuk CF, Stern RC: *Pediatric respiratory therapy,* ed 3, Chicago, 1985, Year Book Medical. Used by permission.

4. Plan a timeline to measure the patient's progress.
5. Document the patient's response to care and the final outcome.

3. Make a recommendation to insert a chest tube into the patient. (IIIC10f) [R, Ap, An]

A pleural chest tube should be inserted into the pleural space of any patient with more than a 10% pneumothorax. A pericardial chest tube should be inserted into the pericardial space of any patient with a pneumopericardium. A mediastinal chest tube should be inserted into the mediastinal space posterior to the heart of any patient with excessive mediastinal blood. This is most commonly seen in open heart surgery patients. (See Section 17 for more information.)

Module K. Record in the patient's chart and interpret the patient's response to respiratory care.

1. Record and interpret the patient's response to the procedure or therapy and attitude toward it. (IIIA1a and IIIA2a4) [An]

This would need to be done for each procedure or therapy that is discussed in the succeeding sections. Hopefully, the patient benefits from what has been performed. The patient should feel better if a procedure to help correct a breathing problem was effective. Make a note of what the patient has to say about how he or she now feels. If there is a problem with the procedure or therapy and the patient has a complaint, it too should be recorded in the chart.

2. Record and interpret the patient's heart rate and rhythm, respiratory rate, and blood pressure. (IIA2a1) [An]

3. Record and interpret the patient's breath sounds. (IIIA2a2) [An]

4. Record and interpret the patient's cough, sputum production, and its qualities. (IIIA2a3) [An]

All the preceding items were discussed earlier in this section and/or in other respiratory care textbooks.

BIBLIOGRAPHY

Aloan CA: *Respiratory care of the newborn: a clinical manual*, Philadelphia, 1987, JB Lippincott.

Avery GB: *Neonatology: pathophysiology and management of the newborn*, ed 2, Philadelphia, 1981, JB Lippincott.

Barnes TA: The respiratory care plan. In Barnes TA, editor: *Respiratory care practice*, Chicago, 1988, Year Book Medical.

Bates B: *A guide to physical examination and history taking*, ed 4, Philadelphia, 1987, JB Lippincott.

Bennington JL, editor: *Saunders dictionary and encyclopedia of laboratory medicine and technology*, Philadelphia, 1984, WB Saunders.

Burgess WR, Chernick V: *Respiratory therapy in newborn infants and children*, ed 2, New York, 1986, Thieme.

Burton GG: Patient assessment procedures. In Barnes TA, editor: *Respiratory care practice*, Chicago, 1988, Year Book Medical.

Carlo, Chatburn: *Neonatal respiratory care*, St. Louis, Mosby–Year Book.

Cherniack RM, Cherniack L: *Respiration in health and disease*, ed 3, Philadelphia, 1983, WB Saunders.

Daily EK, Schroeder JS: *Techniques in bedside hemodynamic monitoring*, ed 4, St. Louis, 1989, Mosby–Year Book.

Des Jardins TR: *Cardiopulmonary anatomy and physiology: essentials for respiratory care*, Albany, NY, 1989, Delmar.

Des Jardins TR: *Clinical manifestations of respiratory disease*, ed 2, Chicago, 1990, Year Book Medical.

DiPietro JS, Mustard MN: *Clinical guide for respiratory care practitioners*, Norwalk, Conn, 1987, Appleton & Lange.

Eubanks DH, Bone RC: *Comprehensive respiratory care*. St. Louis, 1985, Mosby–Year Book.

Kacmarek RM, Mack CW, Dimas S: *The essentials of respiratory therapy*, ed 3, Chicago, 1990, Year Book Medical.

Kenner CV, Guzzetta CE, Dossey BM: *Critical care nursing: body-mind-spirit*. Boston, 1981, Little, Brown.

Koff PB, Eitzman DV, Neu J, editors: *Neonatal and pediatric respiratory care*, St. Louis, 1988, Mosby–Year Book.

Lehrer S: *Understanding lung sounds*, Philadelphia, 1984, WB Saunders.

Levitsky MG, Cairo JM, Hall SM: *Introduction to respiratory care*, Philadelphia, 1990, WB Saunders.

Lillington GA: Roentgenographic diagnosis of pulmonary disease. In Burton GG, Hodgkin JE, Ward JJ, editors: *Respiratory care: a guide to clinical practice,* ed 3, Philadelphia, 1991, JB Lippincott.

Lough MD, Doershuk CF, Stern RC: *Pediatric respiratory therapy,* ed 3, Chicago, 1985, Year Book Medical.

Oblouk Darovic G: *Hemodynamic monitoring: invasive and noninvasive clinical monitoring,* Philadelphia, 1987, WB Saunders.

Peters RM: *Chest trauma.* In Moser KM, Spragg RG, editors: *Respiratory emergencies,* ed 2, St. Louis, 1982, CV Mosby.

Prior JA, Silberstein JS, Stang JM: *Physical diagnosis,* ed 6, St. Louis, 1981, CV Mosby.

Rau JL, Pearce DJ: *Understanding chest radiographs,* Denver, 1984, Multi-Media Publishing.

Shapiro BA, Kacmarek RM, Cane RD, Peruzzi WT, Hauptman D: *Clinical application of respiratory care,* ed 4, St. Louis, 1991, Mosby–Year Book.

Sheldon RL, Dunbar RD: Systematic analysis of the chest radiograph. In Scanlan CL, Spearman CB, Sheldon RL, editors: *Egan's fundamentals of respiratory care,* ed 5, St. Louis, 1990, Mosby–Year Book.

Sills JR: *Respiratory care certification guide,* St. Louis, 1991, Mosby–Year Book.

Swartz MH: *Textbook of physical diagnosis,* Philadelphia, 1989, WB Saunders.

Thompson JM, McFarland GK, Hirsch JE, Tucker SM, Bowers AC: *Clinical nursing,* St. Louis, 1986, Mosby–Year Book.

Tilkian SM, Conover MB, Tilkian AG: *Clinical implications of laboratory tests,* St. Louis, 1983, Mosby–Year Book.

White GC: *Basic clinical lab competencies for respiratory care,* ed 2, Albany, NY, 1993, Delmar.

Wilkins RL, Burton GG: History and physical examination of the respiratory patient. In Burton GG, Hodgkin JE, Ward JJ, editors: *Respiratory care: a guide to clinical practice,* ed 3, Philadelphia, 1991, JB Lippincott.

Wilkins RL, Hodgkin JE, Lopez B: *Lung sounds, a practical guide,* St. Louis, 1988, Mosby–Year Book.

Wilkins RL, Sheldon RL, Krider SJ: *Clinical assessment in respiratory care,* ed 2, St. Louis, 1990, Mosby–Year Book.

Williams JL: Radiographic evaluations. In Koff PB, Eitzman DV, Neu J, editors: *Neonatal and pediatric respiratory care,* St. Louis, 1988, Mosby–Year Book.

SELF-STUDY QUESTIONS

1. An adult patient with a cardiothoracic ratio of .7 (70%) would most likely:
   A. Be normal
   B. Have emphysema
   C. Have pneumonia
   D. Have left ventricular failure
   E. None of the above

2. A tension pneumothorax is identified by all of the following:
   I. Chest x-ray showing a shift of the mediastinum toward the affected lung
   II. Chest x-ray showing an elevation of the hemidiaphragm on the affected side
   III. Sudden deterioration of the patient's vital signs
   IV. Chest x-ray showing a depression of the hemidiaphragm on the affected side

    V.   Chest x-ray showing a shift of the mediastinum away from the affected lung
  VI.   Essentially unchanged vital signs
     A.   I, II, VI
     B.   III, IV, V
     C.   I, II, III
     D.   I, III, IV
     E.   II, V, VI

3. Your patient is complaining of localized pain over the lower right area of the chest when breathing. When auscultating her you hear a rasping noise on both inspiration and expiration at her point of pain. This is most likely:
    A.   Pleural friction rub
    B.   Normal breath sounds
    C.   Wheeze
    D.   Rhonchi

4. Your patient has elevated external jugular veins even though her head and body are raised 45° above her legs. This would indicate that she:
    A.   Is hypotensive
    B.   Is hypertensive
    C.   Is fluid overloaded
    D.   Has emphysema
    E.   Is dehydrated

5. Tactile fremitus would be decreased in all these conditions EXCEPT:
    A.   Pneumothorax
    B.   Chronic obstructive pulmonary disease
    C.   Pulmonary edema
    D.   Pleural effusion
    E.   Thick chest wall

6. You are assisting with the delivery of a high-risk infant. After evaluating the infant, you give him a 1-minute APGAR score of 8 and recommend that the assisting nurse and physician:
    A.   Give the infant supplemental oxygen
    B.   Give the mother supplemental oxygen
    C.   Begin bag-mask rescue breathing on the infant
    D.   Begin full CPR on the infant
    E.   Give the infant to the mother as soon as possible for bonding

7. You are called to the emergency room to help in the evaluation and care of a 4-year-old girl who has been sick the last 2 days. The nurse shows you a lateral neck x-ray of the child and asks for your opinion. You notice a clear air column through the upper airway but some haziness of the tracheal air column below the larynx. You would tell the nurse that you suspect the child has:
    A.   A head cold
    B.   Aspirated a foreign body
    C.   Epiglottitis
    D.   Laryngotracheobronchitis
    E.   Pneumonia

8. You would suspect a patient is fluid overloaded if the following signs are found:
    I.   Tachycardia
   II.   Bradycardia

III.   High urine specific gravity
IV.   Peripheral edema in the dependent parts of the body
V.   Low urine specific gravity
   A.   I, IV, V
   B.   III, IV
   C.   I, III
   D.   II, V
   E.   III, IV

9.   All of the following would result in an elevated left hemidiaphragm and decreased left diaphragmatic excursion:
   I.   Obesity
   II.   Left sided atelectasis
   III.   Enlarged liver
   IV.   Left sided pleural effusion
   V.   Paralysis of the left hemidiaphragm
      A.   I, III
      B.   II, V
      C.   II, III
      D.   II, IV, V
      E.   III, IV

10.   To best evaluate a suspicious upper lobe shadow seen on an anteroposterior chest x-ray, the following radiographic projection would be recommended:
   A.   Posteroanterior
   B.   Lateral
   C.   Lordotic
   D.   Lateral decubitus
   E.   Repeat the anteroposterior x-ray under a stronger power

11.   Which of the following could result in a mediastinal shift on a chest x-ray?
   I.   Right hemothorax
   II.   Bilateral lower lobe pneumonia
   III.   Left tension pneumothorax
   IV.   Right lower lobe atelectasis
   V.   Fibrosis of the left lung
      A.   III
      B.   II
      C.   IV, V
      D.   I, II, III
      E.   I, III, IV, V

12.   The radiologist remarks to you during the viewing of a patient's posteroanterior chest x-ray film that the patient has a silhouette sign on the right side of the heart. This would indicate to you that:
   A.   The patient has a normal chest x-ray
   B.   The patient needs an anteroposterior chest x-ray taken
   C.   The patient has an abnormal heart
   D.   The patient has a right middle lobe consolidation, infiltrate, or mass
   E.   The patient has a right lower lobe consolidation, infiltrate, or mass

13.   A patient who is suffering respiratory distress would exhibit all the following EXCEPT:
   A.   A normal respiratory rate
   B.   Nasal flaring

C. Intercostal retractions
D. Use of accessory muscles of inspiration

14. You are reviewing the leukocyte count and analysis of your adult patient who is suspected of having bacterial pneumonia. Which of the following findings would support that conclusion?
     I. Leukocyte count of 3,000 per cubic mm
    II. Leukocyte count of 7,000 per cubic mm
   III. Leukocyte count of 16,000 per cubic mm
    IV. Increased number of neutrophils
     V. Decreased number of neutrophils
        A. I, V
        B. II, IV
        C. III, V
        D. I, IV
        E. III, IV

15. Which serum electrolyte is the most important to monitor because of its affect on the proper functioning of the nerves and conduction through the heart?
    A. Chloride
    B. Potassium
    C. Bicarbonate
    D. Calcium
    E. Sodium

16. The preferred radiographic projection to minimize distortion of the heart is:
    A. Anteroposterior
    B. Posteroanterior
    C. Lateral
    D. Oblique
    E. Lordotic

Answer Key

1. D; 2. B; 3. A; 4. C; 5. C; 6. E; 7. D; 8. A; 9. B; 10. C; 11. E; 12. D; 13. A; 14. E; 15. B; 16. B.

2 | Blood Gas Analysis and Monitoring

Module A. Obtain arterial blood for analysis, interpret the results of its analysis, and perform quality control procedures.

1. Make a recommendation for arterial puncture to obtain a blood sample for analysis. (IA2g) [An]

Note: Throughout this section and in all other sections, the common phrase "arterial blood gas" (ABG) is used when talking about drawing a sample of blood from a patient's artery for the purposes of determining the arterial pressures of oxygen and carbon dioxide, acid-base status (pH), and related values.

There are three broad, general indications for this recommendation:

1. To check a patient's oxygenation status (PaO_2)
2. To check a patient's acid-base status (pH)
3. To check a patient's ventilation status ($PaCO_2$)

A number of authors have written extensively on these and other indications. No attempt is made to include every possible indication; broad areas are listed with some common examples. It is very important to evaluate the patient's vital signs and physical condition as described in Section 1 to help determine if an ABG is indicated.

A. Cardiac failure
   1. Congenital defect
   2. Heart attack (myocardial infarct)
   3. Congestive heart failure with or without pulmonary edema
B. Chronic obstructive pulmonary disease (COPD)
   1. Asthma
   2. Emphysema
   3. Bronchitis
   4. Bronchietasis
C. Any pneumonia causing hypoxemia
D. Trauma
   1. Broken ribs
   2. Flail chest
   3. Pneumothorax
   4. Hemothorax
   5. Upper airway trauma

E. Ventilatory failure
   1. Overdosage of sedatives or pain relievers
   2. Stroke or head (brain) injury
   3. Spinal cord injury
   4. Neuromuscular diseases such as myasthenia gravis or Guillain Barré syndrome
F. Airway obstruction
   1. Foreign body aspiration
   2. Laryngotracheobronchitis (croup)
   3. Epiglottitis
G. Miscellaneous
   1. Smoke inhalation
   2. Carbon monoxide poisoning
   3. Near drowning
   4. Infant respiratory distress syndrome (IRDS)/hyaline membrane disease
   5. Adult respiratory distress syndrome (ARDS)
   6. No indwelling arterial line
   7. A shunt or $P(A-a)O_2$ calculation must be made
   8. Cardiopulmonary resuscitation

2. Perform an arterial puncture to obtain a blood sample for analysis to evaluate a patient's response to respiratory care. (IIIAik) [An]

A number of possible variations in the technique exist. The following is a general but thorough listing of the steps and any important related information. (Note: The topic of obtaining a capillary blood sample for gas analysis is discussed in Module D.)

1. Check for a valid physician order.
2. Check the patient's chart for pertinent information on supplemental oxygen being used and bleeding disorders such as hemophilia. It is important to check the patient's clotting time because a hematoma will result if extra time is not spent holding the puncture site. The normal activated partial thromboplastin time (APTT or PTT) is 16 to 25 seconds. The normal prothrombin time (PT) is 11 to 16 seconds. If the patient is receiving coumarin (Coumadin), his PT will be significantly increased; heparin therapy may prolong the PT slightly. Be prepared to hold the site for a longer than normal time if the APTT or PT times are increased or the patient is receiving either of these medications.
3. Collect necessary equipment:
   a. Ice water in a cup
   b. 3 to 5 ml glass or plastic syringe
   c. Syringe and needle
   d. Anticoagulant, if needed
   e. Seventy percent isopropyl alcohol and/or iodophor swabs to clean the puncture site; a sterile 4 × 4 inch gauze pad to hold over the puncture site to aid in clotting
   f. Seal for the needle or syringe to prevent room air contamination
   g. Clean gloves to protect both hands of the practitioner from any contact with spilled blood
4. Introduce yourself and your department to the patient. Explain what you are there to do. Gain the patient's confidence so that he or she will cooperate as fully as possible.
5. Select the puncture site. The following choices are listed in order from most to least favorable: radial, brachial, dorsalis pedis, and femoral. If the

radial is selected, try to puncture the left wrist if the patient is right handed or vice versa.

6. If the radial or pedal sites are selected, the *modified Allen's test* must be performed to ensure that there is adequate collateral flow in case the artery becomes clotted as a result of the procedure.

   a. Radial artery site (see Fig. 2-1 for the basic procedure): Circulation is stopped to the hand by pressing closed both the radial and ulnar arteries. Releasing the pressure over the ulnar artery should result in the hand flushing within 10 to 15 seconds. This is a *positive* test and proves that the ulnar artery has adequate circulation to the hand. Do not confuse this with a positive Allen's test that would indicate poor circulation through the ulnar artery. The key point is that if the hand flushes when the ulnar artery is released, there is good flow through it and radial puncture is safe to perform. If the hand does not flush within 15 seconds of the release of the ulnar artery, the circulation is inadequate and the radial artery of that wrist must *not* be punctured. Another site must be evaluated for puncture.

   b. Dorsalis pedis artery site: Press down on the dorsalis pedis artery to occlude it. Press on the nail of the great toe so that it blanches. Release the pressure on the nail and watch for the rapid return of color. This *positive* test confirms that there is good blood flow through the posterior tibial and lateral plantar arteries; it is safe to draw a sample from the site. A slow return of blood flow indicates poor circulation, which means another site must be chosen.

7. Prepare the equipment and the puncture site using sterile technique.

   a. Wash your hands.

   b. If necessary, draw up the heparin solution, flush the syringe with it, and discard the excess.

   c. If a radial or brachial site is selected, the joint should be hyperextended with a folded towel to help stabilize it.

   d. Clean the site by wiping with the alcohol and/or iodophor swab in a widening spiral that starts at the desired puncture site.

   e. Put on your gloves and eye glasses or goggles.

   f. Some prefer to anesthetize the puncture site with a 0.8 to 1.0 ml injection of 2% lidocaine (Xylocaine) into the skin. Others believe that this is unnecessary because the injection will cause pain by itself.

8. Draw the blood sample.

   a. Hold the syringe like a pencil. The radial and dorsalis pedis arteries should be entered from a 45° angle; the brachial and femoral arteries should be entered from a 90° angle (see Fig. 2-2). Use the first two fingers of your free hand to palpate the pulse and hold the artery still. The bevel of the needle should be up as it enters the skin.

   b. The needle should enter the skin quickly to minimize pain. Carefully advance the needle into the artery when a pulsatile flow will be seen with each heartbeat. If unsuccessful, withdraw the needle to the skin, change the angle as needed, and reinsert into the artery.

   c. Two to four milliliters of blood is sufficient.

   d. Press the sterile gauze onto the puncture site for 2 to 5 minutes. Check the site to ensure that clotting has occurred. Hold longer if needed. An assistant may help with this and step e.

   e. While holding the site, seal the needle,* roll the syringe to mix the heparin, and place the syringe in the ice water. (Failure to put the blood

---

* Some department protocols say to leave the needle unsealed and uncapped to minimize the risk of accidental technician puncture. This is to reduce the risk of spreading hepatitis or AIDS.

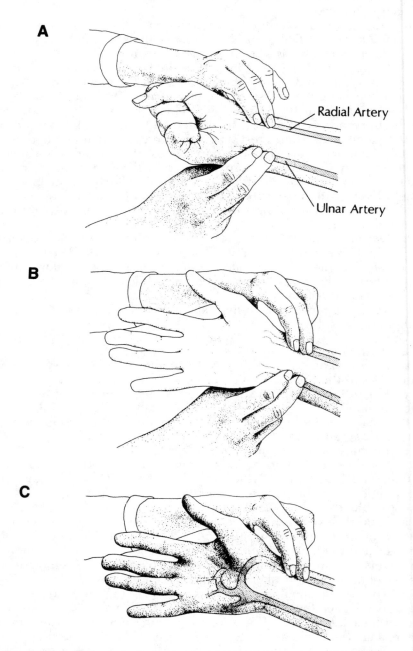

Fig. 2-1 The modified Allen's test. **A,** The hand is clenched into a tight fist and pressure is applied to the radial and ulnar arteries. **B,** The hand is opened (but not fully extended); the palm and fingers are blanched. **C,** Removal of the pressure on the ulnar artery should result in flushing of the entire hand. (From Shapiro BA, Peruzzi WT, Templin R: *Clinical application of blood gases,* ed 5, St. Louis, 1994, Mosby–Year Book. Used by permission.)

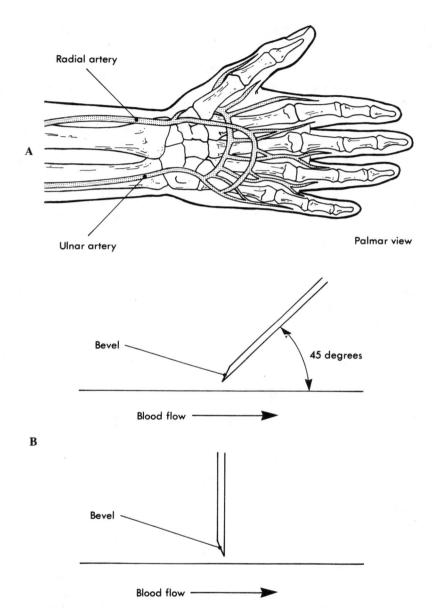

Fig. 2-2 A, Radial arterial position in the lower arm and wrist. **B,** Bevel and needle positioning for radial arterial puncture and other arterial punctures, respectively. (From Lane EE, Walker JF: *Clinical arterial blood gas analysis.* St. Louis, 1987, Mosby–Year Book. Used by permission.)

sample in ice water will result in a decrease in the PaO_2 value, an increase in the $PaCO_2$ value, and a decrease in the pH value.)

f. Label the syringe with the patient's name, oxygen percentage, and the patient's temperature if abnormal. Some departments may also add the patient's age and position when the sample was drawn because of the effects they may have on oxygenation.

g. Have the sample analyzed as soon as possible.

3. Recommend the insertion on an arterial line or umbilical artery line into a patient to get additional data. (IA2h) [R, Ap, An]

An arterial line is a short catheter that is placed into a peripheral artery for the purposes of sampling blood and/or continuously monitoring the patient's blood pressure. Arterial blood for gas analysis or other laboratory values can be easily and painlessly taken from the patient. The procedure is explained in the next discussion. With the addition of pressure monitoring equipment, the patient's blood pressure can be measured and observed continuously. Section 4 contains the discussion on blood pressure monitoring and illustrations on how the system is assembled. The radial artery is the most common site to insert a catheter into an adult. Alternate sites include the brachial, dorsalis pedis, or femoral arteries. A newborn with a severe cardiopulmonary problem should have the catheter inserted into either of the umbilical arteries. This long catheter is then advanced into the aorta. If indicated, this should be done as quickly as possible after birth before arterial spasm prevents the catheter from being advanced. Besides getting blood and monitoring the blood pressure, the newborn can be given glucose or a blood transfusion through the catheter.

4. Obtain a blood sample from an arterial line. (IIIA1m) [R, Ap]

The commonly followed steps for obtaining an arterial blood sample include:

1. Tell a conscious adult that you are going to take a blood sample from the arterial catheter.
2. Remove the dead-ender cap from the sideport on the 3-way stopcock between the catheter and the IV tubing.
3. Screw a sterile 5 to 10 ml syringe to the sideport for removing the IV solution from the catheter. (A smaller syringe would be used with a neonate.)
4. Turn the stopcock off to the IV tubing.
5. Pull a waste sample of IV solution and blood into the syringe. (The amount to be withdrawn and discarded depends on the dead space volume from the tip of the catheter to the sideport. Studies indicate that between 2.5 and 6 times this volume should be removed. Typically, in an adult, about 5 ml; less in a neonate.)
6. Attach a preheparinized sterile syringe to the sideport and withdraw 3 to 5 ml of arterial blood to be analyzed. Cap off the syringe to seal it.
7. Place the blood sample into an ice water bath.
8. Turn the stopcock toward the catheter. Fast flush the IV solution so that any blood left in the sideport is forced out into a sterile gauze pad.
9. Turn the stopcock toward the sideport so that the IV solution will run into the catheter.
10. Fast flush any blood in the catheter back into the patient.
11. Screw the dead-ender cap onto the sideport.

5. Perform quality control procedures for a blood gas sampling device. (IIB3c) [R, Ap, An]

See the next discussion.

6. Fix any problems with a blood gas sampling device. (IIB2g4) [R, Ap, An]

By performing the previous arterial puncture steps properly there should be no problems with the sample of blood that is obtained; however, there are problems that can occur with the blood gas sampling device. (Sampling of blood through an arterial catheter or pulmonary artery catheter is discussed in Section 4. Quality control and correcting problems with the blood sampling device are discussed there also.) The following are quality control procedures for an arterial sampling device and steps that can be taken to correct a problem:

a. Make sure that there is not an air bubble in the syringe. A bubble of room air will result in the oxygen level and the pH being too high and the carbon dioxide level too low. If an air bubble is found in the syringe, tilt it so that the needle is up. The bubble will rise by itself or may be raised by tapping the syringe. Push the plunger into the syringe to eject the air bubble. Cap off the hub of the syringe or needle to prevent air from entering the syringe.

b. Use the proper amount of heparin. This is only a concern when liquid heparin is added to a needle and syringe. Aspirate about 1 ml of 10 mg/ml or 1000 units/ml sodium heparin through the needle into the syringe. Pull the plunger back to coat the inside of the syringe. Push the plunger forward to squirt the excess heparin out through the needle. A 2 to 4 ml sample of blood should not have its values affected by this concentration. Remember that inadequate heparin could result in the blood sample clotting. Excessive heparin can alter the blood gas values by lowering the pH and the carbon dioxide level and raising the oxygen level.

c. Promptly cool down the blood gas sample. If the sample cannot be analyzed within 10 minutes of it being drawn, it should be placed in an ice water bath. Failure to do so will result in the living blood consuming the available oxygen and producing carbon dioxide. Obviously, this will result in the measured values being incorrect.

7. Interpret the results from a standard blood gas analyzer. (IC2b) [An]

A number of authors have written extensively on how to interpret arterial blood gases. The examinee must find a system of interpretation that works best for him or her. After reviewing a number of works, I found the system proposed by Shapiro, Peruzzi, and Templin (1994) in the fifth edition of *Clinical Application of Blood Gases* to be both practical and relatively easy to understand. Most of the following discussion and tables are based on this system. This does not mean that if you have learned another system you are at any disadvantage for taking the NBRC exams. The NBRC may include questions on blood gas interpretation and may also include blood gas results in other questions that relate to any respiratory care technique or procedure.

Assessment of Oxygenation

Hypoxemia/hypoxia can be rapidly life threatening. Because of this, most authors agree that it should be the first blood gas value to be interpreted. Table 2-1 shows the normal PaO_2 values for the adult and child, newborn, and the older adult when room air (21% oxygen) is inhaled at sea level. These values will decrease progressively as the altitude increases. However, under most clinical conditions this is not a factor (unless you work in a hospital in Denver or another high altitude city).

A general rule is that any patient is seriously hypoxemic if his or her PaO_2 is less than 60 mm Hg on room air (See Table 2-2 for guidelines on judging the seriousness of hypoxemia.) Once hypoxemia is recognized it must be corrected. The most obvious way is to give supplemental oxygen. The clinician must realize that oxygen alone will not correct the hypoxemia if the patient is hypoventilating

Table 2-1. Age-Based Acceptable PaO_2 Levels When Breathing Room Air (21% oxygen) at Sea Level

Age	PaO_2
Newborn	
Acceptable range	50 to 70 mm Hg
Child to Adult	
Normal	97 mm Hg
Acceptable range	>80 mm Hg
Hypoxemia	<80 mm Hg
Older Adult	
60 years old	>80 mm Hg
70 years old	>70 mm Hg
80 years old	>60 mm Hg
90 years old	>50 mm Hg

Modified from Shapiro BA, Harrison RA, Cane RD et al: *Clinical application of blood gases,* ed 4, Chicago, 1989, Year Book Medical.

(increased $PaCO_2$), has heart failure, or is unable to carry or make use of the oxygen. (See Table 2-2 for guidelines on giving supplemental oxygen so as to not undersupply or oversupply what the patient needs.) In general, try to keep the patient's PaO_2 between 60 and 100 mm Hg.

Table 2-3 lists general guidelines for the relationship between inspired oxygen and PaO_2 in the normal person. However, because most patients receiving respiratory care do not have normal lung physiology, it can be anticipated that their PaO_2 values will not increase as expected in the face of increased inspired oxygen. Shapiro et al (1994) suggest the following formula for determining if the patient will be hypoxemic on room air: "If PaO_2 is less than $FIO_2 \times 5$, the patient can be assumed to be hypoxemic on room air."

Fig. 2-3 shows a normal oxyhemoglobin dissociation curve. The saturation value is important to know because it shows how much hemoglobin is saturated with oxygen. It is best to directly measure the saturation on a CO-oximeter-type blood gas analyzer. Calculated saturation values can be misleadingly high if the patient has inhaled carbon monoxide. There are several points of correlation between the SaO_2 and the PaO_2 as listed here and shown in Fig. 2-3:

SaO_2 (%)	PaO_2 (mm Hg)	
100	150	Hemoglobin is fully saturated.
90	60	The patient who is *acutely* ill with cardiopulmonary disease should not be allowed to have the oxygenation values fall below these levels.
85	50	The patient who is *chronically* ill with cardiopulmonary disease should not be allowed to have the oxygenation values fall below these levels.
75	40	These are the normal mixed venous blood gas values as obtained from a pulmonary artery (Swan-Ganz) catheter. It is possible to obtain similar values from an attempted arterial puncture that sampled venous blood. If these values are obtained from a true arterial sample, the patient is in serious trouble. Fast action must be taken to correct this life-threatening hypoxemia.

Table 2-2. Evaluation of Hypoxemia

Conditions: Room air is inspired; the patient is less than 60 years old.*

Hypoxemia	PaO_2
Mild	<80 mm Hg
Moderate	<60 mm Hg
Severe	<40 mm Hg

Conditions: Supplemental oxygen is inspired; the patient is less than 60 years old.

Hypoxemia	PaO_2
Uncorrected	Less than room air acceptable limit
Corrected	Within the room air acceptable limit; <100 mm Hg
Excessively corrected	>100 mm Hg; less than the minimal level predicted in Table 2-3

Modified from Shapiro BA, Harrison RA, Cane RD et al: *Clinical application of blood gases,* ed 4, Chicago, 1989, Year Book Medical.
* Subtract 1 mm Hg of oxygen to limits of mild and moderate hypoxemia for each year over 60. A PaO_2 of less than 40 mm Hg indicates severe hypoxemia in any patient at any age.

Fig. 2-4 shows a number of factors that can influence the oxyhemoglobin dissociation curve and how oxygen loads and unloads from hemoglobin. In the patient with normal oxygenation, these factors are not clinically significant; however, when the PaO_2 is less than 60 mm Hg and the SaO_2 is less than 90%, these factors can become an important consideration. As can be seen in Fig. 2-4, a left-shifted oxyhemoglobin

Table 2-3. General Relationship Between Inspired Oxygen Percentage and PaO_2

Oxygen Percentage or F_IO_2	Minimal Predicted PaO_2 (mm Hg)
30	150
40	200
50	250
60	300
70	350
80	400
90	450
100	500

This table is for estimation purposes. It is not as accurate as calculating the patient's $P(A-a)O_2$.
Modified from Shapiro BA, Harrison RA, Cane RD et al: *Clinical application of blood gases,* ed 4, Chicago, 1989, Year Book Medical.

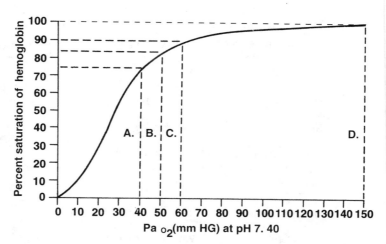

Fig. 2-3 The oxygen (oxyhemoglobin) dissociation curve plots the relationship between hemoglobin saturation (y-axis) and plasma PaO_2 (x-axis). **A,** 75% saturation and a PaO_2 of 40 mm Hg are normally seen in venous blood. **B,** 85% saturation and a PaO_2 of 50 mm Hg are the minimal levels that should be allowed in a *chronically* hypoxemic patient. **C,** 90% saturation and PaO_2 of 60 mm Hg are the minimal levels that should be allowed in an *acutely* hypoxemic patient. **D,** Hemoglobin in the pulmonary capillaries adjacent to normal alveoli will become 100% saturated when the PaO_2 reaches 150 mm Hg. (Modified from Lane EE, Walker JF: *Clinical arterial blood gas analysis*, St. Louis, 1987, Mosby–Year Book.)

dissociation curve results in a lower PaO_2 at any given saturation. This would result in even less oxygen being delivered to the tissues.

Assessment of Carbon Dioxide and pH

The pH is the next most important value to interpret because extreme acidemia/acidosis and alkalemia/alkalosis can be life threatening. The carbon dioxide value is important to interpret because it has a direct effect on the pH and indirectly affects the oxygen level. A high or low $PaCO_2$ level by itself is not life threatening.

Table 2-4 shows normal values for pH and $PaCO_2$ and the acceptable ranges around the mean or average. The most widely acceptable therapeutic range for pH is 7.30 to 7.50. For patients with an acute change, the $PaCO_2$ range is 30 to 50 mm Hg. (This $PaCO_2$ range does not apply to patients with long-standing disease, such as COPD, who may have $PaCO_2$ values greater than 50 mm Hg.) Values that fall outside of these pH and $PaCO_2$ ranges present a progressively greater risk to the patient.

Table 2-5 shows the definitions of Shapiro et al (1994) for alkalemia and acidemia from a respiratory cause. Strictly speaking, a pH greater than 7.4 is alkalemia and a pH less than 7.4 is acidemia. Also, a $PaCO_2$ less than 40 mm Hg would cause a respiratory alkalosis, and a $PaCO_2$ greater than 40 mm Hg would cause a respiratory acidosis. However, Shapiro and colleagues would argue that such narrow values are clinically unnecessary.

Table 2-6 shows the relationships among $PaCO_2$, pH, and bicarbonate. An *acute*

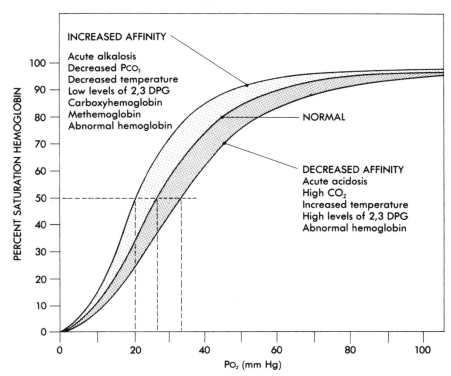

Fig. 2-4 Conditions associated with altered affinity of hemoglobin for O_2. P_{50} is the PaO_2 at which hemoglobin is 50% saturated, normally 26.6 mm Hg. A lower than normal P_{50} represents increased affinity of hemoglobin for O_2; a high P_{50} is seen with decreased affinity. Note that variation from the normal is associated with decreased (low P_{50}) or increased (high P_{50}) availability of O_2 to tissues (dotted lines). The shaded area shows the entire oxyhemoglobin dissociation curve under the same circumstances. (From Lane EE, Walker JF: *Clinical arterial blood gas analysis,* St. Louis, 1987, Mosby–Year Book. Used by permission.)

change in the patient's ventilation will cause the following when starting from a $PaCO_2$ of 40 mm Hg:

a. If the $PaCO_2$ increases by 20 mm Hg, the pH will decrease by .10.
b. If the $PaCO_2$ decreases by 10 mm Hg, the pH will increase by .10.

From this, it can be seen that the body is better able to compensate with metabolic buffers for a respiratory acidosis than a respiratory alkalosis. Changes

Table 2-4. Normal Laboratory Ranges for $PaCO_2$ and pH

	Mean	1 Standard Deviation	2 Standard Deviations
$PaCO_2$	40	38-42 mm Hg	35-45 mm Hg
pH	7.40	7.38-7.42	7.35-7.45

Modified from Shapiro BA, Harrison RA, Cane RD et al: *Clinical application of blood gases,* ed 4, Chicago, 1989, Year Book Medical.

Table 2-5. Naming Unacceptable Values for $PaCO_2$ and pH

$PaCO_2$ greater than 50 mm Hg	Respiratory acidosis/alveolar hypoventilation/ventilatory failure
pH less than 7.30	Acidemia
$PaCO_2$ less than 30 mm Hg	Respiratory alkalosis/alveolar hyperventilation
pH greater than 7.50	Alkalemia

Modified from Shapiro BA, Harrison RA, Cane RD et al: *Clinical application of blood gases*, ed 4, Chicago, 1989, Year Book Medical.

inside or outside of these values will be from *chronic* respiratory conditions and/or metabolic conditions.

Metabolic effects are evaluated by interpreting either the bicarbonate (HCO_3^-) value of base excess/base deficit (BE/BD) value. Both will reveal if there is any metabolic effect on the pH. Normal values are as shown:

HCO_3^- BE/BD
24 mEq/L   0 mEq/L; plus or minus 1 mEq/L is often listed as the normal
                range

Values indicating metabolic alkalosis of a primary or secondary nature are as follows:

Bicarbonate greater than 24 mEq/L
BE greater than 0 or greater than plus 1 mEq/L

Values indicating metabolic acidosis of a primary or secondary nature are as follows:

Bicarbonate less than 24 mEq/L
BE less than 0 or less than minus 1 mEq/L. Some laboratories report this as
    a BD or negative BE.

Tables 2-7 to 2-9 show definitions of terms and classifications of the various acid-base states. This is a complex subject because of all the variables. The reader should study these tables and practice their application on arterial blood gases from real-life situations.

Table 2-6. Approximate Relationships Among $PaCO_2$, pH, and Bicarbonate

$PaCO_2$ (mm Hg)	pH	Bicarbonate/HCO_3^- (mEq/L)
80	7.20	28
60	7.30	26
40	7.40	24
30	7.50	22
20	7.60	20

Modified from Shapiro BA, Harrison RA, Cane RD et al: *Clinical application of blood gases,* ed 4, Chicago, 1989, Year Book Medical.

8. **Perform quality control procedures for a blood gas analyzer (IIB3c) [R, Ap, An]; and fix any problems with the unit (IIB2g4) [R, Ap, An].**

Quality Control (QC).—Quality control refers to creating a measurement and documentation system to confirm the accuracy (precision) and reliability of all blood gas measurements. Accuracy or precision means that the measured physiologic values truly reflect the actual physiologic values. Reliability means that there is a high degree of confidence that the accuracy of the measured values represents the patient's actual physiologic values. Both are critically important if the blood gas results are to be used to make correct clinical decisions.

Quality Assurance (QA).—Quality assurance refers to the broader concern that the results of the blood gas measurement are not only accurate and reliable but also clinically useful. To help ensure this, the Clinical Laboratory Improvement Amendments of 1988 (CLIA '88) require that the department have written policies and procedures on items including record keeping, equipment maintenance, staff training, and the correction of errors.

Calibration.—Calibration is the systematic standardization of the graduations of the blood gas analyzer against known values to ensure consistency. Proper calibration of the electrodes is essential to the accuracy of the blood gas values. Some

Table 2-7. Clinical Terminology for Arterial Blood Gas Measurements

Clinical Terminology	Clinical Finding
Respiratory acidosis/alveolar hypoventilation/ventilatory failure	PaCO$_2$ >50 mm Hg
acute ventilatory failure	PaCO$_2$ >50 mm Hg; pH <7.30
chronic ventilatory failure	PaCO$_2$ >50 mm Hg; pH between 7.30 and 7.50
Respiratory alkalosis/alveolar hyperventilation	PaCO$_2$ <30 mm Hg
acute alveolar hyperventilation	PaCO$_2$ <30 mm Hg; pH >7.50
chronic alveolar hyperventilation	PaCO$_2$ <30 mm Hg; pH between 7.40 and 7.50
Acidemia	pH <7.40*
Acidosis	Pathophysiologic condition in which the patient has a significant base deficit (plasma bicarbonate below normal)
Alkalemia	pH >7.40*
Alkalosis	Pathophysiologic condition in which the patient has a significant base excess (plasma bicarbonate above normal)

* Some authors prefer wider limits such as 7.35-7.45 or 7.30-7.50.
Modified from Shapiro BA, Harrison RA, Cane RD et al: *Clinical application of blood gases*, ed 4, Chicago, 1989, Year Book Medical.

Table 2-8. Evaluation of Ventilatory and Metabolic Effects on Acid-Base Status

Evaluation of PaCO$_2$

PaCO$_2$ >50 mm Hg	Respiratory acidosis/alveolar hypoventilation/ventilatory failure
PaCO$_2$ between 30 and 50 mm Hg	Acceptable alveolar ventilation
PaCO$_2$ <30 mm Hg	Respiratory alkalosis/alveolar hyperventilation

Evaluation of PaCO$_2$ in conjuction with pH

1. Acceptable alveolar ventilation (PaCO$_2$ between 30 and 50 mm Hg)
   a. pH >7.50   metabolic alkalosis
   b. pH 7.30-7.50   acceptable ventilatory and metabolic acid-base status
   c. pH <7.30   metabolic acidosis
2. Alveolar hypoventilation (PaCO$_2$ >50 mm Hg)
   a. pH >7.50   *partially compensated* metabolic alkalosis
   b. pH 7.30-7.50   *chronic* ventilatory failure
   c. pH <7.30   *acute* ventilatory failure
3. Alveolar hyperventilation (PaCO$_2$ <30 mm Hg)
   a. pH >7.50   *acute* alveolar hyperventilation
   b. pH 7.40-7.50   *chronic* alveolar hyperventilation
   c. pH 7.30-7.40   *compensated* metabolic acidosis
   d. pH <7.30   *partially compensated* metabolic acidosis

Some authors use a more narrow pH range for these classifications.
Modified from Shapiro BA, Harrison RA, Cane RD et al: *Clinical application of blood gases,* ed 4, Chicago, 1989, Year Book Medical.

general calibration steps are discussed later. The manufacturer's guidelines must be followed for the specific steps in calibration.

Quality Control Materials

A variety of quality control materials are available to calibrate the electrodes for PO$_2$, PCO$_2$, and pH. Their use varies. Each of the following materials has its advantages, disadvantages, and limitations. The manufacturer of a particular brand

Table 2-9. Primary Blood Gas Classifications

	PaCO$_2$	pH	Bicarbonate	Base Excess
Ventilatory Imbalance				
1. Acute alveolar hypoventilation	I	D	N	N
2. Chronic alveolar hypoventilation	I	N	I	I
3. Acute alveolar hyperventilation	D	I	N	N
4. Chronic alveolar hyperventilation	D	N	D	D
Metabolic Imbalance				
1. Uncompensated acidosis	N	D	D	D
2. Partially compensated acidosis	D	D	D	D
3. Uncompensated alkalosis	N	I	I	I
4. Partially compensated alkalosis	I	I	I	I
5. Compensated acidosis or alkalosis	I or D	N	I or D	I or D

Key: I, Increased; D, Decreased; N, Normal range
Modified from Shapiro BA, Harrison, RA, Cane RD et al: *Clinical application of blood gases,* ed 4, Chicago, 1989, Year Book Medical.

or model of blood gas analyzer may require that a specific type of material be used in its units.

Aqueous buffers are water based and used to check pH and PCO_2 measurements; they cannot be used to check PO_2 measurements. Commercially prepared *gases* are used to check PO_2 and PCO_2 measurements; they cannot be used to check pH. The following CO_2 mixes may be used: 0%, 5%, 10%, and 12%. The following O_2 mixes may be used: 0%, 12%, 20%, 20.95% from room air, 21%, and 100%. *Tonometered liquids* are exposed in the laboratory to known oxygen and carbon dioxide gas mixes until the liquids are saturated and have the same partial pressures as the gases. There are three types of tonometered liquids. First, *human or animal serum or whole blood.* This is the most accurate method available and is mainly used for PO_2 and PCO_2. While whole human blood cannot be used for pH, a bovine blood product can be used for all three values. Second, *assayed liquids* are nonwater-based liquids that are pretonometered by the manufacturer and available in sealed glass vials. They can be used for PO_2, PCO_2, and pH. These are very popular because of the advantages of speed and simplicity. Third, *oxygenated fluorocarbon-based emulsions* (perfluorinated compounds) can be used for PO_2, PCO_2, and pH measurement. They are considered to be as accurate as whole blood without its associated risks.

Levey-Jennings Charts

The Levey-Jennings charts (also known as Shewhart/Levey-Jennings or Quality Control charts) are used to record the results of each calibration procedure. They are similarly designed with time plotted on the horizontal scale and the analyte (PO_2, PCO_2, or pH on the vertical scale. The vertical scale for each analyte has a central value for what is normally expected. On both sides of this normal value are standard deviation (SD) points showing movement away from what is expected. When an analyte electrode is operating within the acceptable limits it is said to be *in control*. In general, if an analyte is within two standard deviations of the normal value it is considered to be in control.

An *out-of-control* situation exists whenever a single or a series of calibration values are outside of established limits. A *random error* is an unpredictable aberation in precision that occurs when the quality control material is sampled. An example of a random error is shown in Fig. 2-5, **A.** The practitioner likely made a simple error in introducing the material or running the analyzer. Common problems include an air bubble injected into the unit or incomplete flushing of the previous sample. Usually the problem can be corrected by flushing out any residual blood and then carefully injecting more of the current patient blood sample. Run the analyzer again to get new patient values. Also, you can run the same patient sample through another analyzer to compare the two sets of results for closeness.

A *systematic error* shows an accuracy problem and is much more serious. It must be investigated, corrected, and documented. An example of a systematic error is shown in Fig. 2-5, **B.** Westgard has established rules for determining whether the error is random or systematic (see Table 2-10 for descriptions). Examples of systematic errors include misanalyzed CO_2 or O_2 standards for calibration; contaminated quality control materials; or deteriorated oxygen, carbon dioxide, or pH electrode function. Each of these must be investigated until the problem is found and corrected. The unit cannot be used again until after it is proven to work properly and to give accurate results.

Review the discussion on one-, two-, and three-point calibration of the oxygen, carbon dioxide, and pH electrodes if necessary. This topic is covered in *Respiratory*

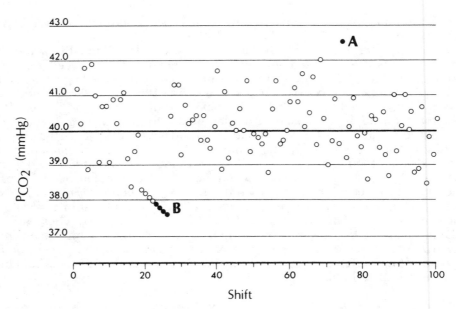

Fig. 2-5 Levey-Jennings quality control chart for PaCO$_2$. The central horizontal line represents the mean value of 40 mm Hg. The next lower and higher horizontal lines show 1 standard deviation (SD) value from the mean. The second most distant lower and higher horizontal lines show 2 SD values from the mean. The most distant horizontal lines show 3 SD values from the mean. The bottom number scale represents 8-hour work shifts. Open circles represent calibration values that are within 2 SDs of the mean value. They are considered to be in control. The black circles represent calibration values that are out-of-control. *A* represents a random error; *B* represents a systematic error. (From Shapiro BA, Peruzzi WT, Templin R: *Clinical application of blood gases,* ed 5, St. Louis, 1994, Mosby–Year Book. Used by permission.)

Care Certification Guide (Sills, 1994) and other sources. In addition, the CLIA '88 guidelines require that all analyzers be enrolled in an approved external quality control program. This involves the unit running five "control" samples three times per year. Failure to accurately analyze the control samples can result in serious

Table 2-10. Westgard's Rules for Determining When an Analyzer Is Not Functioning Properly

Rule Name	Levey-Jennings Chart
Random Error	
1-2s*	The measurement is more than 2 standard deviations (SDs) but not more than 3 SDs from the mean.
1-3s	The measurement is more than 3 SDs from the mean.
R†-4s	Two consecutive measurements are 4 SDs or more apart.
Systematic Error	
2-2s	Two consecutive measurements are either 2 SDs above or 2 SDs below the mean.
4-1s	Four consecutive measurements are either 1 SD above or 1 SD below the mean.
7-trend	Seven consecutive measurements are on only one side of the mean. Each measurement is progressively more out of control.
10-mean	Ten consecutive measurements are on only one side of the mean.

Based on a table in Lane EE, Walker JF: *Clinical arterial blood gas analysis,* St. Louis, 1987, Mosby–Year Book.
* S = standard deviation.
† R = repeat.

consequences. These include not being reimbursed by medicare and medicaid until the problem is corrected.

Module B.   CO-oximetry.

1.   Get the necessary equipment to perform CO-oximetry. (IIA1d4) [R, Ap]

Most hospitals will have a CO-oximeter in addition to a blood gas analyzer. A CO-oximeter should be used to analyze a blood gas sample whenever carbon monoxide poisoning is known or suspected. In addition, a CO-oximeter will give a complete analysis of the relative amounts of the different types of patient hemoglobin.

CO-oximeters are also called spectrophotometric oximeters and are the most accurate method available to measure the four different hemoglobin moities (species or variations in the hemoglobin molecule). These hemoglobin species include: 1) oxyhemoglobin (HbO_2 or O_2Hb), which carries oxygen to the tissues, and reduced hemoglobin (HbR or RHb), which has given up its oxygen and picked up carbon dioxide; 2) carboxyhemoglobin (HbCO or COHb), which is nonfunctional because of the tightness with which carbon monoxide binds to the hemoglobin; 3) methemoglobin (HbMet or MetHb), which is nonfunctional because the Hb molecule is unable to combine reversibly with oxygen; and 4) sulfhemoglobin (HbS or SHb), which is similar to the HbMet and also nonfunctional. In addition, a CO-oximeter can measure the fetal hemoglobin (HbF or FHb) found in a newborn infant instead of adult oxyhemoglobin.

Each of these hemoglobin moities has a spectroscopic "fingerprint" of absorbed lightwave frequencies that is unique to it (see Fig. 2-6 for the spectral analysis of the various forms of hemoglobin).

The principle of operation of a CO-oximeter is the comparison of the relative absorbances of four wavelengths of light by oxyhemoglobin, reduced hemoglobin, and carboxyhemoglobin. This is done by comparing the absorptions at the three isosbestic points (where the moities being compared have equal absorption) and a wavelength point where there is the greatest difference in absorption between the two moities. By computer integration of the data based on Beer's law, the relative proportions of oxyhemoglobin, reduced hemoglobin, and carboxyhemoglobin are determined. If the total is less than 100% of the hemoglobin present, the difference has to be methemoglobin (or, rarely, sulfhemoglobin). The unit then provides data on total hemoglobin; percentages for oxyhemoglobin, reduced hemoglobin, carboxyhemoglobin, and methemoglobin; and total amounts for them in gm/dl blood. Some units will also calculate O_2 content.

2.   Put the CO-oximeter together, make sure that it works properly, and identify any problems with the equipment. (IIB1e4) [R, Ap]

The unit will come preassembled by the manufacturer. Practical experience with a unit is recommended to understand how to add a patient blood sample and perform calibration duties. (See Fig. 2-7 for a schematic drawing of a CO-oximeter). A thallium-neon hollow cathode lamp emits light in the infrared-visible range. A device called a monochromator contains four filters and rotates through the light beam. Each filter will allow only one specific wavelength to pass through it. These four monochromatic wavelengths correspond to the three isosbestic points discussed earlier (shown in Fig. 2-6) and 626.6 nm. This last wavelength is poorly

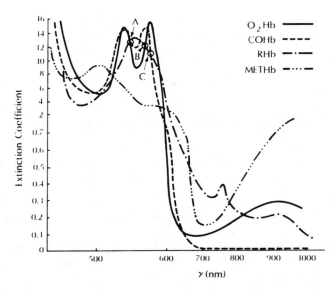

Fig. 2-6 Spectral analysis of the hemoglobin moities (species). O₂Hb is oxyhemoglobin, COHb is carboxyhemoglobin, RHb is reduced hemoglobin, MetHb (METHb) is methemoglobin. Point A shows the triple isosbestic point at 548 nm for O₂Hb, COHb, and RHb. Point B shows the double isosbestic point at 568 nm for O₂Hb and RHb. Point C shows the double isosbestic point at 578 nm for RHb and COHb. A fourth wavelength at 626.6 nm is used for comparison purposes. (From Shapiro BA, Peruzzi WT, Templin R: *Clinical application of blood gases,* ed 4, St. Louis, 1994, Mosby—Year Book. Used by permission.)

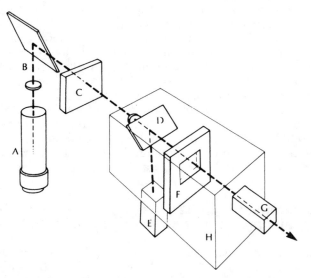

Fig. 2-7 CO-oximeter basic components. *A,* thallium-neon hollow cathode light source; *B,* lens and mirror; *C,* monochromator with four specific wavelength filters; *D,* light beam splitter that diverts half of the light to the reference detector and half to the cuvette; *E,* reference wavelength detector; *F,* patient sample cuvette, *G,* sample wavelength detector; and *H,* temperature regulated block set at 37°C. (From Shapiro BA, Peruzzi WT, Templin R: *Clinical application of blood gases,* ed 5, St. Louis, 1994, Mosby—Year Book. Used by permission.)

absorbed by all four hemoglobin moities. It is used to find the maximal difference in absorption so that the relative amounts of the hemoglobin species can be determined.

When a blood sample is placed into the cuvette, the same four wavelengths are passed through it. The amount of absorbance at each wavelength is measured and compared to the absorbance at each wavelength by a reference sample solution (see the next discussion). The computer integrates the data and calculates the total hemoglobin and amounts of the four hemoglobin moities.

3. Perform quality control procedures on the CO-oximeter. (IIB3e) [R, Ap, An]

Total hemoglobin should be calibrated when the unit is installed, at regular intervals suggested by the manufacturer, after the sample tubing is changed, after the cuvette is disassembled or changed, or whenever there is a suspicious reading. This is done by filling the cuvette with a special dye produced by the manufacturer and analyzing it following the prescribed steps.

Routine calibration is done every 30 minutes. The unit obtains and stores absorbance readings at the four different wavelengths from a "blank" solution in the reference detector. When the same "blank" solution is added to the sample cuvette the same four wavelengths are measured. Normally, they are identical in absorption. The same procedure is done after every patient sample is analyzed.

4. Fix any problems with the equipment. (IIB2g5) [R, Ap, An]

Following are examples of common problems and their solutions:

a. Incomplete hemolysis of the blood sample causes the light to scatter off of cell fragments and lipids. Sickle cells (as in sickel cell anemia) are difficult to disrupt and may cause false oxyhemoglobin and carboxyhemoglobin readings if extra time is not taken for hemolysis. Follow manufacturer's guidelines on the procedure for hemolysing the red blood cells.

b. Greater than 10% methemoglobin may cause errors in the measurement of all hemoglobin moities. Sulfhemoglobin will also cause false readings. Additional information may need to be gathered from the chart or laboratory on the patient's levels of these abnormal hemoglobin moities. CO-oximetry should probably not be performed on blood samples with abnormal levels of methemoglobin or sulfhemoglobin.

c. Intravenous dyes such as methylene blue, Evans blue, and indocyanine green used in various cardiac studies can absorb the same wavelengths of light as used to identify the various forms of hemoglobin. Their presence will result in a lower than actual level of oxyhemoglobin being measured. Check the patient's chart for a record of these dyes being used. CO-oximetry should probably not be used for blood gas analysis on patients who have these dyes in their systems.

d. Failure to reprogram the analyzer for fetal hemoglobin instead of adult hemoglobin may produce false results. Remember to check the chart for the patient's age. Reprogram the analyzer for fetal hemoglobin on any infant who is only a few days old.

e. The presence of lipid particles in the blood will cause light scattering and result in a reading that is falsely high in total hemoglobin and percent of methemoglobin, and falsely low in percent oxyhemoglobin and percent carboxyhemoglobin. Follow the laboratory's guidelines for when a patient's blood lipid value is too high for accurate use of the CO-oximeter.

f. Air bubbles or incomplete hemolysis of blood in the cuvette will cause an absorbance error. Air bubbles need to be flushed out and the blood sample inserted again and reanalyzed. Make sure that all blood samples are hemolysed according to the manufacturer's guidelines.

g. Blood clot(s) in the sample tubing will prevent blood from flowing through to the cuvette. If a sample cannot be inserted into the unit, suspect and check for a blood clot. Obviously, remove any clotted tubing, replace it and confirm that the CO-oximeter is working properly.

5.   Perform CO-oximetry and interpret the results to evaluate the patient's response to respiratory care. (IC1a and IIIA1f) [R, Ap, An]

Follow the manufacturer's guidelines on rewarming the blood sample to body temperature, hemolyzing the sample, and inserting it into the measurement cuvette. Failure to do so could result in incorrect patient values.

The CO-oximeter gives values for oxyhemoglobin (HbO_2), reduced hemoglobin (HbR), carboxyhemoglobin (HbCO), and methemoglobin/sulfhemoglobin (HbMet/HbS). Each hemoglobin moity can be displayed in terms of grams per deciliter, percentage of the whole, and added together for a total hemoglobin (THb) (see Table 2-11 for the normal adult hemoglobin values). The amount of carboxyhemoglobin and methemoglobin should be subtracted from the total hemoglobin to find the amount of functional hemoglobin. Any increase in the carboxyhemoglobin and/or methemoglobin level above those listed is abnormal and results in even less normal hemoglobin to carry oxygen. The patient who suffers from carbon monoxide poisoning is at greatest risk. A HbCO level of 30% saturation or greater can be rapidly fatal. By subtraction, the HbO_2 (SaO_2) level can be no greater than 70% with a resulting PaO_2 of less than 40 mm Hg.

Calculate the amount of functional hemoglobin and saturation as shown here:

Example 1
A patient with normal HbCO and HbMet levels:

15.0 gm total Hb
−.225 gm HbCO

14.775 gm
−.225 gm HbMet

14.550 gm functional Hb

100% potential saturation of oxyhemoglobin in arterial blood
−1.5% saturation of COHb

98.5%
−1.5% saturation of MetHb

97% saturation of arterial blood (SaO_2 of 97%)

Table 2-11. Normal Hemoglobin Values for Adults

Total hemoglobin (THb)	Men: 13.5-18.0 g/dl
	Women: 12.0-16.0 g/dl
	15.0 g/dl is often listed as an average for both.
Oxyhemoglobin (HbO_2) (arterial sample)	94%-100% of Thb (Reported as an SaO_2 of 94%-100%.)
Carboxyhemoglobin (HbCO)	Nonsmokers: less than 1.5% (.225 g/dl) of THb
	Smokers: 5%-10% of THb
Methemoglobin (HbMet)	.5%-3% (.075%-.45% g/dl) of Thb
O_2 content (arterial sample)	15-23 vol %

Example 2

A patient with an elevated COHb and a normal MetHb level:

15.0 gm total Hb
−3.0 gm HbCO
12.0 gm
−.225 gm HbMet
11.775 gm functional Hb

100% potential saturation of oxyhemoglobin in arterial blood
−20% saturation of HbCO
80%
−1.5% saturation of HbMet
78.5% saturation of arterial blood (SaO_2 of 78.5%)

Module C. Mixed venous blood gases.

1. Review the patient's chart for mixed venous blood gas results. (IA1c3) [R]

A mixed venous blood sample can be taken from the pulmonary artery of any patient who has a pulmonary artery (Swan-Ganz) catheter. This is a true mixed venous sample and should not be confused with a blood sample taken from an arm or other vein. The symbol $P\bar{v}$ is the prefix for venous blood gas values of oxygen and so forth. In general, a typical patient will have mixed venous blood gas values of: $S\bar{v}O_2$, 75%, $P\bar{v}O_2$ 40 mm Hg, $P\bar{v}CO_2$ 46 mm Hg, and pH 7.35 (see Table 2-12 for details on normal venous blood gas values and their interpretation in patients with cardiovascular disease.)

2. Interpret the results of mixed venous blood gas analysis to evaluate the patient's response to respiratory care. (IC2e, IB8g and IIIA1o) [R, Ap, An]

In the critically ill patient, it is just as important to measure the mixed venous blood gases as it is to measure the arterial blood gases. The venous blood gas values reveal what has happened as the arterial blood has passed through the body. Oxygen has been extracted and carbon dioxide has been added to the blood. The difference

Table 2-12. Normal and Abnormal Mixed Venous Blood Gas Values

Normal Values
Average: $S\bar{v}O_2$ 75%, $P\bar{v}O_2$ 40 mm Hg, $P\bar{v}CO_2$ 46 mm Hg, pH 7.35
Range: $S\bar{v}O_2$ 76%-70%, $P\bar{v}O_2$ 43-37 mm Hg, $P\bar{v}CO_2$ 46-44 mm Hg, pH 7.36-7.34

Critically Ill Patient	$P\bar{v}O_2$ (mm Hg)		$S\bar{v}O_2$ (%)	
	Average	Range	Average	Range
Excellent cardiovascular reserves	37	40-35	70	75-68
Limited cardiovascular reserves	32	35-30	60	68-56
Failure of cardiovascular reserves	<30	<30	<56	<56

Based on a table in Shapiro BA, Peruzzi WT, Templn R: *Clinical application of blood gases*, ed 5, St. Louis, 1994, Mosby—Year Book.

between the arterial and venous oxygen levels reflects oxygen consumption by the body as well as cardiac output. (These topics are discussed in more detail in Section 4.)

Because of this, the most critical venous blood gas values to measure are the $S\bar{v}O_2$ and $P\bar{v}O_2$ (review Table 2-12 for normal and abnormal values). It is generally accepted that a $P\bar{v}O_2$ value of less than 30 mm Hg or $S\bar{v}O_2$ of less than 56% indicates that the patient has tissue hypoxia. Both values can be obtained by analyzing a mixed venous blood sample taken through a pulmonary artery catheter. If the patient has a fiberoptic catheter, the $S\bar{v}O_2$ value can be monitored continuously. This is extremely helpful if the patient is unstable or having frequent changes in inspired oxygen or ventilator settings. (Pulmonary artery catheters are discussed in more detail in Section 4.)

Module D.   Capillary blood gases.

1.   Perform capillary blood gas sampling. (IIIA1l) [R, Ap]

It is occasionally necessary to obtain a sample of capillary blood from an infant for blood gas analysis. Usually this is because the infant has a pulmonary problem that warrants evaluation, but it would too difficult or traumatic to draw an arterial sample. If the infant were in danger, an arterial sample would be taken or an arterial line inserted for regular, easy sampling.

Following are the steps and key points to keep in mind during the sampling procedure:

1. Select a highly vascularized and well-perfused site. Usually the heel is selected, but the great toe, earlobe, or finger are also acceptable.
2. Warm the heel (or other site) with a warm towel or heat lamp for about 5-10 minutes; 45°C is ideal. Warming vasodilates the vessels and "arterializes" the capillary blood supply.
3. After warming, unwrap the site and wipe it with an antiseptic pad.
4. Use a pediatric lance to deeply puncture the outer edge of the heel (see Fig. 2-8). Blood should flow freely without squeezing the area. The blood will be "de-arterialized" if it is squeezed out and the sample will be useless for blood gas analysis.
5. Insert a preheparinized capillary tube (.075–10 ml) deeply into the drop of blood. The blood should easily flow through the tube. Ideally, a second sample tube is filled.
6. Seal both ends of the tubes.
7. Place the sealed tubes immediately into an ice water bath.
8. Send the samples off to the laboratory for analysis along with the proper paperwork.
9. Apply pressure to stop the bleeding. Complications include infection, bone spurs, and laceration of the posterior tibial artery.

2.   Interpret the results of capillary blood gas analysis to evaluate the patient's response to respiratory care. (IIIA1n) [R, Ap, An]

As mentioned in the previous set of steps, the sampling site must be well perfused. A hypotensive or vasoconstricted infant should not have this procedure done for blood gas analysis. Squeezing the sampling site to force blood from the wound will result in venous blood being forced out along with arterialized blood. This will also render the sample useless for blood gas analysis.

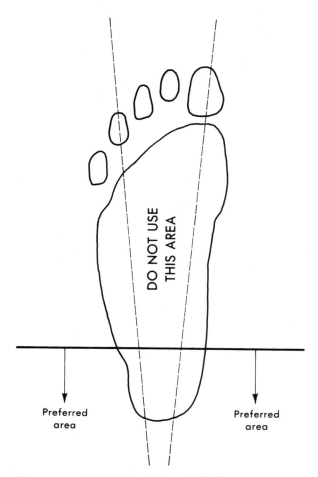

Fig. 2-8 Puncture sites on an infant's heel for obtaining an arterialized capillary blood sample. Avoid the posterior tibial artery that runs through the center of the foot. (From Czervinske MP: Arterial blood gas analysis and other cardiopulmonary monitoring. In Koff PB, Eitzman D, Neu J: *Neonatal and pediatric respiratory care,* ed 2, St. Louis, 1993, Mosby–Year Book. Used by permission.)

Assuming the infant is well perfused and the listed set of steps are followed, the blood sample can be analyzed. Because this is not a true arterial blood gas sample, the following limitations are placed on interpreting the results:

    a. The capillary pH (c pH) will have a good correlation with the arterial pH.
    b. The capillary CO_2 ($PcCO_2$) will correlate with the $PaCO_2$ about 50% of the time.
    c. The capillary O_2 (PcO_2) will *not* correlate well with the $PaCO_2$.

Based on these limitations, an arterialized capillary blood pH value can be clinically useful. The capillary CO_2 value should be viewed with suspicion. It should not be the only parameter followed to judge the infant's ability to ventilate; however, the combination of a low pH and elevated CO_2 would both indicate hypoventilation. Evaluate the infant's vital signs, breathing efforts, chest x-ray, and so on to determine his or her respiratory status.

Unfortunately, the capillary O_2 value is practically useless for judging the infant's oxygenation. Some infants may have a fairly close correlation with the PaO_2 whereas others will not. Unfortunately, there is no way to predetermine those that will match and those that will not; all that can be said is that many practitioners view a low capillary oxygen level as a sign of clinical hypoxemia. The AARC Clinical Practice Guideline "Oxygen Therapy in the Acute Care Hospital" makes mention that a PcO_2 of less than 40 mm Hg documents neonatal hypoxemia. An arterial blood gas sample remains the best way to determine a patient's respiratory status.

Module E.   Alveolar-arterial difference in oxygen pressure ($P[A-a]O_2$).

1.   Perform the $P(A-a)O_2$ procedure. (IB8h and IC1j) [R, Ap, An]

Do not be confused when reading about different abbreviations for the same procedure and calculation. The NBRC uses the abbreviation $P(A-a)O_2$; however, a review of the literature reveals the use of $A-aDO_2$, $D(A-a)O_2$, and $AaDO_2$.
The following must be done to perform the $P(A-a)O_2$ procedure:

1. Note the patient's inspired oxygen percentage.
2. Draw and analyze an arterial blood gas sample. Note the patient's PaO_2 and $PaCO_2$.
3. Note the patient's temperature. This is needed to determine the patient's pulmonary water vapor pressure (PH_2O). The value of 47 mm Hg is used if the patient's temperature is normal. Check published tables for the pulmonary water vapor pressure if the patient's temperature is higher or lower than normal.
4. Measure the local barometric pressure (P_B) in mm Hg.
5. If possible, calculate the patient's respiratory exchange ratio. If this cannot be done use the standard value of 0.8.

2.   Calculate the patient's $P(A-a)O_2$. (IB8h, IC1j, and IIIA1s2) [R, Ap, An]

See the following equation.

3.   Interpret the results of the $P(A-a)O_2$ to evaluate the patient's response to respiratory care. (IB8h, IC1j, and IIIA1s2) [R, Ap, An]

There are a number of possible variations in the formula for calculating the pressure of alveolar oxygen. The formula presented here is the most commonly used and understood.

$$PAO_2 = [(P_B - PH_2O) \, F_IO_2] - \frac{PaCO_2}{.8}$$

Where:

PAO_2 = Pressure of alveolar oxygen.
P_B = Barometric pressure of air. This is 760 mm Hg (torr) at sea level; it decreases as the altitude increases.
PH_2O = Pressure of water vapor in the lungs. This is 47 mm Hg (torr) at the normal temperature of 98.6°F/37°C. Remember that water vapor

pressure increases if your patient has a fever and decreases if your patient is hypothermic.

F_IO_2 = Fractional concentration (percentage) of inspired oxygen. Use whatever percentage of oxygen your patient is breathing in.

$\dfrac{PaCO_2}{.8}$ = Calculates the effect of carbon dioxide and the patient's metabolism. The factor of .8 is based on how much oxygen a normal person uses and how much carbon dioxide is produced in a minute. The symbols for this metabolic value are R for Respiratory Exchange Ratio and RQ for Respiratory Quotient. The following calculation is based on a normal person's metabolism:

$$R \text{ or } RQ = \frac{\dot{V}CO_2}{\dot{V}O_2} = \frac{200\,ml/min}{250\,ml/min} = .8$$

Because many sick patients do not react as would be expected, the factor has a range of .6 to 1.1 depending on oxygen consumption and carbon dioxide production. Assume the factor is .8 unless you are told otherwise or measure otherwise.

The following are two other ways that this metabolic factor is calculated in some references:

1. $PaCO_2 (1.25)$ (This gives the same answer as the previous equation if the factor is .8.)
2. $PaCO_2 \left[FIO_2 + \dfrac{(1 - F_IO_2)]}{.8} \right.$ (This will give a slightly different answer.)

The NBRC may ask the examinee to identify which one of several offered versions of the alveolar oxygen equation is correct. It would be helpful to review the various derivations. If an NBRC question asks the examinee to calculate the pressure of alveolar oxygen, any of the various derivations will result in an answer that is close enough to the best one offered to you. It is possible that none of the offered answers will be exactly correct. Select the closest one.

Example 1

You are working in a major teaching hospital in Miami. The patient's physician asks you to calculate the alveolar-arterial difference in oxygen on a 30-year-old patient. The following conditions exist:

P_B = 760 mm Hg
PH_2O = 47 mm Hg because your patient's temperature is 98.6°F/37°C
F_IO_2 = .21 because the patient is breathing room air
$PaCO_2$ = 40 mm Hg from ABGs
PaO_2 = 90 mm Hg from ABGs
Respiratory Exchange Ratio = .8

1. $PAO_2 = [(P_B - PH_2O)\, F_IO_2] - \dfrac{PaCO_2}{.8}$
2. $PAO_2 = [(760 - 47)\,.21] - \dfrac{40}{.8}$
3. $PAO_2 = [(713)\,.21] - 50$
4. $PAO_2 = [150] - 50$
5. $PAO_2 = 100$ mm Hg
6. $P(A-a)O_2 = 100 - 90 = 10$ mm Hg

Interpretation: A P(A−a)O$_2$ of 10 mm Hg is normal for a patient of this age. It is normal to see a difference between the alveolar and arterial oxygen levels that starts out in the range of 4 to 12 mm Hg and slowly increases with age (see Fig. 2-9).

Example 2:

You are working in a major teaching hospital in Denver. You are asked to calculate the alveolar-arterial difference in oxygen on a 40-year-old patient. The following conditions exist:

P$_B$ = 710 mm Hg
PH$_2$O = 50 mm Hg because your patient's temperature is 100°F/38°C
F$_I$O$_2$ = .35 because the patient is breathing 35% oxygen by mask
PaCO$_2$ = 55 mm Hg from ABGs
PaO$_2$ = 65 mm Hg from ABGs
Respiratory Exchange Ratio = .85

1. $PAO_2 = [(P_B - PH_2O)\, F_IO_2] - \dfrac{PaCO_2}{.85}$

2. $PAO_2 = [(710 - 50)\,.35] - \dfrac{55}{.85}$

3. $PAO_2 = [(660)\,.35] - 65$
4. $PAO_2 = [231] - 65$
5. $PAO_2 = 166$ mm Hg
6. $P(A-a)O_2 = 166 - 65 = 101$ mm Hg

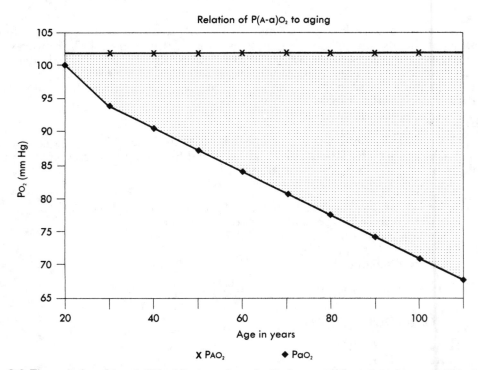

Fig. 2-9 The relationship of P(A-a)O$_2$ to aging. As PaO$_2$ naturally falls with age, P(A-a)O$_2$ increases at the rate of approximately 3 mm Hg per decade beyond 20 years. (From Lane EE, Walker JF; *Clinical arterial blood gas analysis*, St. Louis, 1987, Mosby–Year Book. Used by permission.)

Interpretation: The difference of 101 mm Hg is elevated even though this patient is older than in Example 1.

The following are examples of some conditions in which the measurement of the $P(A-a)O_2$ aids in the diagnosis or treatment:

1. Patients who are hypoxemic because they are hypoventilating (increased CO_2) will have a normal $P(A-a)O_2$ when breathing room air. The hypoxemia can be corrected by increasing their ventilation. Supplemental oxygen results in an expected increase in PaO_2.
2. Any condition where there is a low ventilation to perfusion ratio reveals an elevated $P(A-a)O_2$ when breathing room air. Supplemental oxygen results in an increase in PaO_2; however, it will not be as dramatic as that seen in the hypoventilating patient. Examples include asthma, bronchitis, emphysema, or any other condition where there is unequal distribution of air into and out of the lungs but relatively normal perfusion.
3. Any shunt producing disease or condition. Examples include adult respiratory distress syndrome (ARDS) and right to left anatomic shunt such as seen in a ventricular septal defect. The $P(A-a)O_2$ will become greater as the oxygen percentage is increased. It is commonly accepted that a $P(A-a)O_2$ of greater than 350 mm Hg, when 80% to 100% oxygen is administered, indicates that the patient is experiencing refractory hypoxemia. The patient will need to be supported by a mechanical ventilator. Commonly, positive end-expiratory pressure (PEEP) is administered so that the oxygen percentage can be reduced to a safer level.
4. Any disease producing a diffusion defect. Pulmonary fibrosis from any cause will result in a wider than normal $P(A-a)O_2$. Supplemental oxygen will result in an increase in the PaO_2 but not as great an increase as expected.

Module F.   Pulse oximetry.

1.   Recommend pulse oximetry for additional data. (IA2v) [An]

Pulse oximetry is indicated in the following situations: during anesthesia and intraoperative monitoring of oxygenation, postoperatively when the patient is still sedated, when a patient is receiving sedatives or analgesics that can blunt the airway protective reflexes, during bronchoscopy, during a sleep study, and to evaluate the effectiveness of oxygen therapy.

2.   Interpret the patient's pulse oximetry value. (IB9a and IC2c) [An]

The previously healthy patient who develops cardiopulmonary failure should have the SpO_2 kept at 92% or greater to ensure adequate oxygenation. The patient with chronic obstructive pulmonary disease can probably tolerate a SpO_2 of as low as 87%. The full-term neonate should have the SpO_2 kept between 92% and 96%. Saturations below these values indicate hypoxemia in most patients. See Table 2-13 for a comparison of SpO_2 and arterial blood gas values.

Note the site where the saturation was measured. This is especially important in neonates who may have congenital heart defects. A higher saturation seen in the right fingers or right earlobe compared to the rest of the body is seen with a patent ductus arteriosus. A higher saturation seen in the fingers and earlobes as compared to the toes is seen with a coarctation of the aorta.

The patient with carbon monoxide poisoning should not be evaluated with a pulse oximeter because the units are unable to distingish oxyhemoglobin from

Table 2-13. Recommended Clinical Ranges for True SaO$_2$ Values, SpO$_2$ Values,* and Their Correlation with PaO$_2$ Values

	SaO$_2$	SpO$_2$	Approximate PaO$_2$
Adult			
Acute hypoxemia	90%-95%	92%-95%†	60-95 torr
Chronic hypoxemia	85%-90%	87%-92%	50-60 torr
Neonate			
<1500 gm or in the first week of life	about 97%	92%-96%	60-70 torr
>1500 gm or after the first week of life	90%-96%	90%-96%	50-70 torr
>1 month of age with chronic lung disease	85%-90%	87%-92%	50-60 torr

Note: The clinical goal with most neonates is to prevent both hypoxemia, defined as a PaO$_2$ of less than 45 torr, and hyperoxemia, defined as a PaO$_2$ of greater than 90 torr.
* Based on the patient having normal COHb and MetHb levels. Elevated level(s) will result in an erroneously high SpO$_2$ reading and unsuspected hypoxemia.
† African-American patients should have an SpO$_2$ of 95% maintained to ensure adequate oxygenation.

carboxyhemoglobin. They will read only the functional hemoglobin and report a higher than true O$_2$Hb saturation. These patients should only be evaluated for oxygenation by an arterial blood gas that is analyzed in a CO-oximeter blood gas analyzer.

3.   Perform quality control measures for a pulse oximeter. (IIB3d) [R, Ap]

See the next discussion.

4.   Correct any problems with a pulse oximeter. (IIB2g7) [An]

Follow the manufacturer's suggestions for the set up of the various light-emitting diode (LED) sensors and how to apply them to the various measurement sites. The newer pulse oximetry systems will give a visual display of the strength of the pulse so that the best place for the sensor can be found. The signal will not be strong if the patient is hypothermic, hypotensive, or receiving vasoconstricting medication. Suspect the measured values if the pulse strength is not strong. Keep bright light out of the patient measurement site as it may interfere with the signal. (See Table 2-14 for some common sources of error and their solutions.)

Module G.   Transcutaneous monitoring.

Note: Transcutaneous monitoring (TCM) involves the continuous monitoring of oxygen, carbon dioxide, or both gases as they diffuse through the skin. There are individual electrodes for each gas as well as a combined electrode for both.

Transcutaneous Oxygen Monitoring

Transcutaneous oxygen monitoring (PtcO$_2$, tcPO$_2$, or TcO$_2$) enables the patient's oxygenation status to be followed on a continuous basis.

Table 2-14. Sources of Error in Pulse Oximetry

Source of Error	Remedy
Light interference: xenon lamp, fluorescent light, infrared (bilirubin) light, probe fell off of patient	Cover the probe with an opaque wrap; put the probe back in place on the patient
Low perfusion: low blood pressure, hypothermia, vasoconstricting drugs	Use earlobe, bridge of nose, or forehead instead of finger or toe; discontinue use if still unreliable
Motion artifact	Secure the probe site; ensure that the SpO_2 reading is synchronized with the heart rate
Darkly pigmented patient	Use lightly pigmented site such as tip of finger or toe; SpO_2 value may overestimate PaO_2; discontinue use if still unreliable
Artificial or painted fingernails	Remove acrylic nails; remove black, blue, green, metallic, or frosted nail polish; use a different site
Venous pulsation being read as an arterial pulsation	Loosen a tight sensor; change the finger sensor site every 2-4 hours; loosen the cause of a tourniquet-like effect
The following vascular dyes will cause low SpO_2 readings: methylene blue, indigo carmine, indocyanine green	Do not use pulse oximetry

1. Review the patient's chart for a transcutaneous oxygen ($PtcO_2$) value. (IA1d5) [R]

Transcutaneous oxygen monitoring is done on any patient when it is clinically useful to continuously evaluate his or her oxygenation. In practice, neonates are monitored much more often than adults. Check the chart for a record of the patient's transcutaneous oxygen values. It is particularly important to correlate these values with any arterial blood gas values. As it is explained in the next discussion, this will allow you to compare the PaO_2 with the $PtcO_2$. In addition, note what the $PtcO_2$ values are when the inspired oxygen is changed, the patient is suctioned, or changes are made in CPAP or mechanical ventilation. Avoid clinical situations that resulted in earlier hypoxemia.

2. Recommend transcutaneous oxygen ($PtcO_2$) monitoring for additional data. (IA2w) [R, Ap, An]

Transcutaneous oxygen monitoring has been used for the following purposes:

a. Monitoring oxygenation during transportation of an unstable infant within the hospital or between two hospitals.

b. Intraoperative and postoperative monitoring of oxygenation.

c. Monitoring oxygenation during changes in the inspired oxygen, during changes in the mechanical ventilator parameters, and to identify hypoxemia during an equipment or oxygen delivery failure.

d. To help detect a right-to-left shunt. When a neonate has a patent ductus arteriosus, the $PtcO_2$ will be higher in the right upper chest than in the left upper chest, abdomen, or thighs.

e. To help detect a coarctation of the aorta. When this defect is present, the $PtcO_2$ will be higher in the right and left upper chest than in the abdomen or thighs.

3. Get the necessary equipment to perform transcutaneous oxygen monitoring. (IIA1d5) [R, Ap]

Manufacturers of transcutaneous oxygen (and carbon dioxide) monitors include American Scientific Products, Corometrics Medical Systems, Inc, Kontron Instruments, Novametrix Medical Systems, Inc, Radiometer American, Inc, and SensorMedics Corporation.

The electrode used for monitoring the patient's transcutaneous oxygen level is a miniaturized and modified Clark-type polarographic electrode similar to that used in the blood gas analyzer (see Fig. 2-10). Some authors describe it as a Huch or Hellige electrode after two researchers who modified the original Clark electrode for their work with pediatric patients.

4. Put the transcutaneous oxygen monitor together, make sure that it works properly, and identify any problems with it. (IIB1e5) [R, Ap]

5. Fix any problems with the equipment. (IIB2g6) [R, Ap, An]

6. Perform quality control procedures on a transcutaneous oxygen monitor. (IIB3d) [R, Ap]

Always follow the manufacturer's recommendations for the assembly and care of the equipment. Select the proper electrode for the monitor based on the physician's order for evaluating transcutaneous oxygen, carbon dioxide, or both together.

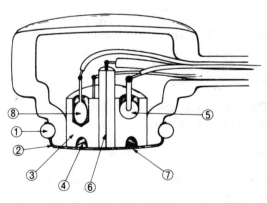

Fig. 2-10 Schematic drawing of the modified Clark electrode used to monitor transcutaneous oxygen tension. *1*, O-ring to hold the membrane to the electrode; *2*, polypropylene membrane permeable to oxygen; *3*, silver anode that surrounds the platium cathode; *4*, electrolyte chamber with solution held in place by the polypropylene membrane; *5*, heating element; *6*, platinum cathode; *7*, electrolyte solution of sodium bicarbonate and sodium chloride held between the membrane and electrode, and *8*, negative temperature coefficient (NTC) resistor that serves to regulate the temperature of the sensor. (From Shapiro BA, Peruzzi WT, Templin R: *Clinical application of blood gases*, ed 5, St. Louis, 1994, Mosby–Year Book. Used by permission.)

Calibration

Two-point calibration must be performed with oxygen percentages that will cause PO_2 values beyond the clinical range that can be expected. Usually the first calibration point is a "zero" point because the electrode is exposed to 0% oxygen in a nitrogen-filled chamber. This point is usually quite stable. The second calibration point is found when the electrode is exposed to room air (20.9% or 0.209 oxygen). Always follow the manufacturer's written procedures during the calibration process. Generally, when environmental conditions include a fairly stable room temperature of 25°C and 50% relative humidity, the following equation can be used to predict the room air calibration point:

$$\text{calibration } PtcO_2 = P_B \times 0.209$$

Where:

P_B = local barometric pressure
0.209 = oxygen fraction found in room air

Expose the electrode to room air to determine if it matches the calculated calibration value. Adjust the instrument to match the calibration $PtcO_2$ if necessary. It is recommended that the room air calibration point be rechecked every 24 hours when in continuous use, after changing the membrane, or after changing the electolyte solution. A variation of up to ±5 mm Hg is acceptable and can be corrected by adjusting the reading on the instrument. If the variation is greater than ±5 mm Hg, the zero-point and room air calibration procedures should be repeated. Problems usually associated with too much electrode drift include electrode or membrane surfaces contaminated by debris like blood or sweat, an improperly applied membrane, a worn-out membrane, an air bubble beneath the membrane, improper gas exposed to the membrane during the calibration, exhausted electrolyte solution in the electrode, or inaccurate calibration values.

Site Selection

Care must be taken to select the best site for the electrode. A bad site will give incorrect information that could lead to mistakes in patient care (see Table 2-15 for a listing of site selection guidelines).

Skin and Electrode Preparation and Application of the Skin Electrode

An airtight seal is necessary between the skin and electrode for accurate readings. An air leak will result in an increase in the $PtcO_2$ reading (and a fall in the $PtcCO_2$ reading). The following steps should be taken to ensure that the skin site and electrode are prepared and an airtight seal is ensured:

1. Clean the skin. Usually cleaning with an alcohol swab is enough to remove perspiration. Oily skin should be cleaned with soap and water.
2. Adults may need to have hair shaved off of the site.
3. Adults may have some of the dead skin cells removed by placing sticky adhesive tape against the site and pulling it off.
4. Prepare the electrode according to the manufacturer's guidelines. Commonly this includes placing a drop of the electrolyte solution on the electrode surface and placing a gas permeable membrane with a double adhesive ring over the electrode.

Table 2-15. Optimal Sites and Sites to Avoid with Transcutaneous Monitoring

Optimal Neonatal Sites
  Upper part of the chest
  Right upper chest if a preductal PtcO$_2$ value is desired
  Abdomen
  Inner aspect of either thigh
Optimal Adult Sites
  Upper part of chest
  Inner aspect of the upper arm
Sites to Avoid
  Large fat deposit
  Bony prominence
  Pressure point
  Thick skin
  Skin edema
  Hands and feet
Conditions When Transcutaneous Monitoring Should Not Be Used
  Locally cold skin or general, deep hypothermia
  Locally decreased peripheral perfusion or general hypotension
  Patient receiving vasoconstricting drugs such as tolazoline or dopamine
  Cardiac index less than 1.9 l/min/m^2 of body surface area
  Halothane anesthesia will give erroneously high PtcO$_2$ values unless a teflon membrane is used

5. The other side of the adhesive ring is pressed against the monitoring site so that there is an airtight seal.
6. As the electrode warms the skin the patient values will fluctuate. Stabilization usually requires several minutes, after which the patient values should be clinically useful.

Limitations and Patient Precautions

Because the electrode is heated it will have to be rotated to a different skin site on a routine basis. The general manufacturer's guidelines for site rotation are every 4-6 hours for neonates between 1000-2500 grams; every 3-5 hours for neonates between 2500-3500 grams; and 2-4 hours for neonates larger than 3500 grams, pediatric patients, and adult patients. As a safety precaution, change the electrode on any patient at least every 4 hours or at least every 3 hours if the patient is hypothermic. The manufacturers' range in times is based on the relative thickness of the patient's skin and the different electrode temperatures. It is important to adjust the site rotation times on an individual patient basis. Some may tolerate longer times whereas others will need more frequent rotations.

Care must be taken when removing the adhesive ring and electrode. It is possible to tear the thin, delicate skin of a premature neonate. Loosen the adhesive by running the edge of an alcohol wipe along the side that is being gently pulled up. After the electrode is removed, it is important to look at the skin; it is normal to see a red circle. This warmed, vasodilated area will stay red for some time and gradually fade away. There will be no scarring or permanent injury. Rarely, the skin will have been overheated and a blister will be seen; this is a second degree burn. Obviously, future site rotations will have to be made more frequently. Do not use this site again. Treat it as a burn and avoid any further injury that would break the skin and lead to an infection.

7. Perform and interpret transcutaneous oxygen (PtcO₂) monitoring to evaluate the patient's response to respiratory care. (IB8b and IIIA1e) [R, Ap, An]

It has been found that heating the electrode speeds up the diffusion of oxygen through the skin. This enables a practitioner to more quickly see changes in the patient's condition. Heating also provides a closer correlation with the patient's PaO_2 values. It must be remembered that the $PtcO_2$ value is *not* the same as the PaO_2 value. However, current recommendations are that any unit should give $PtcO_2$ values that are within ±15% of the PaO_2 over the operating range of the instrument. The values should then correlate within ±15% as the patient's condition changes. This should always be confirmed.

An arterial blood gas should be drawn for PaO_2 every time transcutaneous oxygen monitoring is started. The PaO_2-$PtcO_2$ gradient can then be calculated as the difference between the two. For example, if the patient's PaO_2 is 100 torr, the $PtcO_2$ should be no less than 85 torr. If the $PtcO_2$ decreases to 70 torr, the PaO_2 should have decreased to no lower than 85 torr. Because of this close correlation, the patient can be trend monitored with some assurance of accuracy. In addition, arterial blood gases will not need to be drawn as frequently for the PaO_2. This trending relationship holds true for changes in the patient's pulmonary condition. It does not, however, hold true when the patient has cardiovascular problems such as hypotension, hypothermia, peripheral vascular disease, or cardiogenic shock with decreased tissue perfusion.

When oxygen molecules from the patient (or air) diffuse through the electrode's membrane, they are consumed in an electochemical reaction. This causes electrons to flow through the cathode in proportion to the oxygen level. This electrical flow is measured, amplified, and displayed on the monitor as a number that represents the amount of oxygen at the electrode-membrane interface.

As mentioned earlier, the electrode is heated. Always follow the manufacturer's recommendations for the proper electrode temperature. In general, the temperature ranges from 42.5°C for a 1000 gm infant to 44°C for a 3500 gm infant. A pediatric patient can tolerate a temperature of 44°C, whereas an adult can have an electrode temperature of 45°C. The higher temperatures are needed in older patients because their skin is thicker. Heating the skin and underlying blood vessels results in a number of physiologic changes. The lipid structure of the surface layer of skin (stratum corneum) changes so that the oxygen diffuses to the skin's surface more quickly. The metabolism of the heated skin is increased and more local oxygen is consumed. The heated capillaries in the skin vasodilate, which is said to "arterialize" the capillary blood because so much more blood is made available than needed by the hypermetabolic skin. The heating of the blood shifts the oxyhemoglobin dissociation curve to the right. This causes the blood to release its oxygen to the heated skin more readily.

In preterm neonates, these four effects nearly cancel each other. The PaO_2 and $PtcO_2$ have the closest correlation because they have the thinnest skin. This thin skin allows oxygen to diffuse relatively easily and does not increase its local metabolism when heated as much as the thicker skin of a mature child or adult. Nonetheless, studies have shown that when the neonate's PaO_2 is greater than 100 torr, the $PtcO_2$ value will underestimate it. This can lead to dangerous hyperoxemia. For this reason it is recommended that the $PtcO_2$ be kept at less than 90 torr. In the adult there is less correlation between the PaO_2 and $PtcO_2$ because of the thicker skin. $PtcO_2$ can still be used in the adult to follow trends in oxygenation, but the practitioner must realize that a drop in the $PtcO_2$ value can be from hypoxemia, a decreased cardiac output, or cutaneous vasoconstriction. An arterial blood gas would have to be drawn to further evaluate the patient's status.

Correlation of $PtcO_2$ and Local Power Consumption

As mentioned earlier, the electrode is heated to above body temperature. The amount of electrical current needed to keep the electrode at a constant temperature depends on the temperature of the blood and the speed with which the blood passes below the electrode. This is known as the local power consumption or simply local power (LP). Cardiac output, seen as the heart rate and blood pressure, is the most likely reason to see a change in LP unless the patient's temperature is unstable. Therefore, once the electrode is set up and working properly, the LP should be stable if the patient's heart rate and blood pressure are stable. The LP read-out should then be set at zero to establish this baseline value. From then on whenever there is a change in the patient's cardiac output, the LP will change. For example, if the cardiac output increases, the blood will flow more quickly beneath the electrode; it will require more electricity to maintain the set temperature. The LP reading will show an increased value from the baseline. If the cardiac output decreases, the opposite will occur and the LP value will decrease. Either situation is worth noting.

A change in the LP value and $PtcO_2$ can be used to indicate what is happening to the patient. For example:

a. A normal LP seen with a decreased $PtcO_2$ would indicate that the patient's pulmonary problem has worsened.

b. A normal LP seen with an increased $PtcO_2$ would indicate that the patient's pulmonary problem has improved.

c. A decreased LP seen with a decreased $PtcO_2$ would indicate that the patient's cardiac output has worsened.

d. An increased LP seen with an increased $PtcO_2$ would indicate that the patient's cardiac output has improved.

Transcutaneous Carbon Dioxide Monitoring

Transcutaneous carbon dioxide monitoring ($PtcCO_2$, $tcPCO_2$, or $TcCO_2$) enables the patient's ventilation status to be followed on a continuous basis.

8.   Review the patient's chart for a transcutaneous carbon dioxide ($PtcCO_2$) value. (IA1d5) [R]

Transcutaneous carbon dioxide monitoring is done on any patient when it is clinically useful to continuously evaluate his or her ventilation. In practice, neonates are monitored much more often than adults. Check the chart for a record of the patient's transcutaneous carbon dioxide values. It is particularly important to correlate these values with any arterial blood gas values, which will allow you to compare the $PaCO_2$ with the $PtcCO_2$. In addition, note what the $PtcCO_2$ values are when changes are made in CPAP or mechanical ventilation. Avoid clinical situations that resulted in earlier hypoventilation.

9.   Recommend transcutaneous carbon dioxide ($PtcCO_2$) monitoring for additional data. (IA2w) [R, Ap, An]

Transcutaneous carbon dioxide monitoring has been used for the following purposes:

a. Monitoring ventilation during transportation of an unstable infant within the hospital or between two hospitals.

b. Intraoperative and postoperative monitoring of ventilation.

c. Monitoring ventilation during changes in mechanical ventilator parameters such as tidal volume, rate, minute volume, and mechanical dead space.

d. Detecting hypoventilation during an accidental disconnection of the mechanical ventilator.

10. Get the necessary equipment to perform transcutaneous carbon dioxide monitoring. (IIA1d5) [R, Ap]

The electrode used for monitoring the patient's transcutaneous carbon dioxide level is a miniaturized and modified Stow–Severinghaus–type electrode similar to the arterial blood gas electrode (see Fig. 2-11). A partial list of manufacturers was given earlier.

11. Put the transcutaneous carbon dioxide monitor together, make sure that it works properly, and identify any problems with it. (IIB1e5)[R, Ap]

12. Fix any problems with the equipment. (IIB2g6)[R, Ap, An]

13. Perform quality control procedures on a transcutaneous carbon dioxide monitor. (IIB3d) [R, Ap]

Much of the material presented earlier in the discussion on transcutaneous oxygen monitors applies here as well. Additional information that relates just to this electrode is given.

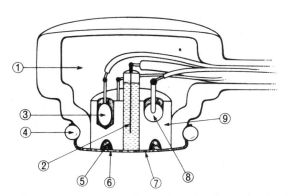

Fig. 2-11 Schematic drawing of the modified Stow-Severinghaus electrode used to monitor transcutaneous carbon dioxide tension. *1*, epoxy resin; *2*, glass electrode with a chlorinated silver wire, a buffer solution (the inner liquid), and a pH sensitive glass membrane; *3*, negative temperature coefficient (NTC) resistor that serves to regulate the temperature of the sensor; *4*, O-ring to hold the membrane to the electrode; *5*, electrolyte chamber with solution held in place by the polypropylene membrane; *6*, electrolyte solution of sodium bicarbonate and sodium chloride held between the membrane and electrode; *7*, polypropylene membrane permeable to carbon dioxide; *8*, heating element, and *9*, silver/silver chloride reference electrode. (From Shapiro BA, Peruzzi WT, Templin R: *Clinical application of blood gases,* ed 5, St. Louis, 1994, Mosby–Year Book. Used by permission.)

Calibration

Two-point calibration must be performed with carbon dioxide percentages that will cause PCO_2 values beyond the clinical range that can be expected. Usually the electrode is exposed to 5% and 10% carbon dioxide from prepared cylinders. Always follow the manufacturer's written procedures during the calibration process. Generally, when environmental conditions include a fairly stable room temperature of 25°C and 50% relative humidity, the following equation can be used to predict the two calibration points:

calibration $PtcCO_2 =$
$$(P_B \times CO_2\% \text{ used}) - (X\ CO_2 \times \text{electrode temperature factor})$$

Where:

P_B = local barometric pressure
$CO_2\%$ = carbon dioxide fraction exposed to the electrode; either 10% (.10) or 5% (.05).
$X\ CO_2$ = Correction factor to equilibrate the $PtcCO_2$ to $PaCO_2$. (This is discussed later.)
Electrode temperature factor = This is a factor determined by the manufacturer based on the electrode's temperature. It is usually heated to 44°C.

Expose the electrode to 10% carbon dioxide in a sealed chamber to determine if it matches the calculated calibration value. Adjust the instrument to match the calibration $PtcCO_2$ if necessary. Next, expose the electrode to 5% carbon dioxide in the sealed chamber. Again, adjust the instrument to match the calibration $PtcCO_2$ if necessary. It is recommended that the two-point calibration points be rechecked every 24 hours when in continuous use, after changing the membrane, or after changing the electolyte solution. A variation of up to ± 4 mm Hg is acceptable and can be corrected by adjusting the reading on the instrument. If the variation is greater than ± 4 mm Hg, the two-point calibration procedures should be repeated. Problems usually associated with too much electrode drift include electrode or membrane surfaces contaminated by debris such as blood or sweat, membrane applied improperly, worn-out membrane, air bubble beneath the membrane, improper gas exposed to the membrane during the calibration, exhausted electrolyte solution in the electrode, or inaccurate calibration values.

14. Perform and interpret transcutaneous oxygen ($PtcO_2$) monitoring to evaluate the patient's response to respiratory care. (IB8b and IIIA1e) [R, Ap, An]

As with the transcutaneous oxygen electrode, it has been found that heating the electrode speeds up the diffusion of carbon dioxide through the skin. This enables a practitioner to more quickly see changes in the patient's condition. It must be remembered that the $PtcCO_2$ value is *not* the same as the $PaCO_2$ value. An arterial blood gas should be drawn for $PaCO_2$ every time transcutaneous carbon dioxide monitoring is started. Unlike transcutaneous oxygen monitoring, the correlation between $PaCO_2$ and $PtcCO_2$ is equally as good in adult as neonatal patients. In addition, it is not as influenced by changes in the patient's skin blood flow.

When carbon dioxide molecules from the patient (or air) diffuse through the electrode's membrane they chemically react with the water in the electrolyte solution to form carbonic acid. This breaks down to release hydrogen ion that acidifies the pH of the solution. This is measured as a voltage change that is proportional to the PCO_2 value. It is displayed on the monitor as a number that represents the amount of carbon dioxide at the electrode/membrane interface.

As mentioned earlier, the electrode is heated. Always follow the manufacturer's recommendations for the proper electrode temperature. In general, the temperature is 44°C in both neonates and adults. Heating the skin and underlying blood vessels results in several physiologic changes. The lipid structure of the surface layer of skin (stratum corneum) changes so that the carbon dioxide diffuses to the skin's surface more quickly. The metabolism of the heated skin is increased and more carbon dioxide is produced locally. The heated blood has a decreased solubility of carbon dioxide, which increases the CO_2 tension. The net effect of these three factors is discussed next.

Correction of $PtcCO_2$ Values to $PaCO_2$ Values

The net effect of the three factors results in the $PtcCO_2$ readings being 1.2 to 2 times (120% to 200%) greater than the $PaCO_2$ values. Commonly, an average multiplier of 1.6 is found. The actual value will vary among patients and can be found by dividing the $PtcCO_2$ by the $PaCO_2$. For example: Your patient has a $PaCO_2$ of 40 torr and a $PtcCO_2$ of 64 torr. Calculate the gradient between the arterial and transcutaneous values.

$$\text{Gradient} = \frac{PtcCO_2}{PaCO_2} = \frac{64}{40} = 1.6$$

As long as the patient's cardiovascular status is fairly stable, the $PaCO_2$ can be calculated by dividing the $PtcCO_2$ by 1.6. For example, if the patient's $PtcCO_2$ increases to 80 torr, calculate the $PaCO_2$.

$$PaCO_2 = \frac{PtcCO_2}{1.6} = \frac{80}{1.6} \times 50 \text{ torr}$$

Rather than perform these calculations every time there is a change in the patient's status, some practitioners divide the CO_2 values found during the calibration procedure by 1.6. This results in "real" $PaCO_2$ values being given continuously on the monitor. This change must be clearly communicated to all staff members to avoid confusion between the original $PtcCO_2$ values and values that have been reduced to "arterialize" them.

This ends the general discussion on blood gas analysis and monitoring. The following module relates to other aspects of care that the therapist must be aware of when evaluating the blood gas results and the overall care of the patient. The general discussion of patient assessment was presented in Section 1 and should be reviewed as it relates to this section. Some additional comments are made as indicated.

Module H. Patient Assessment.

These technologies allow for the analysis of arterial, venous, and capillary blood samples for PaO_2, $PaCO_2$, and pH, as well as the continuous monitoring of oxygen saturation and transcutaneous oxygen and carbon dioxide levels. They offer the practitioner many choices in patient care. The challenge is in selecting what is needed for the patient.

Arterial blood gas analysis remains the "gold standard" by which all other values are judged. Typically the arterial sample is analyzed through a standard blood gas analyzer. A CO oximeter is needed if the patient has carbon monoxide poisoning. Mixed venous and capillary blood sample analysis is limited in clinical application but very helpful in the right patient situation. However, these offer only momentary insight into the patient's condition.

Pulse oximetry and transcutaneous oxygen monitoring offer continuous information on the patient's oxygenation. Transcutaneous carbon dioxide monitoring allows continuous monitoring of the patient's ventilation. As with all technology, these units have advantages, disadvantages, and limitations. It is up to the practitioner to make the correct choices. Some unstable patients can best be monitored through the combination of periodic evaluation of arterial blood gases and these noninvasive continuous monitoring systems.

As part of the patient care team, you may need to evaluate the patient's blood gas values and other parameters to make a recommendation. For example, if the patient has carbon monoxide poisoning, it is best treated by giving the patient 100% oxygen by a nonrebreather mask. Pure oxygen reduces the half-life of COHb to 60 to 90 minutes. A pulse oximeter should *not* be used to measure this patient's saturation of oxyhemoglobin. These units are unable to identify COHb and will give misleadingly high saturation values for O_2Hb.

Be prepared to make a recommendation on adjusting the patient's inspired oxygen based on the PaO_2 (or related) value. Also be prepared to make a recommendation on adjusting the patient's mechanical ventilation settings for tidal volume, rate, minute volume, and/or mechanical dead space based on the $PaCO_2$ (or related) value.

BIBLIOGRAPHY

AARC Clinical Practice Guideline: Oxygen therapy in the acute care hospital, *Respir Care* 36(12):1410-1413, 1991.

AARC Clinical Practice Guideline: Pulse oximetry, *Respir Care* 36(12):1406-1409, 1991.

AARC Clinical Practice Guideline: Sampling for arterial blood gas analysis. *Respir Care* 37(8):913–917, 1991.

AARC Clinical Practice Guideline: In-vitro pH and blood gas analysis and hemoximetry. *Respir Care* 38(5):505–510, 1993.

American Academy of Pediatrics: Task force on transcutaneous oxygen monitors, *Pediatr* 83(1):122-126, 1989.

Bennington JL, editor: *Saunders dictionary and encyclopedia of laboratory medicine and technology,* Philadelphia, 1984, WB Saunders.

Bickford L, Bickford C, Hodgkin JE: Methodology of arterial blood gas analysis. In Burton GC, Hodgkin JE, editors: *Respiratory care: a guide to clinical practice,* ed 2, Philadelphia, 1984, JB Lippincott.

Blanchette T: Appropriate use of pulse oximetry, *RT,* 3(6):35-40, 1991.

Blanchette T, Dziodzio J, Harris K: Pulse oximetry and normoximetry in neonatal intensive care, *Respir Care* 36(1):25-32, 1991.

Bohn DJ: Ask the expert, the Respiratory tract, 9, Feb 1988.

Czervinske MP: Arterial blood gas analysis and other cardiopulmonary monitoring. In Koff PB, Eitzman D, Neu J: *Neonatal and pediatric respiratory care,* ed 2, St. Louis, 1993, Mosby–Year Book.

Daily KE, Schroeder JS: *Techniques in bedside hemodynamic monitoring*, ed 4, St. Louis, 1989, Mosby–Year Book.

Elser RC: Quality control of blood gas analysis: a review, *Respir Care* 31(9):807-815, Sep 1986.

Federal government releases CLIA '88 final regulations, *AARC Times* 16(4):76-86, 1992.

Fell WL: Sampling and measurement of blood gases. In Lane EE, Walker JF, editors: *Clinical arterial blood gas analysis*, St. Louis, 1987, Mosby–Year Book.

Instrumentation Laboratories, Operator's Manual for the IL282 CO-oximeter.

Jubran A, Tobin MJ: Reliability of pulse oximetry in titrating supplemental oxygen therapy in ventilator-dependent patients, *Chest* 97:1420, 1990.

Lane EE, Walker JF: *Clinical arterial blood gas analysis*, St. Louis, 1987, Mosby–Year Book.

Levitzky MG, Cairo JM, Hall SM: *Introduction to respiratory care*, Philadelphia, 1990, WB Saunders.

Martin RJ: Transcutaneous monitoring: instrumentation and clinical applications. *Respir Care* 35(6):577-583, 1990.

McPherson SP: *Respiratory therapy equipment*, ed 4, St. Louis, 1990, Mosby–Year Book.

Mohler JG, Collier CR, Brandt W et al: Blood gases. In Clausen JL, editor: *Pulmonary function testing guidelines and controversies*, Orlando, 1984, Grune & Stratton.

Moran RF: Assessment of quality control of blood gas/pH analyzer performance, *Respir Care* 26(6):538-546, 1981.

Moran RF: CLIA regulations. I. The cure might be worse than the disease, *AARC Times* 14(11):41-43, 50-51, 1990.

Moran RF: CLIA regulations. II. An analysis of some technical requirements, *AARC Times* 14(12): 25-32, 1990.

Nelson CM, Murphy EM, Bradley JK et al: Clinical use of pulse oximetry to determine oxygen prescriptions for patients with hypoxemia, *Respir Care* 31(8):673-680, 1986.

Peters JA, Hodgkin JE, Collier CA: Blood gas analysis and acid-base physiology. In Burton GG, Hodgkin JE, Ward JJ, editors: *Respiratory care: a guide to clinical practice*, ed 3, Philadelphia, 1991, JB Lippincott.

Plunkett PF: Blood gas interpretation. In Barnes TA, editor: *Respiratory care practice*, Chicago, 1988, Year Book Medical.

Product literature on the model 4701A ear oximeter, Hewlett-Packard, Medical Products Group, 175 Wyman Street, Waltham, MA 02154.

Product literature on Oxisensors, Nellcor Incorporated, 25495 Whitesell Street, Hayward, CA 94545.

Product literature on transcutaneous monitoring, Novametrics Medical Systems, Inc., Wallingford, Conn.

Ruppel G: *Manual of pulmonary function testing*, ed 6, St. Louis, 1994, Mosby–Year Book.

Salyer JW: Pulse oximetry in the neonatal intensive care unit, *Respir Care* 36(1):17-20, 1991.

Shapiro BA, Peruzzi WT, Templin R: *Clinical application of blood gases*, ed 5, St Louis, 1994, Mosby–Year Book.

Sills JR: *Respiratory care certification guide: the complete review resource for the entry level exam*, ed 2, St. Louis, 1994, Mosby–Year Book.

Sonnesso G: Are you ready to use pulse oximetry? *Nursing* 60-64, Aug 1991.

Tilkian SM, Conover MB, Tilkian AG: *Clinical implications of laboratory tests*, ed 3, St. Louis, 1983, Mosby–Year Book.

Uhing M, Dziedzic K: Pulse oximetry in neonatal management. *Respir Management* 20(5):116-120.

Walton JR, Shapiro BA: Value and application of temperature-compensated blood gas data, *Respir Care* 25(2), 1980.

Welch JP, DeCesare R, Hess D: Pulse oximetry: instrumentation and clinical applications, *Respir Care* 35(6):584-601, 1990.

Whitaker K: *Comprehensive perinatal and pediatric respiratory care*, Albany, NY, 1992, Delmar.

Yelderman M, New W: Evaluation of pulse oximetry. *Anesthesiology* 59(4):349-352, 1983.

Note: A copy of the final CLIA regulations can be purchased with a check for $3.50 sent to:

Government Printing Office
Attn: New Order
P.O. Box 371954
Pittsburgh, PA 15250-7954

Be sure to request stock #069-001-0042-4 Final Clinical Laboratory Regulations, February 28, 1992.

SELF-STUDY QUESTIONS

You are ordered to calculate your patient's $P(A-a)O_2$. The following conditions exist:

P_B = 750 mm Hg. Normal is 760 mm Hg for sea level.
PH_2O = 55 mm Hg because your patient's temperature is 104°F/40°C. Normal is 47 mm Hg for a normal temperature.
F_IO_2 = .5 for 50% inspired oxygen. Normal is .21 for room air.
$PaCO_2$ = 35 mm Hg from ABGs. Normal is 40 mm Hg.
PaO_2 = 60 mm Hg from ABGs. Normal is 90 mm Hg.
Respiratory Exchange Ratio = .8

$$PAO_2 = [(P_B - PH_2O) F_IO_2] - \frac{PaCO_2}{.8}$$

1. Based on the previous conditions, your patient's PAO_2 is what?
    A. 309 mm Hg
    B. 102 mm Hg
    C. 313 mm Hg
    D. 96 mm Hg
    E. 304 mm Hg

2. Based on the previous conditions, your patient's $P(A-a)O_2$ is what?
    A. 244 mm Hg
    B. 249 mm Hg
    C. 42 mm Hg
    D. 223 mm Hg
    E. 6 mm Hg

3. All of the following are appropriate steps in the procedure for obtaining a capillary heel stick blood sample on an infant EXCEPT:
    A. Making sure that the puncture site is well perfused.
    B. Chilling the heel area with ice water.

C.   Wiping the puncture site with an antiseptic swab.
D.   Putting the blood sample into an ice water bath.

4.   Which of the following would indicate that a patient's tissues are adequately oxygenated?
A. PaO_2 85 mm Hg
B. $P\bar{v}O_2$ 30 mm Hg
C. $S\bar{v}O_2$ 75%
D. SaO_2 90%

5.   Calibration values are considered to be in control if they are:
A.   Within 1 SD of the norm
B.   Within 2 SDs of the norm
C.   Within 3 SDs of the norm
D.   Within 4 SDs of the norm
E.   A and B

6.   A 45-year-old patient has been admitted through the emergency room after suffering smoke inhalation from a house fire. He is wearing a nonrebreather mask set at 10 l/min of oxygen. The most appropriate way to evaluate his oxygenation status is by:
A.   Pulse oximetry.
B.   Transcutaneous oxygen probe.
C.   Running an arterial blood gas sample through the blood gas analyzer.
D.   Running an arterial blood gas sample through the CO-oximeter.
E.   Running a mixed venous blood gas sample through the CO-oximeter.

7.   Thirty minutes into a weaning attempt on a Briggs adapter (aerosol T), a 50-year-old patient with emphysema seems to be tiring. The best way to evaluate her ventilatory status is by:
A.   Checking her PaO_2 value.
B.   Measuring a transcutaneous CO_2 value.
C.   Monitoring her end-tidal CO_2.
D.   Checking her $PaCO_2$ value.
E.   Performing a bedside vital capacity and tidal volume.

8.   Your patient has Guillain-Barre syndrome and pneumonia. The patient has just been placed on 35% oxygen by mask. The physician asks for your suggestion on the best way to evaluate the patient's overall ability to breathe. You would recommend:
A.   Doing a full set of pulmonary function tests.
B.   Drawing an arterial blood sample for analysis.
C.   Performing pulse oximetry.
D.   Getting a chest x-ray.
E.   Performing pulse oximetry and a force vital capacity measurement.

9.   You are working with a neonate who has $PtcO_2$ electrodes placed on her right upper chest and right thigh. The nurse calls your attention to the patient because the right upper chest value is 75 mm Hg and the right thigh value is 55 mm Hg. What would explain this difference?
A.   The patient has pneumonia.
B.   The patient is not receiving the prescribed oxygen percentage.
C.   The patient has a patent ductus arteriosus.
D.   The patient has a ventricular septal defect.
E.   The patient has a right sided pneumothorax.

10. You are called to evaluate a patient who is using a pulse oximeter. Upon entering the room you notice an African-American woman with an oximeter probe on her right earlobe. The monitor shows a weak pulse signal and fluctuating SpO_2 value. Which of the following would you evaluate to correct the problem?

   I.   Try monitoring from a fingertip.
   II.   Switch to a probe over the bridge of the nose.
   III. Cover the probe with an opaque wrap.
   IV.   Switch the probe to the left earlobe.
   V.   Try monitoring from the toe tip.
   A.   II
   B.   I, III, V
   C.   II, IV
   D.   IV
   E.   III

11. To follow the treatment of a neonate with a patent ductus arteriosus, a $PtcO_2$ monitor electrode should be placed on the:

   I.   Left upper chest.
   II.   Left thigh.
   III. Right hand.
   IV.   Right upper chest.
   V.   Right thigh.
   A.   II, IV
   B.   I
   C.   III
   D.   IV
   E.   I, V

12. You notice that the $PtcO_2$ value on your neonatal patient has decreased from 80 torr to 65 torr. The local power consumption value has not changed. The most likely cause for this is:

   A.   The patient's cardiac output has improved.
   B.   The patient's pulmonary condition has worsened.
   C.   The patient's cardiac output has decreased.
   D.   The patient's pulmonary condition has improved.
   E.   Either A or C.

13. You are working with a postanesthesia patient who has on a transcutaneous carbon dioxide monitor. The correlation factor between the $PaCO_2$ and $PtcCO_2$ is 1.4. The patient's previous $PtcCO_2$ was 63 torr. The nurse has called you because it is now 75 torr. The patient's approximate $PaCO_2$ would be calculated as:

   A.   63 torr
   B.   75 torr
   C.   54 torr
   D.   105 torr
   E.   88 torr

Answer Key

1. A; 2. B; 3. B; 4. C; 5. E; 6. D; 7. D; 8. B; 9. C; 10. B; 11. A; 12. B; 13. C.

3

Pulmonary Function Testing

Note: This section contains equations for determining normal pulmonary function values. They should prove helpful for the therapist student who is now learning advanced pulmonary function testing. However, to date, the NBRC has not expected an examinee to perform any of these advanced calculations on either Registry Exam. Therefore, focus on definitions, normal values, and the interpretation of abnormal values.

Module A.   Review the patient's records for data on the following tests.

1.   Ventilation to perfusion scan. (IA1i20) [R]

A ventilation scan (V scan) is performed to verify or refute the clinical suspicion that a patient has an area of the lung(s) that is underventilated. Abnormal ventilation would be seen in a bronchial obstruction from a tumor or foreign body or an alveolar problem such as atelectasis, consolidation, or emphysema. Radioactive xenon (^{133}Xe) is mixed with oxygen and inhaled to show the lung fields. A special scanner is used to "pick up" the radioactivity through the chest wall. Areas of normal ventilation will appear dark against a bright background. Underventilated areas will be lighter whereas unventilated areas will appear as bright as the background.

A perfusion scan (Q scan) is performed to verify or refute the clinical suspicion that a patient has an area of the pulmonary circulation that is underperfused. Abnormal perfusion would be seen in a pulmonary embolism, tumor, or vascular problem such as pulmonary hypertension. Radioactive technetium (^{99m}Tc) is injected into the patient's venous system where it is filtered out by the pulmonary circulation. As above, a special scanner is used to "pick up" the radioactivity through the chest wall. Areas of normal perfusion will appear dark against a bright background. Underperfused areas will be lighter whereas unperfused areas will appear as bright as the background.

The two tests can be done singly or as a set. Comparing both results side by side enables the physician to look for areas of ventilation and/or perfusion mismatching. Normally, ventilation and perfusion match fairly closely to result in a 1 : 1 mix of air and blood at the alveolar capillary membrane. A pulmonary embolism would result in a V : Q ratio of 2 (or greater) : 1 (or less) because normal ventilation would be present and perfusion reduced or absent. An obstructed airway with atelectasis would result in a V : Q ratio of 1 (or less) : 2 (or greater) because ventilation would be reduced or absent and perfusion would be normal.

2.   Spirometry and pulmonary mechanics tests. (IA1d4) [R]

Spirometry tests include flows and volumes. Pulmonary mechanics tests include maximal inspiratory pressure (MIP) and maximal expiratory pressure (MEP). The following wave forms should also be reviewed: flow volume loops from a spirometer and volume and airway resistance loops from a plethysmograph. These test results are discussed in the next module.

Module B.   Recommend lung mechanics tests to obtain additional data. (IA2x) [R, Ap, An]

Different authors include various tests in the category of lung mechanics tests. In general, the following are included:

a. Lung volumes and capacities except for those requiring the residual volume. These values are important but are needed also to calculate functional residual capacity and total lung capacity. They are needed to differentiate between obstructive and restrictive lung disease.

b. Spirometry for forced vital capacity (FVC) and flow values derived from the FVC. These values are needed to determine the degree of impairment with the obstructive diseases patient.

c. Spirometry for flow-volume loop. This test is used to determine obstructive problems in the lungs or upper airway.

d. Maximum inspiratory pressure (MIP) and maximum expiratory pressure (MEP). These values indicate the patient's overall respiratory muscle strength.

e. Airway resistance to determine the extent of obstruction.

f. Lung compliance to differentiate between obstructive and restrictive lung disease.

g. Maximum voluntary ventilation as a general indication of the functioning of the lungs and thorax.

Module C.   Interpret the following spirometry and lung mechanics tests from the bedside procedure.

1.   Tidal volume. (IB9b) [An]

The tidal volume (V_T) is the volume of gas breathed out with each respiratory cycle. It is important to realize that individual tidal volumes are rarely identical; normally there is some variation (see Fig. 3-1 for several tidal volume breaths before a forced vital capacity effort). The average predicted tidal volume for a resting, afebrile, alert adult should be about 3 ml/lb or 6 to 7 ml/kg.

A tidal volume that is larger or smaller than expected for the patient's size requires further evaluation. A small tidal volume may be seen in patients who have a low metabolic rate, who are asleep or in a coma, who have a neuromuscular disease that does not allow them to breathe deeply, or who are alkalotic. A large tidal volume will be seen in patients with a high metabolic rate, a fever, a dead space producing disease, an increased intracranial pressure, or who are acidotic.

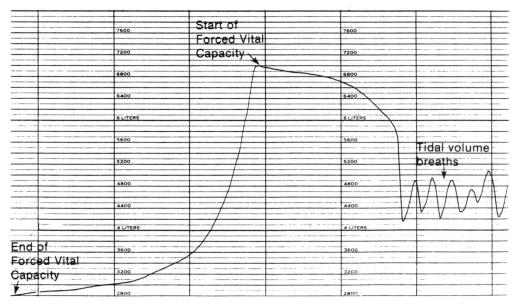

Fig. 3-1 Tracing of tidal volumes and forced vital capacity.

2. Inspiratory to expiratory ratio. (IB9b) [An]

The inspiratory to expiratory (I : E) ratio is the ratio of the inspiratory time to the expiratory time. It can be measured simply at the bedside with a stopwatch. Again, make sure that the patient is relaxed and breathing in the normal pattern to get an accurate timing. Measure several of the patient's inspiratory times and expiratory times to figure an average for each. A spirometer that gives a printout will be needed if a more complete analysis of the patient's breathing pattern and I : E ratio is needed. Remember that a patient breathing normally (eupnea) will have a ratio of about 1 : 2. A patient with obstructed inspiration will usually have a longer inspiratory than expiratory time. A patient with obstructed expiration, as seen with bronchitis, emphysema, and asthma, will have a longer than normal expiratory time. Unusual I : E ratios will be seen in patient's with Kussmaul's respiration, Cheyne-Stokes respiration, and Biot's respiration.

The NBRC is known to test the examinee's ability to calculate: a) inspiratory time (T_I) and expiratory time (T_E) from a given I : E ratio and respiratory rate, or b) I : E ratio from a given inspiratory time and expiratory time. Examples are given in *Respiratory Care Certification Guide* (1994) if they need to be reviewed.

3. Minute volume. (IB9c) [An]

The minute volume ($\dot{V}_E$) is the volume of gas exhaled in 1 minute. The minute volume is usually a more stable value than individual tidal volumes. It is found by adding up the accumulated tidal volumes for 1 minute. If the patient cannot perform the test for a minute, do it for 30 seconds and double the value. The predicted range for a minute volume in a resting, afebrile, alert adult should be 5 to 10 l/min.

The wide range is found in part because it is made up of two factors: tidal volume and respiratory rate. It is possible for either one or both of these factors to be normal, abnormally high, or abnormally low. For these reasons, the minute volume must be evaluated along with the tidal volume and respiratory rate to reach any conclusion about the patient's condition. The same factors that have an impact on the tidal volume will affect the patient's minute volume. (See the following discussion for the calculation of minute volume.)

4. Alveolar ventilation. (IB9c) [An]

Alveolar ventilation (V_A) is the amount of tidal volume that reaches the alveoli. It is calulated by subtracting the physiologic dead space (anatomic plus alveolar dead space) from the measured exhaled tidal volume. For a bedside test, it is only possible to subtract the approximate anatomic dead space. This is estimated at 1 ml/lb or 2.2 ml/kg of lean body weight. For example:

A 154 lb/70 kg person would have an estimated anatomic dead space of about 154 ml. The measured tidal volume is 500 ml.
Calculated alveolar ventilation = 500 ml − 154 ml = 346 ml

The amount of gas that reaches the alveoli in 1 minute is defined as the minute alveolar ventilation ($\dot{V}_A$). The following example shows how it can be calculated:

Normal patient: f = 12, tidal volume = 500 ml, anatomic dead space = 154 ml
minute volume ($\dot{V}_E$) = 12 × 500 ml = 6000 ml
minute alevolar ventilation ($\dot{V}_A$) = 12 (500 ml − 154 ml)
= 12 (346 ml)
= 4152 ml

A larger than normal tidal volume will result in a larger than normal alveolar ventilation. This will cause a respiratory alkalosis. A respiratory acidosis would result from a smaller than normal tidal volume and smaller than normal alveolar ventilation.

5. Maximum inspiratory pressure. (IB9i) [An]

The maximum inspiratory pressure (MIP) is the greatest amount of negative pressure that the patient can create when inspiring from residual volume against an occluded airway. Black and Hyatt (1969) published the following MIP prediction formulas for spontaneously breathing nonintubated subjects breathing from residual volume. The values are in centimeters of water pressure.

Lower Limits of Normal

Males: 143 − (0.55 × age)   −75
Females: 104 − (0.51 × age)   −50

These would be predictive for patients who are 20 to 86 years old. As can be seen, the older the patient is, the lower the predicted maximum inspiratory pressure would be. Some advocate having the procedure done from the functional residual capacity instead of residual volume. This is how the procedure would have to be performed if the patient is unconscious and uncooperative. In these cases, it would probably be necessary to occlude the airway for several breathing efforts to obtain a realistic maximum inspiratory pressure. The prediction formulas by Black and Hyatt (1969) would not be useful. Branson, Hurst, Davis et al (1989) found that this method of MIP measurement underestimated the value compared to when a one-way valve system was used. This is because patients breathing through the one-way valve system tended to exhale and then inspire from nearer their residual volume.

Patients of either sex and any age should be able to generate at least -60 cm water pressure. This is enough to offer assurance that the patient has enough strength and coordination to protect the airway, take a deep breath, and cough effectively. Patients with neuromuscular diseases, diseases of the respiratory muscles, thoracic injury or abnormality, and chronic obstructive lung diseases tend to have decreased strength. The patient who cannot generate at least -20 cm water pressure is at risk. This patient probably does not have the strength to cough effectively. Depending on the blood gas values and other physical parameters, the patient may need to be intubated and maintained on a mechanical ventilator.

6. Maximum expiratory pressure. (IB9d) [An]

The maximum expiratory pressure (MEP) is the greatest amount of positive pressure that the patient can create when expiring from total lung capacity against an occluded airway. Normal people of either sex and any age should be able to generate at least 80 cm water pressure. Patients with neuromuscular diseases, thoracic injury or abnormality, and COPD will tend to have decreased strength. An MEP value of 40 cm water is probably enough to offer assurance that the patient has enough strength and coordination to cough effectively to clear secretions; however, depending on the blood gas values and other physical parameters, the patient may need to be intubated and maintained on a mechanical ventilator.

Black and Hyatt (1969) have published the following MEP prediction formulas for spontaneously breathing nonintubated subjects breathing from total lung capacity. The values are in centimeters of water pressure.

Lower Limits of Normal

Males: $268 - (1.03 \times \text{age})$	140
Females: $170 - (0.53 \times \text{age})$	95

These would be predictive for patients who are 20 to 86 years old. As can be seen, the older the patient is, the lower the predicted maximal expiratory pressure would be.

7. Forced vital capacity. (IB9k) [An]

The forced vital capacity (FVC) is the greatest volume of gas that the patient can exhale as rapidly as possible after the lungs have been completely filled. Careful instructions, demonstrations, and coaching are needed to ensure that the patient's efforts are the best possible. At least *three* proper efforts must be obtained and the largest reported.

If the measurement instrument does not give a printout, simply record the patient's efforts in the chart. If the measurement instrument does give a printout, include copies of the efforts. See Fig. 3-1 for the tracing of a FVC that shows a graphic display of flow over time. The tracing enables us to compare the volumes exhaled in a series of 1-second time periods. Notice that the start of the effort is smooth and without interuption. The initial fast flow of gas from the upper airway is seen as the nearly vertical part of the tracing. The rest of the tracing is smooth without any coughing or other interuptions in the patient's effort. The tracing becomes progressively more horizontal as the end of the effort is reached. Encourage the patient to try to push out as much air as possible as the end approaches. Current guidelines require that the patient keeps pushing so that the total effort lasts at least 6 seconds.

Fig. 3-1 was made on a chain-compensated, water-seal spirometry system made by Warren E. Collins, Inc. Notice how the tracing progresses from right to left. This company also makes the Stead-Wells water-seal spirometry system. The Stead-Wells system shows the same tracing "upside down" compared to the chain-compensated system. The tracing starts on the left and moves to the right (see Fig. 3-2). Other systems could show either the chain-compensated or Stead-Wells tracings in a mirror image or opposite shape. This is an important point because the NBRC can show an FVC tracing from any system and expect it to be interpreted. The start of each effort can be determined by the near vertical portion of the tracing and the relatively small expiratory reserve volume (ERV) compared to the inspiratory reserve volume (IRV).

There are normally racial differences in the FVC that must be taken into consideration. Most modern pulmonary function systems will automatically adjust the measured values for racial differences when so programmed by the operator. If not, the predicted values should be mathematically adjusted by the therapist. The predicted Caucasian patient normal values in liters for the forced vital capacity* were reported by Morris, Koski, and Johnson (1971) as:

Men: [(0.148 × height in inches) − (0.025 × age)] − 4.24 (SD [1 standard deviation] 0.58)

Women: [(0.115 × height in inches) − (0.024 × age)] − 2.85 (SD 0.52)

Example
Calculate the predicted forced vital capacity of a 50-year-old Caucasian male who is 6 feet (72 inches) tall.

$$
\begin{aligned}
FVC &= [(0.148 \times \text{height in inches}) - (0.025 \times \text{age})] - 4.24 \\
&= [(0.148 \times 72) - (0.025 \times 50)] - 4.24 \\
&= [10.656 - 1.25] - 4.24 \\
&= 9.406 - 4.24 \\
&= 5.166 \text{ l}
\end{aligned}
$$

The following adjustments should be made for an African-American patient:

Predicted FVC for Caucasians × .89 = Adjusted FVC for African Americans (11% less)

Adjustments for Hispanic and Asian populations are not as well documented. It has been reported that the predicted FVC values should be adjusted down by 20% to 25% for Asians.

It has been commonly accepted that a measured FVC that is at least 80% of the predicted FVC is considered to be within normal limits for adults of all races. In addition, the forced expiratory volume in 1 second and total lung capacity measurements have also been included in this 80% of predicted rule. More recent studies by Knudson, Kaltenborn, Knudson et al (1987), and Paoletti, Viegi, Pistelli et al (1985) suggest that normal values for most tests should be determined by

---

* The body, temperature, pressure, saturated (BTPS) correction has been calculated into these equations. Note: These and some other researchers have already calculated a standard patient and room temperature and barometric pressure into their formulas.

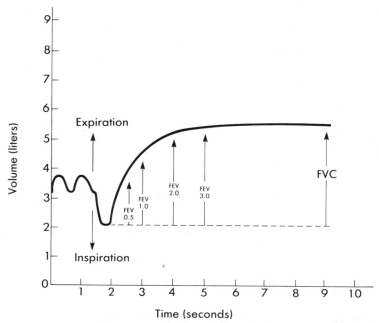

Fig. 3-2 One method of determining the $FEF_{200-1200}$ value from a FVC tracing. First, mark the 200- and 1200-ml points from the start of the effort. Second, draw a line through these two points to intersect the dashed time lines at points A and B. Horizontal dashed lines are added from A and B to cross the volume scale. The $FEF_{200-1200}$ value is read as the distance between A and C or about 3 l/sec. BTPS correct this measured value. (From Ruppel G: *Manual of pulmonary function testing,* ed 5, St. Louis, 1991, Mosby–Year Book. Used by permission.)

finding the percent of predicted above which 95% of the population would be seen (the so-called "normal 95th percentile"). Even though this method will find 5% (1 in 20) of healthy nonsmokers to be abnormal, it offers more realistic predicted values. It is normal to see a decline in the FVC with age.

Restrictive problems such as advanced pregnancy, obesity, ascites, neuromuscular disease, sarcoidosis, and chest wall or spinal deformity can result in a small FVC. Patients with chronic obstructive lung diseases such as emphysema, bronchitis, asthma, cystic fibrosis, and bronchiectasis commonly have a small FVC. (See Fig. 3-12 for a comparison of the spirometry tracings of a normal, obstructed, and restricted patient.)

It is beyond the scope of this text to discuss back extrapolation to find the start of a less than perfect effort or the calculations for converting volumes and flows from ATPS to BTPS. However, most pulmonary function textbooks discuss these topics.

8. Peak flow. (IB9j) [An]

The peak flow (PF) is the fastest instantaneous expiratory flow of gas. It is usually seen at the beginning of an acceptable FVC effort. The patient does not need to completely empty the lungs to residual volume.

The patient's effort is easily directly measured from a handheld peak flow meter. Usually at least three efforts are required to find two that are acceptably close. Peak flow values that are consistent and low despite variable patient efforts probably indicate a malfunctioning unit that should not be used.

Cherniack and Raber (1972) have published the following formula* for predicting peak flow in liters/second:

Males: $[(0.144 \times \text{height in inches}) - (0.024 \times \text{age})] + 2.225$

Females: $[(0.090 \times \text{height in inches}) - (0.018 \times \text{age})] + 1.130$

It is reasonable to record the patient's effort in liters/second because the effort takes place in about that much time. However, do not be confused by some measurement instruments and other prediction equations giving the value in liters/minute. Simply multiply or divide by 60 to convert your patient's effort from one time frame to the other. For example, the predicted normal for a young man is 10 l/sec or 600 l/min.

The peak flow is a rather nonspecific measurement of airway obstruction. It measures flow through the upper airways and would be reduced in patients with an upper airway problem such as a tumor, vocal cord paralysis, or laryngeal edema. However, the test is often given to patients having an asthma attack as a quick and easy measurement of small airways obstruction and to evaluate the patient's response to an inhaled bronchodilator. A 15% to 20% increase in the peak flow and/or $\text{FEV}_{1\%}$ shows that the patient is responding to the medication. Peak flow would be expected to decrease with age.

9.   Timed, forced expiratory volumes. (IB9f) [An]
a.   Forced expiratory flow $_{200\text{-}1200}$ ($\text{FEF}_{200\text{-}1200}$).

The $\text{FEF}_{200\text{-}1200}$ is the mean forced expiratory flow between 200 ml and 1200 ml of an acceptable FVC (see Fig 3-2). The measurement is usually recorded in liters/second but may be recorded in liters/minute.

When interpreting the $\text{FEF}_{200\text{-}1200}$ value, the respiratory therapist and physician must be ensured that the patient did his or her best effort. The results are effort dependent and will not be valid if the patient did not make a full effort. The results normally decline with age and are lower in women than men. A patient with a restrictive lung disease may have a normal or increased value. The patient with obstructive lung disease or with an upper airway, tracheal, or large bronchial obstruction will have a low value. A normal 150 lb/68 kg young man will have values of 6 to 7 l/sec or 360 to 420 l/min. The following formulas* have been developed by Morris, Koski, and Johnson (1971) to calculate predicted values in liters/second:

Men: $[(0.109 \times \text{height in inches}) - (0.047 \times \text{age in years})] + 2.010$ (SD 1.66)

Women: $[(0.145 \times \text{height in inches}) - (0.036 \times \text{age in years})] - 2.532$ (SD 1.19)

b.   Forced expiratory flow $_{25\% \text{ to } 75\%}$ ($\text{FEF}_{25\% \text{ to } 75\%}$).

The $\text{FEF}_{25\%\text{-}75\%}$ is the mean forced expiratory flow during the middle half of an acceptable FVC (see Fig. 3-3). The FVC effort to use for this test is the one that has the greatest combination of FVC volume and FEV_1. The measurement is usually recorded in liters/second but may be recorded in liters/minute.

As mentioned earlier, the patient must give his or her best effort. The results are normally less than in the $\text{FEF}_{200\text{-}1200}$ and peak flow tests because the flow being measured comes from medium-size and small airways (less than 2 mm in diameter). The results should decline with age and be lower in women than men. A

---

* The BTPS correction has been calculated into these equations.

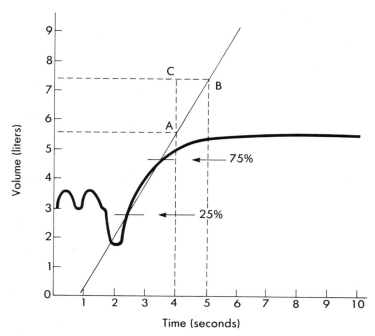

Fig. 3-3 On method of determining the $FEF_{25\%-75\%}$ value from a FVC tracing. First, mark the 25% and 75% points from the start of the effort. These are found by multiplying the FVC value by .25 and .75, respectively, and measuring from the start of the effort. Second, draw a line through these two points to intersect the dashed time lines at points A and B. Horizontal dashed lines are added from A and B to cross the volume scale. The $FEF_{25\%-75\%}$ value is read as the distance between A and C or about 2 l/sec. BTPS correct this measured value. (From Ruppel G: *Manual of pulmonary function testing,* ed 6, St. Louis, 1994, Mosby–Year Book. Used by permission.)

patient with a restrictive lung disease may have a normal or increased value whereas a low value will be seen in the patient with obstructive lung disease. A small $FEF_{25\%-75\%}$ value when the FVC, FEV_1, and $FEF_{200-1200}$ values are normal is often taken to indicate early small airways disease. A normal 150 lb/68 kg young man will have values of 4 to 5 l/sec or 240 to 300 l/min. The following formulas* have been developed by Morris, Koski, and Jonnson (1971) and can be used to calculate the predicted values in liters/second:

Men: [(0.047 × height in inches) − (0.045 × age in years)] + 2.513 (SD 1.12)

Women: [(0.060 × height in inches) − (0.030 × age in years)] + 0.551 (SD 0.80)

c. Forced expiratory volume, timed (FEV_T).

The FEV_T is the volume of air exhaled from an acceptable FVC in the specified time. The time increments are .5, 1, 2, and 3 seconds or more and are listed as $FEV_{.5}$, FEV_1, FEV_2, FEV_3, and so on. It is important that the FVC have a good start and a maximum effort to the end.

The FEV_1 is the most commonly used measurement along with the FVC value

---

* The BTPS correction has been calculated into these equations.

to judge the patient's response to inhaled bronchodilators, for inhalation challenge testing to sceen for asthmatic tendencies, to detect exercise-induced asthma, and for simple screening. BTPS correct all the measured values.

The timed forced expiratory volumes ($FEV_{.5}$, FEV_1, FEV_2, FEV_3) effectively "cut" the FVC into sections based on how much volume the patient forcibly exhales in .5, 1, 2, and 3 seconds. Some patients with severe obstructive lung disease will require several more seconds to completely exhale. In these cases, simply keep measuring the volume exhaled in each additional second. (See Fig. 3–4 for a FVC tracing that is subdivided at .5, 1, 2, and 3 second intervals.)

Some bedside units will give a numerical value for some or all the timed intervals; however, it is best to have a spirometer that produces a printed copy of the patient's FVC effort. The individual volumes can be determined by marking the vertical distance on the volume scale from the baseline (total lung capacity) to the respective arrow tips.

The FEV_T values will often be reduced in both restrictive and obstructive lung diseases. The patient with a severe restrictive lung disease will exhale almost all of his or her small FVC within the first second. The patient with severe obstructive lung disease will show low values at all time intervals with the volumes at $FEV_{2, 3, etc.}$ becoming progessively smaller. However, the most commonly used are the FEV_1 and the $FEV_{1\%}$. The following formulas* have been developed by Morris, Koski, and Johnson (1971) and can be used to calculate the predicted values for FEV_1 in liters:

Men: $[(0.092 \times \text{height in inches}) - (0.032 \times \text{age in years})] - 1.260 \ (\text{SD} \ .55)$

Women: $[(0.089 \times \text{height in inches}) - (0.024 \times \text{age in years})] - 1.93 \ (\text{SD} \ 0.47)$

d. Forced expiratory volume/forced vital capacity ratio (FEV_T/FVC or $FEV_{T\%}$).

The FEV (timed) to FVC ratio compares by division the volume exhaled at .5, 1, 2, and 3 (or more) seconds to the FVC. This results in a series of decimal fractions. These are multiplied by 100 to convert the answers to percentages.

It must be obvious that every person will exhale different volumes for the FEV time intervals because their FVCs are all different. This procedure mathematically standardizes the results regardless of the patient's FVC. Therefore these percentage values can be standardized for all individuals despite different FVCs. The predicted values for normal patients are:

$FEV_{.5}$ = 50% to 60% of the FVC
FEV_1 = 75% to 85% of the FVC
FEV_2 = 94% of the FVC
FEV_3 = 97% of the FVC

These values will normally decrease slightly in the elderly patient. Most patients with normal lungs and airways will still be able to completely exhale their FVC within 4 seconds. Patients with restrictive lung diseases will likely exhale their FVC more quickly than expected. Patients with obstructive lung disease will take longer than expected to exhale their FVC.

---

* The BTPS correction has been calculated into these equations.

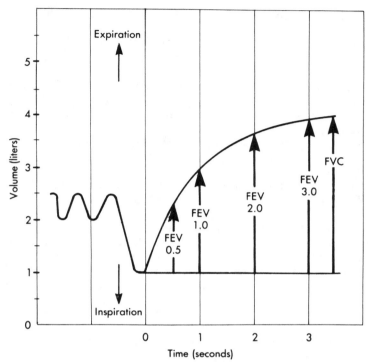

Fig. 3-4 Tracing of a forced vital capacity divided into $FEV_{.5}$, FEV_1, FEV_2, and FEV_3, (From Ruppel G: *Manual of pulmonary function testing,* ed 4, St. Louis, 1986, Mosby–Year Book. Used by permission.)

Module D. Special purpose pulmonary function tests.

1. Spirometry before and after an aerosolized bronchodilator has been inhaled.

a. Recommend the procedure for additional data. (IA2n) [An]

The following are common indications of the procedure:

1. Patient is known to have asthma or another type of chronic obstructive lung disease.
2. The patient has an $FEV_{1\%}$ of less than 70% (unless elderly).
3. The effectiveness of a new bronchodilator is being evaluated.

b. Interpret the results of the procedure. (IC2a) [An]

The most commonly administered tests are the peak flow and $FEV_{1\%}$ from a FVC. Either one or both should be measured before the medication is given to determine the patient's initial airway condition. The medication can be given by intermittent positive pressure breathing (IPPB), hand-held nebulizer, or metered dose inhaler as long as the method is done properly. Wait about 10 to 15 minutes for the medication to take effect and the patient's blood gas values to return to normal. Then, repeat the peak flow and/or $FEV_{1\%}$ test.

The percentage of improvement is calculated by using this formula:

$$\% \text{ of change} = \frac{\text{after-drug air flow} - \text{before-drug air flow}}{\text{before-drug air flow}} \times 100$$

The medication is shown to be effective if the patient has a 15% to 20% improvement in peak flow and/or $FEV_{1\%}$. It is not uncommon to see patients with asthma improve much more than this. Other patients may not have this much improvement but do show increases in air flow and FVC and say that they feel better. In these cases, the physician may decide to continue the medication.

2. Flow-volume loops.
a. Recommend the procedure for additional data. (IA2m) [R, Ap, An]

The flow-volume loop is a graphic display of the flow and volume generated during a forced expiratory vital capacity (FEVC) that is immediately followed by a forced inspiratory vital capacity (FIVC). It is used to identify inspiratory or expiratory flow at any lung volume. As discussed next, it has gained wide popularity because the shape of the tracing can indicate a pulmonary and airway problem.

b. Perform the procedure. (IC1e) [R, Ap, An]

As with the FVC test, the patient should be coached to inhale completely and blast the air out until he or she is completely empty. When you are sure that the patient has exhaled to residual volume, coach him or her to inhale as quickly as possible until the lungs are completely full. There should not be any hesitation at the start, leaks, glottis closing, or coughing throughout the entire procedure.

The expiratory half of the curve is called the maximal expiratory flow-volume (MEFV) curve. It begins at total lung capacity and ends at residual volume. The inspiratory half of the curve is called the maximal inspiratory flow-volume (MIFV) curve. It begins at residual volume and ends at total lung capacity. Ideally, the two halves of the loop meet at the total lung capacity. Flow is recorded in liters/second and graphed on the vertical (ordinant or Y) axis. Volume is recorded in liters and graphed on the horizontal (abscissa or X) axis. Both flow and volume should be BTPS adjusted.

c. Interpret the results from the procedure. (IC1e) [R, Ap, An]

Flow-volume loops have gained great popularity because the shape of the curve is diagnostic of the patient's condition. In addition, peak inspiratory and peak expiratory flows can be determined. If the effort can be timed, all the parameters found on the previously discussed volume-time curves can be found on the flow-volume loop. The following examples will show a normal flow-volume loop and representative abnormal loops.

Normal

A normal flow-volume loop is shown in Figs. 3-5 and 3-6. Let us look first at Fig. 3-5 where the various volumes are measured on the horizontal scale. The tidal volume (V_T) of 500 ml is the small loop within the larger vital capacity loop. The expiratory reserve volume (ERV) and inspiratory reserve volume (IRV) are shown

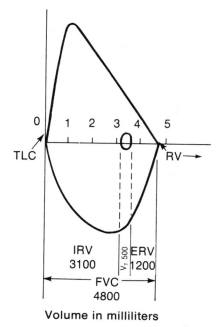

Fig. 3-5 Flow-volume loop tracing of a normal adult showing the positions and values of the lung volumes.

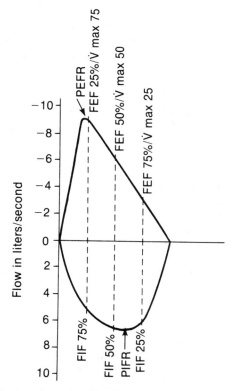

Fig. 3-6 Flow-volume loop tracing of a normal adult showing the positions and values of the various inspiratory and expiratory flows.

on both sides of the tidal volume. The FVC is shown as the total of all three volumes. Finally, total lung capacity (TLC) and residual volume (RV) are marked.

Fig. 3-6 shows the same normal flow-volume loop where the various flows are measured on the vertical scale. Starting from TLC with the FEVC, the peak expiratory flow rate (PEFR) is seen as the greatest flow that is generated; it is about 9 l/sec. Starting from RV with the forced inspiratory vital capacity, the peak inspiratory flow rate (PIFR) is seen as the greatest flow that is generated; it is about 7 l/sec. It is normal for the PEFR to be greater than the PIFR.

To find the instantaneous flow at any FVC lung volume, the FVC must be divided by 4 to find the 25th, 50th, and 75th percentile points. In this example, the FVC is 4800 ml. Dividing by 4 gives 1200 ml per quarter of the FVC. These points are marked on the horizontal volume scale. If a vertical (dashed) line is drawn through these three points to the flow-volume tracing, the instantaneous flows at these volumes can be found. *Expiratory flows* are reported as:

a. Flow at 75% of the FEVC = $\dot{V}_{max75}$ (maximum flow with 75% of the FVC remaining) or $FEF_{25\%}$ (forced expiratory flow with 25% of the FVC exhaled)
b. Flow at 50% of the FEVC = $\dot{V}_{max50}$ (maximum flow with 50% of the FVC remaining) or $FEF_{50\%}$ (forced expiratory flow with 50% of the FVC exhaled)
c. Flow at 25% of the FEVC = $\dot{V}_{max25}$ (maximum flow with 25% of the FVC remaining) or $FEF_{75\%}$ (forced expiratory flow with 75% of the FVC exhaled)

Inspiratory flows are reported as:

a. Flow at 25% of the FIVC = $FIF_{25\%}$ (forced inspiratory flow with 25% of the FVC inhaled)
b. Flow at 50% of the FIVC = $FIF_{50\%}$ (forced inspiratory flow with 50% of the FVC inhaled)
c. Flow at 75% of the FIVC = $FIF_{75\%}$ (forced inspiratory flow with 75% of the FVC inhaled)

The PEFR and $FEF_{25}/\dot{V}_{max75\%}$ values should be about the same because they all measure flow through the large upper airways. Either test is a good gauge of the patient's effort because it will be low if the patient is not trying hard and the rest of the values will also be low. It is normal for the FIF_{50} to be greater than the FEF_{50}. The $FEF_{50}/\dot{V}_{max50\%}$ values should approximate the $FEF_{25\%-75\%}$ values because they both show flow though the medium to small airways in the middle half of the FVC effort. The $FEF_{75}/\dot{V}_{max25\%}$ values are the best indicator of early small airways disease because both show flow through the small airways as the patient approaches the residual volume. Note that the tracing from the $FEF_{25}/\dot{V}_{max75\%}$ point to the residual volume is a straight line. In normal people, the flow decreases in proportion to the decreasing lung volume resulting in the straight line tracing. Cherniack and Raber (1972) have published formulas for predicting adult MEFV flows in liters/second; see the bibliography.

Small Airways Disease

Examples of conditions resulting in small airways disease (less than 2 mm in diameter) include asthma, chronic bronchitis, bronchiectasis, cystic fibrosis, and emphysema. The obstruction can be from bronchospasm, mucus plugging, or damage to the alveoli and small airways leading to their collapse on expiration.

Fig. 3-7 shows representative flow-volume loops of asthma and emphysema superimposed over a normal flow-volume loop. Notice that both loops are shifted

Pulmonary mechanics

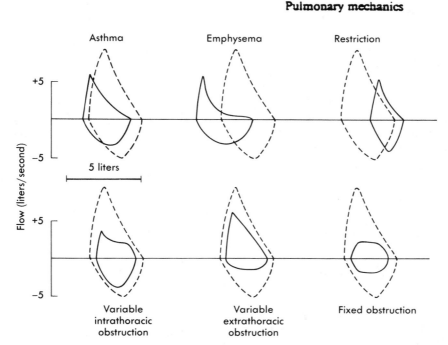

Fig. 3-7 A series of abnormal flow-volume loop tracings superimposed over a dashed line tracing of a normal loop. (From Ruppel G: *Manual of pulmonary function testing*, ed 6, St. Louis, 1994, Mosby—Year Book. Used by permission.)

to the left toward the total lung capacity because the residual volumes are increased. Also notice that the flows are decreased more than normal as the patient exhales closer to the residual volume. This "scooped out" appearance is very characteristic of small airways disease. Having the patient inhale a bronchodilator and repeating the flow-volume loop will show the degree of reversibility. Some computer-based systems allow the before and after bronchodilator loops to be superimposed to further show the amount of improvement.

Restriction

A restriction can be caused by a pulmonary condition such as fibrosis; a thoracic condition such as pleural effusion, pneumo or hemothorax, or kyphoscoliosis; or obesity, advanced pregnancy, or ascites pushing up on the diaphragm. Only fibrosis and kyphoscoliosis are permanent. Fig. 3-7 shows a representative flow-volume loop for a patient with restrictive lung disease. Notice that the volume is small and shifted to the right toward the small residual volume.

Variable Intrathoracic Obstruction

A variable intrathoracic obstruction could be caused by a tumor or foreign body partially blocking a bronchus. Fig. 3-7 shows a representative flow-volume curve.

Note that the forced vital capacity volume is almost normal and there is a greatly decreased peak expiratory flow rate.

Variable Extrathoracic Obstruction

A variable extrathoracic obstruction could be caused by vocal cord paralysis, laryngeal tumor, or a foreign body partially obstructing the upper airway. Fig. 3-7 shows a representative flow-volume curve. Note that the forced vital capacity volume is almost normal with a greatly reduced inspiratory flow. This same pattern is commonly seen in patients with obstructive sleep apnea. The $FEF_{50\%}$ will be greater than the $FIF_{50\%}$.

Fixed Large Airway Obstruction

A fixed large airway obstruction is usually caused by a tumor in the trachea or a mainstem bronchus. Fig. 3-7 shows a representative flow-volume loop. Again, the forced vital capacity volume is close to normal. Note the abnormally reduced inspiratory and expiratory flow rates. The tracing looks almost "squared off" with the $FEF_{50\%}$ and $FIF_{50\%}$ values being about the same.

3.   Maximum voluntary ventilation.
   **a.   Recommend the procedure for additional data. (IA2f)
   [R, Ap, An]**

The maximum voluntary ventilation (MVV) is the volume of air exhaled in a specified period during a repetitive maximal respiratory effort. It is most commonly done to evaluate a patient's ability to perform a stress test. It may also be used as a preoperative screening test to help determine the patient's chance of pulmonary complications.

   b.   Perform the procedure. (IC1g) [R, Ap, An]

The patient should breathe at a volume that is greater than the tidal volume but less than the vital capacity with a rate between 70 and 120 per minute. The minimal time for the test is 5 seconds with a recommended time of 12 seconds (see Fig. 3-8 for two different tracings of the MVV effort). The total volume exhaled in the given time period is mathematically adjusted for 1 minute so that the derived value is in liters/minute. This is done by multiplying a 5-second effort by 12 or a 12-second effort by 5. The derived value is then BTPS corrected to give the final value.

   c.   Interpret the results from the procedure. (IC1g) [R, Ap, An]

The results of the MVV test are among the more difficult to evaluate. This is because the patient's effort, the condition of the respiratory muscles, lung-thoracic compliance, neurological control over the drive to breathe, and airway and tissue resistance all have an influence. Abnormalities in any of these can cause the MVV value to be decreased. Also, because more than one problem can exist, a decreased MVV value does not pinpoint the exact difficulty. A healthy young man can have an MVV of 150 to 200 l/min. Women tend to have smaller values, and the values for both sexes decline with age. Because of the many factors involved in the MVV, normal predicted values may vary by as much as ± 30%. Therefore unless a patient

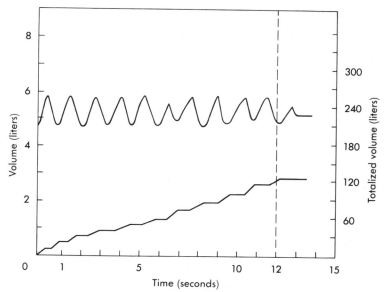

Fig. 3-8 Two tracings of the same maximum voluntary ventilation (MVV) effort. The saw-toothed tracing shows each individual volume effort and the respiratory rate. The stair-stepped tracing shows the cumulative volume during the effort. (From Ruppel G: *Manual of pulmonary function testing*, ed 6, St. Louis, 1994, Mosby–Year Book. Used by permission.)

has an MVV value that is less than 70% of predicted, he or she cannot really be considered abnormally low. Cherniack and Raber (1972) have published the following equations* for predicting the MVV in liters/minute:

Males: [(3.03 × height in inches) − (0.816 × age in years)] − 37.9

Females: [(2.14 × height in inches) − (0.685 × age in years)] − 4.87

When evaluating an abnormally low MVV result the following considerations must be made:

a. Did the patient try his or her best? The respiratory therapist must make a professional judgment that the patient made his or her best effort. An objective way of judging this is to multiply the patient's FEV_1 × 35 to estimate the MVV. They should be close to the same volume. For example, if the patient's FEV_1 is 3 l, the estimated MVV is 105 l/min (3 l × 35). An MVV value that is much less than this would indicate that the patient did not try very hard. Conversely, an MVV value that is much greater than this would indicate that the FEV_1 value is too low and should be repeated.

b. What is the condition of the patient's respiratory muscles? Patients with neuromuscular abnormalities probably will not be able to breathe much deeper than the normal tidal volume or keep up the great effort required for the duration of the test. Because of this their results will be low.

c. What is the patient's lung-thoracic compliance? Patients with low compliance probably will not be able to sustain the greater than normal work load required by the MVV test. However, some patients are able to compensate for a small tidal

---

* The BTPS correction has been calculated into these equations.

volume by increasing their respiratory rate enough to generate an MVV value within normal limits. A printout of the MVV test would show a smaller than expected volume moved at a higher than expected respiratory rate.

d. What is the patient's neurological control over the drive to breathe? Patients who have had an injury to the brain may have an abnormal drive to breathe. Because of this they produce a low MVV result.

e. What is the patient's airway and tissue resistance? Patients with increased airway resistance will usually have a low MVV result. This problem may also cause air trapping and force the patient to stop the effort. Increased tissue resistance such as seen in pulmonary edema, obesity, and ascites will also result in a low MVV value.

Despite these difficulties in determining the cause of a decreased MVV value, it has proven helpful in preoperative evaluation and cardiopulmonary stress testing. Any patient with a lower than normal MVV value is at an increased risk of postoperative atelectasis and pneumonia. The risks of pulmonary complications related to MVV are low when the patient reaches 75% to 50% of predicted, moderate when the patient reaches 50% to 33% of predicted, and high when the patient reaches less than 33% of predicted. Patients with known moderate to severe COPD will usually have to stop exercise testing due to their inability to breathe. An MVV value of less than 50 l/min is a good predictor of this.

4. Single-breath nitrogen washout (SBN₂) test.
a. Recommend the procedure for additional data. (IA2s) [R, Ap, An]

The single-breath nitrogen washout (SBN_2) test is used to measure two things: 1) the evenness of the distribution of ventilation into the lungs during inspiration, and 2) the emptying rates of the lungs during exhalation. It would be a helpful diagnostic test in any adult patient who is known or suspected of having obstructive airways disease. The NBRC uses the phrase "nitrogen washout distribution test" for this exam. This is also known as the single-breath oxygen (SBO_2) test and Fowler's test.

b. Perform the procedure. (IC1b) [R, Ap, An]

The SBN_2 test is done by analyzing the nitrogen (N_2) percentage that is exhaled after an inspiratory vital capacity of 100% oxygen. It is beyond the scope of this book to go into detail on all the steps of the procedure; however, the general steps include instructing the patient to perform an inspiratory vital capacity while inhaling oxygen. Without any breath holding, tell the patient to slowly and evenly exhale until his or her lungs are empty again. The exhaled gases are sent through a rapid N_2 analyzer to measure the percentage, a spirometer to measure the volume, and a graphing device.

c. Interpret the results from the procedure. (IC1h) [R, Ap, An]

Refer to Fig. 3-9 for a normal tracing showing these phases:

Phase I.—Phase I shows gas exhaled from the anatomic dead space of the upper airway. Because it is made up of 100% oxygen the nitrogen percentage shows a zero reading.

Phase II.—Phase II shows a mix of dead space gas and alveolar gas. The nitrogen percentage rises rapidly as the pure oxygen is exhaled and nitrogen rich

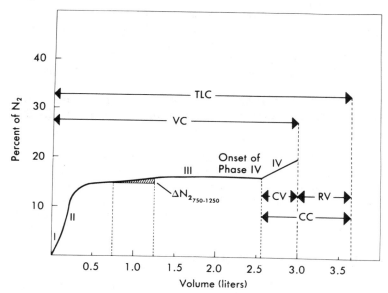

Fig. 3-9 Tracing of a normal single-breath nitrogen washout (SBN₂) test showing the four phases and other features. (From Ruppel G: *Manual of pulmonary function testing,* ed 6, St. Louis, 1994, Mosby–Year Book. Used by permission.)

gas from the alveoli is brought out. The first 750 ml of gas that includes these first two phases is not used in the evaluation of the distribution of ventilation.

Phase III.—Phase III shows a fairly level plateau as alveolar gas when a stable mix of oxygen and nitrogen is exhaled. Phase III is further evaluated in the following two ways.

$\Delta N_{2\ 750\text{-}1250}.$—$\Delta N_{2\ 750\text{-}1250}$ looks at the increase in the nitrogen percentage found in the 500 ml of gas exhaled between 750 ml and 1250 ml of the vital capacity. It is normally no more than 1.5% in healthy young adults. It increases to about 4.5% in healthy older adults. Patients with severe airways and lung disease, such as emphysema, may have a finding of 6% to 10% or more.

Slope of Phase III.—The slope of phase III is found by drawing a straight line from the point where 30% of the vital capacity is exhaled to the point where phase IV begins. It is normally no more than .5% to 1% per liter of exhaled volume in healthy young adults but may vary widely.

Phase IV.—A sharp increase in the nitrogen percentage is seen and continues to residual volume. This is seen when the nitrogen rich gas from the upper airways continues to be exhaled as the basilar airways became compressed and close off near the end of the vital capacity effort. The start of phase IV is called the closing volume (CV). It marks the lung volume when small airway closure begins and is an early indicator of small airways disease. Healthy young adults will not have the closing volume occur until after about 80% to 90% of the vital capacity has been exhaled. The closing capacity (CC) is found by adding the closing volume to the residual volume (found by another test). Healthy young adults will have a closing capacity that is about 30% of their total lung capacity.

Increases in the ΔN_2 750-1250, slope of phase III, and especially early onset of phase IV; increased closing volume; and increased closing capacity can indicate a number of problems. Included in the problems are small airways disease, restrictive processes where the functional residual capacity (FRC) is less than the closing volume, congestive heart failure with pulmonary edema, or obesity.

5. Functional residual capacity (FRC) by the helium dilution method.
a. Recommend the procedure for additional data. (IA2p) [R, Ap, An]

The functional residual capacity (FRC) is the volume of gas left in the lungs at the end of a normal expiration. It cannot be measured through spirometry. An FRC is needed to calculate a patient's total lung capacity (TLC). This procedure is discussed in the following section. It is necessary to know a patient's FRC and TLC to diagnose and determine the severity of obstructive lung disease and restrictive lung disease.

b. Perform the procedure. (IC1b) [R, Ap, An]

Because the FRC cannot be directly measured, this, the following technique, and the body plethysmograph have been devised to discover it.

The helium (He) dilution method basically involves diluting the resident gases in the lungs (mainly nitrogen and oxygen) with helium to mathematically determine the FRC. It is also called the closed-circuit method because the patient and circuit are sealed off. Fig. 3-10 shows a schematic drawing of the components that make up the circuit. This includes a two-way valve to switch the patient from breathing room air to the helium mix, soda lime to absorb the patient's exhaled carbon dioxide

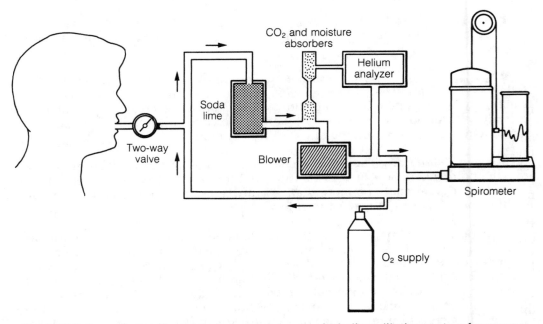

Fig. 3-10 Schematic drawing of the key components of a helium dilution system for measuring functional residual capacity. (From Beauchamp RK: Pulmonary function testing procedures. In Barnes TA, editor: *Respiratory care practice*, Chicago, 1988, Year Book Medical. Used with permission.)

from the circuit, a combined CO_2 and water vapor absorber to prevent these gases from entering the helium analyzer, the helium analyzer, a variable speed blower to move the gases through the circuit, a spirometer for monitoring tidal volumes, attached kymograph to trace out the patient's breathing pattern, and an oxygen supply to meet the patient's needs. The helium supply is not shown.

It is beyond the scope of this text to cover all the steps in the test; however, the following features of the procedure are important to know. Add enough helium to the room air in the circuit to create a 10% to 15% He mix. At the end of a normal exhalation, the patient is switched to breathing the mix so that the functional residual capacity can be determined. The patient breathes the gas mix until the helium is evenly distributed throughout the lungs and the helium percentage is stable. Typically, the test is performed for up to 7 minutes if needed to reach an equilibrium point. Extending the test longer may help to reach a stable equilibrium point in abnormal patients. The calculation of residual volume is rather complex and is usually done through the computer built into the pulmonary function system. Spirometry must also be performed because the expiratory reserve volume is subtracted from the functional residual capacity to find the residual volume. Commonly the test is repeated. The patient should be allowed to breathe room air for 5 minutes between tests to clear the helium from the lungs. Patients with severe obstructive lung disease may need more time.

Bates, Macklem, and Christie (1971) have published the following equations* for calculating the normal FRC in liters:

$$\text{Males} = (0.130 \times \text{height in inches}) - 5.16$$

$$\text{Females} = (0.119 \times \text{height in inches}) - 4.85$$

Goldman and Becklake (1959) have published the following equations* for calculating the normal RV in liters:

$$\text{Males} = [(0.069 \times \text{height in inches}) + (0.017 \times \text{age in years})] - 3.45$$

$$\text{Females} = [(0.081 \times \text{height in inches}) + (0.009 \times \text{age in years})] - 3.90$$

6. Interpret the results from the procedure. (IC1b) [R, Ap, An]

The normal young man would have an FRC volume of about 2400 ml. As shown in Fig. 3-11, it is composed of the expiratory reserve volume (ERV) and the residual volume (RV). The FRC and RV values are invaluable in diagnosing obstructive and restrictive lung diseases. Fig. 3-12 shows the relative volumes and capacities for a normal patient, a patient with an obstructive pattern, and a patient with a restrictive pattern. Note that the obstructive patient has a disproportionate increase in the residual volume with a resulting decrease in the FVC. The total lung capacity may be normal, as shown, or, more commonly, increased. The patient with restrictive disease has a proportionate decrease in all the lung volumes and capacities. It is commonly accepted that the normal limits of total lung capacity are about ± 20% of the predicted value. This ± 20% of the normal limit applies to the FRC and RV values as well. In other words, obstructive lung disease can be diagnosed by an RV, FRC, and/or TLC that is more than 120% of the predicted value. Common examples of obstructive diseases include asthma, bronchitis, and emphysema. Restrictive lung disease can be diagnosed by an RV, FRC, and/or TLC that is less than 80% of the predicted value. Examples of restrictive diseases include fibrotic

---

* The BTPS correction has been calculated into these equations. Predicted normals can be calculated for any patient by filling in the height as shown in the equation.

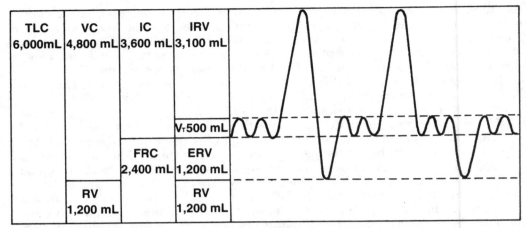

TLC 6,000mL	VC 4,800 mL	IC 3,600 mL	IRV 3,100 mL
			V_T 500 mL
		FRC 2,400 mL	ERV 1,200 mL
	RV 1,200 mL		RV 1,200 mL

Fig. 3-11 Lung volumes and capacities for a normal young man. (From Sills JR: *Respiratory care certification guide,* St. Louis, 1991, Mosby–Year Book. Used by permission.)

lung disease, air or fluid in the pleural space, obesity, kyphoscoliosis, pectus excavatum, and neuromuscular weakness or paralysis.

The following considerations should be accounted for to have faith that the measured values are accurate:

a. There should be no leaks in the system. A leak could result in an overestimation of the FRC because the lost helium would result in a lower final helium percentage. Or, a leak could result in failure of the final helium percentage to stabilize as expected.

b. The patient must be breathing on the system long enough for the helium to reach all of the lung units and reach equilibrium. Usually this takes about 7

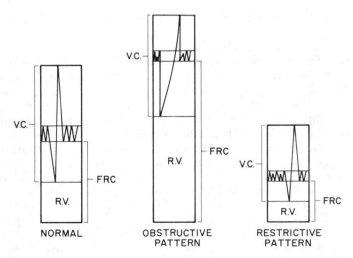

Fig. 3-12 Spirometry tracings of a normal, obstructed, and restricted patient. Note how the obstructed and restricted patients' volumes and capacities are out of proportion compared to the normal patient. (From Cherniack RM: *Pulmonary function testing,* Philadelphia, 1977, WB Saunders. Used by permission.)

minutes; however, patients with severe obstructive lung disease will need more time and may never reach an equilibrium state. This would result in an underestimation of the FRC.

7. Functional residual capacity (FRC) by the nitrogen washout method.
a. Recommend the procedure for additional data. (IA2p) [R, Ap, An]

As discussed in the helium dilution method, the nitrogen (N_2) washout method is used to find the functional residual capacity so that the residual volume can be derived from it.

b. Perform the procedure. (IC1b) [R, Ap, An]

The nitrogen washout method basically involves having the patient breathe in 100% oxygen until all the resident nitrogen is removed from the lungs. It is also called the open-circuit method because the patient inspires as much oxygen as needed to displace the nitrogen to a reservoir for measurement.

Fig. 3-13 shows a schematic drawing of the components that make up the automated nitrogen washout system and circuit. This includes a solenoid valve to switch the patient from breathing room air to pure oxygen, an oxygen source with demand valve, a nitrogen analyzer with recorder, a pneumotachometer, and a microprocessor that directs all the necessary activities for the test. It is beyond the scope

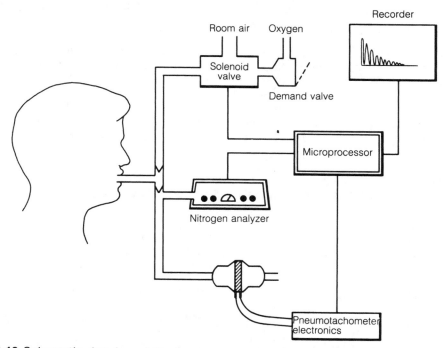

Fig. 3-13 Schematic drawing of the key components of the automated nitrogen washout system for measuring functional residual capacity. (From Beauchamp RK: Pulmonary function testing procedures. In Barnes TA, editor: *Respiratory care practice*, Chicago,1988, Year Book Medical. Used by permission.)

of this text to go into the complete procedure for the test; however, the following features should be known. The circuit is filled with pure oxygen. The patient is switched from room air to oxygen at the end of a normal exhalation so that the nitrogen in the functional residual capacity can be determined. Typically, the test is performed for up to 7 minutes or until the nitrogen percentage falls below a target level. This target percentage has been reported by various authors as 1% (best results), 1.2%, 1.5%, 2%, 2.5%, and 3%. Extending the test longer may help to reach a target level in patients with increased airway resistance or an increased lung volume. As before, the calculation of residual volume is rather complex and is usually done through the computer built into the pulmonary function system. Spirometry must also be performed because the expiratory reserve volume is subtracted from the functional residual capacity to find the residual volume. Commonly the test is repeated. The patient should be allowed to breathe room air for at least 15 minutes between tests to clear the oxygen from the lungs. Patients with severe obstructive lung disease may need more time.

c.   Interpret the results from the procedure. (IC1b) [R, Ap, An]

As discussed earlier about the helium dilution test, the FRC and RV values are invaluable in diagnosing obstructive and restrictive lung diseases. When done properly, the helium dilution and nitrogen washout tests reveal similar patient values. If the nitrogen percentage is graphed over time, the shape of the washout curve can also be helpful in evaluating the degree of airway obstruction. Both the normal and abnormal tracings show rapid nitrogen washout from the upper airway dead space. However, as the test continues, the patient with obstructive lung disease shows a progressive slowing of the nitrogen washout rate.

The following considerations should be accounted for to have faith that the measured values are accurate:

a. There should be no leaks in the system. A leak would be noticed as a sudden increase in the nitrogen percentage after a steady decrease. This would result in an overestimation in the FRC value.

b. The patient must be breathing on the system long enough for the nitrogen to be washed out of all the lung units. Usually this takes less than 7 minutes; however, patients with severe obstructive lung disease will need more time and may never reach the targeted percentage. This would result in an underestimation of the FRC.

8.   Total lung capacity.
a.   Recommend the procedure for additional data. (IA2t) [R, Ap, An]

Total lung capacity is the volume of air in the lungs after inhaling a vital capacity. As discussed earlier, it is necessary to determine a patient's total lung capacity (TLC) to diagnose obstructive or restrictive lung disease.

b.   Perform the procedure. (Ic1l) [R, Ap, An]

Refer to Fig. 3-11 for the relationships of the lung volumes and capacities to each other. As can be seen, total lung capacity (TLC) can be found by adding several combinations of volumes and capacities. Most commonly it is calculated by adding the FRC (determined by the helium dilution or nitrogen washout methods or in a body plethysmograph) to the inspiratory capacity (IC) found through spirometry. However, be prepared to add or subtract various combinations of volumes and capacities to find the TLC.

c.   Interpret the results from the procedure. (IC1I) [R, Ap, An]

The total lung capacity results cannot be interpreted without looking at the volumes and capacities that compose it. See Fig. 3-11 for the normal relationships of the volumes and capacities to themselves and the TLC. The following list shows the lung volumes and capacities seen in a normal 150 lb/68 kg young man:

Tidal volume (V_T) = 500 ml (Tidal volume is normally about 10% of the total lung capacity [TLC].)

Inspiratory reserve volume (IRV) = 3100 ml (Inspiratory reserve volume is normally about 50% of the TLC.)

Expiratory reserve volume (ERV) = 1200 ml (Expiratory reserve volume is normally about 20% of the TLC.)

Residual volume (RV) = 1200 ml (Residual volume is normally about 25% of the TLC.)

Inspiratory capacity (RC) = 3600 ml (made up of the V_T and IRV) (Inspiratory capacity is normally about 60% of the TLC.)

Functional residual capacity (FRC) = 2400 ml (made up of the ERV and RV) (Functional residual capacity is normally about 40% of the TLC.)

Vital capacity (VC) = 4800 ml (made up of the V_T, IRV, and ERV) (Vital capacity is normally about 80% of the TLC.)

Total lung capacity (TLC) = 6000 ml (made up of the V_T, IRV, ERV, and RV)

Fig. 3-12 shows representative TLC patterns for a normal patient and patients with an obstructive pattern and a restrictive pattern. Note that with the abnormal patterns, the FRC and its components, the expiratory reserve volume and residual volume, are out of proportion. Patients with emphysema, bronchitis, and/or asthma often show the obstructive pattern with its large FRC of trapped gas. Patients with fibrotic lung disease, thoracic deformities, or obesity often show the restrictive pattern with its decreased FRC and other lung volumes.

Some practitioners use the general rule that a TLC that is more than 120% of predicted indicates an obstructive pattern, and a TLC that is less than 80% of predicted indicates a restrictive pattern. However, this may be an oversimplification. It is more reliable to calculate the residual volume : total lung capacity ratio (RV : TLC). This takes into account the interrelationship of the two. Normal healthy adults have a RV : TLC ratio that is .20 to .35 (20% to 35%). An increased RV : TLC ratio is commonly seen in patients with emphysema and an increased residual volume. However, if the patient's TLC is increased in proportion to the residual volume, the ratio may be within normal limits. A decreased RV : TLC ratio is commonly seen in patients with fibrotic lung disease. The ratio will be normal, however, if the patient's TLC is decreased in proportion to the residual volume. Table 3-1 shows the relationships of the lung volumes and capacities, TLC, and the RV : TLC ratio found in a number of conditions.

9.   Body plethysmography.

The body plethysmography unit (sometimes called the body box) is a sealable chamber large enough for an adult to sit inside. Auxiliary equipment includes a differential pressure pneumotachometer, monitor/storage oscilloscope, computer, and recording device (see Fig. 3-14). The plethysmograph can be used to measure: 1) the FRC and, from that, the RV and total lung capacity; 2) lung compliance; and 3) airway resistance.

Table 3-1. Lung Volumes and Capacities Seen in Various Disorders

Disorder	VC	IC	ERV	FRC	RV	TLC	RV : TLC
Asthma/airway disease	D	N	D	N,I	I	N,I*	I
Emphysema	N	N	N	I	I	I	N,I
Diffuse parenchymal disease							
Early	N	N	N	D	N	N	N
Advanced	(All volumes and capacities are equally reduced.)						
Space-occupying lesions	N	N	N	N	D	N	D
Obesity	N	N	D	N,I†	N	N	I
Thoracic/skeletal disease	D	D	D	D	N	D	I

Key: N, normal; I, increased; D, decreased
* When airway resistance is greater than about 3.5 cm $H_2O/l/sec$.
† When the weight : height (pounds : inches) ratio is greater than 5 : 1.
Based on a table in Snow MG: Determination of functional residual capacity. In *Respir Care* 34(7):586-596, 1989.

a. Thoracic gas volume.
i. Perform the procedure for additional data. (IC1n) [R, Ap, An]

The volume of gas measured in the lungs at the end of exhalation by a plethysmograph is termed thoracic gas volume (TGV or VTG). When the unit is accurately calibrated and the test properly performed, the plethysmograph provides a more accurate FRC volume measurement than either the helium dilution or nitrogen washout methods.

It is not possible to go into a complete discussion of the procedure; however, the following steps are important. The unit must be sealed so that it is airtight during the patient's breathing. The patient is instructed to breathe a normal tidal volume through the pneumotachometer. At the end of exhalation (FRC), a shutter

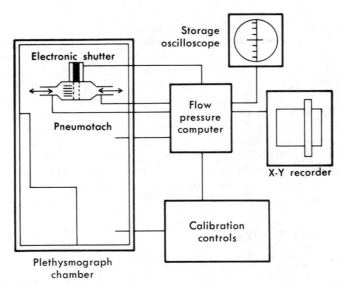

Fig. 3-14 Schematic drawing of the layout of a body plethysmograph with its components. The patient sits within the sealed plethysmograph chamber for the tests. (From Ruppel G: *Manual of pulmonary function testing*, ed 6, St. Louis, 1994, Mosby–Year Book. Used by permission.)

is closed on the pneumotachometer so that no air leaks. The patient is instructed to continue to make tidal volume breathing efforts. The computer integrates the following two pressure changes: 1) a drop in mouth pressure as the patient attempts to inhale, and 2) an increase in plethysmograph chamber pressure as the patient's chest expands. The patient's thoracic gas volume (TGV) is then determined at functional residual capacity. Fig. 3-15 A shows a normal TGV loop on the oscilloscope. Through spirometry the patient's expiratory reserve volume, residual volume, and total lung capacity can be calculated.

ii. Interpret the results from the procedure. (IC1n) [R, Ap, An]

The interpretation of the TGV and TLC results from a body plethysmograph would be about the same as the interpretation of the FRC and TLC results from the helium dilution or nitrogen washout methods. (Review the earlier discussions if needed.) The only difference would be if the TGV was significantly larger than the FRC. This would indicate that the patient has trapped gas that was only measured in the plethysmograph. The TGV is commonly larger than the FRC measured by the above two methods when the patient has chronic obstructive pulmonary disease (COPD). This is because it includes *all* the gas found in the thorax. That gas may be found in normal alveoli connected by a patent airway to the atmosphere, but it may also include gas trapped in emphysematous blebs and bullae, pneumothorax, pneumomediastinum, and so forth.

b. Lung compliance.
i. Perform the procedure for added data. (IC1f) [R, Ap, An]

Lung compliance (C_L) is the volume change per unit of pressure change in the lungs. It is recorded in liters or milliliters per centimeter of water pressure. Following are the key steps in its measurement: The patient must swallow a 10-cm long balloon to the midthoracic level. A catheter connects the proximal end of the balloon to a pressure transducer outside of the patient. Air is injected into the balloon and the transducer is calibrated to accurately measure changes in intrathoracic pressure as the patient breathes. The patient is then placed into a body plethysmograph that is sealed. He or she is told to breathe through the differential pressure pneumotachometer to measure lung volumes. The patient is then instructed to slowly inhale from the resting level (FRC) to total lung capacity. As this is being done the pneumotachometer shutter is periodically closed to measure the intrathoracic pressure drop at the increasing volumes (see Fig. 3-16). As the patient slowly exhales from TLC the shutter is again periodically closed to measure the increasing intrathoracic pressure as the patient returns to FRC volume. Lung compliance is usually calculated from the pressure and volume points of FRC and FRC + 500 ml (for a tidal volume).

ii. Interpret the results from the procedure. (IC1f) [R, Ap, An]

Normal lung compliance (C_L) in an adult is 0.2 l/cm water. Through other methods the normal adult's thoracic compliance (C_T) has been determined to also be .2 l/cm water. However, because the lungs tend to collapse smaller and the thorax cage tends to expand out, the two opposing forces tend to offset each other somewhat. Because of this, the lung-thoracic compliance (C_{LT}) is calculated as 0.1 l (or 100 ml)/cm water.

A number of diseases and conditions can affect the lung, thoracic, and lung-

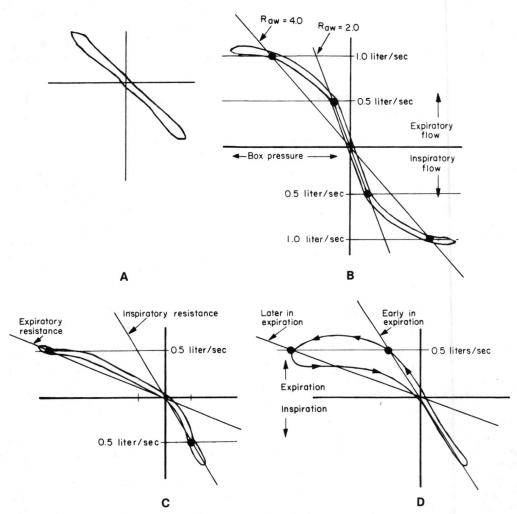

Fig. 3-15 Examples of body plethysmography tracings. Tracing **A** shows a normal thoracic gas volume loop. Tracing **B** shows a normal inspiratory and expiratory loop for airway resistance (Raw). Note that it is symmetrical. This patient has a Raw of 2 cm H_2O/l/sec at the standard flow of 0.5 l/sec. As the flow increases, the Raw increases as a result of the increased turbulence. So, the Raw of 4 cm H_2O/l/sec seen at the flow of 1 l/sec should not be recorded as the patient's value. Tracing **C** shows a patient who has an expiratory resistance that is greater than inspiratory resistance. In this case, either both resistances should be recorded in the chart or just the inspiratory resistance if only one can be recorded. Tracing **D** shows a significant difference between early and late expiratory resistance. This is commonly seen in patients with obstructive airways disease such as emphysema. Record the late resistance because it better represents the patient's disease condition. (From Zarins LP, Clausen JL: Body plethysmography. In Clausen JL, editor: *Pulmonary function testing guidelines and controversies,* Orlando, 1984, Grune & Stratton. Used by permission.)

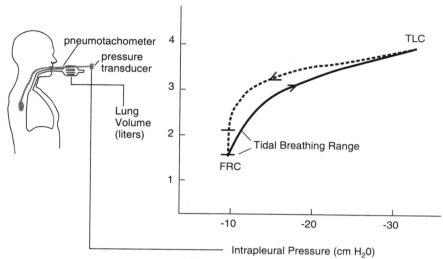

Fig. 3-16 Measurement of lung compliance (C_L) with the esophageal balloon technique. A balloon is swallowed to the midthoracic level, filled with air, and connected to a pressure transducer to measure intrapleural pressure. The patient sits within a body plethysmograph to measure inspiratory and expiratory volumes. (From Ruppel G: *Manual of pulmonary function testing,* ed 6, St. Louis, 1994, Mosby–Year Book. Used by permission.)

thoracic compliance. Patients with emphysema are known to have a higher than normal lung compliance. Their lungs are overly distended. Decreased lung compliance is seen in pulmonary fibrosis (from sarcoidosis, silicosis, or asbestosis), lung tumor, pulmonary edema, atelectasis, pneumonia, or decreased surfactant. Decreased thoracic compliance is seen in patients with kyphoscoliosis, pectus excavatum, obesity, enlarged liver, or advanced pregnancy. All these conditions result in small, stiff lungs.

c. Airway resistance.
i. Perform the procedure for added data. (IC1m) [R, Ap, An]

Airway resistance (Raw) is the difference in pressure between the alveoli and the mouth that develops as air flows into and out of the lungs. It is recorded in centimeters of water pressure per liter of gas moved per second (cm water/l/sec). This test is also performed in a body plethysmograph. The key steps in the procedure are as follows: The patient is placed into a plethysmograph that is sealed. He or she is instructed to breathe through a differential pressure pneumotachometer. With the pneumotachometer shutter open, the patient is told to pant several tidal volumes of about 500 ml at a rate of 1 breath per second. Data on flow rate, tidal volume, mouth pressure changes, and chamber pressure changes are recorded and graphed (see Fig. 3-17). Then, at the patient's resting FRC volume, the shutter is closed. The patient is told to continue panting at the same volume and rate. Again, flow rate, tidal volume, mouth pressure changes, and chamber pressures are recorded and graphed. The computer integrates the data to calculate the patient's airway resistance during tidal volume breathing.

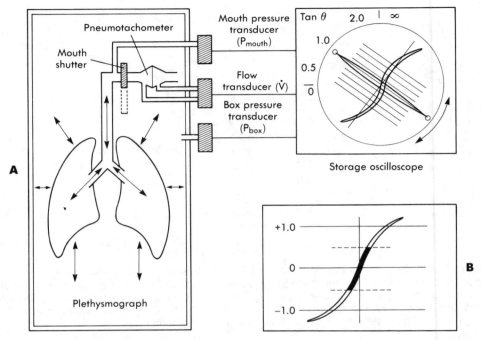

Fig. 3-17 Measurement of airway resistance (Raw). **A,** This represents the body plethysmograph that the patient sits within during the test. Tidal volume panting against an open and then closed pneumotachometer shutter is displayed on the storage oscilloscope. **B,** This represents a printout of the pressure changes as the patient pants a tidal volume of 500 ml/sec. (From Ruppel G: *Manual of pulmonary function testing,* ed 6, St. Louis, 1994, Mosby–Year Book. Used by permission.)

ii. Interpret the results from the procedure. (IC1m) [R, Ap, An]

Airway resistance is the pressure difference developed per unit of flow. This pressure is required to overcome the friction of moving the tidal volume through the airways to the lungs. It can be thought of as the ratio of alveolar pressure to air flow. It is calculated by this formula:

$$Raw = \frac{atmospheric\ pressure - alveolar\ pressure}{flow}$$

Ruppel (1991) reports the normal adult's airway resistance to range from 0.6 to 2.4 cm H_2O/l/sec. The standard inspiratory and expiratory flow rate during the test is .5 l/sec (500 ml/sec). This is to standardize air turbulence during the test. The usual components of airway resistance found in an adult are as follows:

Upper airway including the nose and mouth = 50%

Trachea and bronchi larger than 2 mm in diameter = 30%

Airways less than 2 mm in diameter = 20%

An increased airway resistance is abnormal. It will be most readily noticed if the problem is in the upper airway, trachea, or major bronchi because most resistance is normally found there. Patients with asthma, bronchitis, and emphysema have most of their resistance in the airways that are 2 mm or less in diameter. Because of this, significant disease must be present before a large enough airway resistance will be noticed to alert the therapist or physician to the problem. Fig. 3-15 B, C, and D show normal and increased expiratory resistance curves. Madama (1993) lists the following airway resistance values and their severity:

Raw (cm $H_2O/l/sec$)	*Severity*
2.8-4.5	mild
4.5-8	moderate
>8	severe

10. Diffusing capacity.
a. Recommend the procedure for additional data. (IA2o) [R, Ap, An]

The diffusing capacity (D_L or $D_{L\,CO}$) tests look at the capacity for carbon monoxide to diffuse through the lungs into the blood. This test is also known as the carbon monoxide transfer factor. Carbon monoxide is used because its high affinity for hemoglobin virtually eliminates blood as a barrier to diffusion. The measured value can then be correlated to the ability of oxygen to diffuse through the lungs. This test is indicated when it is important to know the extent of lung disability causing hypoxemia. This is most common with patients having emphysema, but it is also important in patients with fibrotic lung disease.

b. Perform the procedure for added data. (IC1k) [R, Ap, An]

At the time of this writing the single breath carbon monoxide diffusing capacity test ($D_{L\,CO}$ SB) is the only version that has a widely adopted standard technique for administration. The procedure is also known as the modified Krogh technique. It is recorded in milliliters of carbon monoxide (CO) per minute per millimeter of mercury at 0° C, 760 mm Hg, and dry (STPD).

The following are key steps in the procedure: A reservoir or spirometer is filled with a mix of .3% CO, 10% Helium (He), 21% O_2, and the balance of nitrogen (N_2) (see Fig. 3-18). The patient is connected to the apparatus and breathes room air while being instructed in the test. After the patient is told to exhale completely (to residual volume), the practitioner switches the patient to the gas mix. The patient is instructed to rapidly inhale an inspiratory vital capacity. A shutter automatically closes so that the patient cannot exhale for 10 seconds. This allows time for some of the carbon monoxide to diffuse into the patient's blood stream. After the breath hold the shutter opens and the patient is told to exhale to resting volume. The equipment is designed to automatically let 750 to 1000 ml of exhaled gas pass through to the spirometer. The next 500 ml of gas is diverted into the end-tidal gas sampler. This sample is then analyzed for He% and CO%. The remainder of the patient's exhaled volume is passed through into the spirometer. The various measured parameters are integrated into the equations in the computer to give the patient's $D_{L\,CO}$ SB value.

This test is only done after the patient has been measured for both residual volume and total lung capacity. That is because the patient's lung volume directly affects the diffusability of carbon monoxide.

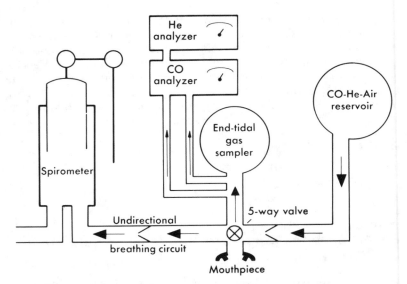

Fig. 3-18 Schematic drawing of the components and breathing circuit used when performing a single breath lung diffusion test ($D_{L\,CO}$SB). Analysis of the patient's exhaled helium (He) and carbon monoxide (CO) percentages is critical to the test. (From Ruppel G: *Manual of pulmonary function testing*, ed 6, St. Louis, 1994, Mosby–Year Book. Used by permission.)

c.   Interpret the results from the procedure. (IC1k) [R, Ap, An]

Interpretation will be limited to the results of the $D_{L\,CO}$ SB test. Ruppel (1991) reports the average resting normal adult $D_{L\,CO}$ SB as 25 ml CO/min/mm Hg STPD. (All diffusing capacity values are reported in standard temperature pressure dry conditions.) Gaensler and Wright (1966) report the following $D_{L\,CO}$ SB prediction equations with values in ml CO/min/mm Hg STPD:

Males: [(0.250 × height in inches) − (0.177 × age in years)] + 19.93

Females: [(0.284 × height in inches) − (0.177 × age in years)] + 7.72

It should be noted that a number of other authors have developed their own prediction equations. In general, patients who show $D_{L\,CO}$ SB results within ±20% of the predicted values (80% to 120% of predicted) are considered to be within normal limits. A patient who has actual results that are significantly below the predicted values has a problem with lung diffusion. Fig. 3-19 shows a number of common conditions that can lead to poor lung diffusion. The following factors should also be taken into consideration when interpreting the measured values:

a. Increased hematocrit and hemoglobin values result in an increased $D_{L\,CO}$ whereas decreased values result in a decreased $D_{L\,CO}$. An actual value should be used to calculate a patient's $D_{L\,CO}$.

b. An increased carboxyhemoglobin level will result in a decreased $D_{L\,CO}$ value. Patients who smoke should be instructed not to smoke from the night before the test so that the COHb level will drop to normal.

c. An increased alveolar carbon dioxide level results in a lowered alveolar oxygen level. This, in turn, results in an increased $D_{L\,CO}$ value. A decreased alveolar carbon dioxide level results in a decreased $D_{L\,CO}$ value.

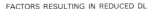
FACTORS RESULTING IN REDUCED DL

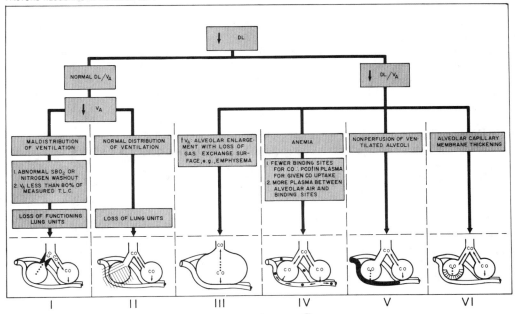

Fig. 3-19 Six factors that can cause a decreased lung diffusion. Factors I and II result in a decrease in D_L that is in proportion to the decrease in alveolar volume. Factors III, IV, V, and IV result in a decrease in D_L that is greater than the decrease in alveolar volume. Therefore these later conditions are more harmful to the patient's pulmonary function and well-being. (From Ayers LN, Whipp BJ, Ziment I: *A guide to the interpretation of pulmonary function tests,* ed 2, New York, 1978, Roerig. Used by permission.)

d. Increased altitude results in an increased $D_{L\,CO}$. This is probably only a concern if the patient is tested in a mountainous area.

e. An increased pulmonary capillary blood volume will result in an increased $D_{L\,CO}$.

f. The patient should breathe room air for at least 4 minutes before the test is repeated.

It is well known that diffusability is directly related to lung volume. This is the reason that African-Americans have lower diffusion rates than Caucasians. To eliminate this as a factor in interpreting the D_L value, it is necessary to divide the diffusion value by the total lung capacity. African-Americans have the same normal values as Caucasians when this calculation is performed.

Module E.   Pulmonary Function Equipment.

1.   Pressure transducers.
a.   Get the necessary equipment for the procedure. (IIA1h) [R, Ap]

Pressure transducers are used in the body plethysmograph for measuring mouth pressure and chamber pressure. They come with the unit and are supplied by the manufacturer. Another type of transducer would be used with an esophageal balloon when performing a lung compliance measurement. Follow the balloon manufacturer's recommendations for the proper transducer.

b. Fix any problems with the equipment. (IIB2k1) [R, Ap]

All these different types of pressure transducers must be able to keep an airtight seal for an accurate reading to be measured. The most common way to confirm a transducer's accuracy is to compare it to a water or mercury manometer. When pressure is applied both to the manometer and transducer they should read identically. Any leakage will cause the measured transducer values to be lower than the manometer values. Tighten any loose connections with the transducer or any patient connections to stop the air leak.

2. Pneumotachometer respirometers.
a. Get the necessary equipment for the procedure. (IIA1i1) [R, Ap]
b. Put the equipment together, make sure that it works properly, and identify any problems with it. (IIB1j1) [R, Ap]

All pneumotachometers convert one type of physical information or signal to another. Two common types are discussed next. Either type should be acceptable for performing bedside spirometry. Make sure that the unit you select is capable of performing the ordered test. Be sure that you select a unit that is capable of printing out a hard copy of the patient's test results and spirometry tracings if they are required for the chart.

Differential-Pressure Pneumotachometer

Some articles refer to a differential pressure pneumotachometer as a Fleisch-type device. These units have a resistive element (tubes or mesh screen) in the flow tube. The faster the flow of gas through the flow tube the greater the pressure difference there is before and after the resistance. Hoses connect the flow tubes before and after the resistive element to the differential pressure transducer. The transducer converts this pressure difference into an electrical difference. A microprocessor calculates the various patient values from this information (see Fig. 3-20).

Assembly requires the addition of the patient's mouthpiece to the inspiratory port so that there is no air leak. The expiratory port should be kept completely open so that the only obstruction to the patient's air flow is from the resistive element. A volume calibration check is performed by forcing a known amount of air from a super-syringe (certified-volume standard syringe) through the pneumotachometer. Minimally, several repetitions of a known 3-l volume should reveal identical measured volumes. As long as the measured volumes are within ±3% or 50 ml (whichever is less) the unit is acceptably accurate. Common problems with accuracy include an air leak around the mouthpiece, cracked, disconnected, or obstructed pressure relaying hoses, water condensation or mucus on the resistive element, or obstructed upstream or downstream port. The resistive element is usually heated to minimize any condensation.

Heat-Transfer Pneumotachometer

Some articles refer to a heat-transfer pneumotachometer as a thermister-type device or hot wire anemometer. These units have a heated thermister that is cooled as the gas flows past it. The temperature transducer automatically increases and measures the flow of electricity to the thermister to keep it at the required temperature. A microprocessor calculates the various patient values from this information.

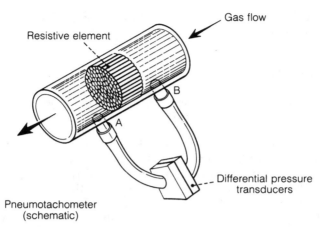

Fig. 3-20 Cutaway view of a differential pressure pneumotachometer. Flow is measured as the pressure drops between A and B, which are ports leading to a differential pressure transducer. The resistive element may consist of a mesh screen, a network of parallel capillary tubes, or other devices. (From Beauchamp RK: Pulmonary function testing procedures. In Barnes TA, editor: *Respiratory care practice,* Chicago, 1988, Year Book Medical. Used by permission.)

The earlier discussion on assembly, calibration, and trouble shooting applies to the heat-transfer–type pneumotachometers except that there are no pressure relaying hoses (see Fig. 3-21).

3. Positive-displacement respirometers.
  a. **Get the necessary equipment for the procedure. (IIA1i2) [R, Ap]**
  b. **Put the equipment together, make sure that it works properly, and identify any problems with it. (IIB1j2) [R, Ap]**

Positive-displacement respirometers are mechanical devices. They are called positive-displacement respirometers because the patient's exhaled gas fills and moves a sealed bell or accordion-like bellows. These systems are self-contained and sealed rather than being open to room air as the other devices. They are the standard in most pulmonary function testing laboratories because they can have residual volume and lung diffusion test hardware added on. There are three general

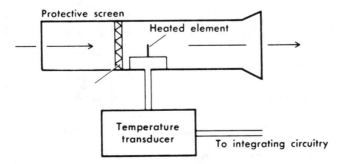

Fig. 3-21 Cutaway view of a heat-transfer pneumotachometer. (From Ruppel G: *Manual of pulmonary function testing,* ed 5, St. Louis, 1991, Mosby–Year Book. Used by permission.)

catagories that are discussed here: water-seal spirometers, dry-rolling–seal spirometers, and wedge-type spirometers.

Water-Seal Spirometers

Water-seal spirometers are the commonly found chain-compensated and Stead-Wells units made by Warren E. Collins, Inc. (see Fig. 3-22 for the cutaway appearance of the chain-compensated type). The bell lowers and rises as the patient breathes in and out. A pulley system attached to the bell and the marking pens permit the recording of the patient's efforts on the rotating kymograph paper. Note that the tracing is inverted from the patient's actual breathing effort. The Stead-Wells units have the marking pen attached directly to the bell, therefore the tracing directly shows the patient's breathing efforts (see Fig. 3-23). The newer chain-compensated and Stead-Wells units also have microprocessors for calculating patient information.

Gas analyzers for helium, nitrogen, carbon monoxide, and other extra equipment can be added for residual volume and lung diffusion measurements. The carbon dioxide absorber should be left out of the breathing circuit for forced vital capacity tests because it will interfere with the fast flow of gas; however, it must be put in line for any testing that will last more than 15 seconds and involves breathing repeatedly into the closed system. Supplemental oxygen must be added to the circuit for any tests that require the patient to breathe repeatedly from the closed system. Take the opportunity to work with one of these units if at all possible. The following is a checklist for set-up and where to look when problem solving:

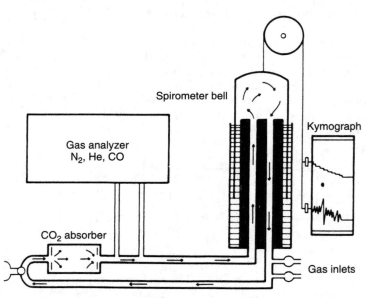

Fig. 3-22 Cutaway view of a chain-compensated water-seal spirometer. (From Ruppel G: *Manual of pulmonary function testing,* ed 5, St. Louis, 1991, Mosby–Year Book. Used by permission.)

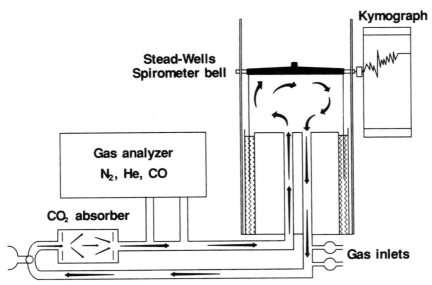

Fig. 3-23 Cutaway view of a Stead-Wells water-seal spirometer. (Courtesy Warren E. Collins, Inc, Braintree, Mass.)

a. Make sure the water level is correct—not too high or too low.

b. Use a 7-l bell for children and a 14-l bell for adults.

c. Make sure all circuit tubing and one-way valve connections are tight.

d. Check the following kymograph features: paper on correctly; pens contain ink; kymograph speeds are adjustable to 32, 160, and 1920 mm/sec.

e. The carbon dioxide absorber should be out of the circuit for FVC tests; it should be in the circuit for residual volume and lung diffusion tests.

f. Oxygen should be added to the system for residual volume and lung diffusion tests.

g. Make sure the various gas analyzers are calibrated properly.

h. As discussed earlier, do not be confused by the various ways the tracing is presented. Always find the start of the FVC by the near vertical slope of the tracing.

Dry-Rolling–Seal Spirometers

Dry-rolling–seal spirometers are sometimes called piston spirometers. As can be seen in Fig. 3-24, these units use a flexible silastic or teflon-coated rubber seal instead of water. The large volume piston moves in and out as the patient breathes. The patient's efforts can be directly recorded by pen on paper. Newer units also have microprocessors for calculating the information. Manufacturers include OHIO Medical Products and SRL.

They are still rather large and are best suited for the pulmonary function laboratory. These units can also be outfitted with a carbon dioxide absorber and various gas analyzers. So, they too, can be used for the full range of lung function tests. The previous checklist for set-up and problem-solving ideas would apply here except for those items that are specific to the chain-compensated and Stead-Wells systems.

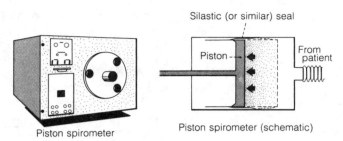

Fig. 3-24 Outside and cutaway views of a dry-rolling–seal or piston spirometer. (From Beauchamp RK: Pulmonary function testing procedures. In Barnes TA, editor: *Respiratory care practice*, Chicago, 1988, Year Book Medical. Used by permission.)

Wedge-Type Spirometers

Wedge-type spirometers are sometimes called bellows spirometers (see Fig. 3-25). Note that these units have plastic or rubber bellows that are fixed on one side and are accordion-like flexible on other sides. The bellows move in and out as the patient breathes. The patient's efforts can be directly recorded by pen on paper. Newer units also have microprocessors for calculating the information. Vitalor and Med Science are manufacturers.

All the earlier information on the dry-rolling–seal spirometers applies here except what is specific to those units. The same set-up and problem-solving ideas apply here also.

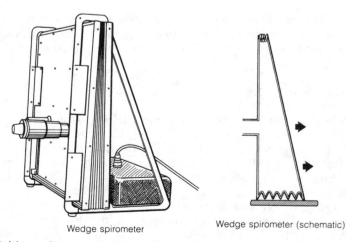

Fig. 3-25 Outside and cutaway views of a wedge-type spirometer. (From Beauchamp RK: Pulmonary function testing procedures. In Barnes TA, editor: *Respiratory care practice,* Chicago, 1988, Year Book Medical. Used by permission.)

4. Perform quality control procedures on pulmonary function equipment. (IIB3a) [R, Ap, An]

Spirometry Equipment

The positive-displacement respirometers should have the following quality control procedures performed on a regular basis:

a. A super-syringe with at least a 3-l capacity should be pumped repeatedly into and out of the unit. A reading that is accurate to within ± 3% or ± 50 ml must be measured. The flow rates should be varied to ensure that they do not have any influence on the measured volumes. It is recommended that 1- and 2-l volumes also be pumped into the unit to check for linearity.

b. To check for leaks in the circuit perform the following:

1. Pump a 3-l volume into the bellows.
2. Close the mouthpiece to atmosphere to seal the circuit.
3. Add a weight to the bell to speed up any small leaks.
4. Turn on the kymograph at a slow speed and put the pen on the paper to record any drop in volume.
5. If a leak is noted it must be discovered and sealed.

c. Turn on the kymograph to its various speeds and check its accuracy with a stopwatch. The manufacturer's literature should tell how far the kymograph will travel at its set speeds.

d. The thermometer reading should be compared to that of a laboratory quality unit.

Replace or repair any component that fails to meet the manufacturer's or established American Thoracic Society-American College of Chest Physicians (ATS-ACCP) standards.

Nitrogen Washout Equipment for Measuring Functional Residual Capacity

See Fig. 3-13 for the basic set up and breathing circuit of a nitrogen washout system. Review the troubleshooting of positive-displacement spirometers; they are used with the nitrogen washout procedure to find the functional residual capacity. The nitrogen washout type residual volume test uses an emission spectroscopy ionization chamber analyzer for nitrogen. It is more commonly called a Giesler tube ionizer. It employs a vacuum pump to draw a gas sample into the ionization chamber. The intensity of the light spectrum given off by the ionized nitrogen directly relates to its percentage in the sample. A two-point calibration check should be performed at least every 6 months to check for linearity. It involves the following steps:

1. Draw a room air sample into the unit and check the nitrogen meter reading. It should read about 78% nitrogen.
2. Adjust the meter reading, if necessary, to the manufacturer's specified value.
3. Turn off the needle valve so that no air can be drawn into the unit.
4. Check to see that the nitrogen meter reading drops to 0% nitrogen as the vacuum pump removes all gas from the ionization chamber.

Linearity (three-point calibration) can be checked by introducing from 5% to 10% nitrogen into the unit to see if the nitrogen meter measures that value. Do not use an analyzer that is inaccurate.

Helium Dilution Equipment for Measuring Functional Residual Capacity

See Fig. 3-10 for the basic set up of the helium dilution equipment and breathing circuit. Again, review the troubleshooting of positive-displacement spirometers; they are used with the helium dilution procedure to find the functional residual capacity. Both the helium dilution FRC test and the lung diffusion tests require the analysis of helium in the gas mixture. A thermal conductivity analyzer is typically used. It operates under the principal of a Wheatstone bridge, where differences in gas density lead to different cooling rates of heated thermister beads. The different rates of cooling change electrical resistances and cause different electrical currents to flow. In a helium analyzer, the greater the helium concentration there is the faster the thermister bead cools and the more electricity flows through the circuit. This is then read off a meter as the helium percentage.

The thermal conductivity helium analyzer should be linear over the clinically used range of helium to an accuracy of ± .2% He. Minimally a two-point calibration should be performed. A room air sample can be drawn into the analyzer and should read 0% helium. A known helium concentration may then be added and analyzed, for example, heliox, which contains 80% helium and 20% oxygen. A third point can be checked if needed by analyzing another known helium percentage.

Body Plethysmography

The plethysmograph chamber must be airtight when the door is closed and all vents are closed. This can be confirmed by attaching a pressure manometer to a chamber port and applying a known volume or pressure into the sealed chamber. The pressures should be identical between the chamber pressure gauges and outside pressure manometer. The differential-pressure pneumotachometer must also read accurately when a known volume is pumped through it. Most manufacturers will have a series of calibration check procedures listed in the equipment literature.

Module F.   Patient Assessment.

1.   Examine all the data to determine the patient's pathophysiological condition. (IC3a) [R, Ap, An]

Even though a physician must legally determine the patient's diagnosis, a therapist must be able to understand the etiology, pathophysiology, diagnosis, treatment, and prognosis for patients with cardiopulmonary disorders. Interpretation of patient data that is tested by the NBRC was discussed earlier. The following is a brief categorization of the conditions that may be diagnosed by pulmonary function testing.

Obstructive Airways Disease

The patient with severe obstructive lung disease will show low gas flow at all time intervals. However, a decreased FEV_3 and the $FEF_{25\%-75\%}$ are early markers of small airways disease. Quite commonly the residual volume is increased due to air trapping. This increases the functional residual capacity and often the total lung capacity. Examples of conditions that cause obstructive lung disease include asthma, emphysema, bronchitis, and bronchiolitis. Excessive mucus, foreign body, and airway tumor will also cause bronchospasm and air trapping.

Restrictive Lung Disease

In restrictive lung disease, all lung volumes and capacities are reduced and lung diffusion is reduced. Expiratory flows such as FEV_1 are increased. Examples of conditions that cause restrictive lung disease include fibrosis, pulmonary edema, hemothorax or pneumothorax, adult or infant respiratory distress syndrome, chest wall deformities, obesity, and various neuromuscular disorders.

2. Participate in the development of the patient's respiratory care plan. (IC3c) [An]

Obviously the patient's care plan depends on the diagnosis and the degree of limitation of the patient. If the patient has reversible small airways disease, he or she should be counseled to stop smoking and avoid all airborne irritants. Inhaled and/or parenteral bronchodilators should be prescribed to relax the airways as much as possible.

If the patient has restrictive lung disease, he or she should also be counseled to avoid any airborne irritants. Whether any medications or other procedures can be performed to offer some relief depends on the specific cause of the patient's disorder.

BIBLIOGRAPHY

AARC Clinical Practice Guideline: Spirometry, *Respir Care* 36(12):1414-1417, 1991.

AARC Clinical Practice Guideline: Single-breath carbon monoxide diffusing capacity, *Respir Care* 38(5):511-515, 1993.

AARC Clinical Practice Guideline: Static lung volumes, *Respir Care* 39(8):830-836, 1994.

American Thoracic Society: Standardization of spirometry: 1987 update, *Am Rev Respir Dis* 136:1285-1298, 1987.

Askanazi J, Weissman C, Rosenbaum SH et al: Nutrition and the respiratory system. *Crit Care Med* 10(3):163-172, 1982.

Ayers LN, Whipp BJ, Ziment I: *A guide to the interpretation of pulmonary function tests*, ed 2, New York, 1978, Roerig.

Bates DV, Macklem PT, Christie RV: *Respiratory function in disease*, ed 2, Philadelphia, 1971, WB Saunders.

Beauchamp RK: Pulmonary function testing procedures. In Barnes TA, editor: *Respiratory care practice*, Chicago, 1988, Year Book Medical.

Black LF, Hyatt RE: Maximal respiratory pressures: normal values and relationship to age and sex, *Am Rev Respir Dis* 99:696-702, 1969.

Branson RD, Hurst JM: Nutrition and respiratory function: food for thought, *Respir Care* 33(2):89-92, 1988.

Branson RD, Hurst JM, Davis K Jr, et al: Measurement of maximal inspiratory pressure: a comparison of three methods, *Respir Care* 34(9):789-794, 1989.

Buist SA, Ross BB: Predicted values for closing volumes using a modified single-breath nitrogen test, *Am Rev Respir Dis* 111:405, 1975.

Cherniack RM: *Pulmonary function testing,* Philadelphia, 1977, WB Saunders.

Cherniack RM: *Pulmonary function testing,* ed 2, Philadelphia, 1992, WB Saunders.

Cherniack RM, Raber MD: Normal standards for ventilatory function using an automated wedge spirometer, *Am Rev Respir Dis* 106:38, 1972.

Clausen JL: Maximal inspiratory and expiratory pressures. In Clausen JL, editor: *Pulmonary function testing guidelines and controversies,* Orlando, 1984, Grune & Stratton.

Clausen JL: Clinical interpretation of pulmonary function test, *Respir Care* 34(7):638-650, 1989.

Clausen JL, editor: *Pulmonary function testing guidelines and controversies,* Orlando, 1984, Grune & Stratton.

Crapo RO: Reference values for lung function tests, *Respir Care* 34(7):626-637, 1989.

Epstein J, Gaines J: *Clinical respiratory care of the adult patient,* Bowie, Md, 1983, Robert J. Brady.

Gaensler EA, Wright GW: Evaluation of respiratory impairment, *Arch Environ Health,* 12:146, 1966.

Gardner RM: Pulmonary function laboratory standards, *Respir Care* 34(7):651-660, July 1989.

Gold PM: Single-breath nitrogen test: closing volume and distribution of ventilation. In Clausen JL, editor: *Pulmonary function testing guidelines and controversies,* Orlando, 1984, Grune & Stratton.

Goldman HI, Becklake MR: Respiratory function tests: normal values at median altitudes and the prediction of normal results, *Am Rev Tuberculosis* 79:457, 1959.

Hansen JE: Exercise testing. In Clausen JL, editor: *Pulmonary function testing guidelines and controversies,* Orlando, 1984, Grune & Stratton.

Hess D: Measurement of maximal inspiratory pressure: a call for standardization, *Respir Care* 34:857-859, 1989.

Jalowayski AA, Dawson A: Measurement of lung volume: the multiple breath nitrogen method. In Clausen JL, editor: *Pulmonary function testing guidelines and controversies,* Orlando, 1984, Grune & Stratton.

Jones NL et al: *Clinical exercise testing,* ed 2, Philadelphia, 1983, WB Saunders.

Kacmarek RM, Cycyk-Chapman MC, Young-Palazzo PJ et al: Determination of maximal inspiratory pressure: a clinical study and literature review, *Respir Care* 34:868-878, 1989.

Knudson RJ, Lebowitz MD, Holberg CJ et al: Changes in the normal maximal expiratory flow-volume curve with growth and aging, *Am Rev Respir Dis* 127:725-734, 1983.

Knudson RJ, Kaltenborn WT, Knudson DE et al: The single-breath carbon monoxide diffusing capacity, *Am Rev Respir Dis* 135:805-811, 1987.

Kory RC, Callahan R, Syner JC: The Veterans Administration-Army cooperative study of pulmonary function. I. Clinical spirometry in normal men, *Am J Med* 30:243, 1961.

Krider TM, Meyer R, Syvertsen WA: *Master guide for passing the respiratory care credentialing exam,* ed 2, Clarement, Calif, 1989, Education Resource Consortium.

Lough MD: Pulmonary responses to exercise, *Respir Care* 34(6):517-523, 1989.

MacIntyre NR: Diffusing capacity of the lung for carbon monoxide, *Respir Care* 34(6):489-499, 1989.

Madama VC: *Pulmonary function testing and cardiopulmonary stress testing,* Albany, NY, 1993, Delmar.

Morris JF, Koski A, Johnson LC: Spirometric standards for healthy nonsmoking adults, *Am Rev Respir Dis* 103:57, 1971.

Neu J, Szidon JP: Exercise testing in pulmonary patients, *Choices in Respiratory Management* 21(3):64-70, 1991.

Paoletti P, Viegi G, Pistelli G et al: Reference equations for the single-breath diffusing capacity, *Am Rev Respir Dis* 132:806-813, 1985.

Ruppel G: *Manual of pulmonary function testing*, ed 5, St. Louis, 1991, Mosby-Year Book.

Sills JR: *Respiratory care certification guide*, St. Louis, 1991, Mosby–Year Book.

Single breath carbon monoxide diffusing capacity (transfer factor): recommendations for a standard technique, *Am Rev Respir Dis* 136:1299-1307, 1987.

Snow MG: Determination of functional residual capacity, *Respir Care* 34(7):586-596, 1989.

Sue D: Exercise testing and the patient with cardiopulmonary disease. In Goldman AL, editor: *Problems in Pulmonary Disease* 2(1):1-7, Spring 1986.

Van Kessel AL: Pulmonary diffusing capacity for carbon monoxide. In Clausen JL, editor: *Pulmonary function testing guidelines and controversies*, Orlando, 1984, Grune & Stratton.

Wasserman K: Breathing during exercise, *N Engl J Med* 298(14):780-785, 1978.

Zamel N, Altose MD, Speir WA: Statement on spirometry, *Chest* 3:547-550, 1983.

Zarins LP, Clausen JL: Body plethysmography. In Clausen JL, editor: *Pulmonary function testing guidelines and controversies*, Orlando, 1984, Grune & Stratton.

SELF-STUDY QUESTIONS

1. Which of the following statements are true of the Maximum Expiratory Pressure (MEP) test?
    - I. −20 to −25 cm water is usually adequate
    - II. +20 to +25 cm water is usually adequate
    - III. +40 cm water is usually adequate
    - IV. It is a good indicator of the patient's ability to cough.
    - V. The patient should hold the effort for 1 to 3 seconds.
    - A. I
    - B. II
    - C. III, IV
    - D. III
    - E. III, IV, V

2. The predicted forced vital capacity (FVC) value for African-Americans is:
    - A. 11% larger than Caucasians
    - B. The same as Caucasians
    - C. 11% less than Caucasians
    - D. 20% to 25% less than Caucasians
    - E. The same as Asians

3. An order is received to perform the following bedside spirometry tests on a patient: tidal volume, FVC, and peak flow. Which device would you take with you to perform the tests?
    - A. Stead-Wells water-seal spirometer
    - B. Dry-rolling–seal spirometer
    - C. Differential pressure pneumotachometer
    - D. Vane-type respirometer
    - E. Bourns/Bear LS-75 electronic respirometer

4. Which of the following test results are needed to calculate total lung capacity (TLC)?
    - I. Functional residual capacity (FRC)
    - II. Residual volume (RV)
    - III. Tidal volume
    - IV. Expiratory reserve volume (ERV)
    - V. Inspiratory capacity (IC)

VI. Vital Capacity (VC)
  A. I and III
  B. II and VI
  C. I and VI
  D. II and V
  E. I and V or II and VI

5. A normal maximal expiratory flow-volume (MEFV) loop test would show:
  A. $FEF_{50\%}$ less than $FIF_{50\%}$
  B. $FEF_{50\%}$ equal to $FIF_{50\%}$
  C. $FEF_{50\%}$ greater than $FIF_{50\%}$
  D. It varies unpredictably in a normal subject.

6. Patient flow rates should be reported at:
  A. ATPS
  B. BTPS
  C. STPD
  D. ATPD
  E. BTPD

7. Your patient is performing a residual volume test on a Collins system in the pulmonary function laboratory. After breathing on the system for 1 minute he takes out the mouthpiece and complains of being short of breath. What is the most likely problem in the pulmonary function system?
  A. The one-way valve was turned the wrong way.
  B. There is too much water around the spirometer bell.
  C. The carbon dioxide absorber has been left out of the circuit.
  D. Nose clips were left off of the patient.
  E. The carbon dioxide absorber was accidentally left in the circuit.

8. Which of the following studies would produce the most accurate determination of the TLC in a patient with severe emphysema?
  A. Helium dilution
  B. Single-breath nitrogen washout
  C. Seven-minute nitrogen washout
  D. Single-breath oxygen dilution
  E. Body plethysmography

9. A patient has been scheduled for a battery of pulmonary function tests. He tells you that he is so nervous about the testing that he has smoked four cigarettes in the last 2 hours. Which of the following tests is most likely to be adversely affected by this?
  A. Functional residual capacity
  B. Forced vital capacity
  C. Airway resistance
  D. Lung diffusion

10. Before having a patient do a forced vital capacity test, the water-sealed spirometer should have all the following done EXCEPT:
  A. Make sure that the circuit is airtight.
  B. Place a carbon dioxide absorbing material in line with the circuit.
  C. Pump a 3-l volume into and out of the circuit to check for leaks.
  D. Check the kymograph speeds.

11. A properly performed FVC test will not have
  I. Any coughing or leaks

II.   A weak patient effort
III. An unsatisfactory start to the test
IV.   Excessive variability among test results
A.   I, II
B.   II, III
C.   I, II, IV
D.   I, II, III, IV
E.   II, IV

12.   To help in the diagnosis of asthma you would recommend all the following tests EXCEPT:
A.   Diffusion study
B.   Flow-volume loop
C.   Before and after bronchodilator study
D.   Airway resistance

13.   A patient has just been tested for lung-thoracic compliance in a body plethysmograph. Her compliance was determined to be .2 l (200 ml)/cm water. Based on this, she most likely has:
A.   Asthma
B.   Pulmonary fibrosis
C.   Emphysema
D.   Normal lungs

14.   Based on the flow-volume loops that are shown here, which one represents the most severe small airways obstruction?

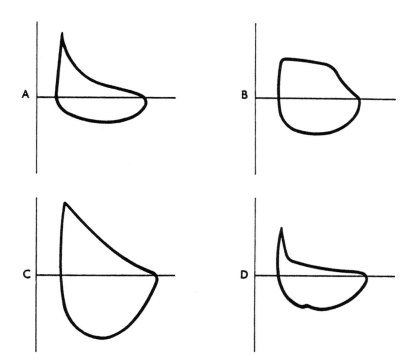

(From Ruppel G: *Manual of pulmonary function testing,* ed 5, St. Louis, 1991, Mosby–Year Book. Used by permission.)

15.   Based on the flow-volume loops that are shown in question 14, which one represents the fixed extrathoracic obstruction?
    A.   Tracing A
    B.   Tracing B
    C.   Tracing C
    D.   Tracing D

Answer Key

1. E; 2. C; 3. C; 4. E; 5. A; 6. B; 7. C; 8. E; 9. D; 10. B; 11. D; 12. A; 13. C; 14. D; 15. B.

4

Advanced Cardiopulmonary Monitoring

Module A. Cardiopulmonary monitoring procedures.

1. Capnography (exhaled CO$_2$ monitoring).
   a. Review capnography data in the patient's chart. (IA1d3) [R]

Capnography is the analysis of graphic and numerical data showing the amount and pattern of exhaled carbon dioxide (CO$_2$). It is wise to look for previous capnography data before measuring the patient's exhaled CO$_2$ level again. Look for numerical values as well as a printout of the tracing of exhaled CO$_2$. Be prepared to compare the previous information with the new data to help evaluate the patient's condition.

   b. Perform the bedside procedure. (IB8e) [R, Ap, An]

The capnometer is a device that measures the concentration of CO$_2$ in a gas sample (usually taken from a patient). Its principle of operation is based on carbon dioxide's absorption of infrared light in a narrow wavelength band (4.3 μ). Infrared light at this wavelength is passed through the gas sample to a receiving unit. The difference between what is sent out and what is received is directly related to how much carbon dioxide is in the gas sample. In other words, the greater the difference between the sent and received infrared light, the greater the concentration of carbon dioxide in the gas sample.

The capnometer is calibrated by drawing a room air sample into it followed by a gas sample containing a known amount of carbon dioxide. Because there is virtually no carbon dioxide in room air, the capnometer should give you a "zero" reading. Adjust the calibration control to zero as needed. The second sample contains a known amount of carbon dioxide, usually 5% to 10%. The capnometer should read out a CO$_2$ level that matches the amount in the known calibration gas. Adjust the calibration control as necessary. The carbon dioxide level can be read as a percent or fraction (F_ACO_2) or as partial pressure (P_ACO_2).

The capnograph is a strip chart recorder that provides a copy of the patient's exhaled carbon dioxide curve. There are at least two paper speeds that are useful for different purposes. The fast speed is most useful for evaluating sudden changes in the patient's condition. Each individual breath is easily seen (see Fig. 4-1). The slow speed is most useful for trend monitoring (see Fig. 4-2).

There are two different gas sampling methods: mainstream and sidestream. The mainstream method involves having the infrared sensing unit at the airway; usually it is attached directly to the endotracheal/tracheostomy tube. If the patient is on a ventilator, the sampling adapter must be placed between the endotracheal

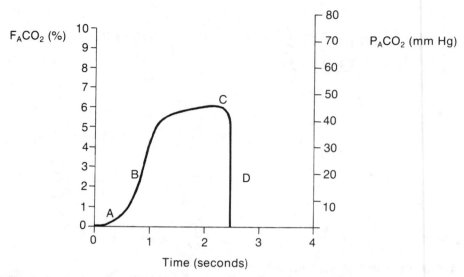

Fig. 4-1 Normal capnograph tracing taken at a fast speed. The percentage of exhaled alveolar CO_2 is shown on the left vertical scale as F_ACO_2. The partial pressure of exhaled alveolar CO_2 is shown on the right vertical scale as P_ACO_2. The tracing of exhaled gas can be divided into these four components: A, the beginning of exhalation, which shows no carbon dioxide in the upper airway anatomic dead space; B, the addition of alveolar gas, rich in carbon dioxide, to the anatomic dead space gas causes a rapid rise in measured CO_2; C, pure alveolar gas with a stable amount of CO_2 causes a plateau—the end-tidal CO_2 point is shown at C just before inspiration; and D, inspiration with a rapid drop in carbon dioxide to zero. A fast-speed tracing is more useful for determining the cause of a patient's changing condition than a slow-speed tracing.

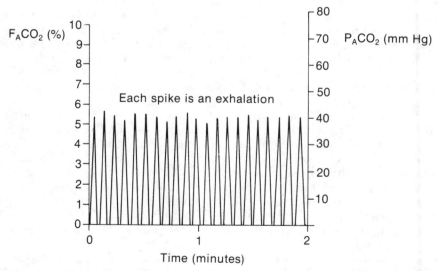

Fig. 4-2 Normal capnograph tracing taken at a slow speed. The percentage of exhaled alveolar CO_2 is shown on the left vertical scale as F_ACO_2. The partial pressure of exhaled alveolar CO_2 is shown on the right vertical scale as P_ACO_2. The slow speed results in a blending of parts A, B, and C of the fast-speed tracing (Fig. 4-1). Each spike is part C of the curve and marks an exhalation. A slow-speed tracing is more useful in trend monitoring of a patient than a fast-speed tracing.

tube and the ventilator circuit (with or without mechanical dead space). All inspired and expired gas passes through the sensor (see Fig. 4-3).

The sidestream method employs a capillary tube placed so that a small sampling of the patient's exhaled gas can be drawn into the capnometer for analysis. It is not necessary for the patient's entire breath to pass through the sampling adapter; therefore it can be used in an unintubated patient by taping the sampling catheter a short distance into a nare. If the patient is on a ventilator, the sampling adapter must be placed between the endotracheal tube and the ventilator circuit (with or without mechanical dead space). Remember that the patient's exhaled tidal volume and minute volume will be reduced by the amount that is drawn into the capnometer (see Fig. 4-4).

c.   Interpret the results from the procedure. (IB8e and IIIA1r5) [R, Ap, An]

As mentioned earlier, capnography is the analysis of graphic and numerical data showing the amount and pattern of exhaled carbon dioxide. Table 4-1 lists normal values and Fig. 4-5 shows the normal physiology behind capnography. Three factors influence capnography's use and the interpretation of the results. First is the patient's metabolism. The average resting adult produces about 200 ml of carbon dioxide per minute. Fever and exercise will increase this value. Hypothermia, sleep, and sedation will decrease the production of CO_2.

Second is the patient's cardiac output; this is not a major factor. Sepsis, which might double a patient's cardiac output, will only reduce the PCO_2 a few mm Hg. Cardiogenic shock, which will reduce the cardiac output, will only raise the PCO_2 a few mm Hg.

Third, and most important, is alveolar ventilation. A doubling of alveolar ventilation, under steady-state conditions for carbon dioxide production, will result in a halving of the PCO_2 in arterial blood and alveolar gas. However, a reduction of

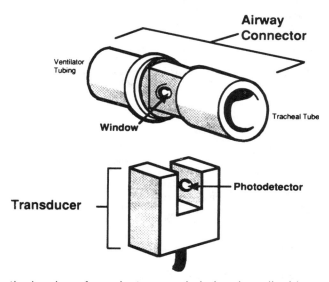

Fig. 4-3 Schematic drawing of a mainstream exhaled carbon dioxide analyzer sensor. The infrared sensor is attached to the patient's airway so that all of the exhaled and inhaled gas passes through it. (From Szaflarski NL, Cohen NH: Use of capnography in critically ill patients, *Heart Lung* 20:363-374, 1991. Used by permission.)

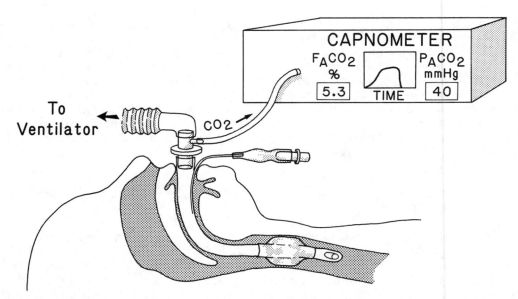

Fig. 4-4 Representation of a sidestream capnometry system. A capillary tube is placed into the ventilator circuit to sample the exhaled and inhaled gases.

alveolar ventilation to half of its previous level will result in the $PaCO_2$ and P_ACO_2 being doubled (see Fig. 4-6).

A number of factors influence alveolar ventilation. Tidal volume and respiratory rate are the most obvious and are directly related to alveolar ventilation. Of the two, tidal volume is more important because it relates to the patient's dead space to tidal volume ratio (V_D/V_T ratio). A decrease in the patient's tidal volume, without a corresponding decrease in the dead space, will result in less alveolar ventilation and a rise in PCO_2. Conversely, an increase in the tidal volume, without a corresponding increase in the dead space, will result in more alveolar ventilation and a drop in the PCO_2.

Capnography is most accurate and correlates best with the $PaCO_2$ if the patient's ventilation and perfusion match. The more ventilation and perfusion mismatching there is, or the more unstable the pulmonary perfusion is, the wider or less reliable

Table 4-1. Normal Blood Gas and Capnography Values (Based on a sea level barometric pressure of 760 mm Hg)

$PaCO_2$ is approximately 40 mm Hg.
$P\overline{v}CO_2$ is approximately 46 mm Hg.
P_ACO_2 ranges from approximately 40 to 46 mm Hg with the breathing cycle. This shows the carbon dioxide level varying between the arterial and mixed venous blood levels.
(end-tidal) P_ACO_2 ranges from 40 to 46 mm Hg and correlates with the $PaCO_2$.
(end-tidal) F_ACO_2 is approximately 5.3% to 6.1% and correlates with the $PaCO_2$.

Both P_ACO_2 and F_ACO_2 may be seen listed in the literature as end-tidal CO_2. End-tidal CO_2 may be seen in the literature abbreviated as ET CO_2, et CO_2, or Pet CO_2.

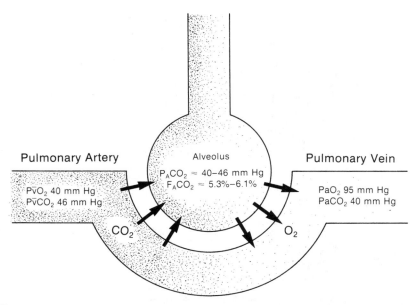

Fig. 4-5 Representation of the alveolar-capillary membrane showing the diffusion of oxygen and carbon dioxide and the arterialization of venous blood. Also shown are alveolar CO_2 values measured by capnography.

the gradient between the patient's arterial carbon dioxide and alveolar carbon dioxide levels.

d. Calculate and interpret the end-tidal alveolar-arterial carbon dioxide gradient (ET A-aCO_a).

The end-tidal alveolar-arterial carbon dioxide gradient is useful because once it is reliably determined, the patient's ventilatory condition can be monitored by capnography alone. There is no need to draw an arterial blood sample to measure the $PaCO_2$ level if the patient is stable.

The normal gradient is 6 mm Hg or less; however, most patients using capnography will not be normal. The possible gradient ranges from -6 to $+20$ mm Hg in unstable patients with cardiopulmonary abnormalities. For example, the patient who is breathing shallowly may have an end-tidal CO_2 that is less than the arterial CO_2. This is because the patient is not exhaling completely to empty alveolar gas. Therefore it is important to determine each patient's own gradient.

Procedure:

1. Simultaneously draw an arterial blood gas sample for $PaCO_2$ measurement and take an end-tidal gas sample for P_ACO_2 measurement.
2. The difference is the ET A-aCO_2 gradient. Most commonly the alveolar sample will show a higher carbon dioxide level than the arterial sample.

Example 1

A patient is seen in the recovery room after surgery and has the following PCO_2 levels:

$$
\begin{aligned}
P_ACO_2 &= 46 \text{ mm Hg} \\
PaCO_2 &= \underline{-40 \text{ mm Hg}} \\
\text{ET A-a } CO_2 &= 6 \text{ mm Hg}
\end{aligned}
$$

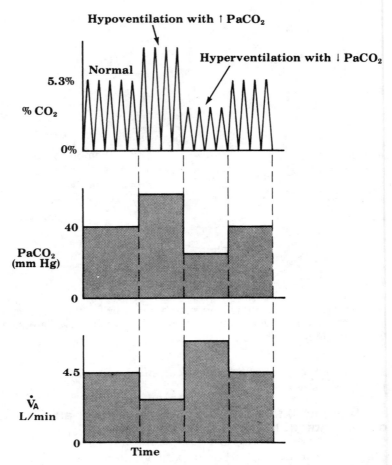

Fig. 4-6 Relationship between alveolar ventilation, $PaCO_2$, and exhaled CO_2 percent. (From Pilbeam SP: *Mechanical ventilation: physiological and clinical applications,* St. Louis, 1986, Multi-Media Publishing. Used by permission.)

The usefulness of this gradient will be seen when monitoring the patient's spontaneous breathing during weaning or making ventilator changes in the tidal volume and/or minute volume. It may be possible to avoid drawing as many arterial blood gas samples.

Example 2

The patient in Example 1 is seen later and has the following capnography reading: $P_ACO_2 = 56$ mm Hg. The patient's $PaCO_2$ can be easily calculated by subtraction:

$$
\begin{aligned}
P_ACO_2 &= 56 \text{ mm Hg} \\
\text{ET A-a } CO_2 \text{ gradient} &= \underline{-6 \text{ mm Hg}} \\
\text{estimated } PaCO_2 &= 50 \text{ mm Hg}
\end{aligned}
$$

It could be concluded that the patient is not breathing as deeply as before. Appropriate action should be taken to awaken the patient, further reverse the anesthesia, or begin artificial ventilation.

Review the components of a fast-speed capnography tracing in Fig. 4-1 to understand a normal person's expiratory pattern. Fig. 4-7 shows eight different abnormal fast-speed capnography tracings. See the figure legend for an explanation of each problem. As the patient returns to normal the tracing should approach that shown in Fig. 4-1.

e. Calculate and interpret the residual volume alveolar-arterial carbon dioxide gradient (RV A-a CO_2).

If the patient is cooperative and will exhale maximally to residual volume, this measurement will provide more clinically useful information. The usual RV A-a CO_2 gradient in a normal person is less than 7 mm Hg. The wider the gradient, the more ventilation to perfusion (V : Q) mismatching there is. A gradient of more than 13 mm Hg is considered to be markedly abnormal. This may be the case in patients with COPD, pulmonary emboli, left heart failure (LHF), or hypotension.

When comparing the normal (solid line) tracing in Fig. 4-8 with the V : Q mismatching (dashed line) tracing, note the increased gradient at end-tidal CO_2. With continued exhalation to residual volume, the left heart failure and COPD patients have a narrowing of the gradient. This could be used clinically to follow these patients' progress and response to treatment. The patient with a large pulmonary emboli will *not* have such a narrowing of the gradient as he or she exhales to residual volume. This patient's gradient will narrow to normal as the embolism is resolved and the physiologic dead space returns to normal.

2. Dead space to tidal volume ratio (V_D/V_T).
a. Review the patient's chart for information on any previously measured dead space to tidal volume ratio tests. (IA1d1) [R]

The dead space to tidal volume ratio (V_D/V_T) is the mathematical comparison of a person's dead space volume to tidal volume. Review previous data before repeating the test to understand if the patient was abnormal. Be prepared to compare the previous information with the new data to help evaluate the patient's current condition.

b. Recommend the dead space to tidal volume test to obtain additional data. (IA2q) [R, Ap, An]

This test is most commonly done to document the amount of dead space (wasted ventilation) in a patient with a pulmonary embolism. There are a number of other clinical situations, discussed next, that can justify the procedure.

c. Perform the bedside procedure. (IB8a and IC1c) [R, Ap, An]

Steps in the procedure (see Fig. 4-9):

1. Determine the *average* exhaled CO_2 ($P_{\overline{E}}CO_2$) value by either of these methods:

   a. Collect the patient's entire exhaled gas sample over a number of breaths in a large airtight bag. Count the number of breaths that occured. Calculate the average tidal breath by dividing the total exhaled volume by the total rate. Put all or part of this gas sample through the blood gas analyzer for the PCO_2 value.

   b. Have the patient's exhaled gas pass through a capnometer that can give you an average value (not end-tidal CO_2). A number of breaths should be averaged

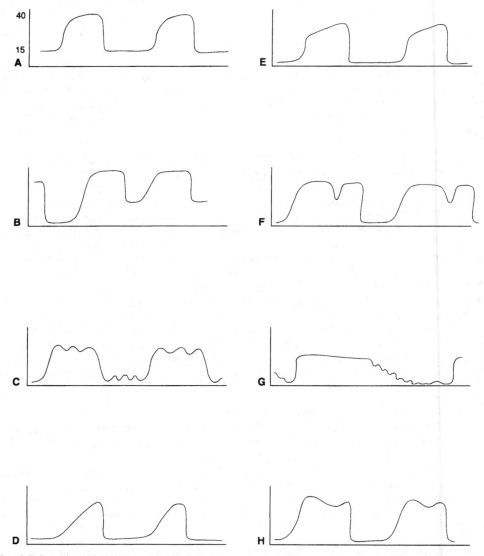

Fig. 4-7 A series of abnormal fast-speed capnography tracings. **A,** A mechanically ventilated patient with a malfunctioning exhalation valve. Note how the baseline CO_2 level is elevated because of the patient's exhaled breath being measured during an inspiration. Correction of the exhalation valve should result in normal inhalation and exhalation. **B,** This rapidly rising baseline gas pressure and failure to return to baseline is usually seen when moisture or secretions block the capillary tube. Clearing the obstruction will enable the patient's gas to again reach the analyzer. **C,** Distortions in the tracing from incomplete exhalation. These could be caused by hiccups, chest compressions during CPR, or inconsistent tidal volume efforts during an asthma attack. **D,** An obstructive lung disease patient with ventilation and perfusion mismatching. There is no alveolar plateau with a stable CO_2 level. Inhaling a bronchodilator should result in the tracing returning closer to normal. **E,** A patient with restrictive lung disease showing no plateau of alveolar gas emptying. This is because the alveoli do not empty evenly. **F,** A sudden drop in carbon dioxide level in the middle of an exhalation indicates the patient attempted inspiration. This "cleft" is usually seen when a patient who has been pharmacologically paralyzed begins to regain movement. **G,** uneven carbon dioxide levels seen at the end of exhalation can be caused by: 1) The patient's heartbeat pumping fresh blood and CO_2 to the emptying lungs. The cardiogenic oscillations should match the heart rate. 2) The ventilator's exhalation valve is fluttering open and closed. **H,** The alveolar plateau is biphasic. This has been seen in patients with lungs that are different in compliance and ventilation/perfusion matching, for example, single lung transplantation.

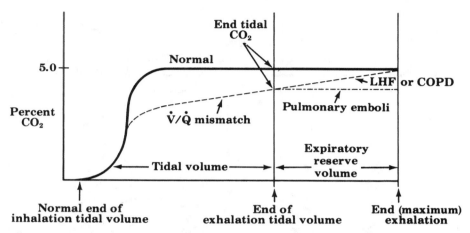

Fig. 4-8 Comparison of several fast-speed capnograph tracings showing how the exhaled carbon dioxide level changes as the patient exhales to residual volume. A normal tracing is matched against abnormal tracings of pulmonary emboli, left heart failure (LHF), and chronic obstructive pulmonary disease (COPD). The normal patient has the same end-tidal CO_2 as residual volume CO_2, showing good matching of ventilation and perfusion. LHF and COPD patients will have a narrowing of the gradient as residual volume is approached. The patient with a pulmonary embolism will keep the same gradient at the residual volume as that found at the end of the tidal volume. (From Pilbeam SP: *Mechanical ventilation: physiological and clinical applications*, St. Louis, 1986, Multi-Media Publishing. Used by permission.)

for greater PCO_2 accuracy. Measure or calculate the patient's average tidal volume over the time of the test.

   2. Draw an arterial sample at the same time that you are performing either step 1a or 1b. Have the blood sample analyzed for $PaCO_2$.

d. Calculate the results. (IIIA1s1) [R, Ap, An]

Place both carbon dioxide values into this formula, which is derived from the original by Bohr:

$$V_D = \frac{(PaCO_2 - P_{\overline{E}}CO_2)}{PaCO_2} \times V_E$$

Where:

V_D = The patient's physiologic dead space
V_E = Average exhaled tidal volume
$PaCO_2$ = The patient's arterial carbon dioxide pressure
$P_{\overline{E}}CO_2$ = The patient's average exhaled carbon dioxide pressure

Example

The following example is based on a normal adult:

V_E = Average exhaled tidal volume = 500 ml
$PaCO_2$ = The patient's arterial carbon dioxide pressure = 40 mm Hg
$P_{\overline{E}}CO_2$ = The patient's average exhaled carbon dioxide pressure = 28 mm Hg

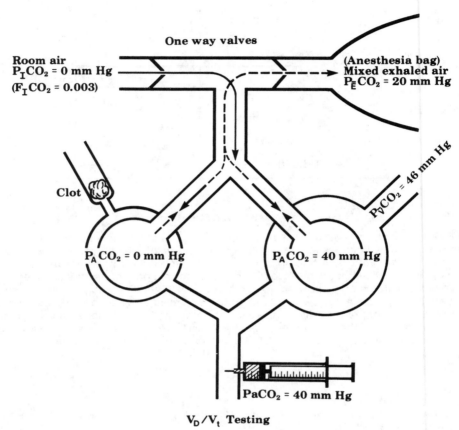

One way valves

Room air
P_ICO_2 = 0 mm Hg
$(F_ICO_2 = 0.003)$

(Anesthesia bag)
Mixed exhaled air
$P_ĒCO_2$ = 20 mm Hg

P_VCO_2 = 46 mm Hg

Clot

P_ACO_2 = 0 mm Hg

P_ACO_2 = 40 mm Hg

$PaCO_2$ = 40 mm Hg

V_D/V_t Testing

Fig. 4-9 A schematic presentation of the procedure for gathering patient samples for calculating the dead space to tidal volume ratio ($V_D : V_T$). An anesthesia or other airtight bag is used to gather all exhaled gas to determine the average exhaled carbon dioxide pressure. An arterial sample is collected for $PaCO_2$. (From Pilbeam SP: *Mechanical ventilation: physiological and clinical applications*, St. Louis, 1986, Multi-Media Publishing. Used by permission.)

$$V_D = \frac{(40 - 28)}{40} \times 500 \text{ ml}$$

$$= \frac{12}{40} = .3 \times 500 = 150 \text{ ml}$$

V_D = The patient's physiologic dead space = 150 ml

The patient's $V_D : V_T$ ratio is $\frac{165}{500}$, .3, or 30% depending on how it is written.

e. Interpret the results. (IB8a, IC1c, and IIIA1s1) [R, Ap, An]

The dead space to tidal volume ratio is the mathematical comparison of a person's dead space volume to tidal volume. The normal adult's dead space to tidal volume ratio range is .2 (20%) to .4 (40%). Anatomic dead space is normally greater in men than in women. The normal 3 kg neonate's dead space to tidal volume ratio is .3 (30%). Physiologic dead space (also known as respiratory dead space) is gas that is ventilated into the lungs but does not take part in gas exhange. This is because the alveoli are not perfused or are underperfused for the amount of gas that they receive.

Physiologic dead space is made up of:

a. Anatomic dead space that is gas in the connecting airways from the nose and mouth to the terminal bronchioles. Generally it is assumed to be about 1 ml/lb of ideal body weight, or 2.2 ml/kg of ideal body weight.

b. Alveolar dead space that is made up of nonfunctioning alveoli that are ventilated but not perfused is minimal in a normal person. The previous "normal" adult example has the expected amount of dead space for his or her weight.

The following conditions or pulmonary disorders can cause the ratio to vary from the normal range:

1. Decreased dead space/tidal volume ratio

a. Lung resection or pneumonectomy because the airways are removed; the patient will maintain his or her tidal volume in the other lung segments.

b. Asthma attack because the airways are narrowed.

c. Insertion of an endotracheal or tracheostomy tube because the upper airway is bypassed.

d. Exercise in the normal person because the increased blood pressure increases perfusion of the apices (Zone 1).

2. Increased dead space/tidal volume ratio

a. Vascular tumor because of decreased perfusion to ventilated alveoli.

b. Pulmonary embolism because the embolism cuts off perfusion of ventilated alveoli. Consider this if the patient is a candidate for a pulmonary embolism and suddenly deteriorates.

3. Increased dead space effect (V > Q)

a. Rapid, shallow ventilations because the upper airway dead space is overventilated compared to the alveoli.

b. Mechanical dead space added to the ventilator circuit. This is an intentional effort to have the patient retain some of his or her carbon dioxide. This is one way to correct for a respiratory alkalosis.

c. COPD (bronchitis, bronchiectasis, cystic fibrosis, emphysema) because varying degrees of bronchospasm, mucus plugging, and tissue destruction lead to increased ventilation and perfusion mismatching.

Many clinicians believe that a dead space/tidal volume ratio of .6 (60%) or more is an indication for mechanically ventilating the patient. A person who is wasting 60% or more of his or her ventilation will soon tire out from the work of breathing and go into ventilatory failure.

3. **Central venous pressure (CVP) monitoring.**
   a. **Review the patient's chart for data on previous central venous pressure measurements. (IA1c1) [R]**

As with the previous procedures, it is wise to review previous patient data to understand if there is an abnormality. Compare the current data with the earlier information to determine if there has been a change in the patient's condition.

b.   Recommend the insertion of a central venous pressure catheter to obtain additional data. (IA2h) [R, Ap, An]

A central venous catheter (also called a CVP line) is inserted into many patients for either of these reasons: 1) to monitor the patient's venous pressure, or 2) to administer intravenous fluids. Of course, it can be used for both reasons. A patient who needs to be monitored for right heart pressure and intravenous fluid level should have a CVP line inserted. Large amounts of fluid can be rapidly infused through the catheter if required to maintain the blood pressure. It is also the preferred route for giving cardiac medications during a CPR attempt.

c.   Perform the bedside procedure and note the results. (IIIA1i and IIIA1j) [R, Ap]

See Fig. 1-22 (Section 1) for a simple drawing of where the catheter is placed. It is usually inserted into the right jugular vein or right subclavian vein and advanced to just above the superior vena cava. When set up for monitoring pressure, it measures the right atrial pressure (see Fig. 4-10 for how to perform the procedure). Note that the stopcock must be kept at the midchest level. Usually a mark is placed there for consistency. Raising the stopcock *above* the mark will result in an incorrectly *low* reading. Lowering the stopcock *below* the mark will result in an incorrectly *high* reading. Clinical practice is very important in learning how to perform this procedure. It is important that the patient breathes spontaneously if at all possible. Peak pressures during inspiration on a mechanical ventilator will artificially raise the CVP reading. Positive end-expiratory pressure (PEEP) may also raise the CVP reading. If the patient cannot be removed from the ventilator, take the reading during exhalation. Make a note of the settings and that the reading was taken with the patient on the ventilator. Record the data in the patient's chart or flow sheet.

d.   Interpret the results. (IB91, IC2h, and IC2k) [R, Ap, An]

As noted earlier, the CVP is a measure of the pressure in the right atrium. The two main factors that influence the right atrial pressure are the blood volume returning to it and the functioning of the right ventricle (see Table 4-2 for the normal CVP readings).

A decreased CVP reading usually means that the patient is hypovolemic. Hypotension will confirm this. An increased CVP could mean one of the following possibilities:

a. Fluid overload: Check for an elevated blood pressure and rales in the bases of the lungs. Unfortunately, an elevated CVP is a late finding with this problem.

b. Right ventricular failure/cor pulmonale: This is seen most commonly in a COPD patient who has pulmonary hypertension.

c. Cardiac tamponade (blood filling the pericardium): Watch for a fall in the blood pressure, tachycardia, and distended jugular veins. This problem can be rapidly fatal if not quickly corrected.

4.   Pulmonary artery pressure (PAP) monitoring.
a.   Review the patient's chart for data on the pulmonary artery pressure. (IA1c1) [R]

The pulmonary artery pressure (PAP) is the systolic and diastolic pressure found in the pulmonary artery. It can only be measured through a pulmonary artery catheter. Normal values and interpretation of abnormal values are presented next.

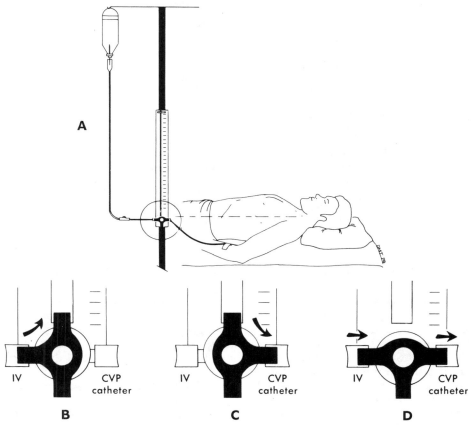

Fig. 4-10 Procedure for determining the central venous pressure (CVP) with a manometer. **A,** Water-column manometer marked in centimeters. IV tubing, and patient in place. **B,** Turn the stopcock so that the manometer fills with fluid above the expected pressure. **C,** Turn the stopcock off to the IV so that the fluid flows from the manometer into the patient. Look at the stable fluid level for the CVP reading. **D,** Turn the stopcock so that the fluid flows from the IV into the patient. (From Daily EK, Schroeder JS: *Techniques in bedside hemodynamic monitoring,* ed 4, St. Louis, 1989, Mosby–Year Book. Used by permission.)

b.   Recommend the insertion of a pulmonary artery catheter for additional data. (IA2h) [R, Ap, An]

The pulmonary artery pressure is important to measure in patients with severe pulmonary or cardiovascular problems. These include pulmonary hypertension, myocardial infarct, congestive heart failure, hypertension, and hypotension.

To read the pulmonary artery pressure, a pulmonary artery catheter (PAC) must be inserted through a vein and passed through the right atrium and right ventricle into the pulmonary artery. The common insertion sites are the basilic vein in either the right or left arm, right internal jugular or subclavian vein, or right or left femoral vein (in decending order of preference). The pulmonary artery catheter is also commonly called a Swan-Ganz catheter after the inventors who lent their names to a particular brand produced by American Edwards Laboratories. The catheters come in different lengths and diameters for pediatric and adult patients.

Table 4-2. Normal Cardiopulmonary
Pressures

Central Venous Pressure (CVP)
Range for a normal adult is 2-8 cm water or 1-6
    mm Hg
Range for a normal infant is 1-5 mm Hg
Range for a normal neonate is 0-3 mm Hg
Pulmonary Artery Pressure (PAP)
Range for a normal adult is 15-28/5-16 mm Hg
    (about 25/10 mm Hg)
Range for a normal adult mean PAP is 10-
    22 mm Hg
Range for a normal child is 15-30/5-10 mm Hg
Range for a normal neonate is 30-60/2-10 mm Hg
Pulmonary Wedge Pressure (PWP)
Range for a normal PWP (mean) is 6-15 mm Hg
    (about 8 mm Hg)

---

c. Perform the bedside procedure. (IIIA1i and IIIA1j) [R, Ap]

Fig. 4-11 is an illustration of a 7 French quadruple lumen thermodilution pulmonary artery catheter. Besides PAP, it is capable of being used to measure cardiac output. Fig. 4-12 shows how a pulmonary artery catheter could be arranged with a pressure transducer and pressure monitor. Fig. 4-13 shows a representation of the series of pressure waveforms seen as the catheter is advanced through the heart and into the wedged position in a branch of the pulmonary artery. Fig. 4-14 shows a larger cutaway view of the heart with a PAC and normal heart chambers and related pressures.

To read the pulmonary artery pressure accurately the equipment must be set up and calibrated properly, the distal lumen of the catheter must be patent and connected to the transducer, and the catheter's balloon must be deflated. Clinical practice is very important in understanding how to perform this procedure. Record the PAP data in the patient's chart or flow sheet.

d. Interpret the results. (IB9m and IC2d) [R, Ap, An)

Again, the PAP is the systolic and diastolic pressure found in the pulmonary artery (see Table 4-2 for normal values). Elevated PAP values are usually seen with these conditions:

a. Left ventricular failure/congestive heart failure, acute myocardial infarction, or fluid overload—to better determine the pathophysiological problem it will be necessary to evaluate the following kinds of clinical information:

1. Known history of heart disease or of sudden illness suggesting a heart attack
2. Hearing rales in the bases of the lungs
3. Decreased static lung compliance
4. Elevated pulmonary capillary wedge pressure
5. Decreased cardiac output and/or low blood pressure
6. The gradient (difference) between the pulmonary artery diastolic pressure (PAD) and the pulmonary capillary wedge pressure (PCWP) is less than 5 mm Hg (normal)

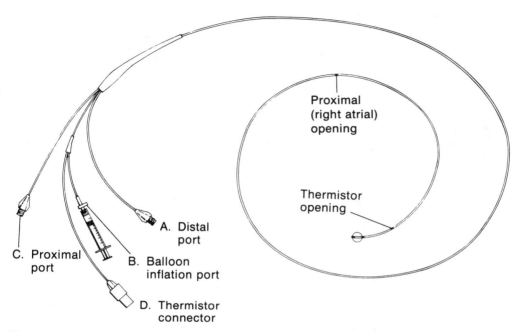

Fig. 4-11 A 7 French quadruple lumen thermodilution pulmonary artery catheter. **A,** Distal port goes to the tip of the catheter. It is used for measuring PAP, PCWP, and sampling blood for $P\bar{v}O_2$. **B,** Balloon inflation port is used to inflate the balloon for inserting the catheter and for obtaining a PCWP reading. **C,** Proximal port is used for measuring central venous pressure and for injecting iced saline for a thermodilution cardiac output study. The iced saline exits from the right atrial opening. **D,** Thermistor connector attaches to the cardiac output computer. A bimetalic wire runs through the catheter to the thermistor opening where it is exposed to temperature changes of the blood and cold injectate. (Note: Not all catheters are capable of measuring cardiac output. Some catheters have other special features such as continuously measuring venous saturation or cardiac pacemaker leads.) (From Oblouk Darovic G: *Hemodynamic monitoring,* Philadelphia, 1987, WB Saunders. Used by permission.)

Example:

PAP is 35/24 mm Hg; PCWP is 22 mm Hg

Pulmonary artery diastolic is:	25 mm Hg
Pulmonary capillary wedge pressure is:	− 22 mm Hg
The PAD-PCWP gradient is normal:	3 mm Hg

   b. Pulmonary hypertension from COPD (usually emphysema)—to better determine the pathophysiological problem it will be necessary to evaluate the following kinds of clinical information:

   1. The patient usually has a known history of COPD.
   2. Systolic PAP may exceed 40 mm Hg if the problem is long standing.
   3. The gradient (difference) between the pulmonary artery diastolic pressure and the pulmonary capillary wedge pressure is greater than 5 mm Hg.

Example:

PAP is 35/25 mm Hg; PCWP is 8 mm Hg

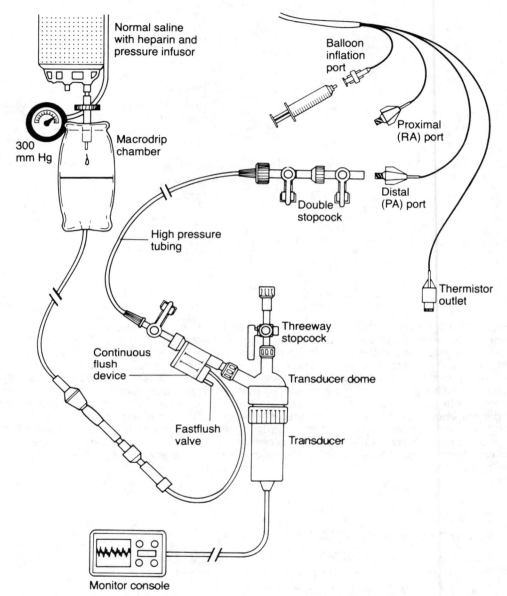

Fig. 4-12 The various components of the pulmonary artery monitoring system. It includes a fluid source such as normal saline that is pressurized to 300 mm Hg to maintain a flow of fluid through the tubing system. The continuous flush device (made by Sorenson) is designed to allow 3 drips of fluid per minute through the tubing system; pulling on the fastflush valve gives a continuous flow of fluid to clear air or blood from the system. The transducer converts a pressure signal to an electrical signal that is sent to the monitor for display as numerical data and a pressure wave form. The high pressure tubing transfers the patient's pressure accurately to the transducer. The double stopcocks are used to close off the tubing system or sample blood from the patient. This then connects to the distal port of the pulmonary artery catheter. This same monitoring system can be used with an arterial catheter for continuous pressure monitoring and blood sampling. (From Oblouk Darovic G: *Hemodynamic monitoring*, Philadelphia, 1987, WB Saunders. Used by permission.)

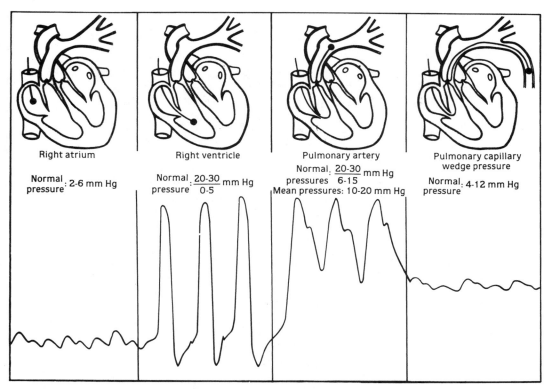

Fig. 4-13 Sequence of pressures and pressure wave forms seen as the pulmonary artery catheter advances through the right atrium, right ventricle, and pulmonary artery until it wedges. Be observant of premature ventricular contractions (PVC) as the catheter is advanced through the right ventricle. (From Wilkins RL, Sheldon RL, Krider SJ: *Clinical assessment in respiratory care,* ed 2, St. Louis, 1990, Mosby–Year Book. Used by permission.)

Pulmonary artery diastolic is:	25 mm Hg
Pulmonary capillary wedge pressure is:	−8 mm Hg
The PAD-PCWP gradient is high:	17 mm Hg

    c. Pulmonary hypertension from a pulmonary embolism—to better determine the pathophysiological problem it will be necessary to evaluate the following kinds of clinical information:

    1. The patient's history will match that of a sudden onset of shortness of breath and other pulmonary problems.
    2. The systolic PAP will be less than 40 mm Hg because the relatively thin-walled right ventricle cannot rapidly increase its muscle mass to increase the driving pressure.
    3. The gradient (difference) between the pulmonary artery diastolic pressure and the pulmonary capillary wedge pressure is greater than 5 mm Hg if the embolism is large.

    d. Pulmonary hypertension in the neonate with persistent pulmonary hypertension of the newborn (PPHN)/persistent fetal circulation (PFC)—this condition is often seen in the premature neonate with the infant respiratory distress syndrome

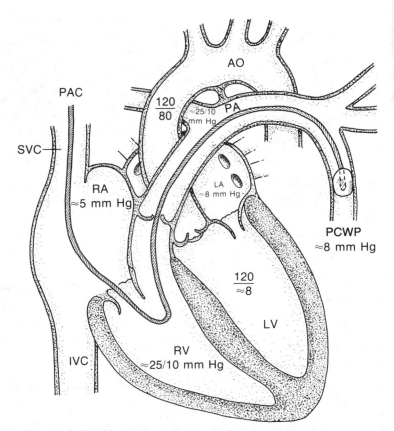

Fig. 4-14 Pulmonary artery catheter (PAC) through a heart with normal chamber pressures. *SVC*, superior vena cava; *IVC*, inferior vena cava; *RA*, right atrium; *RV*, right ventricle; *PA*, pulmonary artery; *PCWP*, pulmonary capillary wedge pressure; *LA*, left atrium; *LV*, left ventricle; and *Ao*, aorta.

(IRDS). When these neonates become hypoxic, the pulmonary vascular bed constricts. This causes the infant to revert back to fetal circulation. Giving 100% oxygen and hyperventilating them usually reverses the processes. The PAP will then return to normal.

Decreased pulmonary artery pressure values are not frequently seen. Patients with hypovolemic shock, anaphylaxis (allergic shock), or excessive use of vasodilating drugs may have a decreased pulmonary artery pressure. The most obvious clinical sign in these patients is a low systemic blood pressure.

5. Pulmonary capillary wedge pressure (PCWP) monitoring.
 a. Review the patient's chart for data on the pulmonary capillary wedge pressure. (IA1c1) [R]

The pulmonary capillary wedge pressure (PCWP) refers to the pressure measured in the pulmonary capillary bed under no-flow conditions. It is important to review previous patient data before doing another pressure measurement. Normal and abnormal values are discussed below.

b. Recommend the insertion of a pulmonary artery catheter for additional data. (IA2h) [R, Ap, An]

A pulmonary artery catheter must be placed into a patient's pulmonary artery for the pulmonary capillary wedge pressure (PCWP) to be measured. It is important to measure the PCWP in patients with severe pulmonary or cardiovascular problems. These include pulmonary hypertension, myocardial infarct, congestive heart failure, hypertension, and hypotension.

c. Perform the bedside procedure. (IB8f, IIIA1i, and IIIA1j) [R, Ap]

The PCWP is obtained by inflating the balloon at the tip of the catheter. This blocks off that branch of the pulmonary artery so that the downstream pressure from the left ventricle is seen on the monitor (see Fig. 4-13). The balloon volume will vary with the diameter of the catheter. The needed volume is printed on the catheter near where the air is injected into the balloon. For example, the 5 French catheter balloon holds .8 ml of air and the 7 French catheter balloon holds 1.5 ml of air. It is important to put in only the required amount. Overinflating may burst the balloon or rupture the pulmonary artery. If the balloon wedges at less than the required volume the catheter is probably too far down into the artery and may need to be withdrawn a short distance. The balloon is only inflated long enough to obtain the PCWP and than the balloon is deflated. Pulmonary infarction will occur if the balloon is left inflated and the blood in the pulmonary artery is stagnant and allowed to clot. Record the PCWP value in the patient's chart or flow sheet.

d. Interpret the results. (IB8f and IC2j) [R, Ap, An]

As noted earlier, the pulmonary capillary wedge pressure (PCWP) refers to the pressure measured in the pulmonary capillary bed under no-flow conditions. This pressure reflects downstream pressure from the left side of the heart. At diastole, in the patient without pulmonary hypertension or mitral valve disease, the PCWP parallels left atrial pressure (LAP) and left ventricular end diastolic pressure (LVEDP). The literature reveals that a variety of terms and initials are used to describe the same physiologic value. Do not be confused by reading about the pulmonary capillary pressure (PCP), pulmonary wedge pressure (PWP), pulmonary artery wedge pressure (PAWP), or wedge pressure.

Elevated PCWP is generally held to be greater than 10 mm Hg and could indicate:

a. Intravascular fluid overload: Look at the patient's history to see if the patient is in renal failure and/or has recently had a large amount of oral or intravenous fluids. Perform a physical exam to see if the patient has edema in the ankles or back if he or she has been lying down. Look for jugular vein distension when the patient lies down. Listen for rales in the bases of the lungs.

b. Left ventricular dysfunction with congestive heart failure: Do the same things as listed in a. In addition, look for a history of chronic heart failure or acute myocardial infarction.

c. Mitral valve insufficiency: Blood regurgitating back into the left atrium is shown as an elevated PCWP.

These conditions result in serious problems for the patient's lung function. When the PCWP reaches 20 to 25 mm Hg, fluid begins to leak into the pulmonary interstitium. This makes the lung less compliant and increases the patient's work of breathing. A PCWP of 25 to 30 mm Hg results in frank pulmonary edema and dramatically decreases the patient's PaO_2.

Decreased PCWP is commonly held to be less than 4 mm Hg and could indicate:

a. Low intravascular volume: Look in the patient's history for an illness resulting in dehydration (vomiting and diarrhea). A physical exam will show tachycardia, low blood pressure, low urine output with a high specific gravity, tenting of the skin when pinched showing poor turger, and flat jugular veins when the patient is lying down.

b. Sepsis: The patient's history will reveal infection; usually a septicemia. The physical exam will reveal tachycardia, hypotension, and oliguria, as noted in a. A major difference is that the patient will appear to be fluid overloaded because of the peripheral edema. This finding is produced when an infectious organism (often *Staphylococcus aureus*) causes a dilation of the peripheral vascular bed and leakage of fluids out of the vascular bed into the tissues. The patient will have weak peripheral pulses and feel warm.

6. Cardiac output (CO).
a. Review the patient's chart for data on cardiac output. (IA1c1) [R]

Cardiac output (CO) is defined as the product of heart rate for 1 minute and stroke volume. It is a measurement of the heart's pumping ability to meet the body's needs. As always, review previous data before repeating the test.

b. Recommend a cardiac output procedure for additional patient data. (IA2j) [R, Ap, An]

A cardiac output measurement is performed on patients with serious cardiovascular disease to assess the patient's condition. A major change in vital signs or new treatment would justify a measurement. The patient must have a pulmonary artery catheter in place that is capable of measuring cardiac output.

c. Perform the bedside procedure. (IB8d, IIIA1i, and IIIA1j) [R, Ap, An]

The bedside procedure involves the use of a four lumen pulmonary artery catheter designed for thermodilution cardiac output studies. Additional hardware and supplies include a computer designed to calculate the CO, injectible saline solution or 5% dextrose, ice water bath, necessary tubing and connections, thermometer, 10 cc syringes, and injector system (see Fig. 4-15). It is beyond the scope of this text to describe all of the steps in the different types of adult and neonatal thermodilution cardiac output procedures. Hands-on experience is necessary. Only the most important and common features are presented here:

a. The usual injectate volume is 10 cc. The neonatal injectate volume may be reduced to 3 cc in an attempt to prevent fluid overloading the patient. The right atrial lumen is used for the injection.

b. The usual injectate temperature is 0 to 4°C. Some clinicians use room air temperature injectate because it is easier to work with. The cold injectate cardiac output result may be more accurate because of the greater difference between it and the patient's body temperature. If the patient is hypothermic the cold injectate must be used for greater accuracy.

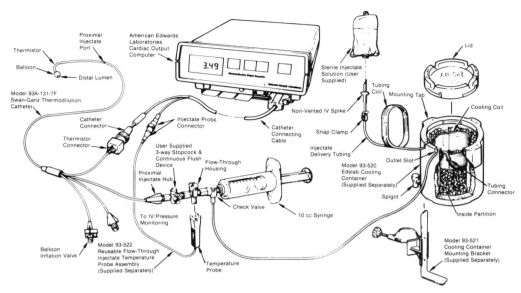

Fig. 4-15 Complete system for performing thermodilution cardiac output studies. (From American Edwards Laboratories, Santa Ana, Calif. Copyright 1985. Used by permission.)

c. Three injections are usually performed. The results are then averaged for the final CO value. Individual CO measurements that vary by more than 10% from each other probably indicate an error in the procedure. A compressed CO_2 "gun" is preferred to hand injection because the injector gun is more smooth and reliable in its injection. The injection must be completed within 4 seconds with the American Edwards Laboratories cardiac output computer.

d. Calculate the patient's value. (IIIAq2) [R, Ap, An]

The following three methods can be used to calculate the patient's cardiac output:

1. A computer calculates the cardiac output (CO) when the thermodilution method is used. As long as the procedural steps are done properly and the patient and catheter variables are programmed into the computer, the results should be reliable. This method is widely used at the bedside. Actual clinical experience is invaluable in understanding the full procedure.
2. The Fick method of measuring cardiac output is the "gold standard" by which all others are measured. Unfortunately, it is difficult to perform at the bedside. The patient's inhaled and exhaled gases must be analyzed for PO_2 to calculate his or her oxygen consumption. In addition, arterial and mixed venous blood samples must be taken and analyzed for oxygen to calculate the arterial-venous oxygen content difference $[C(a-v)O_2]$. The following example shows fairly standard values for an adult:

$$CO \text{ (ml/min)} = \frac{\text{oxygen consumption (ml/min)}}{\text{arterial } O_2 \text{ content (vol\%)} - \text{venous } O_2 \text{ content (vol\%)}}$$

Where:

$$\text{Vol \% = volumes \% or ml of oxygen/100 ml of blood}$$
$$\text{Oxygen consumption} = 250 \text{ ml/min}$$
$$\text{Arterial oxygen content} = 20 \text{ vol \%}$$
$$\text{Mixed venous oxygen content} = 15 \text{ vol \%}$$
$$C(a-v)O_2 = 5 \text{ vol \%}$$

Therefore:

$$CO = \frac{250 \text{ ml/min}}{20 \text{ vol \% } - 15 \text{ vol \%}} = \frac{250 \text{ ml/min}}{5 \text{ vol \%}} = \frac{250}{.05} = 5000 \text{ ml/min} = 5 \text{ l/min}$$

3. The following formula can be used to calculate a predicted cardiac output for the adult patient. This value can then be compared to the actual patient cardiac output.

$$CO = \frac{BSA \times 125}{.045}$$

BSA stands for body surface area and can be calculated mathematically or determined from a data table. See the following discussion on cardiac index for information on calculating BSA.

e. Interpret the patient's cardiac output measurement results. (IB8d, IC2i, and IIIAr2) [R, Ap, An]

Cardiac output is defined as the product of heart rate for 1 minute and stroke volume (CO = HR × SV). The normal, resting adult has a cardiac output in the range of 4 to 8 l/min. A normal, resting neonate has a cardiac output in the range of .6 to .8 l/min.

Cardiac output can increase markedly in a person with a normal heart who is stressed, exercising, has a fever, or has any other reason for an increased metabolism. All these conditions increase the person's demand for oxygen, which is primarily met by increasing cardiac output. (To a lesser extent, the tissues extract more oxygen from the blood.) Sepsis is the one serious condition that results in a high cardiac output.

There are many possible causes of a decreased cardiac output. The most common are hypovolemia, increased peripheral resistance, and heart failure. A patient with low cardiac output often has a low blood pressure. If the cardiac output and blood pressure are too low the patient will develop metabolic acidosis from peripheral hypoxemia. Death can result if this cannot be corrected.

f. Interpret the patient's stroke volume (SV) calculation. (IIIAr4) [R, Ap, An]

Stroke volume (SV) is defined as the volume of blood ejected with each heartbeat. It is the difference between the volume of blood in each ventricle at the end of diastole and the volume left in the ventricles at the end of systole (after ejection). The normal stroke volume is based on a person's age:

Adults: 50 to 120 ml/beat
School-age children: 35 ml/beat
Preschoolers: 15 ml/beat
Neonates: 5 ml/beat

The stroke volume is the same for both ventricles except under pathological conditions. Usually, however, only the left ventricle is of concern. The Frank-Starling curve shows us that as the heart muscle is stretched with greater volume it contracts and pumps more completely resulting in a larger stroke volume. A damaged or overstretched left ventricle will not pump as effectively and the stroke volume will decrease. A drop in stroke volume will result in a drop in cardiac output unless the heart rate can increase to make up the difference. This is seen in many patients with heart disease.

7. Cardiac index (CI).
a. Calculate the patient's value. (IIIAq2) [R, Ap, An]

The cardiac index (CI) is the cardiac output per square meter of body surface area. Cardiac output is usually measured by the thermodilution cardiac output method via a pulmonary artery catheter. The body surface area (BSA) can be determined from the DuBois Body Surface Chart as shown in Fig. 4-16. The body surface area can also be determined with this equation:

$$\text{BSA} = 1 + \frac{\text{weight in kilograms} + (\text{height in centimeters} - 160)}{100}$$

Example

A 166 lb/75 kg, 5'10"/152 cm man has a cardiac output of 6 l/min. According to the DuBois Body Surface Chart, he has a BSA of 1.92 m². His cardiac index is calculated as:

$$\text{CI} = \frac{6 \text{ l/min}}{1.92 \text{ m}^2} = 3.125 \text{ l/min/m}^2$$

b. Interpret the results. (IIIAr2) [R, Ap, An]

A normal, resting cardiac index is 2.5 to 4 l/min/m² of BSA. The cardiac index is a much more accurate way of determining if the patient's oxygen demands are being met than by simply looking at the cardiac output. For example, a resting cardiac output of 4 l/min is considered normal. This cardiac output might be fine for a small adult but not for a large one. The CI takes into account the difference in body sizes. A normal cardiac index indicates that the patient is receiving enough oxygen to meet the body's needs. A low cardiac index should be a cause for concern; it usually indicates that the patient is not getting enough blood and oxygen to his or her tissues. Check to see if the patient's cardiac output and blood pressure are also low and if he or she has hypoxemia and/or acidemia. If these exist, they must be corrected as quickly as possible to prevent dire consequences. A high cardiac index indicates that the patient is pumping more blood than appears necessary. Investigate why. See the earlier discussion on cardiac output and the factors that affect it to understand the factors that affect cardiac index as well.

8. Mixed venous blood sampling.
a. Review the patient's chart for data on mixed venous oxygen values. (IA1c3) [R]

A patient with a functioning pulmonary artery catheter can have a sample of blood withdrawn through it and analyzed for mixed venous oxygen (and the other blood gas values as well). If this has been done the $P\bar{v}O_2$ value(s) should be

DUBOIS BODY SURFACE CHART

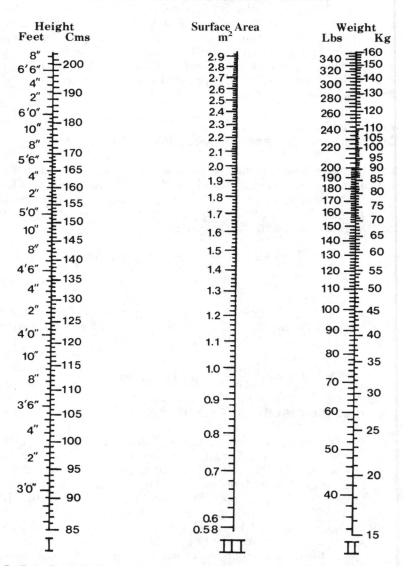

Fig. 4-16 DuBois Body Surface Chart (as prepared by Boothby and Sandlford of the Mayo Clinic). Directions: To find the body surface of a patient, locate the height in inches (or centimeters) on scale I and weight in pounds (or kilograms) on scale II. Place a straight edge (ruler) between these two points, which will intersect scale III at the patient's surface area. (From Pilbeam SP: *Mechanical ventilation: physiologic and clinical applications*, St. Louis, 1986, Multi-Media Publishing. Used by permission.)

reviewed before measuring it again. (See Section 2, Module C, for information on mixed venous blood gas values.)

b.   Perform the bedside procedure. (IB8g and IIIA1m) [R, Ap, An]

There are currently three ways to perform the bedside procedure. They are summarized as follows:

1. The procedure can be done through the distal lumen of a PAC as it is being inserted. This method is employed when trying to determine if there is a ventricular septal defect. The procedure is commonly done on neonates with suspected congenital heart defects but may be used in adults as well. Using sterile technique, blood samples are withdrawn serially from the right atrium, right ventricle, and sometimes from the pulmonary artery.

Normally, the $P\overline{v}O_2$ and $S\overline{v}O_2$ values are the same in all blood samples. The patient with a ventricular septal defect will show an *increase* in $P\overline{v}O_2$ and $S\overline{v}O_2$ values going from the right atrium to the right ventricle and pulmonary artery. This is because the oxygenated blood from the left ventricle is forced though the ventricular septal defect to raise the oxygen value of the right ventricular blood.

2. Use a pulmonary artery catheter with reflectance oximetry capability. These catheters have fiberoptic bundles built into them and utilize technology similar to that used in pulse oximeters. The monitoring unit sends several wavelengths of light down the transmitting fiberoptic bundle to be shined on the passing blood in the pulmonary artery. Oxyhemoglobin in the red blood cells absorbs some of the light. The rest is reflected off. The receiving fiberoptic bundle picks up some of this light and transmits it back to the monitoring unit.

$S\overline{v}O_2$ is determined by the monitoring unit based on the lightwaves that were transmitted and what was received. Care must be taken when using this catheter in patients with elevated carboxyhemoglobin or methemoglobin levels. As with pulse oximetry, COHb and MetHb will be interpreted as oxyhemoglobin. Thus, inaccurately high readings will be seen.

An actual mixed venous blood sample can be taken with this catheter through the distal lumen as described in 3. The advantage of the reflectance oximetry system is that it gives continuous monitoring of your patient's venous oxygen level. In addition, high and low saturation alarms can be set. If the tip should become lodged in the wall of the artery or if a clot should form at the tip, the $S\overline{v}O_2$ will drop or fluctuate dramatically. The alarms should warn the clinician of a problem with the equipment.

3. Distal lumen of a "standard" pulmonary artery catheter. A true mixed venous blood sample is obtained by withdrawing blood from the distal lumen of the catheter. This is the same lumen that is used for the PAP and PCWP readings. Using sterile technique, a 5 to 10 ml syringe is used to pull out the heparinized solution in the lumen until about 1 to 2 ml of blood are removed. A second preheparinized syringe is then used to withdraw about 2 ml of mixed venous blood. It is important to withdraw the IV solution and blood at a rate of no faster than .5 ml per second. Drawing any faster could pull preoxygenated blood back through the capillary bed and give you falsely elevated oxygen values. After sampling the blood, the lumen must be fast-flushed with the heparinized solution to prevent the blood from clotting (see Fig. 4-12). Flush for several seconds until the solution flows freely. This blood sample may be reliably analyzed for $S\overline{v}O_2$, $P\overline{v}O_2$, and $P\overline{v}CO_2$.

c. Interpret the results. (IB8g, IC2e, and IIIA1o) [R, Ap, An]

This topic is discussed in some detail in Section 2, Module C. Briefly, the normal values are:

$P\overline{v}O_2$ of 40 mm Hg (range of 37 to 43 mm Hg)
$S\overline{v}O_2$ of 75% (range of 70% to 76%)

Mixed venous blood oxygen values are useful for following the patient's oxygen consumption. The most accurate methods of calculating percent shunt and cardiac output (Fick method) utilize mixed venous blood oxygen values with arterial blood oxygen values. A $P\overline{v}O_2$ value of less than 30 mm Hg is considered to show tissue hypoxemia. Quick steps must be taken to reverse this. Increase the inspired oxygen percentage as needed. Low stroke volume and cardiac output can be increased by giving digitalis or other inotropic agents. Low blood pressure can be increased by giving vasopressors such as dopamine HCl (Intropin).

9. **Arterial-venous oxygen content difference [$C(a-\bar{v})O_2$].**
   a. **Review the patient's chart for data on any previous arterial-venous oxygen content difference measurements. (IA1c1) [R]**

The arterial-venous oxygen content difference [$C(a-\bar{v})O_2$] is a calculation of oxygen consumption of the body. It is the difference between the oxygen content of arterial blood and the oxygen content of mixed venous blood. Any patient with a functioning pulmonary artery catheter may have this value calculated as shown in the next discussion. As always, check for previous values to compare with present values to understand if the patient's condition has changed.

   b. **Perform the measurement of arterial-venous oxygen content difference. (IC1o) [R, Ap, An]**

The following must be performed to make the arterial-venous oxygen content calculation:

   1. Draw and analyze an arterial blood gas sample.
   2. Simultaneously draw and analyze a mixed venous blood gas sample.
   3. Determine the patient's hemoglobin value.
   4. Place the data into the calculations shown in the next discussion.

   c. **Calculate the patient's value. (IIIA1s3) [R, Ap, An]**

As mentioned in the previous discussion, the arterial-venous oxygen content difference is found by subtracting venous blood oxygen content from arterial blood oxygen content. These two values must first be calculated separately and then subtracted as shown in these three steps:

   1. CaO_2 = The content of oxygen in arterial blood
        = Vol % of oxygen in arterial blood (vol % means ml of oxygen/ 100 ml of blood.)
      $CaO_2 = (Hb \times 1.34 \times SaO_2) + (PaO_2 \times 0.003)$
   2. $C\bar{v}O_2$ = The content of oxygen in mixed venous blood
        = Vol % of oxygen in mixed venous blood
      $C\bar{v}O_2 = (Hb \times 1.34 \times S\bar{v}O_2) + (P\bar{v}O_2 \times 0.003)$
   3. $C(a-\bar{v})O_2 = CaO_2 - C\bar{v}O_2$

Example

Your patient has the following clinical data:

   PaO_2 = 95 mm Hg

   SaO_2 = 97% or .97

   $P\bar{v}O_2$ = 40 mm Hg

   $S\bar{v}O_2$ = 75% or .75

15 g/dl = The patient's hemoglobin concentration

1.34 = ml of oxygen/g Hb in the patient (The value of 1.39 ml of oxygen/g Hb is occasionally used.)

0.003 = the oxygen carrying capacity of blood plasma per mm Hg PO_2

Therefore:

1. CaO_2 = (Hb × 1.34 × SaO_2) + (PaO_2 × 0.003)
   = (15 × 1.34 × .97) + (95 × 0.003)
   = (19.5) + (0.3)
   = 19.8 vol %

2. $C\overline{v}O_2$ = (Hb × 1.34 × $S\overline{v}O_2$) + ($P\overline{v}O_2$ × 0.003)
   = (15 × 1.34 × .75) + (40 × 0.003)
   = (15.1) + (.1)
   = 15.2 vol %

3. $C(a-\overline{v})O_2$ difference = (CaO_2 of 19.8 vol %) − ($C\overline{v}O_2$ of 15.2 vol %)
   = 4.6 vol %

d. Interpret the $C(a-\overline{v})O_2$ results. (IC1o and IIIA1s3) [R, Ap, An]

The normal range of the $C(a-\overline{v})O_2$ difference is 3 to 5.5 vol %. Figures in this range show normal oxygen consumption by the tissues, cardiac output, and cardiopulmonary function. (See Fig. 4-17 for a graphic presentation of $C(a-\overline{v})O_2$ on the oxyhemoglobin dissociation curve.) A $C(a-\overline{v})O_2$ difference of greater than 5.5 to 6 vol % is seen in patients with a low cardiac output. As the blood flows more slowly than normal through the tissues, more oxygen is consumed per ml of blood. The $S\overline{v}O_2$ and $P\overline{v}O_2$ values drop and the $C(a-\overline{v})O_2$ difference widens.

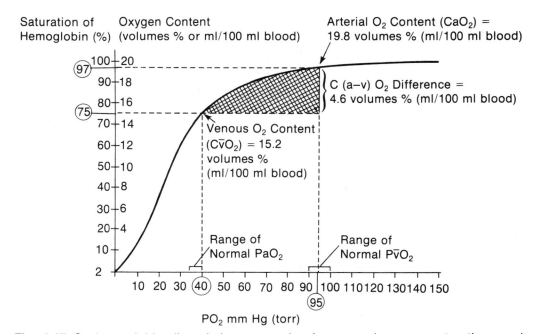

Fig. 4-17 Oxyhemoglobin dissociation curve showing normal oxygen saturations and pressures in arterial and venous blood. From these, the normal C(a–v)O₂ difference of 4.6 vol % can be calculated.

A $C(a-\bar{v})O_2$ difference of less than 4 vol % in the healthy patient commonly indicates good cardiovascular reserve with an increased cardiac output. As the blood flows more quickly than normal through the tissues, less oxygen is consumed per ml of blood. The $S\bar{v}O_2$ and $P\bar{v}O_2$ values increase and the $C(a-\bar{v})O_2$ difference narrows. The septic patient may have a narrowed $C(a-\bar{v})O_2$ difference because of peripheral shunting and decreased oxygen consumption by the tissues caused by the infection. The $C(a-\bar{v})O_2$ difference is necessary to accurately calculate the percent of pulmonary shunting as discussed next.

10. Shunt study ($\dot{Q}s/\dot{Q}t$).
a. Review the patient's chart for data on previous shunt studies. (IA1c1) [R]

Shunt is the amount of blood pumped by the heart that does not participate in gas exchange through the lungs. A pulmonary artery catheter must be inserted into the patient for a shunt study to be performed. Review previous shunt study results and compare to current information to see if there has been a change in the patient's status.

b. Recommend a shunt study for added data. (IA21) [R, Ap, An]

A shunt study is very useful to tell how much ventilation to perfusion mismatch a patient has. Most patients with refractory hypoxemia and requiring mechanical ventilation have an increased amount of pulmonary shunting.

c. Perform the bedside shunt study procedure. (IB8c) [R, Ap, An]

Steps in the bedside shunt procedure:

1. Measure the patient's F_1O_2.
2. Simultaneously draw arterial and mixed venous blood samples.
3. Have both blood samples analyzed for SO_2 and PO_2.
4. Calculate the percent of shunt as shown next.

d. Calculate the patient's shunt percentage. (IIIAq1) [R, Ap, An]

There are a number of possible variations on the methods and equations for calculating shunt percentage. Only the two most commonly used equations are presented here.

Modified Clinical Shunt Equation

$$\dot{Q}_s/\dot{Q}_t = \frac{P(A-a)O_2 \times 0.003}{C(a-\bar{v})O_2 + [P(A-a)O_2 \times 0.003]}$$

Where:

PAO_2 = The partial pressure of oxygen in the alveoli calculated from the alveolar oxygen equation
PaO_2 = The partial pressure of oxygen in the arterial blood
0.003 = The oxygen carrying capacity of blood plasma per mm Hg PO_2
$C(a-\bar{v})O_2$ = The oxygen content of arterial blood minus the oxygen content of mixed venous blood

This formula requires that the patient's hemoglobin be 100% saturated. This does not happen until the PaO_2 reaches 150 torr at any given F_1O_2. An obvious clinical limitation is that very ill patients never reach 100% saturation even on 100% oxygen. Also, putting patients on more than 80% oxygen, even for just the duration of the test, may lead to some denitrogenation absorption atelectasis. This will result in an incorrectly high shunt percentage calculation.

Modified Clinical Shunt Example

The following example shows the modified clinical shunt calculation with the following environmental and patient information:

P_B = Local barometric pressure—760 mm Hg for sea level in this example

PH_2O = 47 mm Hg; water vapor pressure in the lungs at normal body temperature

F_1O_2 = inhaled oxygen percent of 100% or 1.0

PaO_2 = 155 mm Hg

$PaCO_2$ = 40 mm Hg

SaO_2 = 100% or 1.0

$P\overline{v}O_2$ = 40 mm Hg

$S\overline{v}O_2$ = 75% or .75

.8 = The normal respiratory quotient (An exact value can be determined by a metabolic study.)

15 g/dl = The patient's hemoglobin concentration

0.003 = The oxygen carrying capacity of blood plasma per mm Hg PO_2

1.34 = ml of oxygen/g Hb in the patient (The value of 1.39 ml of oxygen/g Hb is occasionally used.)

Preliminary calculations:

1. Oxygen content of arterial blood

$$CaO_2 = (Hb \times 1.34 \times SaO_2) + (PaO_2 \times 0.003)$$
$$= (15 \times 1.34 \times 1.0) + (155 \times 0.003)$$
$$= (20.1) + (0.5)$$
$$= 20.6 \text{ vol \%}.$$

2. Oxygen content of mixed venous blood

$$C\overline{v}O_2 = (Hb \times 1.34 \times S\overline{v}O_2) + (P\overline{v}O_2 \times 0.003)$$
$$= (15 \times 1.34 \times .75) + (40 \times 0.003)$$
$$= (15.1) + (.1)$$
$$= 15.2 \text{ vol \%}.$$

3. Partial pressure of oxygen in the alveoli—the alveolar oxygen equation is used for this. (Review Section 2 if necessary.)

$$PAO_2 = [(P_B - PH_2O) \times F_1O_2] - \frac{PaCO_2}{.8}$$
$$= [(760 - 47) \times 1.0] - \frac{40}{.8}$$
$$= [713] - 50$$
$$= 663 \text{ mm Hg}$$

Final calculation:

$$\dot{Q}_s/\dot{Q}_t = \frac{P(A-a)O_2 \times 0.003}{C(a-\bar{v})O_2 + [P(A-a)O_2 \times 0.003]}$$

$$= \frac{(663 - 155) \times 0.003}{(20.6 - 15.2) + [(663 - 155) \times 0.003]}$$

$$= \frac{(508) \times 0.003}{5.4 + [(508) \times 0.003]}$$

$$= \frac{1.5}{5.4 + 1.5}$$

$$= \frac{1.5}{6.9}$$

$$= .217 \text{ or } 21.7\% \text{ shunt}$$

Classic Shunt Equation

This equation is widely used because of the clinical limitations of the clinical shunt equation.

$$\dot{Q}_s/\dot{Q}_t = \frac{CcO_2 - CaO_2}{CcO_2 - C\bar{v}O_2}$$

Where:

CcO_2 = The content of oxygen in the end pulmonary capillary blood

CaO_2 = The content of oxygen in the arterial blood

$C\bar{v}O_2$ = The content of oxygen in the mixed venous blood

The patient should be inspiring 30% oxygen or more to calculate the oxygen content of end pulmonary capillary blood. This much oxygen should cause the PAO_2 of the ventilated alveoli to reach 150 torr or more. That results in 100% saturation of the hemoglobin of the end pulmonary capillary blood (ScO_2). Most patients who are sick enough to warrant a shunt determination will be on at least 30% oxygen. If not, the ScO_2 will have to be found by using the oxyhemoglobin dissociation curve.

A pulmonary artery catheter will be needed to sample mixed venous blood for $P\bar{v}O_2$ and $S\bar{v}O_2$ in both of these equations. An arterial blood gas sample will also be needed. There will be clinical situations in which either of these equations will work and result in the same answer.

Classic Shunt Example

The following example shows the classic shunt calculation with the following environmental and patient information:

P_B = Local barometric pressure—760 mm Hg for sea level

PH_2O = 47 mm Hg; water vapor pressure in the lungs at normal body temperature.

F_IO_2 = Inhaled oxygen percent of 30% or .3

PaO_2 = 95 mm Hg

$PaCO_2$ = 40 mm Hg

SaO_2 = 97% or .97

$P\bar{v}O_2$ = 40 mm Hg

$S\bar{v}O_2$ = 75% or .75

.8 = The normal respiratory quotient (an exact value can be determined by a metabolic study.)

15 g/dl = The patient's hemoglobin concentration

0.003 = The oxygen carrying capacity of blood plasma per mm Hg PO_2 (The value of 1.39 ml of oxygen/g Hb is occasionally used.)

Preliminary calculations:

1. Oxygen content of arterial blood

$$
\begin{aligned}
CaO_2 &= (Hb \times 1.34 \times SaO_2) + (PaO_2 \times 0.003) \\
&= (15 \times 1.34 \times .97) + (95 \times 0.003) \\
&= (19.5) + (0.3) \\
&= 19.8 \text{ vol } \%
\end{aligned}
$$

2. Oxygen content of mixed venous blood

$$
\begin{aligned}
C\bar{v}O_2 &= (Hb \times 1.34 \times S\bar{v}O_2) + (P\bar{v}O_2 \times 0.003) \\
&= (15 \times 1.34 \times .75) + (40 \times 0.003) \\
&= (15.1) + (.1) \\
&= 15.2 \text{ vol } \%
\end{aligned}
$$

3. Partial pressure of oxygen in the alveoli—the alveolar oxygen equation is used for this.

$$
\begin{aligned}
PAO_2 &= [(P_B - PH_2O) \times F_IO_2] - \frac{PaCO_2}{.8} \\
&= [(760 - 47) \times .3] - \frac{40}{.8} \\
&= [214] - 50 \\
&= 164 \text{ mm Hg}
\end{aligned}
$$

4. Oxygen content of pulmonary capillary blood

$$
\begin{aligned}
CcO_2 &= (Hb \times 1.34 \times ScO_2) + (PAO_2 \times 0.003) \\
&= (15 \times 1.34 \times 1.0) + (164 \times 0.003) \\
&= 20.1 + .492 \\
&= 20.1 + .5 \text{ (Rounded off to one decimal place)} \\
&= 20.6 \text{ vol } \%
\end{aligned}
$$

Final calculation:

$$
\begin{aligned}
\dot{Q}_s/\dot{Q}_t &= \frac{CcO_2 - CaO_2}{CcO_2 - C\bar{v}O_2} \\
&= \frac{20.6 - 19.8}{20.6 - 15.2} \\
&= \frac{.8}{5.4} \\
&= .15 \text{ or } 15\% \text{ shunt}
\end{aligned}
$$

e.   Interpret the results. (IB8c, IC1d, and IIIAr1) [R, Ap, An]

As noted earlier, shunt is the amount of blood pumped by the heart that does not participate in gas exchange through the lungs. It is wasted cardiac output and wasted effort by the heart. The normal person has a shunt of 5% or less. This shunted blood has a low oxygen content and dilutes down the oxygen content of all the blood. The larger the percent of shunted blood, the more the heart and body are stressed. Many clinicians believe that an indication for mechanical ventilation is a shunt of 15% to 20%. The ventilator is used to reduce the patient's work of breathing and oxygen consumption. Also, supplemental oxygen can be more carefully controlled and PEEP may be employed with the ventilator.

11.   Interpret the patient's pulmonary vascular resistance calculations. (IIIAr3) [R, Ap, An]

Pulmonary vascular resistance (PVR) is the total resistance of the pulmonary vascular bed to the blood being pumped through it by the right ventricle. Cardiac output and pulmonary blood pressure determine the PVR. The normal range for PVR in the adult is 1 to 3 mm Hg/l/min. Multiplying this value by 80 gives us the units of dynes $\times$ seconds $\times$ cm^{-5}. PVR is listed this way in some cardiology studies. The normal range of PVR would then range between 80 and 240 dynes $\times$ seconds $\times$ cm^{-5}.

With a normal PVR, the difference between the pulmonary artery diastolic pressure and the pulmonary capillary wedge pressure is 5 mm Hg or less. Any of the following could cause an elevated pulmonary vascular resistance:

1. Decreased oxygen in the lungs
2. Chronic obstructive lung disease (COPD)
3. Adult respiratory distress syndrome (ARDS)
4. Persistent pulmonary hypertension of the newborn/persistent fetal circulation
5. Primary pulmonary hypertension
6. Pulmonary embolism
7. Excessive positive end-expiratory pressure (PEEP)
8. Increased pulmonary blood flow from a left to right intracardiac shunt such as an atrial septal defect or ventricular septal defect

Additional clinical data must be gathered to confirm the diagnosis. An increased PVR is a serious problem because it can lead to right ventricular hypertrophy. The COPD patient is at risk for developing cor pulmonale. This is right ventricular failure secondary to lung disease and increased pulmonary vascular resistance.

12.   Interpret the patient's systemic vascular resistance calculations. (IIIAr3) [R, Ap, An]

Systemic vascular resistance (SVR) is the total resistance of the systemic vascular bed to the blood being pumped through it by the left ventricle. The normal range of SVR in the adult is 15 to 20 mm Hg/l/min. When multiplied by 80, a range of 900 to 1400 dynes $\times$ seconds $\times$ cm^{-5} is usually reported.

Cardiac output and systemic blood pressure determine the SVR. A patient with hypertension will have an elevated SVR. It will also increase if the patient is given a vasoconstricting drug and decrease if the patient is given a vasodilating drug.

Some allergic reactions will result in a dramatic drop in the SVR and blood pressure despite an increase in the cardiac output.

Module B.   Cardiopulmonary monitoring equipment.

1.   Capnography equipment.
a.   Get the necessary equipment for the procedure. (IIA1d3) [R, Ap]

As discussed earlier, a capnograph is used to measure a patient's exhaled carbon dioxide level and expiratory pattern. There are two different types of capnography systems. Their main difference is how the gas is sampled from the patient. Fig. 4-3 shows the patient connection for a mainstream capnograph. Fig. 4-4 shows a sidestream capnograph. Both work well if the patient is intubated as the connector is attached to the endotracheal tube. The patient may or may not be breathing with the aid of a mechanical ventilator. The sidestream unit may also be used with a spontaneously breathing patient because the capillary tube may be taped into a patient's nostril for gas sampling.

b.   Put the capnography equipment together, make sure that it works properly, and identify any problems with it. (IIB1e3) [R, Ap]

Components:

1. Airway attachment: Both the mainstream and sidestream units must have both inhaled and exhaled gas pass through the sensor or connector, respectively. Connections must be airtight and free of obstructions.
2. The gas sampling capillary tube of the sidestream unit must be kept clear of water or secretions.
3. Capnometer: Calibrate the unit with two gases of different CO_2 content. Room air is used for the "zero" value and either 5% or 10% CO_2 in a preanalyzed cylinder is used for the "high" value. Both values should calibrate within the manufacturer's specifications.
4. Capnograph: Check that the paper speeds and marker work properly.

c.   Fix any problems with the capnography equipment. (IIB2g1) [R, Ap, An]

Relatively few things can go wrong with capnography systems. The sidestream capnometer units must be kept dry. An external water trap is located between the capillary tube and the capnometer itself—make sure that the water is drained out periodically. Either capnography system can be disconnected from the patient. This will be seen as a drop in exhaled carbon dioxide to zero. If the alarm has been set it should activate.

d.   Perform quality control procedures on capnography equipment. (IIB3d) [R, Ap]

As presented earlier, both capnography units are calibrated using two points. Room air is for the zero point and either 5% or 10% carbon dioxide from a cylinder is used to set the high point. Follow the manufacturer's guidelines for how much adjustment for low or high point can be tolerated. Do not use a machine that cannot be properly calibrated.

2. **Pressure transducer.**
   a. **Put the strain gauge transducer equipment together, make sure that it works properly, and identify any problems with it. (IIB1i) [R, Ap]**

A strain gauge transducer converts a pressure signal to an electrical signal. The strain gauge is a fine wire screen that bends proportionately to the pressure put against it. Check to see that the wire screen of the transducer is not bent, damaged, or fouled with old blood or other debris. The transducer's wire cable and monitor connecting prongs should not be bent or damaged. Carefully insert the prongs into the receiving jack on the monitor.

A disposible, sterile, clear plastic dome should be firmly screwed onto the transducer. Noncompliant pressure tubing should connect the transducer with the patient's arterial or pulmonary artery catheter. The automatic fluid drip system (Sorenson) should be pressurized to 300 mm Hg. Heparin must be added to the fluid (usually normal saline) to prevent clotting in the patient's catheter. Because this is a continuous fluid "plumbing" system, all connections must be screwed water tight. (See Figs. 4-18 and 4-19.)

The transducer must be kept at the patient's midchest (midheart) level during calibration and measurement. Calibrate the electronics in the monitor by putting known pressures against the fluid system. The electronics should first be adjusted to "zero" pressure by opening the transducer to room air (atmospheric pressure). Adjust the electronic controls as needed. A sphygmomanometer is then used to pressurize the fluid system. A pulmonary artery catheter system is pressurized to relatively low pressures such as 30 and 50 mm Hg. An arterial system is adjusted to higher pressures such as 100 and 150 mm Hg. The monitored pressure should match the sphygmomanometer pressure. If not, adjust the electronic controls on the monitor to match.

   b. **Fix any problems with the equipment. (IIB2k1) [R, Ap]**

As mentioned earlier, all connections must be water tight. If not, the IV solution will drip out when it is pressurized. This could also result in the patient's measured pressures being less than true. Stopcocks must be opened or closed properly to allow the patient's pressure to be measured by the transducer. Electronics that will not calibrate to match the known pressures should not be used.

3. **In-dwelling arterial catheters.**
   a. **Get the necessary equipment for arterial catheterization. (IIA1k1) [R, Ap]**

Following are the general supplies that should be made available for catheterizing an artery for drawing blood gases and continuously monitoring blood pressure:

1. Sterile 20-gauge or 21-gauge needle with a flexible plastic sheath. After placement into the artery the needle is withdrawn and the sheath is left in place.
2. Sterile surgical drape for covering the area surrounding the insertion site.

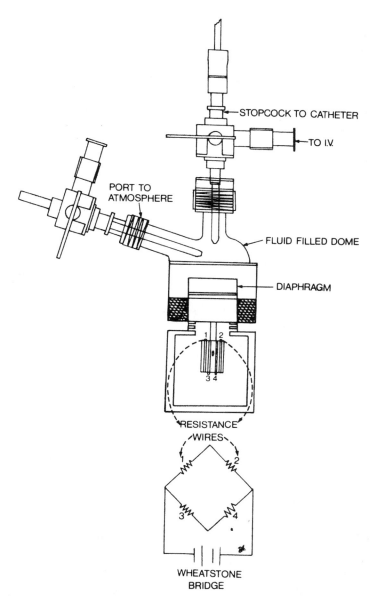

STOPCOCK TO CATHETER

TO I.V.

PORT TO
ATMOSPHERE

FLUID FILLED DOME

DIAPHRAGM

RESISTANCE
WIRES

WHEATSTONE
BRIDGE

Fig. 4-18 Schematic diagram of a strain gauge pressure transducer. The wire mesh resistance wires are arranged like a wheatstone bridge so that a pressure change results in a proportional change in the electrical resistance. (From Armstrong PW, Baigrie RS: *Hemodynamic monitoring in the critically ill*, Philadelphia, 1980, Harper & Row. Used by permission.)

3. Disinfectant such as 70% isopropyl alcohol and/or Betadyne solution.
4. Local anesthetic such as 4% lidocaine in a syringe and needle for injection into the insertion site.
5. One or two sterile 3 ml or 5 ml syringes for blood sampling.
6. Equipment for setting up a pressurized intravenous drip system so that the catheter does not clot.

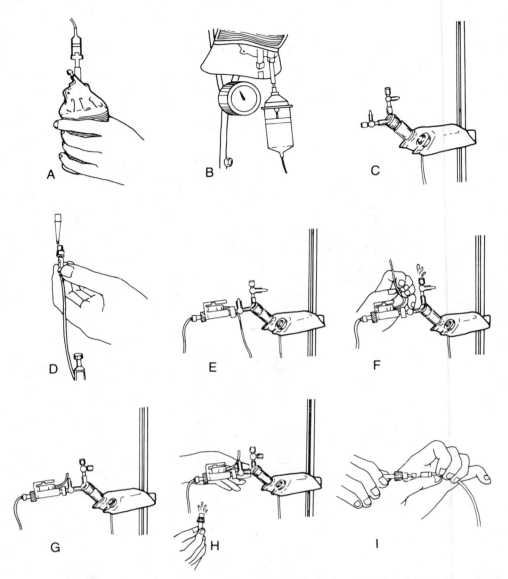

Fig. 4-19 Common steps in the assembly of the tubing circuit and pressure transducer to attach to an arterial or pulmonary artery catheter. Sterile technique must be maintained at all times. (Note: Individual institutions will vary these steps. Clinical practice is very important in this assembly.) **A,** Obtain a 250 to 500 ml bag of sterile, normal saline. Add 1 to 2 units of Heparin per ml of solution. Attach an IV line with a macrodrip chamber. **B,** Insert the solution bag into a pressure bag. Inflate the pressure to about 100 mm Hg to force the fluid through the IV tubing. The pressure bag will be pumped up to 300 mm Hg at the end of this procedure to ensure that 3 drops of fluid flow through the tubing per minute to keep it patent. **C,** Attach the strain gauge pressure transducer to an IV pole. Let it and the monitor warm up. **D,** Attach the IV tubing to the continuous flush device (Sorenson Intraflow). **E,** Screw the continuous flush device into the transducer stopcock. **F,** Backflush the continuous flush device and transducer, with open stopcocks, so that all air is removed and replaced with the saline solution. **G,** Zero and calibrate the pressure transducer and monitor. **H,** Attach high pressure tubing to the continuous flush device. Flush the air out of it. **I,** attach the high pressure tubing to the patient's arterial line or pulmonary artery catheter. Ensure that no air bubbles are present and that there is a continuous saline to blood connection. Accurate patient pressures should now be seen on the monitor. (From Oblouk Darovic G: *Hemodynamic monitoring,* Philadelphia, 1987, WB Saunders. Used by permission.)

b. Put the equipment together, make sure that it works properly, and identify any problems with it. (IIB1k1) [R, Ap]

See Figs. 4-12 and 4-19 for illustrations of how the pressure transducer, connecting tubing, stopcocks, infusion system, and monitoring electronics are assembled. See Fig. 4-20 for a completed system. Clinical experience is needed with these types of systems.

c. Correct any problems with the equipment. (IIB2j1) [R, Ap, An]

Table 4-3 lists problems, causes, prevention, and treatment for inaccurate pressure measurements with arterial or pulmonary artery catheters. Table 4-4 specifically lists problems with arterial lines. Fig. 4-21 shows common problem areas with arterial lines. Pulmonary artery catheters can have problems in the same areas.

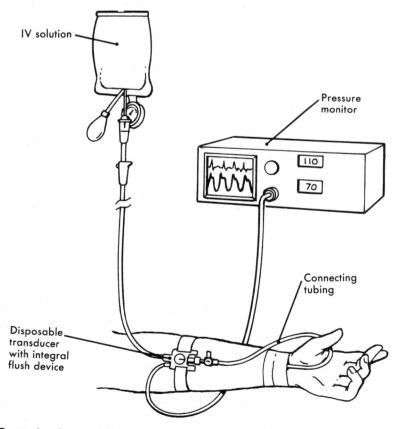

Fig. 4-20 Example of a complete set up for monitoring the arterial pressure. (From Daily EK, Schroeder JS: *Techniques in bedside hemodynamic monitoring,* ed 4, St. Louis, 1989, Mosby–Year Book. Used by permission.)

Table 4-3. Inaccurate Pressure Measurements

Problem	Cause	Prevention	Treatment
Damped pressure tracing or abnormally high reading	Catheter tip against vessel wall	Usually cannot be avoided	Pull back or reposition catheter while observing waveform.
	Partial occlusion of tip by clot	Use continuous drip. May help to use 1 unit heparin/1 ml IV fluid. Occasionally hand flush rapidly and use rapid drip after blood withdrawal. Use heparin-bonded catheter.	Aspirate clot with syringe; flush with heparinized fluid
	Pressure trapped by improper sequence of stopcock operation	Turn stopcocks in proper sequence when two pressures are measured on one transducer.	Thoroughly flush transducers with IV solution; rezero and turn stopcocks in proper sequence.
Inappropriate pressure waveform or measurement	Altered location of catheter tip (e.g., in RV or PAW instead of in PA)	Establish optimal position carefully when introducing catheter initially. Suture catheter at insertion site and tape catheter to patient's skin.	Review waveform on scope. Check position under fluoroscope and/or x-ray after reposition.
	Movement of catheter tip against wall of chamber	Usually cannot be avoided	Reposition catheter.
Negative or inappropriately low pressure	Transducer reference level higher than midchest	Maintain transducer reference at midchest level.	Recheck transducer position.
	Loose connection	Use Luer-Lok stopcocks.	Check connections.
Damped pressure without improvement after catheter flush	Air bubbles in transducer	Set up carefully.	Check system; flush rapidly through transducers.
No pressure available	Transducer not open to catheter	Follow routine, systematic steps for pressure measurement.	Check system, stopcocks.
	Amplifiers still on *cal, zero,* or *off*		
Noise or fling in pressure waveform	Excessive catheter movement, particularly in pulmonary artery	Avoid excessive catheter length in ventricle.	Try different catheter tip position. Purposely damp waveform with damping device.
	Excessive tubing length	Use shortest tubing possible (<3 to 4 feet).	Eliminate excess tubing.
	Excessive stopcocks	Minimize number of stopcocks.	Eliminate excess stopcocks.

From Daily EK, Schroeder JS: *Techniques in bedside hemodynamic monitoring*, ed 4, St. Louis, 1989, Mosby—Year Book. Used by permission.

4. **Pulmonary artery catheters.**
   a. **Get the necessary equipment for the procedure. (IIA1k2) [R, Ap]**

Pulmonary artery catheters come in several diameter sizes. The smallest can be advanced into a pediatric patient's vein. Most adults will have either a 5 French or 7 French catheter inserted. Other than size being a consideration, select a catheter that provides the information that is needed. A standard 5 French catheter can be used to measure pulmonary artery pressure and pulmonary capillary wedge pressure, and a mixed venous blood sample can be withdrawn from it for analysis. A 7 French thermodilution cardiac output catheter can do all these things plus give a central venous pressure and have cardiac output measured through the computer (see Figs. 4-11 and 4-15). A 7 French fiberoptic catheter can measure continuous $S\bar{v}O_2$ as well as PAP, PCWP, CVP, and cardiac output by the thermodilution method. Mixed venous blood can also be sampled for analysis.

   b. **Put the equipment together, make sure that it works properly, and identify any problems with it. (IIB1k2) [R, Ap]**

The 5 French and 7 French catheters come self-contained as a single unit. The general assembly of the related tubing circuit and pressure transducer was discussed earlier and illustrated in Figs. 4-12 and 4-19. Clinical experience is needed. Make sure that all connections are water tight, the transducer calibrates accurately, and the balloon inflates and deflates properly.

   c. **Correct any problems with the pulmonary artery catheter equipment. (IIB2j2) [R, Ap, An]**

See Table 4-5 for a listing of the problems seen with pulmonary artery catheters and their causes, prevention, and treatment. Fig. 4-21 shows common problem areas with the related pressure tubing and equipment.

5. **Get the correct cardiac output computer for the procedure. (IIA1k3) [R, Ap]**

Most makers of pulmonary artery catheters (e.g., American Edwards Laboratories) also make thermodilution cardiac output computers. However, the computer is usually only designed for use with their brand of catheter. Make sure that you have a compatable catheter and computer.

Module C.   Patient assessment.

1. **Interpret the information given by the intravascular monitor. (IC2h) [R, Ap, An]**

The process of calibrating the monitor for pulmonary artery pressures or systemic artery pressures was briefly discussed earlier. Regardless of the catheter being placed into a systemic artery, pulmonary artery, umbilical artery, or superior vena cava, the equipment must be properly calibrated to have any faith in the data. When performing two-point calibration, all pressures should read "zero" when exposed to atmospheric pressure. This is the low point. Calibrating a central venous pressure water-column manometer usually involves only making sure that it reads zero at atmospheric pressure. The high point pressure for pulmonary artery pressure

Table 4-4. Problems Encountered with Arterial Catheters

Problem	Cause	Prevention	Treatment
Hematoma after withdrawal of needle	Bleeding or oozing at puncture site	Maintain firm pressure on site during withdrawal of catheter and for 5 to 15 min (as necessary) after withdrawal. Apply elastic tape (Elastoplast) firmly over puncture site. For femoral arterial puncture sites, leave a sandbag on site for 1 to 2 hr to prevent oozing. If patient is receiving heparin, discontinue 2 hr before catheter removal.	Continue to hold pressure to puncture site until oozing stops. Apply sandbag to femoral puncture site for 1 to 2 hr after removal of catheter.
Decreased or absent pulse distal to puncture site	Spasm of artery	Introduce arterial needle cleanly, nontraumatically.	Inject lidocaine locally at insertion site and 10 mg into arterial catheter.
	Thrombosis of artery		Arteriotomy and Fogarty catheterization both distally and proximally from the puncture site result in return of pulse in more than 90% of cases if brachial or femoral artery is used.
Bleedback into tubing, dome, or transducer	Insufficient pressure on IV bag	Maintain 300 mm Hg pressure on IV bag.	Replace transducer.
	Loose connections	Use Luer-Lok stopcocks.	"Fast flush" through system. Tighten all connections.
Hemorrhage	Loose connections	Keep all connecting sites visible. Observe connecting sites frequently. Use built-in alarm system. Use Luer-Lok stopcocks.	Tighten all connections.

Complication	Cause	Prevention	Treatment
Emboli	Clot from catheter tip into bloodstream	Always aspirate and discard before flushing. Use continuous flush device. Use 1 unit heparin/1 ml IV fluid. Gently flush >2 to 4 ml.	Remove catheter.
Local infection	Forward movement of contaminated catheter Break in sterile technique Prolonged catheter use	Carefully suture catheter at insertion site. Always use aseptic technique. Remove catheter after 72 to 96 hr. Inspect and care for insertion site daily, including dressing change and antibiotic or iodophor ointment.	Remove catheter. Prescribe antibiotic.
Sepsis	Break in sterile technique Prolonged catheter use Bacterial growth in IV fluid	Use percutaneous insertion. Always use aseptic technique. Remove catheter after 72 to 96 hr. Change IV fluid bag, stopcocks, dome, and tubing every 24 to 48 hr. Do not use IV fluid containing glucose. Sterilize transducers before use (if nondisposable transducers used). Use sterile dead-ender caps on all ports of stopcocks. Carefully flush remaining blood from stopcocks after blood sampling.	Remove catheter. Prescribe antibiotic.

From Daily EK, Schroeder JS: *Techniques in bedside hemodynamic monitoring*, ed 4, St. Louis, 1989, Mosby–Year Book. Used by permission.

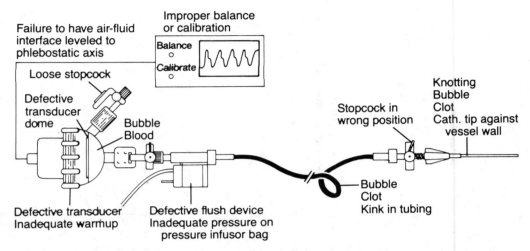

Fig. 4-21 Common problem areas with arterial and pulmonary artery catheters. (From Oblouk Darovic G: *Hemodynamic monitoring,* Philadelphia, 1987, WB Saunders. Used by permission.)

monitoring is commonly 30 mm Hg. The high point pressure for arterial pressure monitoring is commonly 100 mm Hg.

Remember to have the patient lying flat in bed during any pressure monitoring. The patient should also be breathing spontaneously. If the patient must be supported on a ventilator, make a note of it in the charting. High ventilating pressures or positive end-expiratory pressure can artificially increase the patient's actual vascular pressures.

2. Examine all the data to determine the patient's pathophysiological condition. (IC3a) [R, Ap, An]

See Fig. 4-22 for examples of diagnostic pathways. These can be used to help the clinician evaluate all the patient data. The diagnosis or pathophysiologic state can be determined by following the data down a given pathway. Normal values and common conditions associated with abnormal values were discussed earlier in this section.

3. Participate in the development of the patient's respiratory care plan. (IC3c) [An]

Each clinical problem presented in this section requires its own individualized treatment. Be prepared to make recommendations to change the inspired oxygen percentage, give aerosolized bronchodilators, give diuretics to increase urine output, and so forth.

Table 4-5. Problems Encountered with PA Catheters

Problem	Cause	Prevention	Treatment
Phlebitis or local infection at insertion site	Mechanical irritation or contamination	Prepare skin properly before insertion. Use sterile technique during insertion and dressing change. Insert smoothly and rapidly. Change dressings, stopcocks, and connecting tubing every 24 to 48 hr. Remove catheter or change insertion site every 4 days.	Remove catheter. Apply warm compresses. Give pain medication as necessary.
IV fluid infusing poorly Damped waveforms and inaccurate pressures	Partial clotting at catheter tip	Use continuous drip with 1 unit heparin/1 ml IV fluid. Hand flush occasionally. Flush with large volume after blood withdrawal. Use heparin-coated catheters.	Aspirate, then flush catheter with heparinized fluid (not in PAW position).
	Tip moving against wall	Obtain more stable catheter position.	Reposition catheter.
	Improper transducer reference level	Maintain transducer air-reference port at midchest level.	Remeasure level of transducer reference and reposition at midchest level.
	Incorrect zeroing and calibration of monitor	Zero and calibrate monitor properly.	Recheck zero and calibration of monitor.
Ventricular irritability	Looping of excess catheter in right ventricle	Suture catheter at insertion site; check chest x-ray.	Reposition catheter; remove loop.
	Migration of catheter from PA to RV	Position catheter tip in main right or left PA.	Inflate balloon to encourage catheter floatation out to PA.
	Irritation of the endocardium during catheter passage	Keep balloon inflated during advancement; advance gently.	Administer lidocaine if necessary; defibrillate if VF occurs.
Apparent wedging of catheter with balloon *deflated*	Forward migration of catheter tip caused by blood flow, excessive loop in RV, or	Check catheter tip by fluoroscopy; position in main right or left PA.	Aspirate blood from catheter; if catheter is wedged, sample will be arterialized and

(Continued)

Table 4-5. (cont.)

Problem	Cause	Prevention	Treatment
	inadequate suturing of catheter at insertion site	Check catheter position on x-ray film if fluoroscopy is not used. Suture catheter in place at insertion site.	obtained with difficulty or not at all. If wedged, slowly pull back catheter until PA waveform appears. If not wedged, gently aspirate and flush catheter with saline; catheter tip can partially clot, causing damping that resembles damped PAW waveform.
Pulmonary hemorrhage infarction, or both	Distal migration of catheter tip Continuous or prolonged wedging of catheter Overinflation of balloon while catheter is wedged	Check chest x-ray immediately after insertion and 12 hr later; remove catheter loop in RA or RV. Leave balloon deflated with stopcock *open.* Suture catheter at skin to prevent inadvertent advancement. Position catheter in main right or left PA. Pull catheter back to pulmonary artery if it becomes wedged. Do not flush catheter when in wedge position. Inflate balloon slowly with only enough air to obtain a PAW waveform. Do not inflate 7 Fr catheter with more than 1 to 1.5 cc air. Do not inflate if resistance is met.	
"Overwedging" or damped PAW	Overinflation of balloon Eccentric inflation of balloon	Watch waveform during inflation; inject only enough air to obtain PAW pressure. Do not inflate 7 inch French catheter with more than 1 to 1.5 cc air.	Deflate balloon; reinflate slowly with only enough air to obtain PAW pressure. Deflate balloon; reposition and slowly reinflate.

Complication	Cause	Intervention
PA balloon rupture	Overinflation of balloon	Inflate slowly with only enough air to obtain a PAW pressure.	Remove syringe to prevent further air injection.
	Frequent inflations of balloon	Monitor PAD pressure as reflection of PAW and LVEDP.	Monitor PAD pressure.
	Syringe deflation damaging wall of balloon	Allow passive deflation of balloon through stopcock. Remove syringe after inflation.	
Infection	Nonsterile insertion techniques	Use sterile techniques. Use sterile catheter sleeve.	Remove catheter. Use antibiotics
	Fulid contamination through outlet ports of stopcocks	Use sterile dead ender caps on all ports of stopcocks. Change IV solution, stopcock, and tubing every 24 to 48 hr. Do not use IV solution containing glucose.	
	Fluid contamination from transducer through membrane of disposable dome	Check disposable domes for cracks. Sterilize nondisposable transducer before use. Change disposable domes or transducer every 48 hr. Change disposable dome after countershock. Do not use IV solution containing glucose.	
	Exposure of vessel to microorganisms	Use percutaneous insertion technique.	
	Prolonged catheter placement	Change catheter insertion site every 4 days.	
Heart block during insertion of catheter	Mechanical irritation of His bundle in patients with preexisting left bundle branch block.	Insert catheter expeditiously with balloon inflated. Insert transvenous pacing catheter before PA catheter insertion.	Use temporary pacemarker or flotation catheter with pacing wire.

From Daily EK, Schroeder JS: *Techniques in bedside hemodynamic monitoring*, ed 4, St. Louis, 1989, Mosby–Year Book. Used by permission.

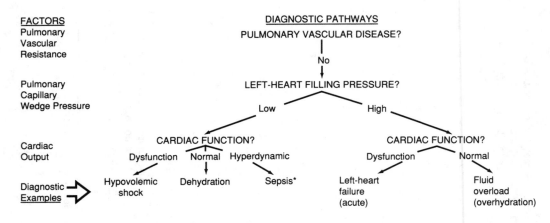

*Sepsis may be associated with normal left-heart filling pressures.

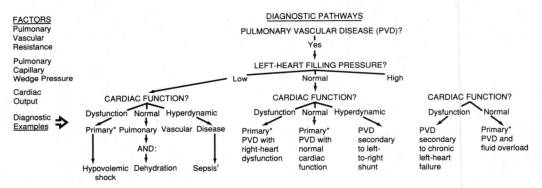

*Primary PVD may be due to pulmonary emboli, pulmonary artery disease (vasculitis, "primary" pulmonary hypertension), respiratory distress syndromes, hypoxic vasoconstriction, or drugs.
†Sepis may be associated with normal left-heart filling pressures.

Fig. 4-22 Possible diagnostic pathways for patients with and without pulmonary vascular disease. In both cases the pulmonary vascular resistance, pulmonary capillary wedge pressure, and cardiac output are measured. High, normal, or low values lead down different pathways. Previous discussions and clinical experience are needed to determine the final diagnosis. (From Osgood CF, Watson MH, Slaughter MS et al: Hemodynamic monitoring in respiratory care, *Respir Care* 29(1):25-34, 1984. Used by permission.)

BIBLIOGRAPHY

Aloan CA: *Respiratory care of the newborn: a clinical manual,* Philadelphia, 1987, JB Lippincott.

Anton WR, Raghu G: Measuring end-tidal carbon dioxide tension at maximal exhalation to improve its utility during T-piece weaning trials, *Respir Care* 35(11):1082-1083, 1990.

Armstrong PW, Baigrie RS: *Hemodynamic monitoring in the critically ill,* Philadelphia, 1980, Harper & Row.

Baele PL, McMichan JC, Marsh HM et al: Continuous monitoring of mixed venous oxygen saturation in critically ill patients, *Anesth Analg* 61(6):513-517, 1982.

Bakow ED: A limitation of capnography, *Respir Care* 27(2):167-168, 1982.

Brainard CA: *Respiratory care: national board review,* Bowie, Md, 1985, Brady Communications.

Carlon GC, Ray C, Miodownik S et al: Capography in mechanically ventilated patients, *Crit Care Med* 16(5):550-556, 1988.

Clark DB, Marshall SG: Mixed venous oxygen saturation measurement. II. General and specific clinical applications, *Respir Ther* 81-86, Nov/Dec 1986.

Daily EK, Schroeder JS: *Techniques in bedside hemodynamic monitoring,* ed 4, St. Louis, 1989, Mosby–Year Book.

Deshpande VM, Pilbeam SP, Dixon RJ: *A comprehensive review in respiratory care,* Norwalk, Conn, 1988, Appleton & Lange.

Divertie MB, McMichan JC: Continuous monitoring of mixed venous oxygen saturation, *Chest* 85(3):423-428, 1984.

Fahey PJ, Harris K, Vanderwarf C: Clinical experience with continuous monitoring of mixed venous oxygen saturation in respiratory failure, *Chest* 86(5):748-752, 1984.

Harris K: Noninvasive monitoring of gas exchange, *Respir Care* 32(7):544-557, 1987.

Hess D: Capnometry and capnography: technical aspects, physiologic aspects, and clinical applications, *Respir Care* 35(6):557-576, 1990

Huang SH, Dasher LA, Larson CA et al: *Coronary care nursing,* Philadelphia, 1983, WB Saunders.

Jaquith SM: The oximetric opticath: what is it and how can it facilitate nursing management of the critically ill patient? *Crit Care Nurse* 55-58, May/June 1984.

Kandel G, Aberman A: Mixed venous oxygen saturation: its role in the assessment of the critically ill patient, *Arch Intern Med* 143:1400-1402, 1983.

Kinasewitz GT: Use of end-tidal capnography during mechanical ventilation, *Respir Care* 25(2):169-171, 1982.

Krider SJ: Cardiac output assessment. In Wilkins RL, Sheldon RL, Krider SJ, editors: *Clinical assessment in respiratory care,* ed 2, St. Louis 1990, Mosby–Year Book.

Krider SJ: Invasively monitored hemodynamic pressures. In Wilkins RL, Sheldon RL, Krider SJ, editors: *Clinical assessment in respiratory care,* ed 2, St. Louis, 1990, Mosby–Year Book.

Marini JJ: Obtaining meaningful data from the Swan-Ganz catheter, *Respir Care* 30(7):572-585, 1985.

McMichan JC: Continuous monitoring of mixed venous oxygen saturation in clinical practice, *Mount Sinai J Med* 51(5):569-572, 1984.

Nuzzo PF, Anton WR: Practical applications of capnography, *Respir Ther* 12-17, Nov/Dec 1986.

Oblouk Darovic G: *Hemodynamic monitoring,* Philadelphia, 1987, WB Saunders.

Osgood CF, Watson MH, Slaughter MS et al: Hemodynamic monitoring in respiratory care, *Respir Care* 29(1):25-34, 1984.

Paulus DA: Invasive monitoring of respiratory gas exchange: continuous measurement of mixed venous oxygen saturation, *Respir Care* 32(7):535-543, 1987.

Pilbeam SP: *Mechanical ventilation, physiological and clinical applications,* St. Louis, 1986, Multi-Media.

Ruppel G: *Manual of pulmonary function testing,* ed 5, St. Louis, 1990, Mosby–Year Book.

Shapiro BA, Harrison RA, Cane RD et al: *Clinical application of blood gases,* ed 4, Chicago, 1989, Year Book Medical.

Shrake KL: Capnography in patients being weaned from mechanical ventilation, *Respir Ther* July/Aug 1980.

Wiedemann HP: Invasive monitoring techniques in the ventilated patient. In Kacmarek RM, Stoller JK, editors: *Current respiratory care*, Toronto, 1988, BC Decker.

Wilkins RL, Sheldon RL, Krider SJ: *Clinical assessment in respiratory care*, ed 2, St. Louis, 1990, Mosby–Year Book.

SELF-STUDY QUESTIONS

1. Your patient has a V_D/V_T ratio of .68. Based on these results, which of the following would you recommend?
   A. Give the patient supplemental oxygen.
   B. Coach the patient in hyperinflation therapy.
   C. Put the patient on a mechanical ventilator.
   D. Give the patient an IPPB treatment.
   E. Put the patient on a CPAP system.

2. Hypovolemia in an adult patient would be indicated by a wedge pressure of:
   A. Greater than 12 mm Hg
   B. 8 mm Hg
   C. 24 mm Hg
   D. 2 mm Hg
   E. None of the above

3. A patient has an end-tidal CO_2 of 30 torr and an A-aCO_2 gradient of 4 torr. His $PaCO_2$ would be estimated as:
   A. 26 torr
   B. 30 torr
   C. 4 torr
   D. 34 torr
   E. 40 torr

4. The wave form sequence seen during the insertion of a pulmonary artery catheter is:
   A. RA, RV, PAP, PCWP
   B. RV, RA, PAP, PCWP
   C. RA, RV, PCWP, PAP
   D. Ao, LV, LA, PAP
   E. Ao, RA, RV, PAP

5. A normal PAP pressure in mm Hg is:
   A. 30/15
   B. 25/10
   C. 20/10
   D. 120/80
   E. 8

6. A 50-year-old patient who has been sick with pneumonia and diarrhea for several days is placed on a mechanical ventilator. Arterial and pulmonary artery catheters are placed for monitoring blood gases and hemodynamic parameters. Arterial blood gas values on 40% oxygen show: PaO_2 70 torr, $PaCO_2$ 39 torr, pH 7.43, bicarbonate 24 mEq/l. Pulmonary artery catheter parameters show: PAP 22/8 torr and PCWP of 3 torr. In addition, serum electrolytes show: sodium 158 mEq/l, potassium 4.3 mEq/l, and chlorine 118 mEq/l. Based on this data, what would you recommend?

A. Administer a diuretic.
B. Increase the oxygen percentage.
C. Administer fluids intravenously.
D. Give a chronotropic agent such as atropine.
E. Restrict fluids.

7. A patient with advanced emphysema is admitted to the respiratory intensive care unit. He is placed on a 24% venturi-type mask and has a pulmonary artery catheter inserted. His initial pulmonary vascular resistance (PVR) is 9 mm/Hg/l/min and PaO_2 is 57 torr. The physician orders him increased to 28% oxygen. The resulting PVR is 5 mm Hg/l/min and PaO_2 is 63 torr. Based on this information, what would you recommend?
   A. Decrease the oxygen back to 24%.
   B. Increase the oxygen to 35%.
   C. Place the patient on a ventilator.
   D. Administer an inotropic agent such as digitalis.
   E. Keep the patient on 28% oxygen.

8. The following capnograph could be interpreted as:
   A. Normal
   B. Ventilation to perfusion mismatching
   C. Decreased physiologic dead space
   D. Pulmonary fibrosis
   E. Cardiopulmonary arrest

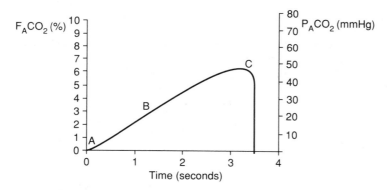

9. A $P\bar{v}O_2$ value of 29 mm Hg would indicate that the patient:
   A. Is normal
   B. Is suffering some tissue hypoxemia
   C. Is not consuming the normal amount of oxygen
   D. Is hypercarbic
   E. Has a normal pH

10. The principle of operation of the capnography monitor is:
    A. The same as the Clark electrode
    B. The same as the Severinhaus electrode
    C. Infrared absorption
    D. Hamburger phenomena
    E. The same as the CO-oximeter

11. Stroke volume:
    A. Is an indicator of the adequacy of perfusion of the body tissues

B.   Is the output of blood for a minute
C.   Is the volume of blood in either ventricle at the end of diastole
D.   Has a range of 60 to 130 ml in the adult
E.   Is the resistance to flow

12.   The normal A-aCO$_2$ gradient is:
A.   Less than 4 torr
B.   About 6 torr
C.   More than 25 torr
D.   More than 40 torr
E.   About 40 torr

13.   Calculate a patient's PAD-PCWP (pulmonary artery diastolic-pulmonary capillary wedge pressure) gradient if the PAP is 30/12 and the PCWP is 8.
A.   38 mm Hg
B.   22 mm Hg
C.   12 mm Hg
D.   8 mm Hg
E.   4 mm Hg

14.   A patient has a PaCO$_2$ of 52 torr and ETCO$_2$ of 66 torr. Calculate her A-aCO$_2$.
A.   118 torr
B.   66 torr
C.   52 torr
D.   40 torr
E.   14 torr

15.   Your patient is in the intensive care unit and is being monitored with a pulmonary artery catheter. She has the following parameters: PAP of 45/20 mm Hg, PCWP of 9 mm Hg, central venous pressure of 9 cm water. You would interpret the data to indicate that she:
A.   Has right ventricular failure/cor pulmonale
B.   Has left ventricular failure
C.   Has increased pulmonary vascular resistance
D.   Is hypervolemic
E.   Is hypovolemic

16.   A patient who was admitted with congestive heart failure is placed on a ventilator and has a S$\bar{v}$O$_2$ measuring pulmonary artery catheter inserted. Her initial S$\bar{v}$O$_2$ was 69%. The physician orders her placed on 10 cm H$_2$O of PEEP. Ten minutes after the PEEP is applied her S$\bar{v}$O$_2$ is 58%. Based on this information, which of the following would you recommend to the physician?
A.   Keep the patient as she is.
B.   Increase the PEEP to 15 cm H$_2$O.
C.   Increase the oxygen by 10%.
D.   Remove the PEEP.
E.   Decrease the oxygen by 10%.

Answer Key

1. C; 2. D; 3. A; 4. A; 5. B; 6. C; 7. E; 8. B; 9. B; 10. C; 11. D; 12. B; 13. E; 14. E; 15. C; 16. D.

5 | Oxygen and Other Gas Therapy

Module A.   Oxygen therapy.

1.   Adjust the inspired oxygen percentage. (IIIC3c) [An]

2.   Adjust the flow of oxygen. (IIIC3b) [An]

3.   Change the method of administering the oxygen. (IIIC3a) [An]

Every patient's oxygen percentage or flow must be tailored to meet his or her clinical goals. Usually this means keeping the PaO_2 between 60 and 100 mm Hg and the SpO_2 between 90% and 97% in patients who are acutely hypoxemic. Exceptions, when the blood oxygen level is kept as high as possible, include cardiopulmonary resuscitation and the treatment of carbon monoxide poisoning.

Another exception is the chronic obstructive lung disease patient who is hypoxemic and hypercarbic. Usually these patients are maintained with a moderate hypoxemia. The PaO_2 should be between 50 and 60 mm Hg and the SpO_2 between 85% and 90%. It is imperative to keep the oxygen in this relatively narrow range. Further hypoxemia will result in pulmonary hypertension and cor pulmonale. Cardiac dysrhythmias or arrest and death can occur if the hypoxemia is severe (less than 40 mm Hg). Oxygen levels in the normal range (greater than 60 mm Hg) may result in blunting of the hypoxic drive. This could result in bradypnea and even greater CO_2 retention with corresponding acidemia. When the $PaCO_2$ exceeds 80 to 90 mm Hg many patients become drowsy. The treatment is to decrease the F_1O_2 and to lower the PaO_2 to 50 to 60 mm Hg. This in turn stimulates the hypoxic drive so that the patient increases his or her ventilation.

The advantages, disadvantages, and possible oxygen delivery ranges for the various oxygen appliances are discussed in *Respiratory Care Certification Guide* (Sills, 1994) and other standard respiratory care textbooks. The general theory of their use is tested on the Entry Level Exam. Review nasal cannulas, catheters, the various oxygen masks, tents, and hoods as necessary. Be prepared to make recommendations to change from one appliance to another.

Module B.   Helium/oxygen (heliux) therapy.

1.   Get the necessary equipment for the procedure. (IIA1g) [An]

The cylinder color code for helium/oxygen mixes (He/O_2) is brown and green. Always read the label to make sure that you have the correct gas in the cylinder. Because helium/oxygen comes in two mixes check the label to tell between an

80% helium and 20% oxygen mix or a 70% helium and 30% oxygen mix. Get the specific regulator to fit the cylinder. If using an E size cylinder the helium/oxygen regulator will have pins in the 2 and 4 locations according to the Pin Index Safety System. If an oxygen flowmeter is used with a helium/oxygen regulator the following adjustments must be made to the flow seen on the flowmeter. This is done because helium is less dense than oxygen.

1. When using an 80% helium and 20% oxygen mix, multiply the observed flow by 1.8. For example, a seen flow of 10 L/min $\times$ 1.8 = 18 L/min actual flow.
2. When using a 70% helium and 30% oxygen mix, multiply the observed flow by 1.6. For example, a seen flow of 10 L/min $\times$ 1.6 = 16 L/min actual flow.

Additional equipment includes a patient face mask, gas delivery tubing, and humidification system. This is discussed further in the next section.

2. Assemble, check for proper function, and identify any problems with the equipment. (IIB1h) [R, Ap]

The type of mask, delivery tubing, and humidifier chosen will depend on whether the patient needs an aerosol delivered or not. If aerosol is not needed, a non-rebreather mask with small bore oxygen tubing is selected. Attach a bubble humidifier with sterile water to the flowmeter. Connect the oxygen tubing to the humidifier nipple and to the non-rebreather mask nipple. If aerosol is required, an aerosol mask with one-way exhalation valves and reservoir will be needed. Screw the nebulizer filled with sterile water to the flowmeter. Make sure that the air entrainment control is set to deliver 100% source gas (no room air should be entrained). Connect the large bore, aerosol tubing to the nebulizer and the mask. Make sure the mask is adjusted to give as tight a fit to the face as practical and comfortable. In either system it is extremely important that all connections be tight because helium will easily leak out of any openings.

3. Adjust the flow on the helium/oxygen gas therapy system. (IIIC4) [R, Ap, An]

Patients who benefit from He/O$_2$ therapy have upper airway obstruction problems such as a laryngeal or tracheal tumor. Because helium atoms are so much smaller than nitogen molecules, patients find that their work of breathing is greatly reduced. Normoxic patients are usually given a mix of 80% helium and 20% oxygen whereas hypoxic patients are given 70% helium and 30% oxygen. If more oxygen is needed, small bore oxygen tubing can be used to add it into the mask or reservoir bag, or a special closed system will have to be assembled from components.

Ideally any helium/oxygen delivery system should have a reservoir bag. Usually the non-rebreathing mask and reservoir are used. The reservoir should be filled with the He/O$_2$ mix before the mask is placed on the patient's face. Again, the fit should be as tight as possible to minimize leaks. Adjust the flow so that the reservoir bag does not collapse by more than one third during an inspiration. If it does, increase the flow. The flow should be increased if the patient complains of shortness of breath. Signs of increased work of breathing include agitation; increased use of accessory muscles of respiration; sweating; and increased respiratory rate, heart rate, and blood pressure.

Module C.   Gas administration equipment.

1.   Fix any problems with air entrainment devices and masks. (IIB2a2) [An]

Air entrainment masks are designed to provide the patient with a controlled oxygen percentage at a flow rate high enough to ensure that all the patient's needs are met. There are two different types of air entrainment devices based on the physical principles seen in the Bernoulli effect: variable jet diameter and variable air entrainment ports. It is important to know about these two types so that you understand what can go wrong with them and how they can be fixed.

Variable Jet Diameter

Manufacturers of variable jet diameter systems include Vickers, OEM, Inspiron, and U-Mid. Notice that the jets have different diameters but the room air entrainment ports are the same size. You will see that the *smaller* the jet diameter is, the *lower* the oxygen percentage is. This is because as the jet becomes smaller the lateral pressure is lower. This results in more room air being brought into the entrainment ports to dilute the oxygen and raise the total flow.

Make sure that the jets are not obstructed by mucus or anything else or the oxygen percentage will be decreased. An obstruction downstream from the jet will prevent as much room air as normal from being brought into the mask. This will result in the oxygen percentage increasing and the total flow decreasing.

Variable Air Entrainment Ports

Manufacturers of variable air entrainment port systems include Hudson and Salter. Notice that the jet size is fixed but the room air entrainment ports are different sizes. You will see that the *smaller* the entrainment ports are, the *higher* the oxygen percentage is. This is because less room air can be entrained to dilute the oxygen. The total flow is also reduced when the entrainment ports are smaller.

Make sure that the entrainment ports are not.obstructed by the patient's sheet or anything else or the oxygen percentage will increase. An obstruction downstream from the jet will also prevent as much room air as normal from being brought into the mask. This will result in the oxygen percentage increasing and the total flow decreasing.

2.   Fix any problems with an oxygen hood. (IIB2a3) [An]

Oxygen hoods are used to provide a warmed aerosol, humidity, and a controlled oxygen percentage to pediatric patients who weigh no more than 18 pounds. In addition, the following procedures should be followed:

1. Use an air/oxygen proportioner with flowmeter to control the oxygen percentage and flow to the hood. The flow should be at least 7 L/min to prevent the buildup of exhaled carbon dioxide. A flow of 10 to 15 L/min is needed to keep a stable oxygen percentage. Keeping the hood sealed as much as possible and minimizing the gap between the infant's neck and the opening to the hood will also help to stabilize the oxygen percentage.

2. A warmed nebulizer is needed to provide a high humidity level and to warm

the oxygen to the infant's body temperature. Care must be taken with infants to ensure that they are neither heated nor cooled by the gas blowing over their heads. A thermometer should be kept in the hood to note the temperature.

3. An oxygen analyzer should be continuously monitoring how much oxygen is inside the hood. The analyzer probe should be placed at the same level as the infant's nose. This is because oxygen is heavier than air and will tend to settle toward the bottom of the hood.

The advantages of the hood over the oxygen tent are that the patient's body is accessible and the head can be reached by lifting the top off the hood. Be aware of the noise level inside the hood to minimize damaging the infant's hearing. The sound level should be monitored and kept well below 65 dB.

3.   Fix any problems with an oxygen tent. (IIB2a3) [An]

Oxygen tents were formerly used for adults but are now only used for children who are too large and active for a hood. The tent is used to control the environment by providing a cooled aerosol, humidity, and controlled oxygen percentage. In addition, the following procedures should be observed:

1. Set an oxygen flowmeter to deliver 8 to 10 L/min to small tents and 12 to 15 L/min to large tents to keep the carbon dioxide level below 1%. Flows of 30 L/min or greater will be needed to keep the oxygen percentage close to the 50% maximum that can be reliably maintained.

2. The oxygen should flow through a nebulizer or ultrasonic unit to provide the needed humidity. Try to keep the relative humidity at 60% or greater to minimize any risk of a spark causing a fire inside the tent. If no mist is seen within the tent check for proper functioning of the nebulizer.

3. The tent must be cooled to prevent the patient from overheating in the enclosed space. Also, if the child has croup, the cooled air is therapeutic. The smaller, simpler units run the oxygen flow through an ice water solution. This can cool the inside about 6 to 8° F below the room's temperature. The larger, more complex units use an electrically powered refrigeration system. This more powerful system can cool the inside about 12 to 21° F below the room's temperature. To some extent the inside temperature of the tent will be moderated by the child's body warmth. It is important to measure the temperature inside the canopy and ensure that the child is not chilled.

4. As with hoods, an oxygen analyzer should be continuously monitoring how much oxygen is inside the tent. The analyzer probe should be placed at the same level as the child's nose. This is because oxygen is heavier than air and will tend to settle toward the bottom of the tent. Keep the tent sealed and the bottom edges tucked under the mattress to try to keep the oxygen percent as high and stable as possible. The child should not be allowed to have any electrically powered toys inside the tent to minimize the risk of a spark and fire.

4.   Fix any problems with an oxygen-conserving device. (IIB2a6) [R, Ap, An]

Oxygen-conserving devices are employed with patients who need long-term oxygen therapy and wish to reduce their costs. There are two different types of conserving devices: reservoir or pendant nasal cannulas and demand-valve nasal cannulas. Two different styles of reservoir nasal cannulas are made by CHAD Therapeutics of Chatsworth, California. Fig. 5-1 shows a reservoir nasal cannula called the Oximizer and how it operates. It has an 18 ml reservoir that fills when

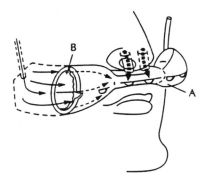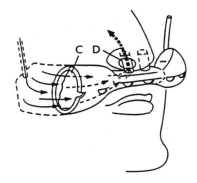

WHILE PATIENT IS EXHALING,
oxygen is accumulating in the reservoir (A) formed by the inflated
diaphragm (B) and the back wall of
the Oxymizer.

WHEN PATIENT INHALES, the
diaphragm (C) collapses, and the
oxygen-enriched air from the reservoir
is released to the patient (D).

Fig. 5-1 Oximizer reservoir nasal cannula and its functions. (Courtesy of CHAD Therapeutics, Chatsworth, Calif.)

the patient exhales and gives up its oxygen bolus during the next inspiration. Fig. 5-2 shows a pendant nasal cannula that is also made by CHAD Therapeutics. Its reservoir is within the pendant that hangs on the chest. Both types can have problems with tubing disconnections or kinks that can happen with any type of cannula. The only problem that is unique to both of these units is that the diaphragm that moves back and forth as the reservoir fills and emptys wears out. This membrane

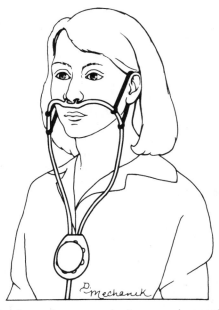

Fig. 5-2 Drawing of a patient wearing a pendant reservoir nasal cannula made by CHAD Therapeutics. (From Wyka KA: Respiratory home care. In Scanlon CL, Spearman CB, Sheldon RL: *Egan's fundamentals of respiratory care,* ed 5, St. Louis, 1990, Mosby–Year Book. Used by permission.)

may wear out after about a week and prevent the reservoir from filling or emptying properly. Watch as the patient breathes to make sure that the diaphragm is moving properly. If not, replace the cannula.

A regular cannula is used with a demand-valve nasal cannula system. It is also known as a demand oxygen delivery system (DODS). The distal end of the cannula is attached to a pressure sensor that senses a drop in pressure as the patient inspires. The sensor triggers a solenoid valve that delivers a burst of oxygen to the cannula. The solenoid can be adjusted to change how long the oxygen is delivered. Make sure that the patient can feel a flow of gas from the cannula after he or she starts to inhale. The gas should stop during exhalation. Adjust the pressure sensor or solenoid if needed to deliver oxygen after the patient inspires. Do not use a system that is malfunctioning and cannot be adjusted. Several companies make demand oxygen delivery systems, including CHAD Therapeutics, Pulsair, John Bann, Co, and Puritan-Bennett.

5.   Transtracheal oxygen catheters.
a.   Put the equipment together, make sure it works properly, and identify any problems with it. (IIB1a) [R, Ap]

The transtracheal oxygen (TTO$_2$) catheter is a 20-cm long flexible plastic tube (see Fig. 5-3, **A**). It is inserted into the trachea via a puncture procedure at the supra sternal notch. This procedure is discussed in Section 17. To date only adults with COPD have had the procedure performed. Oxygen is delivered directly into the trachea. The patient's oxygenation can be maintained at lower oxygen flows than needed by a regular face mask or nasal cannula. The following equipment is needed:

a. 9 French transtracheal catheter (Erie Medical, Milwaukee, Wis. is a manufacturer.)
b. Guide wire/stylet
c. Chain-link necklace to hold the catheter in place
d. Regular small-bore oxygen tubing to connect to the distal end of the catheter
e. Flowmeter and oxygen source
f. Optional bubble humidifier with sterile water for patient comfort

Under normal working conditions the oxygen tubing is used to connect the oxygen source to the catheter. The oxygen flow to the catheter is set high enough to keep a satisfactory PaO$_2$ or SpO$_2$ level. This will be less than previously needed by nasal cannula. When combined with the Linde Walker portable liquid oxygen system or demand oxygen delivery system, the patient has a real opportunity for increased mobility with supplemental oxygen.

b.   Fix any problems with the transtracheal oxygen catheter. (IIB2a5) [R, Ap, An]

The patient needs to be instructed to disconnect the oxygen tubing and flush the catheter with 3 ml of sterile saline twice a day. A cleaning rod can also be pushed through the catheter to make sure that no mucus accumulates. As with any tubing system, the components can become disconnected. Make sure that all connections are tight. If the saline or cleaning rod cannot be pushed through the catheter, an obstruction is likely. The patient should come into the hospital to have the catheter removed and replaced if necessary. It is possible that the proximal catheter tip has twisted into the tracheal mucosa. This can lead to subcutaneous emphysema. The patient should be instructed to identify the signs of this and to

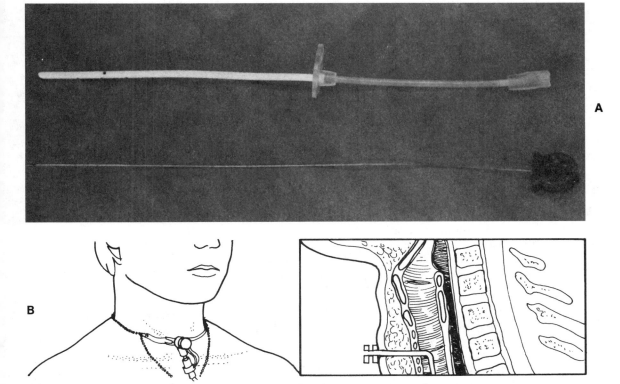

Fig. 5-3 Transtracheal oxygen catheter. **A (top),** Photograph of a flexible, plastic transtracheal oxygen catheter. The part to the left of the flange is inserted into the patient's trachea. The part to the right of the flange is attached to standard oxygen tubing. **A (bottom),** The metal stylet may be used to help keep the catheter stiff during insertion and to clear the catheter of an obstruction. **B (left),** Drawing of a chain-link necklace keeping the external part of the catheter and flange secure. **B (right),** Cutaway drawing showing the catheter inserted into the trachea. (From White GC: *Equipment theory for respiratory care,* Albany, NY, 1992, Delmar. Used by permission.)

turn off the oxygen to the catheter. He or she should go back to using a nasal cannula for oxygen and call the physician for guidance.

6. Oxygen concentrators (enrichers).
a. Get the necessary equipment for the procedure. (IIA1d1) [R, Ap]

There are two different types of oxygen concentrators available for the delivery of continuous low-flow oxygen in the home: molecular sieve and permeable plastic membrane.

Molecular Sieve

Molecular sieve oxygen concentrators use two canisters of zeolite pellets (inorganic sodium-aluminum silicate) to remove nitrogen and water vapor from room air. A pump pulls room air through and the remaining oxygen is delivered to the patient through a flowmeter (see Fig. 5-4). Be aware that with this unit the oxygen percentage varies inversely with the flow that is delivered (see Table 5-1). These units deliver dry gas, therefore a humidification system is frequently added to the flowmeter. That, of course, must be maintained as well. Manufacturers include DeVilbiss and Marx.

Permeable Plastic Membrane

Permeable plastic membrane oxygen concentrators make use of a one-micrometer (μm) thick plastic membrane as a filter. Room air is pulled through it by a vacuum pump. Molecular oxygen and water vapor pass through the membrane faster than nitrogen can. Any excess water vapor is removed by a simple condenser system. There is no need to add an external humidification system to the flowmeter (see Fig. 5-5). The oxygen percentage is fixed at 40% in these units; however, the flow can be varied from 1 to 10 L/min as shown in Table 5-1. Manufacturers include Oxygen Enrichment Company.

When deciding which type of concentrator to use, it is important to know the patient's required oxygen percentage and flow. As can be seen from Table 5-1, the molecular sieve types can deliver a higher oxygen percentage at any liter flow as compared to the permeable plastic membrane units.

b. Put the equipment together, make sure that it works properly, and identify any problems with it. (IIB1e1 and IIIC3e) [R, Ap, An]

In both types of oxygen concentrators it is important to check the air inlet filter on a monthly basis to keep it clean of dust and debris. Follow the manufacturer's requirements for when filters should be replaced. The delivered oxygen concentration should also be checked each month. Both units make use of a vacuum pump to pull room air through them. Follow the manufacturer's guidelines for its preventative maintenance needs. The molecular sieve types will need to have the zeolite pellet canisters replaced on a scheduled basis.

Some units have a visual or audio alarm that warns when there is a problem such as decreased flow. Because this is not a low-oxygen percentage alarm, some home care practitioners have recommended the addition of an external analyzer with alarm systems. This will alert the patient to call the home care company to repair the equipment. If a patient says that he or she cannot feel any gas coming

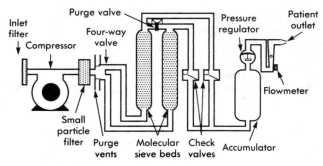

Fig. 5-4 Drawing of the components of a molecular sieve oxygen concentrator. The molecular sieve beds remove nitrogen and pass oxygen through to the patient. (Courtesy of the DeVilbiss Co, Toledo, Ohio.)

Table 5-1. Comparison of Flow Rates and Oxygen Percentages in Oxygen Concentrators

Molecular Sieve Concentrator Flow in L/min	Oxygen Percentage
1-2	>90%
3-5	80%-90%
6	about 74%
8	about 60%
10	50%
Permeable Membrane	
1-10	40%

out of the cannula have him or her place the prongs into a glass of water. If no bubbling is seen have the patient check the tubing for any disconnections. If the concentrator is malfunctioning have the patient turn it off and switch to oxygen from the back-up cylinder until repairs can be made.

7. Portable liquid oxygen systems.
a. Get the necessary equipment for the procedure. (IIA1d2) [R, Ap]

A liquid oxygen (LOX) system is used in the home when it is found to be more cost effective than an oxygen concentrator or battery of oxygen cylinders. An additional advantage is that a smaller portable unit can be carried by the patient in a shoulder bag for added mobility. It is also less conspicuous than wheeling an E cylinder about. The best known unit is the Linde (Union Carbide) Walker System. Fig. 5-6 shows the large reservoir that is kept in the patient's home. Fig. 5-7 shows its smaller companion, the portable Linde Walker (also known as the PCU-500).

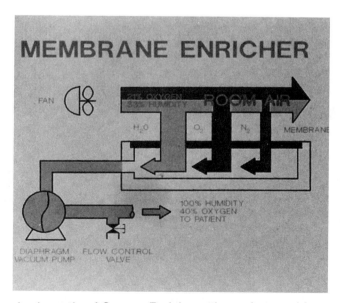

Fig. 5-5 Functional schematic of Oxygen Enrichment's semipermeable membrane oxygen concentrator. The membrane permits more oxygen and water vapor to pass through than nitrogen. (Courtesy of the Oxygen Enrichment Company, Schenectady, New York.)

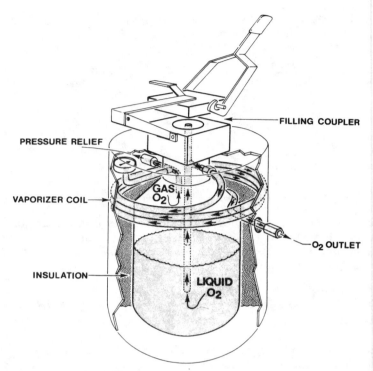

Fig. 5-6 Drawing of the components of a home liquid oxygen supply unit. (From Lampton LM: Home and outpatient oxygen therapy. In Brashear RE, Rhodes ML, editors: *Chronic obstructive lung disease,* St. Louis, 1978, Mosby–Year Book. Used by permission.)

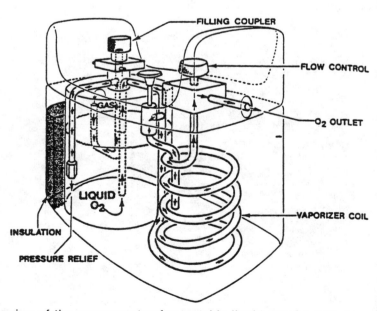

Fig. 5-7 Drawing of the components of a portable liquid oxygen unit. (From Lampton LM: Home and outpatient oxygen therapy. In Brashear RE, Rhodes ML, editors: *Chronic obstructive lung disease,* St. Louis, 1978, Mosby–Year Book. Used by permission.)

Another manufacturer of the portable system is Cryogenics Associates with its Liberator/Stroller.

b. Put the equipment together, make sure that it works properly, and identify any problems with it. (IIB1e2 and IIIC3e) [R, Ap, An]

The Linde Walker reservoir tank weighs about 11 pounds and can be carried over the shoulder by a strap. The full Walker reservoir tank yields about 1025 L of gaseous oxygen. It can be refilled from the larger reservoir tank kept in the home.

Flowrate settings of 1, 2, and 4 L/min can be set by buttons. The flowrates can be combined to offer 3, 5, 6, and 7 L/min maximum. Humidification is provided by the patient's own airway. As with any pressurized system, all fittings must be kept tight to prevent leakage.

The National Fire Protection Agency (NFPA) has established a number of regulations to ensure that home liquid oxygen systems are safely installed. The key safety regulations include:

1. Stabilize the unit to prevent it from being tipped over.
2. The reservoir unit should not be set up near any radiators, steam pipes, or heat ducts to reduce the rate of oxygen loss.
3. There can be no open flames or sources of ignition within 5 feet of the unit.
4. "No smoking" signs must be posted.
5. The patient and family must be instructed in how to use the equipment. This includes how to fill the Walker from the large reservoir tank. The person filling the Walker should wear safety goggles with side shields, loose fitting insulated gloves, and high top boots.
6. If liquid oxygen spills and contacts skin it can cause frostbite. Medical attention should be sought immediately.
7. Avoid contact for at least 15 minutes with any equipment or the floor where liquid oxygen has spilled.

c. Fix any problems with the equipment. (IIB2g2) [R, Ap, An]

Check that all connections are air tight to avoid spills and minimize the loss of oxygen. Make sure that the unit is functioning at its designed working pressure. The Linde unit operates at 90 psig. Make sure that the pressure relief valve operates properly. Use a flowmeter to confirm that the main unit and Walker unit are delivering the proper oxygen flow.

8. Fix any problems with a given oxygen analyzer. (IIB2g3) [An]

Because there are so many different models available it is not practical to discuss all of them here. Consult an equipment book or the manufacturer's literature for details of the various analyzers. All portable, hand-held analyzers fall into one of the following categories: electric, physical/paramagnetic, or electrochemical.

Electric

Mira and OEM are manufacturers of electric oxygen analyzers. Calibration is done on this and all analyzers by sampling room air, adjusting a calibration control to 21% if necessary, sampling 100% oxygen, and adjusting a calibration control to

100% if necessary. In general, always follow the manufacturer's guidelines for set-up and calibration. Failure to calibrate could be caused by a weak battery, plugged capillary line, or a defect in an electrical component.

Physical/Paramagnetic

Beckman is a manufacturer of physical/paramagnetic oxygen analyzers. A silica-gel–filled container is in line with the capillary tube to dry out the sample gas before it gets to the analyzing chamber. Failure to calibrate could be caused by water, a defect in the analyzing chamber, a weak battery, or a plugged capillary line.

Electrochemical

Failure to calibrate an electrochemical analyzer could be caused by a weak battery, exhausted or evaporated supply of chemical reactant in the gas sampling probe, a torn membrane separating the chemical reactant from the gas sample, or an electronic failure. The galvanic units must have their probes kept dry to read accurately. Both polargraphic and galvanic fuel-cell types are pressure sensitive. High altitude will cause them to read a lower-than-true oxygen percentage. High pressure, as seen in a ventilator circuit with PEEP, will cause the units to read a higher-than-true oxygen percentage.

9.   Set up or change air/oxygen proportioners (blenders). (IIIC3d) [An]

Air/oxygen proportioners are designed to change the ratio of oxygen and air so as to blend the specific percent of oxygen from 21% to 100%. To do that, both source gases of pure oxygen and compressed air must be pressurized to 50 psig. Typically, high pressure gas hoses are used to connect both piped gases to the blender. The blended oxygen percentage will remain close to desired even if there is a small drop in either one or both line pressures. Always analyze the oxygen percentage to confirm that the blend is proper. The blended gas can be sent directly to a ventilator or another device that uses 50 psig or through an added flowmeter.

Keep the gas inlets and outlets clear of any debris. All current units give an audible whistle if either one or both of the line pressures drop to an unsafe level (often about 30 psig). If the unit has a water trap, keep it emptied of any condensate. Change to another blender if the original one does not deliver the set oxygen percentage.

10.   Perform quality control procedures for gas metering devices: flowmeters and regulators. (IIB3b) [R, Ap]

Most of the quality control procedures and routine maintenance work are performed by the biomedical department in each hospital. No matter who does the work, it is critical that flowmeters have a known flow sent through them so that they can be checked for accuracy. This should be done without any backpressure. Reducing valves and regulators must have a known pressure directed against them to check for accuracy. When a backpressure is placed against a flowmeter the following will be seen:

a. Non–backpressure-compensated (pressure-uncompensated) Thorpe and kinetic flowmeters will show an inaccurately *low* flow in the face of backpressure. In other words, they will show less flow than is actually being delivered.

b. Bourdon regulators (Bourdon reducing valve and flowmeter) will show an inaccurately *high* flow in the face of backpressure. In other words, they will show more flow than is actually being delivered.

c. Backpressure-compensated (pressure-compensated) Thorpe and kinetic flowmeters will show an accurate flow in the face of backpressure. If the gas flow is restricted, the ball bearing or plunger float will drop to mark the reduced flow. If the flow is completely blocked off, the float will drop to zero showing no flow. These are the preferred flowmeters to use in all situations except for patient transport.

BIBLIOGRAPHY

AARC Clinical Practice Guideline: Oxygen therapy in the acute care hospital, *Respir Care* 36(12):1410-1413, 1991.

AARC Clinical Practice Guideline: Oxygen Therapy in the home or extended care facility. *Respir Care*, 37(8):918-922, 1992.

Aloan C: *Respiratory care of the newborn*, Philadelphia, 1987, JB Lippincott.

Bageant RA: Oxygen analyzers, *Respir Care* 21(5):410-416, 1976.

Bakken E, Desautels DA: Oxygen therapy. In Aloan CA: *Respiratory care of the newborn: a clinical manual*, Philadelphia, 1987, JB Lippincott.

Cleveland DV: Oxygen therapy. In Koff PB, Eitzman DV, Neu J, editors: *Neonatal and pediatric respiratory care*, St. Louis, 1988, Mosby–Year Book.

Eubanks DH, Bone RC: *Comprehensive respiratory care*, ed 2, St. Louis, 1990, Mosby–Year Book.

Eubanks DH, Bone RC: *Principles and application of cardiorespiratory care equipment*, St. Louis, 1994, Mosby–Year Book.

Gaebler G, Blodgett D: Gas administration. In Blodgett D: *Manual of pediatric respiratory care procedures*, Philadelphia, 1982, JB Lippincott.

Lough MD, Doershuk CF, Stern RC: *Pediatric respiratory therapy*, ed 3, Chicago, 1985, Year Book Medical.

McPherson SP: *Respiratory therapy equipment*, ed 4, St. Louis, 1986, Mosby–Year Book.

Scanlan CL, Spearman CB, Sheldon RL, editors: *Egan's fundamentals of respiratory care*, ed 5, St. Louis, 1990, Mosby–Year Book.

Shapiro BA, Harrison RA, Cane RD et al: *Clinical application of blood gases*, ed 4, Chicago, 1994, Year Book Medical.

Shapiro BA, Peruzzi WT, and Templin R: *Clinical application of respiratory care*, ed 3, Chicago, Year Book Medical.

Sills JR: *Respiratory care certification guide: the complete review resource for the entry level exam*, ed 2, St. Louis, 1994, Mosby–Year Book.

Ward JJ: Equipment for mixed gas and oxygen therapy. In Barnes TA, editor: *Respiratory care practice*, Chicago, 1988, Year Book Medical.

White GC: *Basic clinical lab competencies for respiratory care: an integrated approach*, Albany, NY, 1988, Delmar.

White GC: *Equipment theory for respiratory care*, Albany, NY, 1992, Delmar.

SELF-STUDY QUESTIONS

1. Your patient is going home and will require 1 L/min of oxygen when exercising on her stationary bicycle or when she feels short of breath. Which of the following oxygen delivery systems would you recommend?
    A. Molecular sieve oxygen concentrator
    B. Linde Walker portable liquid oxygen system
    C. Semipermeable membrane oxygen concentrator
    D. Piston compressor

2. You are attempting to calibrate a polarographic oxygen analyzer but find that it cannot be done. Possible reasons for this include:
    I.   The membrane is torn on the probe.
    II.   The gas sampling capillary tube is plugged with debris.
    III. The electrode solution has evaporated.
    IV.   The batteries need to be replaced.
    V.   Water has condensed on the membrane.
    A. I, III
    B. II, III
    C. III, IV, V
    D. I, III, IV, V
    E. II, IV

3. A 3-year-old child with bronchitis is being kept in an oxygen tent. He is supposed to be in a 40% oxygen environment. When analyzing the percentage you find the tent to contain 35% oxygen. To increase the oxygen percentage you would do all the following EXCEPT:
    A. Make sure that the bottom edge of the tent canopy is tucked under the mattress.
    B. Increase the flow of oxygen.
    C. Adjust the air entrainment nebulizer to give a more dense mist.
    D. Make sure that all patient access ports are closed.

4. When checking your home care patient's reservoir type nasal cannula you notice that the reservoir does not fill and empty in synchrony with the patient's breathing pattern. Based on this you would:
    A. Increase the oxygen flow to deliver the intended amount.
    B. Replace the cannula.
    C. Decrease the oxygen flow to unstick the reservoir membrane.
    D. Switch the patient to an air entrainment mask at approximately the same oxygen percent as the patient received by cannula.

5. Which of the following would be the best device for giving 35% to 50% oxygen to an alert 2-year-old?
    A. Oxygen tent
    B. Nasal cannula at 3 l/min
    C. Simple mask at 3 l/min
    D. Incubator
    E. Partial rebreather mask

6. You are called to evaluate a patient known to have advanced emphysema. She is wearing a nasal cannula at 6 l/min. The nurse says that she has become drowsy and less responsive since the oxygen was given to her an hour ago. Her ABGs on the oxygen show PaO_2 84 mm Hg, $PaCO_2$ 65 mm Hg, and pH 7.32. You would recommend which of the following?

   I.   Leave her on the cannula.
   II.   Change her to a 24% air entrainment mask and repeat the ABGs in 20 minutes.
   III.   Change her to a simple oxygen mask and repeat the ABGs in 20 minutes.
   IV.   Let her rest undisturbed.
   V.   Monitor her closely for becoming more alert.
   A.   I, IV
   B.   III, IV
   C.   II, V
   D.   II
   E.   III, V

7.   You are assisting with a bronchoscopy to biopsy a suspicious laryngeal node on your patient. Afterward, the patient complains of shortness of breath and a "tight" throat. Which of the following recommendations could you give to the physician?
   I.   Give the patient a 20% oxygen/80% helium mix to breathe.
   II.   Put the head of the bed down 30°.
   III.   Give the patient a 30% oxygen/70% helium mix to breathe.
   IV.   Order a "stat" chest x-ray.
   V.   Do a 7-minute helium dilution residual volume test.
   A.   V
   B.   I, III
   C.   II, IV
   D.   I
   E.   IV, V

8.   You receive a call at the office from one of your home care patients. She reports that she cannot flush out her transtracheal oxygen catheter with saline or push the cleaning rod through it. What should you tell her to do?
   A.   Remove the catheter and put on her nasal cannula at the same flow rate.
   B.   Force the saline through the catheter until the obstruction is cleared.
   C.   Force the cleaning rod through the catheter until the obstruction is cleared.
   D.   Come in to the outpatient area of the hospital to have the catheter replaced.

9.   You are working with a patient who has a tracheal tumor. He is wearing a non-rebreather mask with 20% oxygen and 80% helium. The patient says that it is harder to breathe and has increased his respiratory rate. You notice that the reservoir bag has collapsed. The most appropriate action would be to:
   A.   Decrease the flow of gas.
   B.   Switch to a 24% air entrainment mask.
   C.   Increase the flow of gas.
   D.   Switch to a nasal cannula at 2 lpm.
   E.   Switch to a 30% oxygen/70% helium mix.

10.   You are doing quality assurance on the department's flowmeters. After plugging in a backpressure-compensated Thorpe flowmeter, you set the flow at 10 lpm. The flowmeter outlet is partially and then completely obstructed. You would expect to see the following:
   A.   The float will stay at the 10 lpm mark.
   B.   The float will move upward in the flowmeter.
   C.   The float will move upward and then downward in the flowmeter.
   D.   The float will move downward and then drop to the bottom of the flowmeter showing zero flow.
   E.   The float will move up and down rhythmically when the outlet is completely obstructed.

11. When installing a liquid oxygen system into a patient's home you accidentally tip it over. About a liter of liquid oxygen spills out onto the floor. What should you do?
    A. Soak up the liquid with a clean rag.
    B. Leave the area for at least 15 minutes until it has evaporated.
    C. Turn on a space heater to speed up the evaporation process.
    D. Use a wet/dry vacuum cleaner to suck up the liquid.

Answer Key

1. A; 2. D; 3. C; 4. B; 5. A; 6. C; 7. B; 8. D; 9. C; 10. D; 11. B.

6

Hyperinflation Therapy

Module A. Teach the patient techniques for strengthening the inspiratory muscles. (IIB2a) [An]

Teach the following steps to patients with obstructive airways diseases:

1. The patient should lie in a comfortable supine position; knees can be flexed.
2. Instruct the patient to relax physically as much as possible, especially the shoulders.
3. Soothing music, meditation, or other techniques for mental relaxation should also be used.
4. The practitioner places his or her hands and the patient's hands gently over the area(s) where the patient is to concentrate the breathing effort. Usually this is the abdominal area just below the sternum. This is to encourage the patient to use the diaphragm more effectively as well as to strengthen it. With diaphragmatic breathing, the hands will move out during an inspiration.
5. The same hands-on technique can be used to aid in segmental breathing over an area that is underventilated or atelectatic.
6. Breathing *in* against an obstruction can also increase strength and endurance of inspiratory muscles. One type of device that can be used as an obstruction is a mouthpiece with selectable, variably sized openings at the other end. HealthScan Products is a manufacturer of the Pflex unit seen in Fig. 6-1. The patient breathes in through the largest opening and progresses to smaller openings as tolerated.

Increasing strength and endurance of inspiratory muscles usually requires a training program similar to the following:

1. Plug the nose with nose clips.
2. Inspire a normal tidal volume at a rate of 12 to 15 breaths per minute through the largest opening.
3. Continue for 10 to 15 minutes per day, a total of 3 to 5 times per week for the first week. If the patient notices shortness of breath, a noticeably increased pulse rate, or increased fatigue, the exercise should be stopped until the symptoms are gone. Resume the exercise when comfortable again.
4. Gradually increase the duration to about 30 minutes per session or two 15-minute sessions a day.

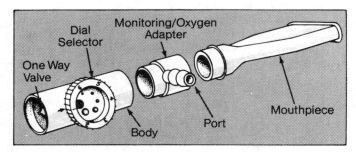

Fig. 6-1 PFLEX Inspiratory Muscle Trainer. The body of the device features a dial selector with inspiratory holes. The 1 setting has the largest opening. The holes range down in size to number 6, which is the smallest. A one-way valve allows the patient to expire. The mouthpiece can be directly attached to the body or have a monitoring/oxygen adapter added between them. This adapter allows oxygen to be added to meet the patient's needs. Or, an inspiratory forcemeter can be added to determine the amount of negative pressure the patient is generating at each of the inspiratory hole settings. (From HealthScan Products, Inc, Cedar Grove, NJ. Used by permission.)

5. When this can be easily tolerated three times per week, switch to the next smallest hole.
6. Continue to repeat steps 1 to 5 as tolerated. For the exercise to be beneficial it is tiring, but not exhausting. The device may be adjusted to the next larger hole setting if the patient becomes too tired. The whole process usually takes 4 to 6 weeks to see positive results.
7. A maintenance program requires the exercise to be done every other day.

HealthScan Products also makes a device called the Threshold. It features a variable spring-loaded valve so that the inspiratory pressure is constant despite changes in the patient's air flow or breathing rate. Other manufacturers of inspiratory muscle training devices include DHD, Instrumentation Industries, and Marquest Medical Products.

Module B.   Increase or decrease the patient's incentive spirometry (IS) goal. (IIC1) [An]

The goal of incentive spirometry is to prevent or treat atelectasis. This is done by having the patient inhale a near normal inspiratory capacity (IC). It is even more beneficial if the patient can hold the inspiratory capacity for several seconds. This is referred to as the sustained maximal inspiration (SMI). The cooperative surgical patient should have his or her IC measured before the operation. It can be measured at the bedside or calculated from any pulmonary function tests. (Review Section 3 for inspiratory capacity information.) The IC is then measured again postoperatively. (See Table 6-1 for incentive spirometry guidelines.) In addition, the following guidelines are suggested:

a. Set the initial inspiratory capacity goal at twice the tidal volume.
b. Increase the goal in 200-ml increments as the patient can tolerate it.
c. Have a final inspiratory capacity goal of greater than 12 ml/kg of ideal body weight, or have a vital capacity goal of greater than 15 ml/kg of ideal body weight.
d. A normal person should have an inspiratory capacity of about 75% of his or her (forced) vital capacity. For example, a predicted FVC of 5.166 L was calcu-

Table 6-1. Guidelines for the Use of Incentive Spirometry

Postoperative Bedside Spirometry	Treatment Modality
Inspiratory capacity (IC) greater than 80% of the preoperative value	No treatment needed unless there is x-ray or clinical evidence of atelectasis
IC at least 33% of the preoperative value; or vital capacity (VC) of at least 10 ml/kg	Incentive spirometry is indicated
IC less than 33% of the preoperative value; or vital capacity (VC) less than 10 ml/kg	IPPB is indicated

lated for a male patient in Section 3. His predicted IC would be calculated as 5.166 L × .75 = 3.875 L. However, due to natural variations in people, he could inhale only 80% of this (3.1 L) and still be considered within normal limits. Use this as a guideline for anticipating a patient's maximum inspiratory capacity. Do not expect your patient to inhale a greater IC than is physically possible.

Consider increasing the IS goal if: 1) the patient is easily able to reach the set goal, or 2) the patient's breath sounds are diminished in the bases. Consider decreasing the IS goal if: 1) the patient cannot reach the set goal because it is too large, 2) the patient is frustrated and discouraged at his or her inability to reach the set goal, or 3) excessive surgical site pain prevents the patient from reaching the set goal.

Module C.   Positive expiratory pressure (PEP) therapy.

1.   Recommend starting positive expiratory pressure (PEP) therapy. (IIIC10m) [R, Ap, An]

Positive expiratory pressure (PEP) therapy involves having a spontaneously breathing patient exhale against a fixed-orifice resistor to create expiratory pressures between 10 and 20 cm water. It is also called PEP mask therapy because many patients use a face mask to deliver the pressure to the airways. Table 6-2 lists indications for its use. The first three are discussed here and the last two are presented in the next discussion.

In patients with air trapping due to small airways disease, PEP therapy seems to act like a pressure splint. The PEP keeps the small airways from collapsing at

Table 6-2. Indications for Positive Expiratory Pressure (PEP) Therapy

To reduce air trapping in patients with
    emphysema, bronchitis, and asthma
To prevent atelectasis
To reverse atelectasis
To help mobilized retained secretions in patients
    greater than 4 years of age who have either
    cystic fibrosis, chronic bronchitis,
    bronchiectasis, and/or bronchiolitis obliterans
To maximize the delivery of aerosolized
    medications such as bronchodilators in
    patients receiving bronchial hygiene therapy

the end of exhalation. Like pursed lips breathing, this allows the trapped alveolar gas to be more completely exhaled.

Patients with atelectasis or at risk for developing atelectasis respond well to PEP therapy. It seems that atelectic areas are opened up by air moving through collateral airways. The air appears to move from open alveoli through the pores of Kohn to adjacent atelectic alveoli to force them open.

Table 6-3 lists relative contraindications to PEP therapy. There are no absolute contraindications. Table 6-4 lists hazards and/or complications of PEP therapy. These should be weighed against the benefits to the patient when making the recommendation to start PEP therapy. Other considerations include the patient's history of pulmonary disease that has responded to postural drainage therapy, ineffective cough to clear retained secretions, and breath sounds and chest x-ray findings of secretions.

2. Initiate positive expiratory pressure (PEP) mask therapy to achieve the removal of bronchopulmonary secretions. (IIB3a) [R, Ap]

PEP therapy has proven effective in helping patients with chronic, copious amounts of secretions. Primarily this includes children 4 years of age or older with cystic fibrosis. It also helps any patient with chronic bronchitis, bronchiectasis, or bronchiolitis obliterans. Clinical evidence indicates that the PEP dilates the small airways so that air is able to get past obstructing secretions. This fills the alveoli and on expiration tends to force the secretions into the larger airways for coughing or suctioning out.

PEP therapy seems also to increase the effectiveness of inhaled aerosolized bronchodilators. As shown in Fig. 6-2, the PEP system can be joined with a small volume nebulizer. The slowed exhalation during PEP breathing should promote better deposition of medication in the small airways. Table 6-5 lists the steps in performing a proper PEP therapy treatment.

3. Alter PEP therapy to modify bronchial hygiene. (IIIC5e) [R, Ap, An]

Be prepared to adjust the expiratory resistance to meet the clinical goal of PEP therapy. The Resistex unit by DC Lung has four fixed orifice settings to choose from. The orifice diameters are 4 mm, 3.5 mm, 3 mm, and 2.5 mm interior diameter. The PEP mask made by Astra Meditec (Molndal, Sweden) uses a series of differently sized pediatric endotracheal tube adapters. They are fitted into an adapter for the

---

Table 6-3. Relative Contraindications to Positive Expiratory Pressure (PEP) Therapy

---

Untreated pneumothorax
Intracranial pressure greater than 20 mm Hg
Active hemoptysis
Recent trauma or surgery to the skull, face, mouth, or esophagus
Patient having asthma attack or acute worsening of COPD who cannot tolerate increased work of breathing
Acute sinusitis or epistaxis
Tympanic membrane rupture or other middle ear pathology known or suspected
Nausea

Table 6-4. Hazards and/or Complications of Positive Expiratory Pressure (PEP) Therapy

Pulmonary barotrauma
Increased intracranial pressure
Myocardial ischemia and/or decreased venous
   return to the heart
Increased work of breathing
Air swallowing that can lead to vomiting
Discomfort from mask or skin breakdown from
   the mask pressure
Claustrophobia

patient to exhale through. With either unit, the patient should be started out with the largest opening to breathe out through. As the training continues the expiratory orifice may be made smaller. Again, the goals are to maintain a positive expiratory pressure of 10 to 20 cm water with an I : E ratio of about 1 : 3. If the pressure is too high or the expiratory time too long the patient will likely become fatigued. If the orifice is too small the pressure will not be high enough to be of any benefit. The patient will probably become tired if the total treatment time lasts longer than 20 minutes.

During the treatment ask the patient if he or she feels dyspnea, pain, or chest discomfort. Also monitor the patient's breath sounds, blood pressure, heart rate, and breathing pattern rate. Monitor oxygenation by pulse oximetry, mental clarity, and skin color. Evaluate sputum for quantity, color, odor, and viscosity. Also monitor the patient's intracranial pressure (ICP) if possible.

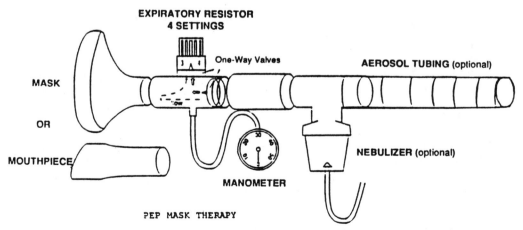

Fig. 6-2 Positive expiratory pressure (PEP) mask components. The basic PEP assembly requires a transparent mask or mouthpiece, expiratory resistor (this shows the Resistex), and pressure manometer with connecting oxygen tubing. If a nebulized medication is added, the following are also needed: small volume nebulizer with T-piece, oxygen tubing to flowmeter, and large bore tubing for an aerosol reservoir. (From Malmeister MJ, Fink JB, Hoffman GL et al: Positive-expiratory-pressure mask therapy: theoretical and practical considerations and a review of the literature, *Respir Care* 36(11):1218-1229, 1991. Used by permission.)

Table 6-5. Steps in Performing Positive Expiratory Pressure (PEP) Therapy

1. Put the equipment together as shown in Fig. 6-2.
2. Have the conscious patient sit up straight, rest elbows on a table, and hold the PEP mask comfortably but tightly over the nose and mouth. The patient may use a mouthpiece and nose clips if preferred.
3. The patient should inhale a deeper than normal breath, but not to total lung capacity, by using the diaphragm. The unconscious patient will only inhale a tidal volume breath.
4. The conscious patient should exhale to functional residual capacity fast enough to generate 10 to 20 cm water pressure in the manometer. Have the patient look at the pressure manometer to judge how fast to exhale. The unconscious patient will exhale passively but still benefit by the increased baseline pressure.
5. The patient should have an expiratory time that is about three times longer than inspiratory time. (An I : E ratio of 1 : 2 to 1 : 4 is acceptable.) This can be accomplished by changing the expiratory resistor and/or having the patient change the force of exhalation.
6. Between 10 and 20 proper PEP breaths should be performed.
7. The patient should now do two or three "huff"-type coughing efforts to raise secretions.
8. Repeat steps 2 to 7 between four and eight times for a full PEP treatment. It should take about 10 to 20 minutes.
   Patients in the intensive care unit can perform PEP therapy as often as every hour or as little as every 6 hours. They should be reevaluated for treatment effectiveness every 24 hours.
   Patients in the acute care or home care settings can perform PEP therapy from two to four times per day. The acute care patient should be reevaluated every 72 hours; the home care patient can be evaluated at longer intervals or when there is a change in pulmonary status.

4. Coordinate the sequence of therapies to modify bronchial hygiene. (IIIC5f) [An]

Coordinate PEP therapy with "huff" coughs, postural drainage therapy (PDT), and/or aerosolized medication delivery. As listed in Table 6-5, PEP breaths should be alternated with huff coughs to clear secretions. Huff coughs are not full, deep coughs; rather, they are performed as follows:

1. Have the patient inhale a slow breath to high or midlung levels but not to total lung capacity.
2. Hold the breath in for 1 to 3 seconds.
3. Perform several quick, forced exhalations with an open epiglottis.
4. Small children may be taught to say "huff" with each quick exhalation. It may also help to have the young patient perform a "chicken breath" by flapping his or her arms against the sides of the chest during the exhalation.

PDT may be used before or after PEP therapy or it may be alternated with PEP therapy to help in the removal of secretions. Likewise, aerosolized medications may be inhaled before or simultaneously with PEP therapy. Bronchodilators and mucolytic agents should be very helpful with PEP therapy to mobilize secretions.

Module D. Positive expiratory pressure (PEP) therapy equipment.

1. Get the necessary PEP mask for the procedure. (IIA1f) [R, Ap]

The PEP mask should be transparent, flexible, and fit the patient's facial contours so that no air will leak out as the pressure is increased. The following equipment is needed for PEP therapy as shown in Fig. 6-2:

a. Appropriate size PEP mask or mouthpiece and noseclips, or universal airway (elbow) adapter for attachment to an endotracheal or tracheostomy tube
b. Expiratory resistor
c. Pressure manometer calibrated in cm water
d. Small bore oxygen tubing to connect the expiratory resistor to the pressure manometer
e. Basin and tissues to collect and dispose of sputum
f. Gloves, mask, goggles, and/or gown for the practitioner

The following *additional* equipment is needed for delivering an aerosolized medication as shown in Fig. 6-2:

a. Small volume nebulizer
b. T-piece and female adapter to connect the nebulizer to the expiratory resistor
c. Large bore aerosol tubing to act as medication reservoir

2. Assemble, check for proper function, and identify any problems with the PEP mask. (IIB1g) [R, Ap]

As shown in Fig. 6-2 the component pieces must be properly put together. Make sure that all connections are air tight. If a leak is present, the desired PEP goal will not be reached or maintained. In addition, if an air leak is present it may be felt or a high-pitched sound may be heard. If a nebulizer is added for aerosolizing medications ensure that it works properly. Connect the small volume nebulizer into the system as shown. Add the medication and run a flow of oxygen or air at 4 to 6 L/min through the nebulizer as is customary.

3. Fix the PEP mask equipment. (IIB2l) [R, Ap, An]

Any leaks in the system will prevent the PEP goal from being reached. Tighten any loose connections. If the one-way valves are put together backwards the patient will inspire against a resistance instead of exhaling against it. Observe the one-way valves in use and ask the patient if he or she finds it easy to inhale but more difficult to exhale. Move the valves to their proper positions if incorrectly placed. If no mist is seen coming from the nebulizer check the capillary tube or baffle for an obstruction; clear it by running tap water or a sterile needle through it. See Section 7 if necessary for more information on fixing problems with small volume nebulizers.

Module E. Patient assessment.

1. Examine all the data to determine the patient's pathophysiological condition. (IC3a) [R, Ap, An]

The indications for PEP therapy are listed in Table 6-2. If the patient has one of these problems, he or she may benefit from receiving PEP therapy.

2. Take part in the development of the respiratory care plan. (IC3c) [An]

Be prepared to look at all of the available data on the patient, evaluate it, and make recommendations for patient care. Raise or lower the PEP level to help the patient without causing fatigue or complications.

3. Maintain records and communication about the patient's cough and sputum production and characteristics. (IIIA2a3) [An]

PEP therapy has been indicated in patients who have retained secretions that are difficult to cough out. If PEP therapy does not increase the amount of sputum produced per day in a patient who already produces more than 30 ml, PEP may not be needed. It does not make sense to continue an ineffective treatment.

BIBLIOGRAPHY

AARC Clinical Practice Guideline: Incentive spirometry, *Respir Care* 36(12):1402-1405, 1991.

AARC Clinical Practice Guideline: Directed cough, *Respir Care* 38(5):495-499, 1993.

AARC Clinical Practice Guideline: Use of positive airway pressure adjuncts to bronchial hygiene therapy, *Respir Care* 38(5): 516-521, 1993.

Campbell TC, Ferguson N, McKinlay RGC: The use of a simple self-administered method of positive expiratory pressure (PEP) in chest physiotherapy after abdominal surgery, *Physiotherapy* 72(10):498-500, 1986.

Douce FH: Incentive spirometry and other aids to lung inflation. In Barnes TA, editor: *Respiratory care practice*, Chicago, 1988, Year Book Medical.

Eubanks DH, Bone RC: *Comprehensive respiratory care: a learning system*, ed 2, St. Louis, 1990, Mosby–Year Book.

HealthScan Products, Inc. Unit B-2. 908 Pompton Avenue, Cedar Grove, NJ 07009-1292.

Hoffman GL, Cohen NH: Positive expiratory pressure therapy, *NBRC Horizons* 19(2):1-7, 1993.

Johnson NT, Pierson DJ: The spectrum of pulmonary atelectasis: pathophysiology, diagnosis, and therapy, *Respir Care* 31(11):1107-1120, 1986.

Larson JL, Kim MJ, Sharp JT: Inspiratory muscle training with a threshold resistive breathing device in patients with chronic obstructive pulmonary disease, *Am Rev Respir Dis* 133:A100, 1986.

Malmeister MJ, Fink JB, Hoffman GL et al: Positive-expiratory-pressure mask therapy: theoretical and practical considerations and a review of the literature, *Respir Care* 36(11):1218-1229, 1991.

Mang H, Obermayer A: Imposed work of breathing during sustained maximal inspiration: comparison of six incentive spirometers, *Respir Care* 34(12):1122-1128, 1989.

Oberwaldner PT, Johannes CE, Zach MS: Forced expirations against a variable resistance: a new chest physiotherapy method in cystic fibrosis, *Pediat Pulmonol* 2(6):358-367, 1986.

Scanlan CL, Spearman CB, Sheldon RL, editors: *Egan's fundamentals of respiratory care*, ed 5, St. Louis, 1990, Mosby–Year Book.

Scuderi J, Olsen GN: Respiratory therapy in the management of postoperative complications, *Respir Care* 34(4):281-291, 1989.

Shapiro BA, Kacmarek RM, Cane RD et al: *Clinical application of respiratory care*, ed 4, Chicago, 1991, Mosby–Year Book.

Wojciechowski WV: Incentive spirometers and secretion evacuation devices. In Barnes TA, editor: *Respiratory care practice*, Chicago, 1988, Year Book Medical.

SELF-STUDY QUESTIONS

1. You are called to evaluate a patient diagnosed as having atelectasis in both bases from the chest x-ray report. You would recommend which of the following to treat the problem?
   - I.   Deep coughing
   - II. Bed rest to minimize oxygen consumption
   - III. 28% air entrainment mask
   - IV. Sustained maximal inspiration therapy
   - V.   Humidity therapy
   - A. I, IV
   - B. II, III
   - C. IV
   - D. III, V
   - E. I, II

2. While instructing a patient in positive expiratory pressure therapy, she complains that it is taking too long to breathe out. What would you do?
   - A. Tell her to blow out harder.
   - B. Change the expiratory resistance to a larger diameter orifice.
   - C. Change the expiratory resistance to a smaller diameter orifice.
   - D. Increase the flow of oxygen to the system.

3. A patient has been using an inspiratory muscle training device. She recently switched to the fourth largest of six settings but has complained that she gets too tired and short of breath when using it. What would you recommend to her?
   - A. Keep breathing through the same inspiratory hole.
   - B. Breathe through the next largest hole.
   - C. Breathe through the smallest hole.
   - D. Breathe through the largest hole.
   - E. Breathe through the next smallest hole.

4. A patient is having his flow displacement incentive spirometry unit replaced with a volume displacement unit. How would you set his therapeutic goal?
   - A. Measure his total lung capacity.
   - B. Measure his inspiratory capacity.
   - C. Measure his inspiratory reserve volume.
   - D. Measure his residual volume.
   - E. Measure his expiratory reserve volume.

5. Your 15-year-old cystic fibrosis patient has copious amounts of secretions. She cannot tolerate postural drainage therapy due to a headache when tipped head down. Aerosolized bronchodilators and mucolytic agents are ordered every 4 hours. What else would you recommend be done?
   - A. Add incentive spirometry.
   - B. Give the aerosolized medications by IPPB therapy.
   - C. Add positive expiratory pressure therapy.
   - D. Modify the postural drainage therapy positions so that the head is not lower than the patient's body.

6. Your patient has an ideal body weight of 130 lb/59 kg. What would be her initial inspiratory capacity goal?
   - A. At least 885 ml

B. Half of her vital capacity
C. At least 700 ml
D. 40% to 50% of her current total lung capacity
E. Her current vital capacity

7. Your patient has been using an inspiratory muscle training device. He is currently on the third largest of six settings and has been comfortably breathing through it 4 days a week for the past 2 weeks. What would you now recommend he do?
A. Keep breathing through the same inspiratory hole.
B. Breathe through the next largest hole.
C. Breathe through the smallest hole.
D. Breathe through the largest hole.
E. Breathe through the next smallest hole.

8. Your are called to evaluate a patient who has been using incentive spirometry for 2 days since undergoing a cholecystectomy. The patient is able to easily inspire the 2 L limit set on the volume displacement unit. What would you recommend?
A. Increase the volume goal to 4 L.
B. Keep the goal as it is.
C. Switch to a flow displacement unit.
D. Incease the volume goal to 2250 ml.
E. Switch to IPPB treatments.

Answer Key

1. A; 2. B; 3. E; 4. B; 5. C; 6. C; 7. E; 8. D.

7

Humidity and Aerosol Therapy

Module A. Aerosol and humidity generators and administrative devices.

Note: It is recommended that the following terms and concepts related to humidity and aerosol therapy be reviewed: humidity, water vapor, absolute humidity, vapor pressure, relative humidity, dew point, dew point line, body humidity, humidity deficit, aerosol, aerosol particle size, factors that influence the deposition of particles, indications for humidity therapy, and indications for aerosol therapy. They are discussed in some detail in *Respiratory Care Certification Guide* (Sills, 1994) and other textbooks.

1. Fix any problems with a bubble humidifier. (IIBf) [An]

Bubble humidifiers are used on patients with normal upper airways who need some supplemental humidity because of the dryness of medical oxygen. These devices are not usually heated and, in fact, deliver gas cooled to below room temperature. They provide approximately 40% relative humidity at the delivered gas temperature; the balance has to be made up by the patient. (see Fig. 7-1). It is possible to add a wrap-around type of heater if it is clinically indicated to raise the temperature of the delivered gas and reduce the patient's humidity deficit.

There are three different types of bubble humidifiers that are designed to add some humidity to dry oxygen delivered through small-bore tubing: traditional bubble humidifiers, jet humidifiers underwater, and jet humidifers. If needed, their basic functions can be reviewed in *Respiratory Care Certification Guide* (Sills, 1994).

The bubble and other types of humidifiers consist of a reservoir jar for the water and a DISS oxygen connector lid that screws on. Turn on the flowmeter and make sure that oxygen flows through the delivery tube and bubbles into the water. Failure to bubble usually indicates that the lid and jar are not screwed together tightly or the delivery tube is plugged. If the tube cannot be cleared it must be replaced.

Most of the newer bubble units have a pop-off type of high pressure relief valve that releases if the pressure builds up to either 40 mm Hg or 2 pounds per square inch (psig). Pinch close the small-bore tubing to build up pressure and test the pop-off valve. Feel for the gas to escape from the valve. Many units will whistle to signal the gas leak. Do not use a unit whose pop-off valve will not open under pressure.

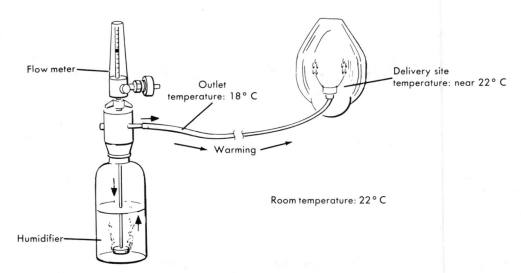

Flow meter

Outlet
temperature: 18° C

Delivery site
temperature: near 22° C

Warming

Room temperature: 22° C

Humidifier

Fig. 7-1 Gases leaving the outlet of the simple bubble humidifier are cooler than room temperature due to evaporation. Warming toward room temperature occurs en route to the patient delivery site. (From Scanlan CL: Humidity and aerosol therapy. In Scanlan CL, Spearman CB, Sheldon RL, editors: *Egan's fundamentals of respiratory care,* ed 5, St. Louis, 1990, Mosby–Year Book. Used by permission.)

2. Fix any problems with a Cascade humidifier. (IIB2f) [An]

It is recommended that a heated humidifier be used with patients who have had their upper airway bypassed. It should be set to deliver 32 to 37°C/90 to 99°F gas to the patient and able to provide 80% to 100% relative humidity in those temperature ranges. All of the following humidity-generating and aerosol-generating devices deliver the conditioned gas to the patient through large-bore (also known as aerosol or corrugated) tubing.

It is beyond the scope of this book to go into detail on all the different models of humidifiers that use large-bore tubing. Instead, some common features are briefly described. All these humidifiers have an adjustable heater so that the water in the reservoir is at or above body temperature. This enables them to provide up to 100% of the patient's body humidity. It is necessary with all these units to measure the temperature of the inspired gas near the patient. The gas temperature is usually kept the same as the patient's temperature or a few degrees cooler.

As the heated gas passes through the large-bore tubing there will be some cooling. This will result in condensation that must be drained out. Water traps placed in the lowest loops in the tubing will help in draining and keeping the tubing clear. Remember to look periodically for water puffing or sloshing back and forth in the low points of the tubing. Even though some of the water vapor condenses out, the relative humidity remains 100% as the gas cools along the dew point line. The absolute humidity, however, will drop (see Fig. 7-2).

The Bennett Cascade is the most well known of these types of humidifers (see Fig. 7-3). It is most commonly used with a mechanical ventilator but can be used with other types of systems for delivering humidity with or without oxygen. Its basic principle of operation is an efficient bubble humidifier. The inspiratory gas must flow through the water for evaporation to occur. A variety of similar devices are now on the market and include the Bourns humidifier, Ohio Heated Humidifier, Monaghan Model 610, Chemetron HR-1 Humidity Center, and Bennett Cascade

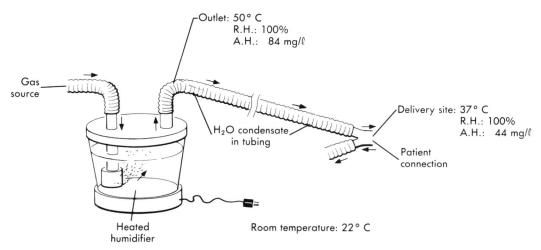

Fig. 7-2 Gases leaving the outlet of a heated humidifier are hot and saturated with water vapor. As cooling occurs in tubing, vapor condenses and absolute humidity (AH) decreases while relative humidity (RH) remains 100% (saturated). Note that almost half the original water vapor is "lost" to condensate in this example. (From Scanlan CL: Humidity and aerosol therapy. In Scanlan CL, Spearman CB, Sheldon RL, editors: *Egan's fundamentals of respiratory care,* ed 5, St. Louis, 1990, Mosby–Year Book. Used by permission.)

II. It is important with the Cascade humidifier and the others discussed later that they be properly assembled. This is especially important when they are used to humidify a mechanical ventilator.

Any loose connections will result in an air leak and loss of tidal volume. Be sure to follow the manufacturer's guidelines for assembly and troubleshooting. Make sure that the heating element and tower are tightly screwed into the lid, that the lid has a rubber O ring in the slot around the edge, and that the base is tightly screwed into the lid.

3. Fix any problems with a wick humidifier. (IIB2f) [An]

A wick type of heated humidifier employs a wick, often made of sponge or paper, to soak up water for evaporation. The water and/or wick are heated so that 100% relative humidity can be delivered. These units are also used with mechanical ventilators or other systems including air entrainment devices. This is because they offer very little resistance to the gas flowing through them as evaporation occurs. Examples include the HLC 37 by Travenol Laboratories, Dual Servo MR500 by Fisher and Paykel Medical, Conchapak by Respiratory Care, and the Bird Humidifier Model 3000.

Follow manufacturer's guidelines for assembly to make sure that all connections are air tight. Make sure that the heating element works properly to avoid overheating or underheating. Keep the water level within the set limits to get the best humidification.

4. Fix any problems with a passover humidifier. (IIB2f) [An]

A passover humidifier simply has the patient gas passing over the surface of a reservoir of hot water. This is sometimes called a "hot pot" and has been used in Emerson ventilators. By itself, this unit is probably the least effective at humidifying

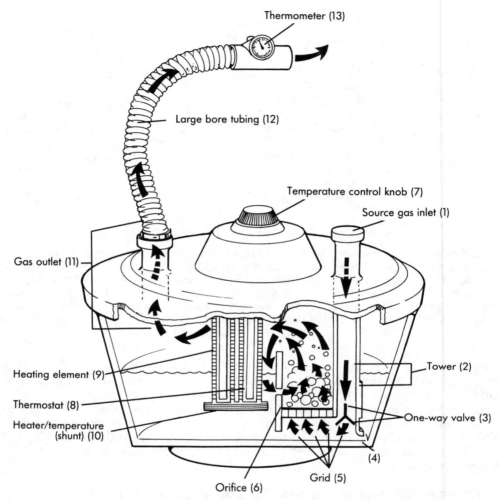

Fig. 7-3 Cascade humidifier. (From Scanlan CL; Humidity and aerosol therapy. In Scanlan CL, Spearman CB, Sheldon RL, editors: *Egan's fundamentals of respiratory care,* ed 5, St. Louis, 1990, Mosby–Year Book. Used by permission.)

gas. When it is used on a ventilator, other features such as copper mesh in a heated inspiratory tube are used to increase the surface area for evaporation.

Again, follow manufacturer's guidelines for assembly to make sure that all connections are air tight. Make sure that the heating element works properly to avoid overheating or underheating. Keep the water level within the set limits to get the best humidification. A thermometer should be kept in line to make sure that the temperature is being kept within the desired range.

5.   Fix any problems with an ultrasonic nebulizer. (IIB2b2) [An]

Always follow the manufacturer's instructions when setting up an ultrasonic nebulizer. There are too many brands and models to discuss here; however, Fig. 7-4 shows the common features of ultrasonic nebulizers and Table 7-1 describes how to troubleshoot many common problems. It seems that many of the clinical

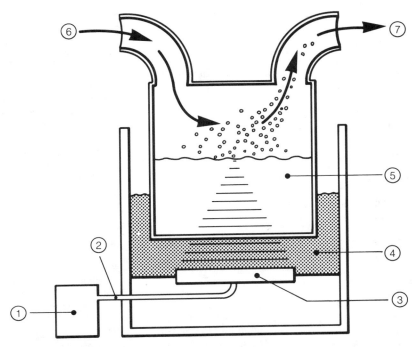

Fig. 7-4 Functional diagram of the ultrasonic nebulizer: *1*, electric current generator; *2*, cable; *3*, piezoelectric crystal; *4*, couplant chamber; *5*, solution cup; *6*, carrier gas inlet; and *7*, aerosol outlet. (From Op't Holt T: Aerosol generators and humidifiers. In Barnes TA, editor: *Respiratory care practice*, Chicago, 1988, Year Book Medical. Used by permission.)

difficulties have to do with keeping the proper fluid levels in the couplant chamber and the solution cup. If the sterile water in the couplant chamber is too low, the vibration cannot reach the solution cup and no aerosol will be produced. If the saline level in the solution cup is either too low or too high the vibrational energy will not focus properly on the surface of the saline and no aerosol will be produced. Water should not be allowed to condense out and fill any low points in the large-bore tubing. If this occurs, the ultrasonic particles will liquify as the carrier gas is forced to pass through the condensate. The exiting gas will be humidified through evaporation but carry no aerosol particles. If the carrier gas is oxygen enriched through a high airflow with oxygen enrichment (HAFOE) system, the backpressure could result in an increase in the oxygen percentage and a decrease in the total flow. Remember to always measure the oxygen percentage near the patient.

6. Fix any problems with aerosol (mist) tents. (IIB2i) [An]

Oxygen tents are discussed in Section 5. The aerosol or mist tents are essentially like the oxygen tents. The main difference is that no supplemental oxygen is used because the patient does not need it. The top of the canopy can be now be left open for better flow-through ventilation. At least 10 L/min of compressed air should still be run through the nebulizer to make sure that there is no carbon dioxide buildup. The nebulizer or ultrasonic system should be cared for as described earlier to ensure that there is enough aerosol to treat the condition.

Aerosol tents are sometimes used to treat upper respiratory problems such as laryngotracheobronchitis (LTB or pediatric croup). A cool aerosol seems to be

Table 7-1. Ultrasonic Nebulizer Troubleshooting

Symptom	Possible Problem	Suggested Check
1. Unit installed and connected as specified, but pilot light does not turn on when switch is turned to the "on" position	Electrical outlet defective Circuit breaker tripped Fuse blown	Check outlet with lamp or other appliance Reset the circuit breaker, or change fuse on the power switch. If the circuit breaker continues to trip or the fuse blows again, service is needed
2. Unit installed and connected as specified. Power pilot light turns on, normal ultrasonic activity visible in nebulizer chamber, but no aerosol output	Nebulizer chamber contaminated	Wash nebulizer chamber, decontaminate
3. Unit installed and connected as specified. Power pilot light turns on, but there is little ultrasonic activity visible in the nebulizer chamber, and aerosol output is low (even when on the no. 10 power setting)	Couplant water excessively aerated Nebulizer module and couplant water too cold Diaphragm distorted, permitting air bubbles to interfere with proper transmission of vibrational energy into the nebulizer chamber Couplant contaminated	Wait for deaeration Use warmer couplant water Check to see that diaphragm is properly shaped and installed. Be sure the concave (recessed) side faces the interior of the chamber Clean couplant compartment and replace couplant water
4. Same as symptom no. 3 but at a lower power setting	Power setting too low to start and establish nebulization	Turn output control knob to maximum power setting, then reduce to desired setting
5. Unit installed and connected as specified. Power pilot light turns on. "Add couplant" light is on, and there is no ultrasonic activity visible in the nebulizer chamber	Insufficient couplant water	Add water to the couplant compartment
6. Unit installed and connected as specified. Power pilot light turns on. "Add couplant" light is off, but there is no ultrasonic activity visible in the nebulizer chamber	Power supply overheated and its thermostatic control opened	The cooling air has been restricted, or cooling fins need cleaning. The switch will reset when the equipment returns to room temperature
7. Liquid reservoir filled and properly connected to nebulizer chamber, but chamber does not fill (for *continuous-feed system only*)	Foreign material or air bubbles in feed tubes Liquid level control in nebulizer chamber plugged with foreign material Air leaks at tube connections or reservoir cap	Flush the system Clean or flush the system Tighten all connections by pushing tubes into fittings

From Op't Holt T: Aerosol generators and humidifiers. In Barnes TA, editor: *Respiratory care practice*, Chicago, 1988, Year Book Medical. Used by permission.

clinically preferred because it reduces airway edema. Never use so much aerosol that the child cannot be seen inside the tent. Also, be wary of fluid overloading the young patient who is in the tent for a prolonged period. Most clinical problems relate to problems with the aerosol-generating system. Review fixing ultrasonic nebulizers; pneumatic nebulizers are discussed next.

7. Fix any problems with a pneumatic nebulizer. (IIB2b1) [An]
a.   Large-volume nebulizers.

It is beyond the scope of this book to cover all of the different brands of large-volume (large-reservoir) and air entrainment nebulizers in detail. However, the following is a list of common features of pneumatic nebulizers:

1. All pneumatic nebulizers are powered by air or oxygen delivered through a flowmeter. As the gas flow drops, the aerosol output decreases. Make sure the flowmeter is functioning properly to send gas through the nebulizer. Make sure that a gas cylinder or oxygen concentrator is working properly to send gas through the flowmeter and nebulizer.

2. All pneumatic nebulizers make use of Bernoulli's principle with a jet that is used to entrain liquid and/or room air into the main gas flow (see Fig. 7-5). Keep the air entrainment ports open so that the proper gas mixing will occur and the desired oxygen concentration will be provided. Always check the oxygen percent with an analyzer.

3. All pneumatic nebulizers have a reservoir jar that can be filled with 250 to 2500 ml of liquid. Overfilling or underfilling will prevent the nebulizer from working properly.

4. All pneumatic nebulizers have a capillary tube that allows the liquid to flow *up* to the jet for nebulization. Keep the capillary tube and jet clear of debris or the aerosol output will drop. (Remember that with the bubble humidifiers the oxygen flows *down* the capillary tube.)

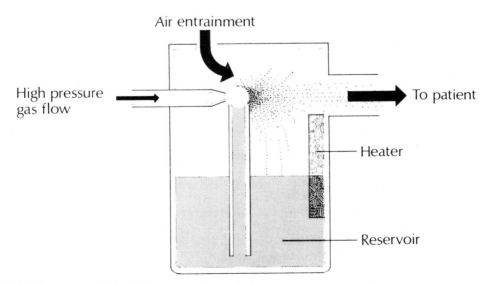

Fig. 7-5 Large reservoir air entrainment nebulizer. (From Shapiro BA, Harrison RA, Kacmarek RM et al: *Clinical application of respiratory care,* ed 3, Chicago, 1989, Year Book Medical. Used by permission.)

5. All pneumatic nebulizers have a baffle that the aerosol is sprayed against to create a more uniform particle size. Keep the baffle free of debris or the nebulizer output will drop and the particles may not be of the intended size.

Many, but not all, pneumatic nebulizers allow for a changeable inspired oxygen percentage. Provided that the jet is powered by oxygen, the air entrainment ports can be opened up more to increase air entrainment (lowering the inspired oxygen) or closed down to decrease air entrainment (raising the inspired oxygen). Closing the entrainment ports completely allows only the powering gas (oxygen or air) to pass through the nebulizer. The reusable units have several fixed oxygen percentages (usually 35% to 40%, 60% to 70%, and 100%). The disposable units are more flexible and usually allow for a continuous dialing from 35% to 100% oxygen. Remember to always analyze the inspired oxygen near the patient because water in the aerosol tubing and back pressure will decrease the entrained air and raise the oxygen percentage.

The largest and oldest group of pneumatic nebulizers look similar to the bubble humidifiers. The key components include a large reservoir jar at the top with a DISS oxygen connector and capillary tube to the jet. Examples include the reusable Puritan All Purpose and Ohio Deluxe units and many disposable types. These allow for variable oxygen percentages. Keep the capillary tube and jet clear of debris or the aerosol output will drop. Keep the air entrainment ports open so that the proper gas mixing will occur and the desired oxygen percentage will be provided. Heating of the water and/or aerosol is accomplished in one of the following ways:

1. A heated metal rod is immersed in the reservoir water through a port in the top of the nebulizer. A dial is used to control how hot the rod gets but it has no automatic shut-off feature. The water temperature varies depending on how deep it is; as the water level drops the remaining water gets hotter. It is very important to measure the gas temperature near the patient and keep the water level stable to prevent burning the airway. The heated rod presents a risk of burns to the practitioner who accidentally touches it while still hot. It must be disinfected between patients and changed as often as the nebulizer. There are other systems that are variations on this idea of directly heating the water in the reservoir jar.

2. A flexible heater is wrapped around the outside of the reservoir. A dial is used to control how hot the heater gets but it has no automatic shut-off feature. The water temperature will increase as the water level drops. Monitor the gas temperature near the patient for safety purposes.

3. A clip-on heating base plate can be added to special reservoir jars with a metal plate. These are preferable to the first two types because they are thermostatically controlled. High and low temperature limits can be set and the unit will shut itself off if the limits are reached. They also ensure a constant temperature to the aerosol as the water level drops. Examples include the Ohmeda Ohio Deluxe nebulizer top and Puritan All-Purpose nebulizer top.

Units making use of the Babington nebulizer are a variation on these types of pneumatic nebulizers. Their main difference is in how the jet is constructed. These units have a more controlled particle size than the types in the list. Examples include the Solo-Sphere, Hydro-Sphere, and Maxi-Cool by Airlife/American Pharmaseal. These untis are quite complex with many parts in comparison to the listed types of nebulizers. Make sure that all components of the jet and baffle are kept free of debris. There is no heating element with these nebulizers.

b.   Small-volume nebulizers.

A small-volume nebulizer (SVN) is designed to hold a relatively small volume of fluid—typically 10 ml or less. It is designed to nebulize liquid medications such as bronchodilators and mucolytics for inhalation. Either compressed air or oxygen can be used to generate the mist. These units operate under the same physical principles as the large-volume nebulizers described earlier. There are two different types: mainstream and sidestream.

Mainstream Nebulizers.—Mainstream nebulizers are designed so that the main flow of gas to the patient flows through the aerosol as it is produced (see Fig. 7-6). A second high pressure gas flow is used to power the jet to create the aerosol. The Bird Corporation makes a reusable type called the Micronebulizer for its IPPB (Intermittent Positive Pressure Breathing) circuit.

Sidestream Nebulizers.—Sidestream nebulizers are designed so that the aerosol is produced out of the main flow of gas and added to it by the jet's gas flow (see Fig. 7-7). The Puritan-Bennett Corporation makes a reusable type called the Slipstream for its IPPB circuits.

Many manufacturers produce disposable medication nebulizers for IPPB circuits or hand-held circuits. Most of these are sidestream nebulizers. Select the nebulizer that produces a particle size that matches the therapeutic target.

See Fig. 7-8 for an illustration of a typical hand-held nebulizer circuit. The nebulizer can be powered by either air or oxygen. Typically, flows of 4 to 6 L/min are used to nebulize 3 to 5 ml of medication in about 10 minutes. The nebulizer finger control allows the patient to power the nebulizer by covering the open hole in the "T." Uncovering the hole permits the gas to exit and the medication is not nebulized and wasted. The reservoir tube serves to hold oxygen and medication for the next inspiration.

A concern has been raised recently about two risks to practitioners related to using SVNs. First, any aerosolized medications that escape into the room air may be inhaled. It is possible that the practitioner, or anyone else who happens be near, may have an allergic or other adverse reaction. Second, nebulized secretions from

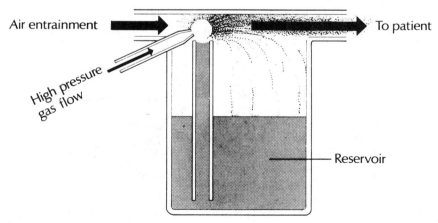

Fig. 7-6 Mainstream medication nebulizer. (From Shapiro BA, Harrison RA, Kacmarek, RM et al: *Clinical application of respiratory care*, ed 3, Chicago, 1985, Year Book Medical. Used by permission.)

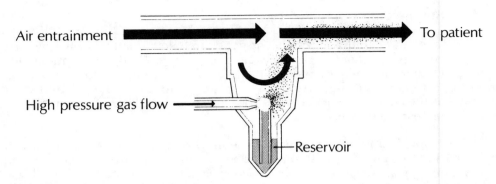

Fig. 7-7 Sidestream medication nebulizer. (From Shapiro BA, Harrison RA, Kacmarek RM et al: *Clinical application of respiratory care,* ed 3, Chicago, 1989, Year Book Medical. Used by permission.)

the patient's airway and lungs may be inhaled. This may place the practitioner or others at risk of acquiring a pulmonary infection from the patient. Although it is unlikely that many actual problems like this occur, it is a possibility. If either of these situations is a concern, a special SVN with a downstream particle filter should be used. This filter will trap any exhaled aerosol droplets.

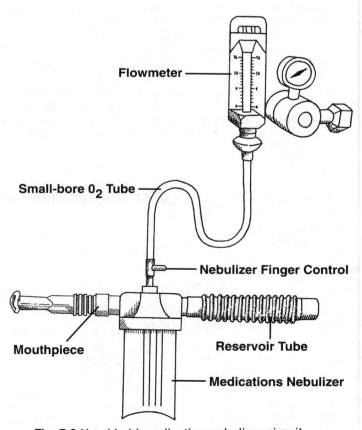

Fig. 7-8 Hand-held medication nebulizer circuit.

Marquest Medical Products manufactures the original Respirgard and newer Respirgard II Nebulizer System (see Fig. 7-9). They have been recommended for use when nebulizing pentamidine isethionate (Pentam). Flows of 5 to 7 L/min are used and the particle size is small enough to reach the alveolar level. The system is different from traditional SVNs in that it has three one-way valves and an exhalation side filter. This ensures that the patient breathes in the medication and that none escapes to the room air. Although designed for nebulizing pentamidine, it could be used for any other antibiotic or medication that should not contaminate the room air. More recently Cadema has manufactured the AeroTech II. Although it differs in basic design from the Respirgard II, it also features one-way valves and an exhalation side filter to prevent any aerosolized particles from reaching room air. Either could be used to ensure that room air contamination is prevented.

If any small-volume nebulizer fails to generate an aerosol, make sure that the jet and capillary tube are not plugged with debris. Sometimes they can be cleared by running them under water or pushing a needle through the channel. Do not use a nebulizer that does not generate an aerosol. Make sure that the medication cup and top are screwed tightly together to prevent aerosol leakage.

8. Fix any problems with a tracheostomy mask or collar. (IIB2a1) [An]

The adult or pediatric tracheostomy mask or collar is shaped to fit over a tracheostomy tube or stoma to provide oxygen and humidity (see Fig. 7-10). A nebulizer or humidifier is commonly added because the patient's upper airway is bypassed. Because this is a low-flow system with no reservoir, it is not possible to guarantee

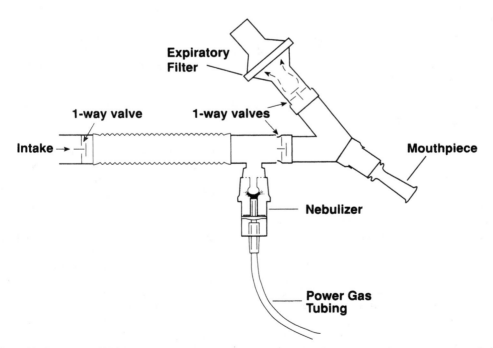

Fig. 7-9 Schematic diagram of the Respirgard II nebulizer and scavenging system useful with pentamidine or other aerosolized antiinfective agents. (From Rau JL Jr: *Respiratory care pharmacology*, ed 4, Chicago, 1994, Mosby–Year Book. Used by permission.)

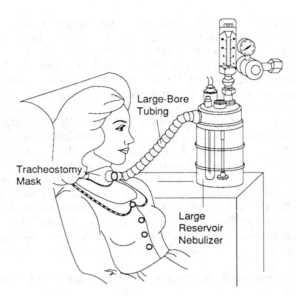

Fig. 7-10 Adult wearing a tracheostomy mask or collar. (From guidelines for disinfection of home equipment, *Respir Care* 33(9):801-808, 1988. Used by permission.)

the patient's inspired oxygen percentage. Gas flows are usually set high enough to make sure that there is a good flow of aerosol and oxygen to meet as much of the patient's needs as possible. Analyze the oxygen percentage from inside the mask to try for as much accuracy as possible. A PaO_2 or SpO_2 level should be checked whenever a change is made in the oxygen percentage or liter flow, or if the patient's condition changes significantly. Any of the previously mentioned humidity or aerosol devices can be used with the mask and powered by air or supplemental oxygen.

9. Fix any problems with a Brigg's adapter or T-adapter. (IIB2a1) [An]

The Brigg's adapter or T-adapter is designed to provide air or supplemental oxygen with humidity. It has one 15 mm inner diameter (ID) opening that fits over any endotracheal or tracheostomy tube adapter. The other two openings are 22 mm outer diameter (OD) so that aerosol tubing can be added (see Fig. 7-11). Any of the previously mentioned humidity or aerosol devices can be used with it and powered by air or supplemental oxygen.

Typically an air entrainment large volume nebulizer is used so that the oxygen percentage can be easily adjusted. The addition of a length of aerosol tubing downstream from the adapter acts as a reservoir so that the inspired oxygen percentage is ensured. A reservoir of 50 to 100 ml of aerosol tubing is commonly needed for an adult. Care must be taken to adjust the gas flow so that it is high enough to meet the patient's peak inspiratory flow rate. Make sure that during inspiration the aerosol is still flowing past the tracheostomy/endotracheal tube and into the reservoir. Inadequate flow could result in the patient rebreathing gas from the reservoir. This gas has just been exhaled and is high in carbon dioxide and low in oxygen.

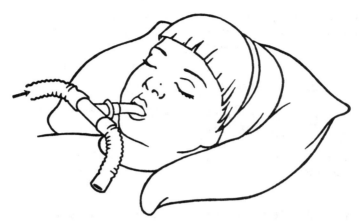

Fig. 7-11 Intubated child with a Brigg's adapter or T-adapter and aerosol tubing added to the endotracheal tube. (From Gaeber G, Blodgett D: Gas administration. In Blodgett D, editor: *Manual of pediatric respiratory care procedures*, Philadelphia, 1982, JB Lippincott. Used by permission.)

Module B. Coach the patient to modify his or her breathing pattern. (IIIC2d) [An]

Patients will breathe in whatever pattern and rate is easiest for them. Although this will have some benefit to a patient because of the minimized work of breathing and fewer calories being burned, it may not be best for the patient's pulmonary condition. Frequently, sick patients breathe in a rapid and shallow pattern because of their weakened condition. With this pattern, any therapeutic aerosol particles will tend to be deposited in the first few airway generations. This may or may not be best for the patient depending on the aerosol target site. Coached breathing patterns will help to get the aerosol where it is intended.

Upper Airway Deposition

Particles 10 micrometers (μm) or larger are more likely to impact on the upper airway when the patient is coached to:

a. Inhale at a normal or faster speed. The flow should be greater than 30 l/min.
b. Inhale a normal tidal volume.
c. Breathe in a normal pattern.

Lower Airway and Alveolar Deposition

Particles 2 to 5 μm in size are more likely to deposit on the smaller airways and in the alveoli when the patient is coached to:

a. Inhale at a slow speed. The flow should be less than 30 L/min.
b. Inhale an inspiratory capacity.
c. Hold the full breath in for 10 to 15 seconds before exhaling.

Obviously, all patients will not be able to perform these techniques perfectly, but to the extent that they can the medication will be deposited where it is needed and the treatment will be more effective.

Module C.   Patient assessment.

1.   Examine all the data to determine the patient's pathophysiological condition. (IC3a) [R, Ap, An]

Look for the reason(s) that humidity or aerosol therapy is needed. Examples of indications include viscous secretions, artificial airway, and croup (laryngotracheobronchitis).

2.   Take part in the development of the respiratory care plan. (IC3c) [An]

Be prepared to look at all the available data on the patient, evaluate it, and make recommendations for patient care.

3.   Modify aerosol therapy based on the patient's response to respiratory care.
a.   Change the type of equipment being used. (IIIC2a) [An]

Be prepared to change the type of humidity and/or aerosol delivery system from among any of those available in respiratory care based on the patient's condition. Review the indications, contraindications, uses, and limitations of the various systems. Change the nebulizer based on the desired aerosol particle size. (See Table 7-2 for particle sizes and likely deposition sites.)

Table 7-2. Aerosol Particle Sizes and Their Likely Deposition Point in the Airways and Lungs

Location	MMAD* Particle Size in Micrometers
Nose or mouth to larynx	10 and larger
Trachea to terminal bronchioles	9-5
Respiratory bronchioles to alveoli	5-2
Likely to be exhaled	Less than 1

* MMAD is mass median aerodynamic diameter. It is defined as the aerosol diameter around which the mass is equally divided. That is, 50% of the aerosol mass is found in particles smaller than the MMAD and 50% of the aerosol mass is found in particles larger than the MMAD.
Note: There is some controversy over what size particles deposit in the airways and lungs. This table lists what seems to be a majority opinion. Aerosol particle diameter sizes are listed in units of micrometers, which are one thousandth of a millimeter. As a point of clarification, most references list the symbol for a micrometer as μ; others use the international system unit of micrometer which is symbolized as μm.

b. Adjust the temperature of the liquid being used in the equipment. (IIIC2c) [An]

In general, a cool humidity or aerosol system is used with patients with the following conditions:

a. Pediatric croup
b. Upper airway irritation such as post-extubation or after a bronchoscopy procedure

In general, a body temperature humidity or aerosol system is used for the following reasons:

a. Bypassed upper airway
b. Viscous secretions
c. Hypothermia
d. With a neonate to maintain a neutral thermal environment

c. Change the output of aerosol by the equipment. (IIIC2e) [An]

Neonates are sensitive to overhydration; therefore long-term aerosol therapy for them should be avoided or minimized. Adult patients with heart failure or pulmonary edema should also not be given long-term aerosol therapy. Instead, a Cascade humidifier can be used.

The adult patient who has viscous secretions may be aided by long-term aerosol therapy of a dense mist at body temperature. The secretions will often be liquified and made easier to cough or suction out. An ultrasonic nebulizer is often used for this purpose. The child with croup is usually given a dense mist of a cool bland aerosol in a mist tent. This therapy is usually only needed for a few days. Be wary of fluid overload if the mist is needed for a longer period of time.

4. Maintain records and communication on the patient's cough and sputum production and characteristics. (IIIA2a3) [An]

For pulmonary secretions to be properly cleared out they must be of the appropriate viscosity and tenacity. Secretions that are too viscous or tenacious cannot be coughed out or suctioned out easily. More humidity or inhaled bland aerosol would help to make the secretions more watery. If not, active mucolytics such as Mucomyst or Pulmozyme would be needed. Secretions that are watery are easy to suction out; however, the patient's mucociliary escalator may not be able to move them as well as mucus of natural consistency.

Record the nature of the patient's secretions as well as his or her cough effort. This information should also be told to other respiratory care practitioners, nurses, and the patient's physician.

BIBLIOGRAPHY

AARC Aerosol Consensus Statement, *Respir Care* 36(9): 916-921, 1991.

AARC Clinical Practice Guideline: Selection of aerosol delivery device, *Respir Care* 37(8):891-897, 1992.

AARC Clinical Practice Guideline: Bland aerosol administration, *Respir Care* 38(11):1196-1200, 1993.

AARC Clinical Practice Guideline: Delivery of aerosols to the upper airway, *Respir Care* 39(8):803-807, 1994.

Dolovich M: Clinical aspects of aerosol physics, *Respir Care* 36(9):931-938, 1991.

Eubanks DH, Bone RC: *Comprehensive respiratory care*, ed 2, St. Louis, 1990, Mosby–Year Book.

Helmholz HF Jr, Burton GG: Applied humidity and aerosol therapy. In Burton GG, Hodgkin JE, editors: *Respiratory care: a guide to clinical practice*, ed 2, Philadelphia, 1984, JB Lippincott.

Kacmarek RM, Hess D: The interface between patient and aerosol generator, *Respir Care* 36:952-976, 1991.

Marquest Medical Products, Inc, Englewood, Colo. Manufactuter's literature on the Respirgard II.

McPherson SP: *Respiratory therapy equipment*, ed 4, St. Louis, 1990, Mosby–Year Book.

Monaghan Medical Corp, Plattsburg, NY. Manufacturer's literature on the AeroVent.

Op't Holt T: Aerosol generators and humidifiers. In Barnes TA, editor: *Respiratory care practice*, Chicago, 1988, Year Book Medical.

Rau JL Jr: Humidity and aerosol therapy. In Barnes TA, editor: *Respiratory care practice*, Chicago, 1988, Year Book Medical.

Rau JL Jr: *Respiratory care pharmacology*, ed 4, Chicago, 1994, Year Book Medical.

Scanlan CL: Humidity and aerosol therapy. In Scanlan CL, Spearman CB, Sheldon RL, editors: *Egan's fundamentals of respiratory care*, ed 5, St. Louis, 1990, Mosby–Year Book.

Shapiro BA, Kacmarek RM, Cane RD et al: *Clinical application of respiratory care*, ed 4, Chicago, 1991, Year Book Medical.

Sills JR: *Respiratory care certification guide: the complete review resource for the entry level exam*, ed 2, St. Louis, 1994, Mosby–Year Book.

Vinciguerra C, Smaldone G: Treatment time and patient tolerance for pentamidine delivery by Respirgard II and AeroTech II, *Respir Care* 35(11):1037-1041, 1990.

SELF-STUDY QUESTIONS

1. Ten minutes into hand-held nebulizer treatment to deliver Alupent, the patient complains of dizziness and tingling fingers. What would you do?
    A. Advise the patient to breathe in the same pattern.
    B. Change the medication.
    C. Tell the patient to breathe more slowly.
    D. Have the patient use pursed lips breathing.
    E. Advise the patient to breathe deeper and faster.

2. Your 30-year-old patient has a face tent on for the delivery of a heated aerosol. Her secretions are still too viscous to be easily coughed out. What would you recommend?
    A. Change to a mist tent.
    B. Change to an aerosol mask.
    C. Change to a simple oxygen mask.
    D. Change to a non-rebreather mask.
    E. Make no change at this time.

3. The physician wants more aerosol inside the mist tent of a 3-year-old child. What would be the best way to do this?
    A. Cut a hole in the top of the tent.
    B. Close the hole on the top of the tent.
    C. Lower the temperature on the refrigeration unit.

D.   Increase the gas flow to the nebulizer.

E.   Remove the dust filter.

4.   Your comatose patient is intubated and receiving 35% oxygen with aerosol by way of a T-adapter. While observing the patient, you notice that during each inspiration the mist disappears from the downstream end of the T-adapter. What would you recommend?

A.   Add 100 ml of aerosol tubing as a reservoir on the T-adapter.

B.   Change the oxygen to 30%.

C.   Change the oxygen to 40%.

D.   Increase the oxygen flow to the nebulizer.

E.   Tell the patient not to breathe as deeply.

5.   A technician calls you when he has analyzed 40% oxygen to an infant inside a mist tent. This is despite his attempt to get the ordered 50% oxygen by setting the nebulizer's entrainment port at 60% and the blender to the nebulizer at 50%. What would you recommend be done?

A.   Increase the flow by 5 L/min.

B.   Set the blender to 100%.

C.   Check the accuracy of the oxygen analyzer.

D.   Get a new equipment set-up.

E.   Set the entrainment port on the nebulizer to 100%.

6.   A humidity or aerosol system delivering body temperature gas would be used in all the following situations EXCEPT:

A.   Patient with a tracheostomy.

B.   Twenty-month-old infant with laryngotracheobronchitis.

C.   COPD patient with viscous secretions.

D.   Newborn receiving oxygen inside an infant hood.

E.   A cold water near-drowning patient.

7.   To prepare a patient for a laryngoscopy procedure the physician wants her to inhale nebulized lidocaine. You would select a nebulizer that generates what size particles?

A.   1 to 3 μm

B.   3 to 5 μm

C.   5 to 7 μm

D.   7 to 10 μm

E.   10 μm or larger

8.   To ensure the best deposition of these particles, what breathing pattern would you coach the patient to follow?

I.   Inhale a tidal volume.

II.   Inhale an inspiratory capacity.

III.   Inhale slowly.

IV.   Inhale quickly.

V.   Hold the breath for at least 10 seconds before exhaling.

VI.   Breathe in a normal pattern.

A.   I, IV, V

B.   II, III, V

C.   I, IV, VI

D.   IV, V

E.   II, IV

9. A physician calls you to evaluate a 40-year old patient with bronchitis and make a recommendation for an aerosol delivery system. The patient's breath sounds indicate the presence of large airway secretions. Despite a good cough effort the patient has great difficulty in raising them. What would you recommend?
   A. Hand-held nebulizer with 3 cc of normal saline every 4 hours
   B. Place the patient in a mist tent
   C. Room temperature nebulizer to a face tent
   D. Continuous ultrasonic to aerosol mask
   E. Heated cascade humidifier to an aerosol mask

10. When doing patient rounds you notice that very little aerosol is going to a new patient's tracheostomy mask. Which of the following could be the problem?
    I. The water level is above the refill line on the nebulizer's reservoir jar.
    II. The nebulizer is not tightly screwed into the DISS connector on the flowmeter.
    III. The nebulizer jet is obstructed.
    IV. The water level is below the refill line on the nebulizer's reservoir jar.
    V. The capillary line is obstructed.
    A. II, III, V
    B. I, II
    C. III, IV
    D. I, IV
    E. III, V

Answer Key

1. C; 2. B; 3. D; 4. A; 5. E; 6. B; 7. E; 8. C; 9. D. 10. A.

8 | Pharmacology

Module A. Change the dilution of a medication used in aerosol therapy. (IIIC2b) [An]

The various saline solutions and sterile water are known collectively as "bland" aerosols because they have no direct pharmacologic effect on the lungs and airways. They are used to increase the volume of liquid in a small volume nebulizer (SVN) after the medication has been added. Most of these nebulizers work most efficiently when they hold about 3 to 5 ml of liquid. Usually normal saline (.9% NaCl) is added.

Adding little or no saline to the medication will result in the patient inhaling a very concentrated solution. The nebulizer will aerosolize the medication(s) within a few minutes. The patient should quickly feel the beneficial effects of the treatment. However, depending on the nature of the medication, the patient might find it to be quite irritating to the airway. Coughing or bronchospasm could result. Side effects, such as tachycardia, should be watched for with sympathomimetic agents because the medication will enter the bloodstream so quickly.

The more saline that is added, the less concentrated the solution will be. The nebulizer will take longer to aerosolize the medication because of the added volume. Relief of symptoms will take longer, but it will be less likely to irritate the airway. Side effects with sympathomimetic agents could be less severe because the drug is given over a longer period of time. However, remember that increasing the amount of saline makes no difference on the total amount of medication that is given to the patient. Tachycardia or other side effects may still be seen if the total amount of medication is given.

Saline-only aerosol treatments, such as for an induced sputum, will be more effective at higher concentrations of saline. (See Table 8-1 for complete information on saline solutions).

Module B. Recommend the use of the following pharmacologic agents.

1.   Inotropic agents. (IIIC11b) [R, Ap, An]

Positive inotropic agents are used to increase the contractility of the heart muscle. There are two classes of drugs that do this. The best-known, older group are called the cardiac glycosides. They are derived from the plants *Digitalis purpurea* and *Digitalis lanata*. This group of medications, in general, is referred to as "digitalis." The newer group includes synthetic catecholamine agents. These two important groups of medications are used in patient's who have a weak or damaged myocardium. They will increase the patient's myocardial contractility. This results

Table 8-1. Saline Solutions Used
as Mucolytics

Normal saline, .9% saline
  Direct instillation into the airway:
    Infants may be given about 1 ml several times
      per day before suctioning.
    Adults may be given about 3-5 ml several
      times per day before suctioning.
  Aerosol:
    Most medication nebulizers hold 3-5 ml that
      are nebulized several times per day.
  Miscellaneous:
    Usually well tolerated because it is isotonic to
      the body.
    Particle size is fairly stable as nebulized.
Hypotonic saline, .45% saline
  Direct instillation into the airway:
    (Same as above.)
  Aerosol:
    (Same as above.) Many practitioners use this
      concentration in ultrasonic nebulizers.
  Miscellaneous:
    Particles tend to shrink due to evaporation.
      This results in smaller particles than
      nebulized that are closer to isotonic.
    Impaction is more likely in the smaller
      airways.
Hypertonic saline, 1.8%-20% saline.
  Aerosol:
    Some practitioners use a large reservoir
      nebulizer with a heater to generate the
      aerosol. Hypertonic saline is most
      commonly used to induce a cough and
      sputum sample for cytology (lung cancer)
      or fungal or mycobacteria (tuberculosis)
      culture. It should not be used for a general
      bacteria culture as the high salt
      concentration inhibits the growth of most
      bacteria.
  Miscellaneous:
    Particles tend to enlarge due to the
      absorption of water vapor.
    This results in larger particles than nebulized
      that are closer to isotonic. Impaction is
      more likely in the upper airway.
      This concentration is the most likely to
      cause bronchospasm in asthmatic patients
      because it is the farthest from isotonic and
      therefore the most irritating.

From Sills JR: *Respiratory care certification guide: the complete review resource for the entry level exam,* ed 2, St. Louis, 1994, Mosby–Year Book.

in an increased cardiac output, increased blood pressure, and increased urine output. Examples of inotropic agents include:

- Cardiac glycosides
    digoxin, Lanoxin (preferred)
    digitoxin, Purodigin
- Catecholamines
    dobutamine hydrochloride, Dobutrex
    isoproterenol hydrochloride, Isuprel
    epinephrine, Adrenaline chloride

These two groups of medications work by different mechanisms. The cardiac glycosides increase the level of intramuscular sodium and calcium to increase the contraction of the heart muscle. Of these, Lanoxin would be the preferred medication in a patient with congestive heart failure. The catecholamine agents are similar to adrenaline and stimulate beta receptors in the heart. Dobutrex is used as a short-term agent in adult patients who have organic heart disease or who had heart surgery. Its use results in an increase in contraction with only a minor increase in heart rate. Isuprel is used to increase the heart rate and contractility in cases of heart block, congestive heart failure, or cardiac arrest. Adrenaline is used during a cardiac arrest to increase heart rate and contractility.

2. Vasoconstrictors. (IIIC11b) [R, Ap, An]

Vasoconstrictors are medications that cause the peripheral blood vessels to constrict so that blood flow is reduced through them. Many medications do this by stimulating the alpha-1 (α_1) receptors on the vessels. There are three common clinical situations where vasoconstrictors are used in the care of patients with cardiopulmonary problems: laryngeal edema or upper airway edema, upper airway procedure, and hypotension.

Laryngeal Edema or Upper Airway Edema

This type of problem requires the administration of a medication that will reduce the swelling of the mucosa of the larynx, epiglottis, or tracheobronchial tree. Agents that stimulate the alpha-sympathomimetic receptors are called for. Inhaled racemic epinephrine (MicroNefrin, Vaponefrin, AsthmaNefrin) has been widely used for many years to treat upper airway edema. Be aware that it also stimulates Beta-1 (β_1) and Beta-2 (β_2) receptors. Because many of these patients also have some bronchospasm, the β_2 effect is beneficial. Watch for signs of tachycardia. Phenylephrine (Neo-Synephrine) is a more pure alpha receptor stimulator. There should be fewer pulmonary or cardiac effects with its use. All these medications will cause vasoconstriction of the mucosal blood vessels. Because of this, the swelling is reduced, the patient's airway is enlarged, and breathing is easier.

The medication nebulizer and breathing pattern to treat upper edema are summarized here:

1. Use a nebulizer that generates particles 10 μm or larger.
2. Have the patient inhale a normal tidal volume.
3. Have the patient inhale at a normal or faster speed (greater than 30 L/min or .5 L/sec).
4. Have the patient breathe in a normal pattern.

Upper Airway Procedure

Procedures where the nasal passage must be entered with a medical instrument include nasotracheal intubation, passage of a fiberoptic bronchoscope, and nasal surgery. Racemic epinephrine or phenylephrine is nebulized into the appropriate nostril. A so-called atomizer is often used for this purpose because it generates relatively large particles.

Hypotension

Hypotension is usually defined as a systemic blood pressure of less than 80 mm Hg in an adult and less than 70 mm Hg in a child. A pressure of less than this is not adequate to perfuse the kidneys. Urine output will drop dramatically or stop altogether. Cerebral blood flow is also greatly reduced and the patient may faint. When hypotension is caused by vasodilation it usually has to be treated by inducing vasoconstriction. Examples of conditions where dangerous vasodilation occur include an anaphylaxis, such as an allergic reaction to a bee sting or penicillin injection, and bacterial septicemia from a species such as *Staphylococcus aureus*. Hypotension from heart failure or a myocardial infarction often must also be treated with a vasoconstrictor.

Common examples of medications that cause vasoconstriction to increase blood pressure include:

- dopamine hydrochloride, Intropin
- norepinephrine, Levophed, Levarterenol

The effects of dopamine are dose related. At relatively low doses of 2 to 5 µg/kg/min there is an increase in renal blood flow. Urine output increases. There is no change in blood pressure. At medium doses of 5 to 30 µg/kg/min there is an increase in myocardial contractility and a progressive peripheral vasoconstriction. These effects raise the blood pressure without decreasing renal blood flow. At high doses of more than 30 µg/kg/min, the total systemic vascular resistance further increases; however, renal blood flow and urine output both decrease. Current practice indicates that dopamine works best in patients with moderate hypotension.

The patient who needs greater than 20 µg/kg/min of dopamine to raise the blood pressure is probably depleted of his or her own natural stores of norepinephrine. This is often seen in patients with congestive heart failure and in neonates. These patients probably need to be given norepinephrine (Levophed or Levarterenol) to raise the blood pressure. Any time a hypotensive patient is given a vasoconstricting agent, the blood pressure, peripheral blood flow, and urine output must be watched closely. The prognosis is grim for patients who do not respond to these medications or attempts to correct the underlying condition.

3. Vasodilators. (IIIC11b) [R, Ap, An]

Hypertension in the adult is defined as a blood pressure of greater than 140 to 150/90 mm Hg. The higher the blood pressure is, the greater a strain it places on the heart. It also increases the risk of vessel rupture and stroke. For these reasons, hypertension is treated to reduce the blood pressure closer to normal.

A wide variety of medications in a number of drug catagories is used to reduce blood pressure. They range from diuretics to reduce blood volume, to calcium and sympathomimetic blockers that reduce heart rate and vasodilate, to angiotensin converting enzyme (ACE) inhibitors. Medications in these catagories are used to treat moderate, chronic hypertension.

The patient in a hypertensive crisis (blood pressure greater than 200/120 mm Hg) must be treated quickly and effectively. The following medications are commonly given by the intravenous route to control severe hypertension:

- nitroprusside, Nipride
- diazoxide, Hyperstat
- trimethaphan, Arfonad

Nitroprusside is also given to reduce the afterload in a patient with left ventricular failure after a myocardial infarct. Any patient who is receiving a powerful vasodilator must have frequent monitoring of his or her blood pressure.

4. Diuretics. (IIIC11e) [R, Ap, An]

Diuretics are most commonly indicated in patients with edema or hypertension. Edema is usually a result of heart failure and/or fluid overload. Examples of diuretics used to treat these problems include:

- furosemide, Lasix
- ethacrynic acid, Edecrin
- chlorthiazine, Diuril

These are some of the most powerful diuretics in use today. They will produce a rapid increase in urine output. They basically prevent the kidneys from retaining sodium (Na^+) so that water is excreted. A side effect of their use is a loss of potassium (K^+) through the kidneys. It is important that the patient be given replacement potassium to avoid dangerous hypokalemia. Triamterene (Dyrenium) is referred to as a potassium sparing diuretic because the patient should not suffer as great a loss of K^+ with its use. It may be a better diuretic in patients who tend to lose too much potassium with the other diuretics listed.

Another catagory of diuretic is used in patients who have an increased intracranial pressure (ICP). The increased ICP is usually due to cerebral edema from a head injury. Examples of medications used to treat an increased intracranial pressure include:

- mannitol, Osmitrol
- sterile urea, Ureaphil, Urevert

These medications have a large molecular weight and through osmosis "pull" fluid from the brain into the bloodstream. Because of this they are sometimes called osmotic diuretics. When the medication crosses into the kidney it prevents the reabsorption of water and increases urine output.

5. Antibiotics.

Antibiotics are drugs derived from microorganisms (bacteria, fungi, or molds) or produced synthetically in a laboratory. They are capable of inhibiting or killing bacteria, viruses, protozoa, or other microorganisms. The terms *antiinfective agents* or *antimicrobial agents* have the same meaning. The NBRC has only listed the following two agents as specifically testable on the advanced practitioner examinations: antiviral and antipneumocystic. Further discussion on common respiratory pathogens and antibiotics is presented in Module E.

a. Antiviral agent: ribavirin (Virazole). (IIIC11b) [R, Ap, An]

Virazole is most commonly used in the treatment of infants and young children who have bronchiolitis or pneumonia from the respiratory syncytial virus (RSV). Patients requiring treatment for their condition usually are very sick and have complicating factors such as prematurity or cardiopulmonary disease. They will require the treatment course of 3 to 7 days of nebulization of the drug for 12 to 18 hours per day. Only the SPAG II (small particle aerosol generator) can be used for the procedure. This is because it is specifically designed to nebulize the 1 to 2 μm size particles needed to penetrate to the alveoli to kill the virus. The usual dose of Virazole is 20 mg/ml. It comes in a 100-ml vial containing 6 g of ribavirin. Sterile water is added to the vial to mix the drug. The solution is added to the large-volume nebulizer in the SPAG II unit. More sterile water is then added to bring the total volume to 300 ml of a 2% solution for nebulization. Virazole is known to also be effective against influenza types A and B viruses and the herpes simplex virus.

b. Antipneumocystic agent: pentamidine isethionate (NebuPent). (IIIC11c) [R, Ap, An]

NebuPent has been approved for the prophylactic treatment of the protozoal organism *Pneumocystis carinii*. Patients with impaired immune systems, such as those with acquired immunodeficiency syndrome (AIDS), are most likely to get pneumocystic carinii pneumonia (PCP). Currently, these patients are given a single 300-mg dose of NebuPent mixed with 6 ml of sterile water once every 4 weeks through the Respirgard II nebulizer. (The AeroTech II unit may also be used.) Some patients will need to be pretreated with an inhaled bronchodilator to prevent bronchospasm before the NebuPent is inhaled. Do not mix the two medications in the Respirgard II or use the Respirgard II for any medication other than NebuPent. Mixing of NebuPent with normal saline or a bronchodilator can result in a precipitation of the medications. Given by the inhalation route there are few systemic side effects.

There is also an intramuscular or intravenous form of pentamidine called Pemtam 300. It is indicated in patients known to have a PCP infection. A dose of 4 mg/kg is indicated once a day for 14 days. An adult would receive a 300-mg dose mixed with sterile water. Given by IM or IV route, pentamidine is known to cause serious side effects, even death, from severe hypotension, cardiac arrhythmias, and hypoglycemia. Patients should be lying down and have their blood pressure monitored regularly during and after its administration until it is stable.

While not specified by the NBRC, a second drug is also used to combat a *Pneumocystis carinii* infection. Bactrim (trimethoprim and sulfamethoxazole) is preferred over systemic pentamidine because there are fewer and less serious side effects. This combination of medications is also used against a wide variety of bacteria that cause urinary tract and other infections. The recommended dose for the treatment of PCP is 20 mg/kg of trimethoprim and 100 mg/kg of sulfamethoxamole per 24 hours given in divided doses every 6 hours for 14 days.

6. Sedatives. (IIIC11f) [R, Ap, An]

Sedatives are medications that affect the brain to induce calming in a patient who can be either simply anxious or very agitated and uncooperative. Examples of when a patient would be given a sedative include: 1) when he or she is struggling against a necessary intubation or the mechanical ventilator so that his or her condition worsens, 2) he or she is displaying self-destructive behavior because of a drug reaction, and 3) before a medical procedure. The effects on the patient are dose related. Low to moderate doses will calm the patient. Higher doses will induce sleep. There are three different groupings of these types of medications. The most widely used are the benzodiazepines because they have fewer side effects, fewer drug interactions, and are less likely to cause addiction than the barbiturate drugs. In addition, the benzodiazepine agents can be pharmacologically reversed. The barbiturates are widely used during general anesthesia to rapidly induce sleep. Commonly used examples of these types of medications include:

- Benzodiazepine minor tranquilizers
    Diazepam, Valium
    Chlordiazepoxide, Librium
    Alprazolam, Xanax
    Trizolam, Halcion
    Flurazepam, Dalmane
- Nonbarbiturate sedative-hypnotics
    Ethylchlorvynol, Placidyl
    Meprobamate, Miltown
    Glutethimide, Doriden
    Chloral hydrate, Noctec
- Barbiturate sedative-hypnotics
    Pentobarbitol sodium, Nembutol
    Seconbarbital sodium, Seconal
    Phenobarbitol, Luminol
    Thiopental, Pentothal

7. Analgesics. (IIIC11f) [R, Ap, An]

Analgesics are medications that control or block pain after injury or a surgical procedure. Morphine and similar drugs that are based on opium can control severe pain. Morphine is indicated to control the pain of a myocardial infarct and to vasodilate the patient with pulmonary edema. In addition, pain-relieving agents, when given in large enough doses, will induce sleep. The patient who is both in pain and agitated may be treated with a combination of an analgesic and a sedative, for example, moderate doses of morphine and Valium. The two drugs potentiate each other. Or the physician may decide to give the patient only Morphine at a larger dose. Examples of commonly used analgesics include:

- Morphine sulfate, Morphine Sulfate injection or tablets, Duramorph
- Codeine phosphate, Methylmorphine
- Hydromorphone, Dilaudid
- Meperidine, Demerol
- Propoxyphene, Darvon

Patients receiving sedatives and/or analgesics must be closely monitored. Both can cause respiratory center depression if given in great enough doses. The patient may hypoventilate and even experience apnea and death. Another concern with these agents is that morphine and these other medications can become habit forming or addictive if used for a prolonged period of time.

8. Neuromuscular blocking agents. (IIIC10e) [R, Ap, An]

Neuromuscular blocking agents are used to cause a pharmacological paralysis. These medications block nerve transmission from reaching skeletal (voluntary) muscles. Complete paralysis will follow. They are used most commonly as part of balanced anesthesia before major thoracic or abdominal surgery. These drugs are also used in the intensive care unit to stop a patient from fighting against an intubation or to prevent the patient from struggling against the mechanical ventilator. All are given intravenously and act rapidly. Obviously, in all these cases the patient must use a manual resuscitator or ventilator. Examples of the commonly used neuromuscular blocking agents include:

- Depolarizing blocker
    Succinylcholine chloride, Anectine, Quelicin
- Nondepolarizing blockers
    Pancuronium bromide, Pavulon (Preferred)
    Vecuronium bromide, Norcuron
    Gallamine triethiodide, Flaxedil
    Atracurium besylate, Tracrium

The nondepolarizing blockers such as Pavulon are preferred for their longer duration of action. Although all these agents will induce complete paralysis of all voluntary muscles, they have little or no affect on the involuntary muscles or autonomic nervous system. Some patients may have a minor, passing change in heart rate and blood pressure. Remember that they are able to hear, feel pain, and are completely awake and alert to their surroundings. Care must be taken to sedate the patient for anxiety and give analgesics for pain. Talk to the patient normally and move the patient periodically to prevent pressure sores.

9. Respiratory stimulants. (IIIC11d) [R, Ap, An]

In theory, respiratory stimulants are supposed to increase a patient's ventilatory drive. In practice, this has met with only limited success. The decision to use any of the medications listed as follows depends on the patient's underlying diagnosis. Respiratory simulatants will have no affect on the patient who is physically unable to breathe more deeply. Patients with central or peripheral nervous system disorders, severe restrictive or obstructive lung disease, or who have overdosed on barbiturates may be unable to breathe despite the use of drugs to stimulate the respiratory center. If the patient cannot be safely stimulated to breathe, he or she should be intubated and placed on a mechanical ventilator. Common examples of the drugs that may stimulate breathing are listed throughout the rest of this discussion.

- Analeptic
    Doxapram, Dopram

Dopram is a general stimulant of the central nervous system and stimulates breathing; however, it only lasts 5 to 10 minutes when given by an intravenous bolus. When given by continuous drip to have a longer affect, the patient runs the risk of an overdose with resulting convulsions.

- Methylxanthines
    Theophylline
    Aminophylline
    Caffeine

The methylxanthines have been tried with some success in neonates with periodic breathing. Care must be taken to measure the peak and trough serum concentrations to maintain a safe level. A toxic level can cause gastrointestinal distress, tachycardia, or seizures. A subtherapeutic level will have no affect on breathing rhythm. A number of other medications and foods affect these serum levels, which makes the methylxanthines challenging to use. These infants should also be wearing an apnea monitor.

- Progesterone
    Protriptyline, Triptin, Vivactil

Protriptyline is similar to the female hormone estrogen. It has been used with some success in patients diagnosed with central sleep apnea. Male patients receiving this medication should be informed of the possible side effects of impotence and developing secondary female sex characteristics.

- Narcotic antagonists
    Naloxone, Narcan (drug of choice)
    Nallorphine, Nalline
    Levallorphan, Lorfan

The narcotic antagonists counteract the effects of narcotic agents such as morphine, heroin, codeine, and so forth. They will not reverse the effects of sedatives such as barbiturates. Narcan may be tried in anonymous suspected drug overdose patients when there is no knowledge of what drug was taken. If the patient begins breathing and wakes up, the overdose was of a narcotic agent. Remember that the patient who received an accidental overdose of morphine given to control pain will feel pain again when Narcan is given to reverse it.

- Benzodiazepine antagonist
    Flumazenil, Mazicon

Mazicon is indicated in the reversal of benzodiazepine agents such as Valium, Librium, and so forth. These patients may have been given the drug for sedation before a medical procedure or may have overdosed. Patients who are unconscious will usually quickly awaken after the proper dose of Mazicon is given. Watch the patient for signs of seizure activity related to the rapid reversal of the benzodiazepine medication. Furthermore, the patient should be observed for 2 hours in case resedation occurs. If it does, Mazicon can be given again.

- Nondepolarizing neuromuscular blocker antagonists
    Neostigmine bromide, Prostigmin (drug of choice)
    Edrophonium, Tensilon

These drugs are used to reverse the affects of the nondepolarizing neuromuscular blockers such as pancuronium bromide (Pavulon), vecuronium bromide (Norcuron), and so forth. They will have no affect on the depolarizing neuromuscular blocker succinylcholine chloride (Anectine, Quelicin, or Sucostrin). Prostigmin is the drug of choice because of its longer duration. Patients will quickly be able to breathe and move about after it has been given. It should be noted that Prostigmin will cause an outpouring of oral and bronchial secretions. Atropine is given to prevent this.

10. Artificial surfactants. (IIIC11g) [R, Ap, An]

Artificial/exogenous surfactants have been approved for the prevention or treatment of infant respiratory distress syndrome (IRDS) in premature neonates. These neonates have immature lungs that lack natural surfactant. As a result they become atelectatic. These two artificial surfactant agents have been approved for instillation into the airways to treat this problem:

- Colfosceril palmitate, cetyl alcohol, and tyloxapol are combined to make Exosurf
- Beractant, Survanta

Doses for both medications are based on the infant's weight. Exosurf must be mixed with sterile water at the bedside. Always follow the manufacturer's guidelines for preparation and the procedure for instilling either drug into the airway. Be prepared to make rapid changes in the neonate's mechanical ventilator settings as the lungs rapidly become more compliant.

At the time of this writing artificial surfactants are being tried experimentally in patients with adult respiratory distress syndrome (ARDS). It may be determined that artificial surfactant is helpful in cases of ARDS where natural surfactant is destroyed or decreased.

11. Nicotine replacement therapy. (IIIC11h) [R, Ap, An]

Nicotine replacement therapy is indicated whenever a patient wishes to stop smoking but finds it difficult to abruptly quit due to nicotine addiction. This patient should be referred to his or her physician. The physician will help make arrangements for a psychological support group as well as give a prescription for a nicotine replacement system. (Section 16 has more discussion on smoking cessation.) Currently these are the two nicotine replacement systems available for weaning a patient off of nicotine and smoking:

- Nicotine gum
     Nicotine polacrilex, Nicorette
- Nicotine transdermal system
     Prostep
     Nicoderm
     Habitrol

Nicotine is a powerfully addictive chemical found in both smoking and chewing tobacco. It is difficult to stop using because of its withdrawal symptoms. The listed nicotine replacement systems can be very helpful in smoking cessation if properly used; they allow the patient to slowly taper off the drug. This avoids the withdrawal symptoms so that the patient will not feel compelled to smoke again.

Of the two, nicotine gum is more difficult to dose properly. This is because the rate of nicotine absorption depends on the pH of the patient's mouth as well as his or her chewing rate. However, it has the advantage of letting the patient feel more in control of the whole situation. The transdermal system (commonly called the patch) has the advantage of being easier to maintain the desired nicotine level. The patch must be placed on a skin area that is clean, dry, and hairless. The trunk and upper arm are common sites. The patch site must be changed each day. The patient must be told to watch for skin inflammation or irritation. In both cases the patient must totally stop smoking when the nicotine replacement is started. A dangerous nicotine overdose can result if the patient continues to smoke while using either the nicotine gum or patch. It will likely take a period of 6 to 10 weeks before the patient is totally weaned off of the nicotine replacement system and no longer nicotine dependent.

Note: A contraindication to nicotine replacement therapy, or any medication, is a hypersensitivity or allergic reaction to it or any preservative or other included component of the medication.

Note: The uses of a variety of other medications have been tested on the Advanced Practitioners' Examinations even though they have not been specified on the Detailed Examination Outline. Sometimes the medications were directly tested and at other times they were used as a foil. It is apparent that the student and examinee must be aware of a wide variety of medications. It would be wise to become familiar with any medication that is currently and widely used in the care of patients with cardiopulmonary diseases. This includes those medications that were tested on the Entry Level Examination.

Module C.   Recommend the delivery of medications during an emergency.

1.   Recommend the instillation of medications through an endotracheal tube during an emergency situation. (IIID8) [R, Ap, An]

Cardiac medications should be instilled down the endotracheal tube when a resuscitation attempt is underway and the patient does not have a functional central or peripheral intravenous (IV) line. The following medications may be instilled: lidocaine, epinephrine, and atropine. In addition, naloxone can be instilled into the airway of a pediatric patient. (See Section 10 for details on the doses and instillation procedure.)

2.   Recommend the administration of bicarbonate during an emergency situation. (IIID3) [R, Ap, An]

Bicarbonate is an alkaline substance that has been used in clinical practice to correct metabolic acidosis from a cardiopulmonary arrest. It is administered intravenously as sodium bicarbonate ($NaHCO_3^-$). According to the most recent guidelines, bicarbonate should be used, if at all, only after other CPR procedures have been instituted. It may then be used if a diagnosis has been made and the patient has a preexisting acidemia. (See Section 10 for details on doses and administration.)

Module D.   Drug dosage calculations.

The NBRC's detailed examination outline does not specifically list drug dosage calculations; however, versions II and III of the Written Registry Examinations for self-assessment have one calculation each.

The problems will be easier to solve if the following is remembered:

a. A milliliter (ml) = a cubic centimeter (cc) = a gram (g).
b. 1000 milligrams (mg) = 1 g
c. Most drug doses are listed in milligrams (mg) instead of grams. Convert grams to milligrams by moving the decimal point three places to the right (the same as multiplying by 1000), for example, 0.5 g equals 500 mg. Also, be able to convert milligrams to grams by moving the decimal point three places to the left, for example, 750 mg = 0.75 g.
d. Know how to interconvert fractions, decimal fractions, and percentages, for example, 1 : 100 = 1/100 = .01 = 1%.

One common way to solve any drug dosage calculation is by the creation of a proportional problem. The first two example problems here deal with calculating the amount of active ingredient in a given volume of medication. To do this, the drug concentration must be converted into fractional form. The proportional problem can then be set up to solve for the unknown.

Example 1

How much active ingredient would be in 0.7 ml of 1 : 200 Isuprel?

A 1 : 200 drug concentration means that there is 1 part of active ingredient in 200 parts of the solution. Or, there would be 1 ml or g of active ingredient in 200 ml or g of the solution. This can be set up in the following proportion:

$$\frac{1 \text{ ml active ingredient}}{200 \text{ ml total solution}} = \frac{\text{unknown active ingredient or X}}{.7 \text{ ml solution}} \quad \text{(Cross multiply)}$$

$$200 \text{ X} = 0.7 \text{ ml} \quad \text{(Divide both sides of the equation by 200.)}$$

$$\text{X} = .0035 \text{ ml} = .0035 \text{ g} = 3.5 \text{ mg active ingredient}$$

Example 2

How much active ingredient would be in 0.5 ml of Alupent? Alupent is 5% active ingredient.

A 5% drug concentration means that there are 5 parts of active ingredient in 100 parts of the solution. So, there would be 5 ml or g of active ingredient in 100 ml or g of the solution. This can be set up in the following proportion:

$$\frac{5 \text{ ml active ingredient}}{100 \text{ ml total solution}} = \frac{\text{unknown active ingredient or X}}{0.5 \text{ ml solution}} \quad \text{(Cross multiply)}$$

$$100 \text{ X} = 0.25 \text{ ml} \quad \text{(Divide both sides of the equation by 100.)}$$

$$\text{X} = 0.025 \text{ ml} = 0.025 \text{ g} = 25 \text{ mg active ingredient}$$

Thus, it can be seen that the amount of active ingredient can be calculated if the drug concentration is given in either a fractional or percentage form. These next two examples deal with calculating the volume of medication needed to deliver a desired amount of active ingredient. With these types it is necessary to convert to consistent units—usually grams to milligrams.

Example 3

How much 1 : 100 strength Isuprel would be needed to give a patient 2.5 mg of active ingredient by IPPB?

A 1 : 100 drug concentration means that there is 1 part of active ingredient in 100 parts of the solution. Or, there would be 1 ml or g of active ingredient in 100 ml or g of the solution. This converts to 1000 mg/100 ml. Set up the following proportion:

$$\frac{1000 \text{ mg active ingredient}}{100 \text{ ml total solution}} = \frac{2.5 \text{ mg}}{\text{X ml needed}} \quad \text{(Cross multiply)}$$

$$250 \text{ ml} = 1000 \text{ X} \quad \text{(Divide both sides of the equation by 1000.)}$$

$$\text{X} = 0.25 \text{ ml of Isuprel should be given.}$$

Example 4

How much 4% Xylocaine would be needed to give a patient 100 mg of active ingredient by hand-held nebulizer before a bronchoscopy?

A 4% drug concentration means that there are 4 parts of active ingredient in 100 parts of the solution. So, there would be 4 ml or g of active ingredient in 100 ml or g of the solution. This converts to 4000 mg/100 ml. Set up the following proportion:

•

$$\frac{4000 \text{ mg active ingredient}}{100 \text{ ml total solution}} = \frac{100 \text{ mg}}{X \text{ ml needed}} \quad \text{(Cross multiply)}$$

10,000 ml = 4000 X   (Divide both sides of the equation by 4000.)

X = 2.5 ml of Xylocaine should be given.

So it can be seen that the volume of medication needed to deliver a given amount of active ingredient can be calculated if the drug concentration is given in either a fractional or percentage form.

This ends the general discussion on pharmacology. Information related to patient assessment can be found in Section 1. Some additional comments are added in Module E.

Module E.   Patient assessment.

1.   Examine all of the data to determine the patient's pathophysiological condition. (IC3a) [R, Ap, An]

Review Modules A-D and other references for the differential diagnosis of cardiopulmonary diseases and conditions. At the minimum, be able to identify bronchospasm, airway edema, pulmonary infection, hypertension, and hypotension. Investigate the uses of medications that would be used in the treatment of these conditions. Review the normal physiology of the pulmonary and cardiovascular systems, renal function, and the central and peripheral nervous system.

2.   Take part in the development of the respiratory care plan. (IC3c) [An]

Following are brief discussions of common conditions that require the use of the correct medication(s):

Bronchospasm.—Recent research indicates that acute, severe bronchospasm, as seen in status asthmaticus, is best treated by inhaled corticosteroids (beclomethasone, Vanceril) and fast-acting β_2 agonists (isoetharine, Bronkosol or metaproterenol, Alupent). If necessary, inhaled parasympatholytic agents (ipratropium bromide, Atrovent), intravenous corticosteroids (prednisone or methylprednisolone), and theophylline ethylenediamine (Aminophylline) are added. Make a recommendation to increase the amount of medication if the patient's bronchospasm is not reversed and there are no adverse side effects. Some patients may require continuous nebulization of a β_2 medication at a level far greater than that recommended by the manufacturer. It is needed to keep them off of a mechanical ventilator. Frequent bedside spirometry measurements of the peak flow, vital capacity, and/or forced expiratory flow in 1 second should be taken. Stop giving the medication when these values are maximized. Frequently or continuously monitor the patient for signs of tachycardia caused by the high doses of medication. Make a recommendation to decrease the amount of medication if the patient is having serious side effects such as tachycardia or palpitations.

The patient with chronic, moderate bronchospasm can usually be managed with inhaled corticosteroids and longer duration β_2 agonists (terbutaline, Brethaire or albuterol, Proventil or Ventolin). Prophyllactic treatment to prevent an asthma attack should include cromolyn sodium and inhaled corticosteroids.

Upper Airway Edema.—This is seen after the removal of an endotracheal tube, in a child with laryngotracheobronchitis (croup), or in an allergic reaction. Inhaled racemic epinephrine (MicroNephrin or Vaponefrin) is the drug of choice. Make a recommendation to increase the dose or repeat the treatment if inspiratory stridor or other signs of edema return. Make a recommendation to decrease the dose or stop the treatment if the patient develops tachycardia.

Pulmonary Infection.—Obtain a mucus sample under sterile conditions. The sample should be promptly sent to the laboratory for culture of the infecting organism(s) and antibiotic sensitivity. The antibiotic(s) that are most effective at killing the pathogen should then be given. It may be necessary to pretreat the patient with a mucolytic such as acetylcysteine (Mucomyst) before giving the aerosolized antibiotic. If mucus is removed, the antibiotic will be better able to penetrate deeply into the lungs.

Many different organisms can cause pneumonia and/or acute bronchitis. The most common pathogens are listed by category in Table 8-2; however, this list is far from complete. Table 8-3 lists some of the types of antibiotics that are used to treat the most common respiratory pathogens. Usually the patient is given antibiotics by either the oral or parenteral route. Sometimes pulmonary infections are also treated by aerosolizing the antibiotic. Besides respiratory syncytial virus and pneumocystis carinii pneumonia, patients with an infectious lung cavity or cystic fibrosis with a gram$^-$ infection are treated with aerosolized antibiotics. The decision to use an aerosolized antibiotic is based on the type of infection, the side effects of the antibiotic, and the risks to the patient and caregiver of nebulizing the drug. A nebulizer with a downstream filter such as the Respirgard II or AeroTech II are recommended with aerosolized antibiotics. Table 8-4 lists antibiotics that have been given by inhalation for treating a pulmonary infection. Watch the patient for signs of intolerance of the medication. Some patients will develop a severe cough or bronchospasm. It may be necessary to pretreat the patient with an inhaled fast onset, short duration sympathomimetic (isoetharine, Bronkosol) before giving the antibiotic.

Be prepared to identify and respond to adverse reactions to any medications. Watch for tachycardia and/or palpitations from an aerosolized bronchodilator. A

Table 8-2. Common Respiratory Pathogens in Approximate Order of Frequency

Bacteria:	Gram Positive	Gram Negative	Cell Wall Deficient
	Streptococcus pneumoniae	*Hemophilus influenzae*	Mycoplasma pneumonia
	*Staphylococcus aureus**	*Klebsiella pneumoniae*	Acid-Fast
	Streptococcus faecalis (*enterococcus*)	*Pseudomonas aeruginosa**	Mycobacterium tuberculosis*
		*Serratia species**	
Viruses:			
	Rhinovirus	Varicella virus*	
	Adenovirus	Herpes simplex virus*	
	Respiratory syncytival virus	Cytomegalovirus*	
Fungi:			
	*Candida albicans**	*Histoplasma capsulatum* (Ohio Valley)	
	*Aspergillus species**	*Coccidioides immitis* (Southwest U.S.)	
Protozoa:			
	*Pneumocystis carinii**		
	*Toxoplasma gondii**		
	*Cryptosporidium**		

* Seen most frequently in debilitated or immunosuppressed hosts.

Table 8-3. Classification of Antibiotic Agents Commonly Used Against Pulmonary Infections

Class or Group	Agents	Spectrum	Major Toxicity
Penicillin	Penicillin G	Staphylococcus aureus often resistant	Allergy
Semisynthetic penicillins	Ampicillin, Omnipen	Gram-positive organisms, Gram negative *Hemophilus influenzae*; variable against gram-negative rods	Diarrhea and rash, especially with viral disease (mononucleosis)
	Oxacillin, Prostaphlin	Like penicillin, with antistaphylococcal effects	Allergy
	Carbenicillin, Geopen	Like penicillin, with antipseudomonas effects	Sodium overload-congestive failure
Cephalosporine	Oephalothin, Keflin	Like penicillin, with antistaphylococcal effects	Renal (usually not severe)
Aminoglycosides	Streptomycin	Primarily tuberculostatic	Vestibular, renal
	Kanamycin, Kantrex	Gram-negative rods, except *Pseudomonas* and some *Proteus*	Auditory, renal
	Gentamicin, Garamycin	Gram-negative rods, including *Pseudomonas* and *Proteus*	Vestibular, renal
Macrolide	Erythromycin, Erythrocin	Like penicillin (used in penicillin allergy); drug of choice for *Mycoplasma*	Gastrointestinal
tetracyclines	Tetracycline, Achromycin	Broad spectrum; useful against *Hemophilus* and *Mycoplasma* infections	Fungal overgrowth in bowel or vagina; hepatic with large IV doses
Chloramphenicol	Chloromycetin	Broad spectrum; used for *Hemophilus* if it is Ampicillin-resistant or if patient is allergic	Bone marrow
Antituberculosis agents	INH, Isoniazid	Used for both prophylaxis and treatment	Hepatic
	Ethambutol, Rifampin	Used for tuberculostatic therapy	Retinal (maculapathy), hepatic
Antifungal agents	Ketoconazole, Nizoral	Major agent for systemic fungal disease	Gastrointestinal upset
	Amphotericin B	Major agent for systemic fungal disease	Renal, gastrointestinal
Antiviral agents	AZT, Retrovir	Stops reproduction in retroviruses. Used against HIV virus.	Anemia
	Ribavirin, Virazole	Same spectrum, used against respiratory syncytial virus; experimental against HIV virus.	
Antiprotozoal agents (Sulfonamides)	Pentamidine isethionate, NebuPent, Pentam 300	Used against *Pneumocystis carinii*	Impaired renal and liver function
	Trimethaprim and sulfamethoxazole, Bactrim	Used against *Pneumocystis carinii*	Impaired renal and liver function

Table 8-4. Aerosolized Antibiotic Agents Used in Respiratory Care

Agent	Antimicrobial Spectrum	Usual Dosage Range*
Amikacin	Gram-negative bacteria	Uncertain
Amphotericin B	Fungal infections	1-20 mg
Bacitracin	*Staphylococci*	5000-20,000 units
Carbenicillin	*Pseudomonas sp.*	125-100 mg
Cephalosporins	Not recommended for use	
Colistin	Gram-negative bacteria	2-300 mg
Gentamicin	Gram-negative bacteria	5-120 mg
Kanamycin	Gram-negative bacteria†	25-300 mg
Neomycin	Gram-negative bacteria	25-400 mg
Nystatin	*Candida Aspergillus spp.*	25,000-50,000 units
Penicillins	Not recommended for use	
Pentamidine	*Pneumocystis carinii*	50-600 mg‡
Polymyxin	Gram-negative bacteria	5-50 mg
Tobramycin	Gram-negative bacteria	50 mg

* Dosages are poorly established. The drug should be dissolved in 2 ml of saline and each dose should be administered two to four times daily after initial bronchodilator therapy.
† Not suitable for *Pseudomonas*.
‡ Treatments given in large dosage daily for treatment and in small dosage once every 1-2 weeks for prophylaxis.
From Ziment I: Drugs used in respiratory therapy. In Burton GG, Hodgkin JE, Word JJ, editors: *Respiratory care: a guide to clinical practice*, ed 3, Philadelphia, 1991, JB Lippincott. Used by permission.

common policy is to stop the treatment if the patient's pulse increases by more than 20% from the initial level. For example, the patient's initial pulse was 100 and is now 120. Make a recommendation to reduce the amount of beta antagonist or switch to one with less β_1 effect. If this does not result in a reduced heart rate, the treatment should be stopped.

Watch for bronchospasm from the bland aerosols (especially hypertonic saline) or Mucomyst. Compare the patient's initial breath sounds with the breath sounds during the treatment. Ask if the patient's breathing is all right or if his or her chest feels "tight." Stop the treatment if the patient develops or has worsening bronchospasm during the treatment.

If any of these problems persist despite changes in the medication doses or the addition of a β_2 agonist to Mucomyst, the treatment should probably be discontinued. Stop a breathing treatment anytime the patient appears to have had an allergic reaction to a medication. Tell the patient's physician and ask for further orders.

BIBLIOGRAPHY

AARC Clinical Practice Guideline: Surfactant replacement therapy. *Respir Care* 39(8):824-829, 1994.

Au JP, Ziment I: Drug therapy and dosage adjustment in asthma, *Respir Care* 31(5):415-418, 1986.

Barnes TA, editor: *Respiratory care practice*, Chicago, 1988, Year Book Medical.

Bills GW, Soderberg RC: *Principles of pharmacology for respiratory care*, Albany, NY, 1994, Delmar.

Blanchard PW, Aranda JV: Drug treatment of neonatal apnea, *Perinatology/Neonatology* 21-28, 1986.

Corkery KJ, Luce JM, Montgomery AB: Aerosolized pentamadine for treatment and prophylaxis of Pneumocystis carinii pneumonia: an update, *Respir Care* 33(8):676-685, 1988.

Emergency Cardiac Care Committee and Subcommittees, American Heart Association: Guidelines for cardiopulmonary resuscitation and emergency cardiac care, *JAMA* 268(15):2184-2281, 28, 1992.

Eubanks DH, Bone RC: *Comprehensive respiratory care,* ed 2, St. Louis, 1990, Mosby–Year Book.

Howder CL: *Cardiopulmonary pharmacology: a handbook for respiratory practitioners and other allied health personnel,* Baltimore, 1992, Williams & Wilkins.

Hughes JR: Combined psychological and nicotine gum treatment for smoking: a critical review, *Substance Abuse* 3:337-350, 1991.

Jones S, Bagg AM: L-E-A-D: drugs for cardiac arrest, *Nursing* 18(1):34-41, 1988.

Kacmarek RM, Mack CW, Dimas S: *The essentials of respiratory care,* ed 3, St. Louis, 1990, Mosby–Year Book.

Lam A, and Newhouse MT: Management of asthma and chronic airflow limitation: are methylxanthines obsolete? *Chest* 98(1):44-52, 1990.

Lehnert BE, Schachter EN: *The pharmacology of respiratory care,* St. Louis, 1980, Mosby–Year Book.

Mathewson HS: Intravenous aminophylline: a dangerous therapeutic weapon, *Respir Care* 27(6):713-715, 1982.

Mathewson HS: Anticholinergic aerosols, *Respir Care* 28(4):467-469, 1983.

Mathewson HS: *Pneumocystis carinii* pneumonia: chemotherapy and prophylaxis, *Respir Care* 89(5):360-362, 1989.

Nett LM: The physician's role in smoking cessation, *Chest* 97(suppl 2):28-32, 1990.

Newhouse MT: Is theophylline obsolete? *Chest* 98(1):1-2, 1990.

Peters JA, Peters BA: Pharmacology for respiratory care. In Scanlan CL, Spearman CB, Sheldon RL, editors: *Egan's fundamentals of respiratory care,* ed 5, St. Louis, 1990, Mosby–Year Book.

Physicians' desk reference, ed 47, Montvale, NJ, 1993, Medical Economics.

Plank CS: Aerosolized pentamidine: a new weapon against PCP, *Nursing* 19(2):48-49, 1989.

Rau JL: *Respiratory care pharmacology,* ed 2, Chicago, 1984, Year Book Medical.

Rau JL: *Respiratory care pharmacology,* ed 3, Chicago, 1989, Year Book Medical.

Rennard SI, Doughton D: Transdermal nicotine for smoking cessation, *Respir Care* 38(3):290-293, 1993.

Sills JR: *Respiratory care certification guide: the complete review resource for the entry level exam,* ed 2, St. Louis, 1994, Mosby–Year Book.

Tashkin DP: Dosing strategies for bronchodilator aerosol delivery, *Respir Care* 36(9):977-988, 1991.

Witek TJ, Schachter EN: *Pharmacology and therapeutics in respiratory care,* Philadelphia, 1994, WB Saunders.

Ziment I: *Respiratory pharmacology and therapeutics,* Philadelphia, 1978, WB Saunders.

Ziment I: Drugs used in respiratory therapy. In Burton GG, Hodgkin JE, Ward JJ, editors: *Respiratory care: a guide to clinical practice,* ed 3, Philadelphia, 1991, JB Lippincott.

SELF-STUDY QUESTIONS

1. You are working the night shift when a 17-year-old patient with status asthmaticus is admitted through the emergency room. The intern on call asks for your recommendation on what medication to give first to treat the patient. You would recommend:
    A. Isoproterenol (Isuprel) by aerosol
    B. Terbutaline sulfate (Bricanyl) tablets

    C.   Isoetharine (Bronkosol) by aerosol
    D.   Acetylcysteine (Mucomyst) by aerosol
    E.   Intravenous theophylline ethylenediamine (Aminophylline)

2.   The preliminary laboratory results of a sputum sample that was sent from your patient indicate that she has a gram positive pulmonary infection. Which of the following medications would you recommend for her?
    A.   Ribavirin (Virazole)
    B.   Penicillin (Ampicillin)
    C.   Ketoconazole (Nizoral)
    D.   Acetylcysteine (Mucomyst) by aerosol
    E.   Gentamicin (Garamycin)

3.   Which of the following have been approved for the treatment of infant respiratory distress syndrome?
    I.   Survanta
    II.   Robinul
    III.   Bactrim
    IV.   Exosurf
    V.   Valium
    A.   II, III
    B.   IV, V
    C.   I, IV
    D.   I, II, IV

4.   You have finished giving your 68-year-old patient an IPPB treatment with 0.5 ml of Alupent. You notice that her heart rate has increased significantly and she is having an arrhythmia that was not there before the treatment. What would you recommend to the physician for her next treatment?
    A.   Give her 0.5 ml of isoproterenol (Isuprel).
    B.   Discontinue her treatments altogether.
    C.   Add more normal saline to the Alupent.
    D.   Decrease the Alupent to 0.3 ml.
    E.   Begin her on nebulized beclomethasone dipropionate (Vanceril).

5.   You are called to the emergency room to assist in the care of an orally intubated patient who was in a car accident. He is having frequent premature ventricular contractions (PVCs). Due to hypotension, the physician cannot start an intravenous line. What would you recommend?
    A.   Instill lidocaine into the endotracheal tube.
    B.   Continue trying to start an intravenous line.
    C.   Instill sodium bicarbonate into the endotracheal tube.
    D.   Perform defibrillation.
    E.   Give the patient intracardiac atropine.

6.   You are called to the recovery room to assist in the care of a patient who returned 2 hours ago from having her bowel resected. The patient is apneic and on a mechanical ventilator. Which of the following medications could be used so that she might be weaned?
    I.   Flumazenil (Mazicon)
    II.   Naloxone (Narcan)
    III.   Dopamine (Intropin)
    IV.   Succinylcholine chloride (Anectine)
    V.   Diazepam (Valium)

A. I, IV
B. V
C. II, III
D. IV
E. I, II

7. Sodium bicarbonate would be indicated during a cardiopulmonary resuscitation attempt under the following conditions:
    A. The patient had a preexisting metabolic alkalosis.
    B. The patient had a normal pH before the cardiac arrest.
    C. The patient is acidotic despite manual ventilation and effective chest compressions having been performed for the previous 10 minutes.
    D. The patient has more than 40% of his or her weight as body fat.

8. All of the following have some stimulating effect on the respiratory center of the brain EXCEPT:
    A. Doxapram (Dopram)
    B. Theophylline
    C. Ethacrynic acid (Edecrin)
    D. Caffeine

9. The physician has ordered a series of induced sputum procedures on a patient. He was unable to cough productively after the first treatment with normal saline. What would you recommend to the physician?
    A. Continue to use normal saline but give it for 5 more minutes.
    B. Switch to half-normal saline.
    C. Nasotracheal suction the patient for the sample.
    D. Switch to hypertonic saline.
    E. Perform a fiberoptic bronchoscopy to obtain the sample.

10. Your 60-year-old patient has been admitted through the emergency room to the coronary care unit. She is diagnosed with a myocardial infarct and pulmonary edema. Her heart rate is 135 beats per minute and blood pressure is 90/50. Which of the following medications would you recommend for her?
    I.   Morphine sulfate (Morphine)
    II.   Furosemide (Lasix)
    III. Digoxin (Lanoxin)
    IV.   Dopamine HCl (Intropin)
    A. III
    B. II, IV
    C. I, II, III
    D. III, IV
    E. I, II, III, IV

11. An 18-month-old boy is admitted with inspiratory stridor and history of an upper respiratory infection. Thirty minutes after giving him a hand-held nebulizer treatment with racemic epinephrine (Vaponephrine), the stridor is almost gone and he lies down to sleep on his left side. You would conclude the following:
    A. He has epiglottitis.
    B. He has subglottic edema (croup).
    C. He has had an adverse drug reaction.
    D. A foreign body has passed from his trachea to the right mainstem bronchus.
    E. A foreign body has passed from his trachea to the left mainstem bronchus.

12. An 18-month-old infant is diagnosed with bronchiolitis from the respiratory syncytial virus. Which medication would you recommend?
    A. Trimethoprin and sulfamethoxazol (Bactrim)
    B. Pentamedine isethionate (NebuPent)
    C. Gentamycin (Garamycin)
    D. Ribavirin (Virazol)
    E. Dobutamine hydrochloride (Dobutrex)

13. Your patient is a 40-year-old man who has been smoking a pack of cigarettes a day for the past 25 years. After recovering from pneumonia he has expressed a desire to stop smoking. Which of the following medications would you recommend to help in the process?
    A. Bactrim
    B. Osmitrol
    C. Habitrol
    D. Nizoral
    E. NicoGum

14. The physician has ordered 0.3 ml of 1 : 100 Isuprel to be given by hand-held nebulizer. How much pure drug is being given.
    A. 3 mg
    B. 0.15 mg
    C. 30 mg
    D. 33 mg
    E. 300 mg

15. How much Alupent would it take to give the patient 20 mg of the active ingredient? Alupent contains 5% active ingredient.
    A. 4 ml
    B. 1 ml
    C. 0.4 ml
    D. 40 ml
    E. 0.1 ml

16. Your patient has the AIDS virus and should be treated for the prevention of *pneumocystis carinii* pneumonia. Which would you recommend?
    A. NebuPent by Respirgard II nebulizer every 4 weeks.
    B. Pentam 300 by intramuscular injection every day for 14 days.
    C. Ribavirin (Virazol) by SPAG II nebulizer for 3 to 7 days.
    D. Gentamicin (Garamycin) by Respirgard II nebulizer.
    E. Bactrim by pill four times a day for 14 days.

Answer Key

1. C; 2. B; 3. C; 4. D; 5. A; 6. E; 7. C; 8. C; 9. D; 10. E; 11. B; 12. D; 13. C; 14. A; 15. E; 16. A.

9 | Postural Drainage Therapy

Module A.   Modify postural drainage therapy in the following ways.

1.   Change the postural drainage therapy position based on the patient's response. (IIIC5a) [R, Ap, An]

Postural drainage therapy (PDT) is also known as chest physiotherapy, chest physical therapy, bronchopulmonary drainage, postural drainage and percussion, and percussion and vibration. Postural drainage is performed to clear secretions or prevent the accumulation of secretions. It is presumed that the user of this book understands the various postural drainage positions and how to perform percussion and vibration. If not, the topics can be reviewed in *Respiratory Care Certification Guide* (Sills, 1994) or another standard respiratory care textbook. See Table 9-1 for the indications for turning, postural drainage, and percussion and vibrating; Table 9-2 for assessing the patient's need for postural drainage therapy; and Tables 9-3 and 9-4 for the contraindications and hazards. The patient is positioned so that the bronchus of a particular segment is as vertical as possible. Gravity will then pull the secretions toward a major bronchus or the trachea. From there the secretions are either coughed or suctioned out.

It may be found during the treatment that the patient's secretions are more effectively drained if he or she is repositioned from what would seem to be the ideal angle. It may be that the patient's airway anatomy is different from what is expected. Patients with chronic lung disease such as cystic fibrosis or bronchiectasis often know what positions and angles are best for draining their lungs. Follow their advice if it produces good results.

Some patients may not tolerate being properly placed because their underlying lung or heart disease is aggravated by the unnatural body position. This is most commonly seen in the head down positions to drain the lower lobes. Watch for signs of hypoxemia and shortness of breath. The patient may have to be put in a better tolerated but less desirable position. As long as there is some downward angle to the bronchus, mucus will drain. Each patient will have to be evaluated on an individual basis.

In addition to Table 9-3, a number of authors have listed the following as contraindications to percussion and vibration:

1. Not over bare skin
2. Not over buttons, zippers, folded clothes, seams of clothing
3. Not over female breast tissue
4. Not over the spine, sternum, or kidneys
5. Not over an area with a known lung tumor

Table 9-1. Indications for Turning, Postural Drainage, and Percussion and Vibration

Turning

The patient is unable to change his or her body position; for example, the patient has a cerebral injury or neuromuscular disease, is being mechanically ventilated, or has been medicated to cause sedation or paralysis.

Atelectasis or the potential for its development exists.

Hypoxemia that is associated with a particular position is present. Commonly, if one-sided lung disease is present, the patient is turned so that the affected lung is superior.

Patient has an artificial airway.

Postural Drainage

Mobilize retained secretions so that they can be coughed or suctioned out. Patient has difficulty in coughing out secretions but produces more than 25-30 ml/day. Evidence or indications that a patient with an artificial airway has retained secretions.

Atelectasis that is known or believed to be caused by mucus plugging is present.

Patient has a diagnosis of cystic fibrosis, bronchiectasis, or cavitating lung disease.

A foreign body is in an airway.

There was removal of an aspirated foreign body or stomach contents.

Percussion and Vibration

A patient is receiving postural drainage who has a large volume of viscous sputum. This suggests that the external manipulation of the thorax would assist gravity in the movement toward a more central airway.

Based on information found in AARC Clinical Practice Guideline: Postural drainage therapy, *Respir Care* 36(12):1418-1426, 1991.

2. Change the length of time of the treatment. (IIIC5b) [An]

In general, individual segments are drained for 3 to 15 minutes. If the patient is tolerating the position and secretions are still being cleared, the position can be held longer. Stop the treatment if the patient is showing any signs of intolerance as listed in Tables 9-3 and 9-4.

Table 9-2. Assessment of the Patient's Need for Postural Drainage Therapy

All of the following should be assessed *together* to evaluate the patient's need for postural drainage therapy (PDT):

Excessive production of sputum

Ineffectiveness of cough

Patient history of PDT being helpful in treating past problem (e.g., bronchiectasis, cystic fibrosis, lung abscess)

Abnormal breath sounds (e.g., decreased sounds, crackles, or rhonchi suggesting airway secretions)

Change in the patient's vital signs

Abnormal chest x-ray finding consistent with infiltrates, atelectasis, and/or mucus plugging

Not all patients will show all the above. The seriousness of the above problems should be used in determining which patients will benefit from PDT.

Based on information found in AARC Clinical Practice Guideline: Postural drainage therapy, *Respir Care* 36(12): 1418-1426, 1991.

Table 9-3. Contraindications of Turning, Postural Drainage, and Percussion and Vibration

Turning and Postural Drainage

All positions are contraindicated* for patients with:
Unstabilized head and/or neck injury (absolute)
Active hemorrhage and hemodynamic instability (absolute)
Intracranial pressure (ICP) greater than 20 mm Hg
Recent spinal surgery, such as a laminectomy, or acute spinal injury
Active hemoptysis
Empyema
Bronchopleural fistula
Pulmonary edema secondary to congestive heart failure
Large pleural effusions
Advanced age, anxiety, confusion, and intolerance for position changes
Fractured rib(s) with or without flail chest
Healing tissue or surgical wound

Trendelenburg position is contraindicated in patients with:
Intracranial pressure (ICP) greater than 20 mm Hg
Sensitivity to increased ICP (e.g., neurosurgery, cerebral aneurysms, eye surgery)
Uncontrolled hypertension
A distended abdomen
Esophageal surgery
Recent gross hemoptysis associated with lung surgery that was recently treated surgically or by radiation therapy
An uncontrolled airway in a patient at risk of aspirating (e.g., recent meal or tube feeding). Many authors list less than 1 hour since eating as a contraindication.

Reverse Trendelenburg position is contraindicated in patients who are:
Hypotensive
Receiving a vasoactive medication

Percussion and Vibrations
All of the previously listed contraindications
Subcutaneous emphysema (Several authors list an untreated pneumothorax as an absolute contraindication.)
Spinal anesthesia or recent epidural spinal infusion for pain control
Recent thoracic skin grafts or skin flaps
Thoracic burns, open wounds, or skin infections
Transvenous or subcutaneous pacemaker that has been recently placed (Especially true if a mechanical percussor/vibrator is to be used.)
Suspicion of pulmonary tuberculosis
Lung contusion
Bronchospasm
Osteomyelitis of the ribs
Osteoporosis
Clotting disorder (coagulopathy)
Patient complains of chest-wall pain

* The positions are relative contraindications except those marked as absolute.
Based on information found in AARC Clinical Practice Guideline: Postural drainage therapy, *Respir Care* 36(12):1418-1426, 1991.

It is generally recommended that the total time of the procedure be no longer than 30 to 40 minutes. This is because the patient may become exhausted by the various position changes. If this is the case, the practitioner must select the worst segments to be drained first. It may take several drainage sessions to get to all of the involved segments.

Table 9-4. Hazards and Complications, with Recommended Actions, and Limitations of Postural Drainage and Percussion and Vibration

Hazards and Complications

Hypoxemia: The patient who is known to be hypoxic or is prone to hypoxemia during the procedure should be given a higher inspired oxygen percentage. Give 100% oxygen to any patient who becomes hypoxic during the procedure. Stop the treatment, return the patient to the original resting position, make sure ventilation is adequate, and consult with the physician before continuing.

Increased intracranial pressure: If this happens, stop the treatment, return the patient to the original resting position, and consult with the physician before continuing.

Acute hypotension during the procedure: If this happens, stop the treatment, return the patient to the original resting position, and consult with the physician before continuing.

Pulmonary hemorrhage: If this happens, stop the treatment, return the patient to the original resting position, and call the physician immediately. Give the patient supplemental oxygen and keep an open airway until the physician responds.

Pain or injury to the patient's muscles, ribs, or spine: Stop the therapy that seems to be causing the problem. Carefully move the patient to a more comfortable position and call the physician before continuing.

Vomiting and aspiration: Stop the treatment, suction as needed to clear the airway, give supplemental oxygen, maintain a patent airway, return the patient to the original resting position, and call the physician immediately.

Bronchospasm: If this happens, stop the treatment, return the patient to the original resting position, give or increase the supplemental oxygen while calling the physician. Give the patient any aerosolized bronchodilators that the physician orders.

Arrhythmias: If this happens, stop the treatment, return the patient to the original resting position, give or increase the supplemental oxygen while calling the physician.

Limitations

Be careful to give PDT only to those patients who would benefit from it. Do not rely on past experiences with other patients when judging current cases.

Patients with ineffective coughs may not be able to clear their airways as well as desired.

Critically ill patients are difficult to position optimally.

Based on information found in AARC Clinical Practice Guideline: Postural drainage therapy, *Respir Care* 36(12):1418-1426, 1991.

3. Change the treatment techniques used. (IIIC5d) [An]

Be prepared to modify the postural drainage, percussion, and/or vibration procedures depending on how the patient tolerates them. For example:

1. Some patients will not tolerate certain positions, especially head down, because of pain, shortness of breath, hypoxemia, or elevated blood pressure.
2. Percussion rate, pressure, and hand position may need to be modified depending on the patient's tolerance, chest size, and secretion clearance.
3. It may not be possible to percuss or vibrate female patients in the right middle lobe and left ligula positions because of breast tissue.
4. Hypoxemia should be prevented with supplemental oxygen in those patients who need it. Pulse oximetry could be performed before and during the procedure to monitor the patient's SpO_2. The SpO_2 should improve as atelectatic areas open up and secretions are removed. Ventilation should then better match with perfusion.
5. Cardiac patients should have their heart rate, heart rhythm, and blood pressure monitored. Check the heart rate before the procedure and with each position change.

6. Postoperative or trauma patients may not tolerate certain positions or percussion or vibration because of pain.
7. Patients with copious secretions that cannot be coughed out should not be put in a compromising situation. Suctioning equipment must be available. This may include patients who are not alert or who have a tracheostomy.
8. Very obese patients may not tolerate any head down positions because of increased shortness of breath.

4. Organize the sequence of drainage positions and treatment techniques. (IIIC5f) [An]

There are differences of opinion as to the sequence in which the segments should be drained. Some authors state that an apices to bases approach is better whereas others state that a bases to apices pattern is preferred.

It makes sense to take an apices to bases approach for a first treatment when all lobes are to be drained. This pattern gives the patient time to get used to the whole procedure. It may also be safer because the practitioner can evaluate the patient through a sequence of positions that progress from the least to the most stressful.

If the patient is known to tolerate all positions without any difficulties, and the lower lobes are the worst in terms of secretions, then choose to drain the lower lobes first. If time permits, work up through the middle lobe and lingula to the upper lobes.

Careful study of the positions will show you that the patient's work can be minimized by sequencing them properly. For example:

1. Drain the upper lobes in a posterior, apical, anterior sequence.
2. Drain the lateral basal and anterior basal segments of either lower lobe.
3. Drain the superior and posterior basal segments of either lower lobe.

It may be found that the patient can cough out more secretions if positive expiratory pressure (PEP) and postural drainage are done sequentially. PEP with or without an aerosolized bronchodilator or mucolytic helps many patients mobilize their secretions. Postural drainage therapy would then help in the draining process. (PEP therapy was discussed in Section 6.)

Module B. Modify mechanical percussors and vibrators used in postural drainage therapy. (IIIC5c) [An]

The terms *percussor* and *vibrator* are sometimes used interchangeably. It is not clear if there is a difference in cycling rate or stroking distance between the two. Check the manufacturer's information for specific details. There are several manufacturers who produce either electrically or pneumatically powered percussors and vibrators. Some are large enough to be wheeled into the patient's room. Obviously, electrically powered units need a standard electrical outlet for power whereas the pneumatically powered units need to be plugged into a 50 psig oxygen or air source. Some electrical units are small enough to fit over the hand and are battery powered.

Pediatric units must be smaller to focus accurately on the much smaller target area of the infant's chest. They are battery powered. The Neocussor produced by General Physiotherapy is an example. Some practitioners find that an electric toothbrush with padded bristles works very well. Manual percussion of infants can be aided by using soft rubber palm cups that come in several pediatric sizes. Some practitioners prefer to make their own infant percussion aids out of a pediatric resuscitation mask, an adapter, and an end cap.

Some electrically powered units use a rubber belt and different size wheels to change gears and produce several vibration rates. Others electrically vary the motor speed to change the vibration rate. Some pneumatically driven units can have their percussion force and rate varied.

General Physiotherapy recommends the following percussion rates for its Vibramatic and other models:

a. Twenty to thirty cycles per second (Hertz) for an average size adult
b. Less than 20 cycles per second for larger adults
c. Greater than 30 cycles per second for smaller adults or children

One author lists an ideal rate of 25 to 35 cycles per second to mobilize secretions. There is no consensus on the ideal rate to use. It seems reasonable that the practitioner should use whatever rate is tolerated by the patient and seems to best help mobilize the secretions.

Some adult percussors and vibrators come with a variety of patient contact pads. Select the one that best fits the patient's chest area that needs to be percussed. For example, a flat pad would be used over a broad area of the patient's back while a U-shaped pad would be used around a patient's side.

It is important that the practitioner use the mechanical percussor or vibrator properly. General Physiotherapy recommends that the patient applicator be held in one place for only 30 to 60 seconds; any longer may cause skin irritation. The applicator should be held loosely in the operator's hand; it is not necessary to press down on the patient. Because the patient applicator moves horizontally and vertically, it must be used properly to help move the secretions. Follow the manufacturer's guidelines for loosened secretions to the drain toward a mainstem bronchus or the trachea.

This ends the general discussion on postural drainage therapy. The following information may be included in the questions offered by the NBRC. The general discussion of these topics was covered in Section 1 and earlier in this section. Some additional comments that relate directly to PDT are included.

Module C.   Patient assessment.

1.   Make the recommendation for a chest x-ray, as needed, to help determine the patient's condition. (Ia2d) [An]

2.   Inspect the patient's chest x-ray as necessary. (IB6b) [R, Ap]

Make a recommendation for a chest x-ray to find specific areas for postural drainage therapy. A white shadow on a chest x-ray over what should be normal lung may indicate areas of atelectasis and/or infiltrates that can be targeted for treatment. Repeat chest x-rays should be performed to look for an improvement in the lungs. The resolution may be slow or dramatic depending on the original problem and how it responds to the various treatments used.

3.   Examine all the data to determine the patient's pathophysiological condition. (IC3b) [An]

The patient's breath sounds should be auscultated before the treatment begins to determine which segments are silent or have secretions. Auscultate each segment after it has been drained and the patient has coughed. Listen for air moving into formerly silent areas or cleared secretions.

The following should be evaluated to determine if PDT is needed:

a. Postural drainage therapy is usually not indicated if an optimally hydrated patient is coughing out less than 25 ml/day with the procedure.

b. A dehydrated patient should have apparently ineffective PDT continued for at least 24 hours after the patient is rehydrated. The combination of rehydration and PDT may help to mobilize previously viscous secretions.

c. PDT is not indicated in a patient who is producing greater than 30 ml of secretions per day if the treatments do not increase the sputum production. This is because the patient is already able to effectively cough out the sputum.

4. Take part in the development of the respiratory care plan. (IC3b) [An]

Postural drainage procedures should not be performed if they are not indicated or if the patient has a contraindicating condition. During the patient evaluation the practitioner may find that different segments need to be drained than originally ordered or indicated. Make note of any treatment modifications that have been started and how the patient tolerated them. Some practitioners believe that PDT should be used as a prophylactic treatment to prevent the accumulation of secretions. Patients who are bedridden, comatose, or have neuromuscular defects may have PDT because of their increased risk of atelectasis and pneumonia. The following poor pulmonary function test results have been used by some practitioners to indicate the need for postural drainage therapy:

a. Tidal volume less than 10 ml/kg of ideal body weight
b. Vital capacity less than 600 ml in an adult
c. Peak flow of less than 200 L/min (3.3 L/sec) in an adult
d. Maximum voluntary ventilation less than 33% of predicted

BIBLIOGRAPHY

AARC Clinical Practice Guideline: Postural drainage therapy, *Respir Care* 36(12):1418-1426, Dec 1991.

Barrascout JR: Chest physical therapy and related procedures. In Burton GG, Hodgkin JE, editors: *Respiratory care*, ed 2, Philadelphia, 1984, JB Lippincott.

Eid N, Buchheit J, Neuling M et al: Chest physiotherapy in review, *Respir Care* 36(4):270-282, April 1991.

Eubanks DH, Bone RC: *Comprehensive respiratory care*, ed 2, St. Louis, 1990, Mosby–Year Book.

Frownfelter DL: Chest physical therapy and airway care. In Barnes TA, editor: *Respiratory care practice*, Chicago, 1988, Year Book Medical.

Meyer CL: Chest physiotherapy in infants requiring ventilatory assistance, *Respir Ther* Jan/Feb 1984.

Rarey KP, Youtsey JW: *Respiratory patient care*, Englewood Cliffs, NJ, 1981, Prentice-Hall.

Scanlan CL: Chest physical therapy. In Scanlan CL, Spearman CB, Sheldon RL, editors: *Egan's fundamentals of respiratory care*, ed 5, St. Louis, 1990, Mosby–Year Book.

Scott AA, Koff PB: Airway care and chest physiotherapy. In Koff PB, Eitzman DV, Neu J, editors: *Neonatal and pediatric respiratory care*, St. Louis, 1988, Mosby–Year Book.

Shapiro BA, Harrison RA, Kacmarek RM et al: *Clinical application of respiratory care*, ed 3, Chicago, 1985, Year Book Medical.

Sills JR: *Respiratory care certification guide: the complete review resource for the entry level exam*, ed 2, St. Louis, 1994, Mosby—Year Book.

White GC: *Basic clinical lab competencies for respiratory care*, Albany, NY, 1988, Delmar.

Wojciechowski WV: Incentive spirometers and secretion evacuation devices. In Barnes TA, editor: *Respiratory care practice*, Chicago, 1988, Year Book Medical.

SELF-STUDY QUESTIONS

1. Your new patient has been admitted with acute bronchitis and has an order for postural drainage therapy. She tells you that she has bronchiectasis in her right lower lobe because she had whooping cough when she was a child. She tells you that she drains herself at home with the help of her husband. She insists that you position her in a way that you know is ideal for draining the lateral and medial segments of the right middle lobe. What would you do?
   A. Refuse to position her that way because you know it will not drain her right lower lobe.
   B. Call the nurse and ask her to sedate the patient so that you can perform postural drainage as you know best.
   C. Call the physician to tell her that the patient is confused and combative.
   D. Position the patient as she desires and evaluate its effectiveness.

2. You are working with a patient who begins to cough up blood after being positioned to drain the superior segment of the left lower lobe. Percussion was provided with a mechanical device. After the patient has coughed out 50 ml of blood you would recommend the following as the best action:
   A. Continue the treatment because the patient has not lost a great deal of blood.
   B. Continue the treatment on only the upper and middle lobes.
   C. Discontinue the treatment, sit the patient up, and call the physician.
   D. Continue the treatment with manual percussion only.
   E. Let the patient rest for 10 minutes and continue the treatment.

3. A patient with bilateral pneumonia is positioned to drain the lateral and medial segments of her right middle lobe. After 5 minutes in this position the patient complains of shortness of breath. The electrocardiogram shows the patient to be a trigeminy rhythm. The most likely cause of this is:
   A. Fatigue
   B. Arterial hypoxemia
   C. A full stomach causing vagal stimulation
   D. Increased intracranial pressure
   E. Increased venous return to the heart

4. You are using a pneumatically powered mechanical percussor on a patient receiving postural drainage therapy. The unit is powered by an E cylinder of oxygen because piped-in oxygen is not available. After a few minutes of operation you notice that the percussor begins to slow down and then stops. What would you do now?
   A. Switch to an electrically powered percussor.
   B. Make sure the cylinder is completely turned on.
   C. Check the unit's batteries.
   D. Check the electrical cord.

5. All the following are contraindications for Trendelenburg position **EXCEPT**:
    A. Distended abdomen
    B. Hypotension
    C. Intracranial pressure of 30 mm Hg
    D. Hypertension
    E. Twenty minutes after a comatose patient has been fed by nasogastric tube

6. A patient is known to have infiltrates in the posterior basal segment of her left lower lobe. What position would you recommend to drain them out?
    A. Face down, pillow under hips, bed flat
    B. Right side down, foot of the bed elevated 15°
    C. Face down, pillow under hips, foot of the bed elevated 18 inches
    D. Left side down, foot of the bed elevated 15°
    E. Supine, pillow beneath the knees, bed flat

7. Postural drainage with percussion and vibration have been performed for 5 days on a cooperative patient with bronchiectasis. During that time he has been treated with antibiotics and well fed and hydrated. He has produced a total of 20 ml of sputum during the last 24 hours. What would you recommend?
    A. Continue the current treatment program for 48 hours.
    B. Continue the current treatment program for 24 hours.
    C. Add ultrasonic nebulizer treatments to the PDT to better liquify the secretions.
    D. Add nasotracheal suctioning to the PDT to remove the secretions.
    E. Discontinue the PDT and follow the patient's progress.

8. A patient has chest x-ray findings that indicate infiltrates in the superior segment of his right lower lobe. What position would you recommend in order to drain them out?
    A. Face down, pillow under hips, bed flat
    B. Right side down, foot of the bed elevated 15°
    C. Face down, pillow under hips, foot of the bed elevated 18 inches
    D. Left side down, foot of the bed elevated 15°
    E. Supine, pillow beneath the knees, bed flat

9. Which of the following should be used to evaluate a pneumonia patient's response to postural drainage and percussion and vibration?
      I. Breath sounds
     II. Chest x-ray findings
    III. Sputum production
     IV. PaO_2
      V. Patient's opinion on the effectiveness of the PDT
    A. I, II
    B. III, IV
    C. IV, V
    D. I, II, III, IV, V
    E. I, II, IV

Answer Key

1. D; 2. C; 3. B; 4. A; 5. B; 6. C; 7. E; 8. A; 9. D.

10 | Cardiopulmonary Resuscitation (Emergency Care)

It is expected that technicians can perform adult and infant cardiopulmonary resuscitation (CPR). These skills and required knowledge are tested of all examinees on the Entry Level Exam. This section will cover only those additional areas tested on the Advanced Practitioner Exams.

Module A. Review the patient's records and recommend diagnostic tests for additional data.

1. Review the results of previous electrocardiogram tests from the patient's chart. (IA1c2) [R]

A patient who has been admitted for a suspected myocardial infarct (MI) or other serious cardiac condition will probably have had an electrocardiogram (ECG). Review the interpretation report to find out if there is a cardiac problem. If the patient did have an MI, he or she will have a series of ECGs performed to follow its progress and response to treatment.

2. Recommend an electrocardiogram for additional patient data. (IA2i) [R, Ap, An]

An ECG is indicated if the patient is suspected of having cardiac problems. Symptoms such as angina pectoris, sudden crushing chest pain, shortness of breath, or unstable heart rate and blood pressure point to a sudden heart problem. An ECG is indicated to document the nature of the cardiac problem or rule out the heart as a source of the symptoms.

Module B. Begin, conduct, and modify CPR-related duties.

1. CPR equipment.
a. Fix any problems with a manual resuscitator (bag-valve). (IIB2cl) [An]

Learners and examinees should disassemble and reassemble as many different models as possible to understand how they function and how to repair them. See Fig. 10-1 for illustrations of a complete set of Laerdal infant, pediatric, and adult manual resuscitators. Most other units have similar features to the Laerdal equipment.

It is beyond the scope of this book to go into detail on all the available units;

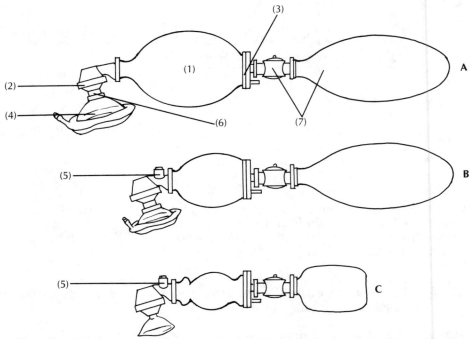

Fig. 10-1 A, Adult Laerdal resuscitator; **B,** pediatric Laerdal resuscitator; **C,** infant Laerdal resuscitator. These features are found on all modern units: *1,* self-filling reservoir bag; *2,* exhalation valve that does not jam at an oxygen flow of 15 L/min or in subfreezing temperatures—it must be clearable of debris within 20 seconds; *3,* intake valve for adding draw room air or supplemental oxygen into the reservoir bag; *4,* transparent mask that easily conforms to the patient's face; *5,* pressure relief (pop-off) valve that is set to open at 40 cm water; *6,* standard 15 mm ID/22 mm OD connector for the endotracheal tube or face mask; *7,* oxygen enrichment/reservoir system. In addition, some units have an adjustable PEEP valve (not shown) attached to the exhalation valve. (From Eubanks DH, Bone RC: *Comprehensive respiratory care,* ed 2, 1990, St. Louis, Mosby–Year Book. Used by permission.)

however, the following steps should be taken when evaluating the function of a manual resuscitator:

1. Squeeze and release the bag to see if the non-rebreathing valve and air/oxygen reservoir intake valve open and close properly.
2. Feel the air leave the outlet port of the non-rebreathing valve when the bag is squeezed.
3. Occlude the outlet port and squeeze the bag. No gas should leak out. If present, the pop-off valve should open at the correct pressure.
4. The face mask should fit onto the 22-mm OD fitting and have its cushion properly inflated.

Check for a reversed or improperly seated one-way valve if the gas does not enter or exit the unit as it should. In clinical use, mucus, vomitus, and blood can foul the non-rebreathing valve system and must be cleared within 20 seconds. Do this by disconnecting the unit from the patient, aiming the adapter into a neutral area, and squeezing the bag to blow out the obstruction. Replace a unit that cannot be promptly cleared.

b.   Pneumatic (demand-valve) resuscitator.
i.   Get the necessary equipment for the procedure. (IIA1a) [R, Ap]

The two most commonly available pneumatic (gas-powered) resuscitators are the Robertshaw Demand Valve and Hudson's Elder Valve (see Fig. 10-2). An advantage of these types of units over manual resuscitators is that they are easier to operate. One hand can be used to activate the actuator/manual control button for an extended period of time without fatigue. The patient outlet has a standard 15-mm ID/22-mm OD connector. It will fit any endotracheal tube adaptor or to a face mask. The operator will deliver tidal volume gas to the patient as long as the button is depressed or until the pressure limit is reached. This may be set as high as 60 cm of water. If possible, select a unit that delivers a constant flow rate of less than 40 L/min (to minimize gastric insufflation) and gives an audible alarm if the pressure limit is reached. Because of the factors of variable inspiratory time and pressure limiting, the delivered tidal volume will vary with the patient's changing pulmonary condition. This is a drawback of these units compared to the manual resuscitators. With them, an experienced rescuer can tell that when it becomes harder to squeeze the bag, when the patient's airway resistance has increased, or when the lungs have become less compliant. The rescuer then squeezes the bag more forcefully to deliver the same tidal volume. Clinical experience is needed to use either type of pneumatic resuscitator to safely deliver a tidal volume to most patients.

A variation on the pneumatic resuscitator is the demand-valve. With it, the spontaneously breathing patient can trigger a breath similar to how the assist mode operates on a mechanical ventilator. The breath is delivered until the rescuer preset pressure is reached or the patient makes an expiratory effort. If the patient should become apneic the rescuer can depress the button to deliver a tidal volume.

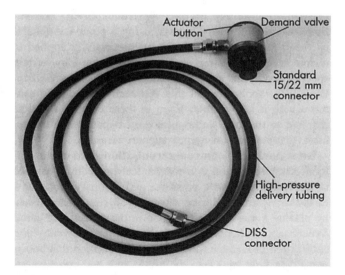

Fig. 10-2 Features of a pneumatic resuscitator with high-pressure hose. (From Scanlan CL: *Emergency life support.* In Scanlan CL, Spearman CB, Sheldon RL, editors: *Egan's fundamentals of respiratory care,* ed 5, St. Louis, 1990, Mosby–Year Book. Used by permission.)

ii. Put the equipment together, make sure that it works properly, and identify any problems with it. (IIB1b) [R, An]

Pneumatic resuscitators come preassembled by the manufacturer. The only added piece of equipment is a length of high pressure oxygen hose with a female DISS connector at both ends. Screw one end of the hose to the inlet of the demand valve as shown in Fig. 10-2. The other end of the hose is then screwed onto either a reducing valve or regulator connected to the hospital's central oxygen source or a flowmeter connected to an oxygen cylinder. Turning on the flowmeter to maximum or inserting the reducing valve into the central oxygen source conducts pure oxygen at 50 psig to the unit. This pressure is reduced by the demand valve to its working pressure (up to 60 cm of water).

When properly assembled and the oxygen source is opened you should feel gas escape from the outlet port when the actuator/manual control button is pushed (see Fig. 10-3). The gas flow should stop when the button is released. By attaching a test lung to the outlet port and starting a breath, you can see that the test lung fills during inspiration and cycles off when the pressure limit is reached. Make sure that the unit properly cycles on and off.

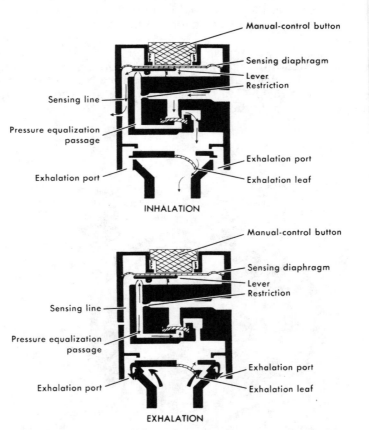

Fig. 10-3 Cut-away drawings of the internal functioning of a Robertshaw Demand Valve during inhalation and exhalation. (From McPherson SP: *Respiratory therapy equipment*, ed 4, St. Louis, 1990, Mosby–Year Book. Used by permission.)

iii.   Fix any problems with the equipment. (IIB2c2) [R, Ap, An)

The following types of problems can be encountered with demand valve units:

a. Foreign body obstruction of the control valve. Remove the unit from the patient, point it into a neutral area, and depress the actuator/manual control button to blow the obstruction clear. Do not use a unit that cannot be cleared of an obstruction or will not cycle on or off properly.

b. A gas leak can be heard or felt. Search out and tighten the loose connection to seal the leak and deliver 50 psig gas pressure to the unit.

c.   Fix any problems with a mouth-to-valve mask resuscitator. (IIB2c3) [An]

Mouth-to-valve mask resuscitators are relatively simple devices. Most have only two or three pieces: face mask, mouthpiece with a one-way valve, and possibly an oxygen T-piece. The male and female connections are designed to fit together only one way. When properly assembled there should be no air leaks when the breath is delivered to the victim. If the breath cannot be delivered, check the one-way valve to make sure that it has not been put together backwards. Reverse it if necessary and ventilate the victim. Keep the oxygen nipple on the mask or T-piece capped off if it is not being used. Air will leak out during the delivered breath if the cap is left off the nipple.

2.   Electrocardiogram (ECG) monitoring.
a.   Get the necessary cardiac electrodes. (IIA1j2) [R, Ap]

Cardiac electrodes or leads pick up the electrical signal from a heart contraction and conduct it to the electrocardiogram machine. There are three different types that are mainly distinguished by their placement on the patient. The first type is called chest leads (or chest electrodes), which consist of four parts: 1) a conducting wire coated with an electrically neutral plastic, 2) an adapter at one end of the wire that plugs into the electrocardiogram (ECG) machine, 3) a different adapter at the opposite end of the wire that plugs into a patient electrode, and 4) the patient electrode.

Basic rhythm monitoring is done with the patient wearing chest leads (see Fig. 10-4). Conducting jelly is added to the surface of the electrode to reduce the skin's resistance to the heart's electrical signal. The adhesive ring holds the electrode tightly to the skin. The conducting wire snaps into the back of the electrode. Three of these chest leads are used for rhythm monitoring.

The second type is called limb leads. These come in a set of four; one for each limb (see Fig. 10-5). They are used during a diagnostic electrocardiogram. The only significant difference between the limb leads and the chest leads is that the limb leads are usually held in place by a rubber strap. Either conducting jelly or an alcohol wipe is used to reduce the skin's resistance.

The third type is called precordial leads. They came in a set of six and are placed on the chest in the positions shown in Fig. 10-6. They are also used during a diagnostic electrocardiogram. These are different from the first two types because they each include a suction cup to get a tight seal. A conducting jelly is also used to reduce the skin's resistance. With all three cardiac leads, bad skin contact, dried conducting jelly, or a disconnected wire results in a distorted or absent electrical signal.

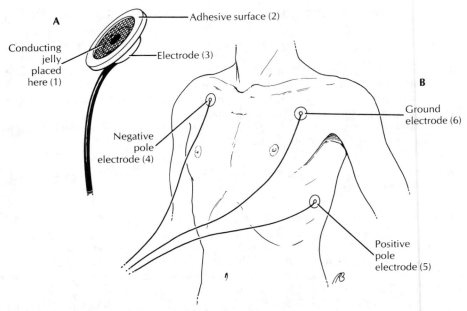

Fig. 10-4 A, Close-up of the features of a prepackaged monitoring electrode or lead. **B,** Standard electrode placements for lead II monitoring. This results in the traditional looking ECG waveform with upright P, QRS, and T waves. (Note: The electrodes are often labeled as right arm (RA) instead of negative pole, left arm (LA) instead of ground electrode, and left leg (LL) instead of positive electrode.) (From Eubanks DH, Bone RC: *Comprehensive respiratory care,* ed 2, St. Louis, 1990, Mosby–Year Book. Used by permission.)

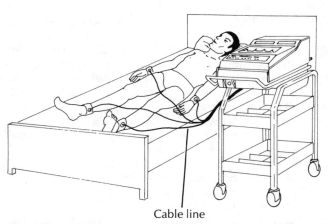

Cable line

Fig. 10-5 Limb electrodes or leads properly placed on all four of the patient's limbs. Make sure that the right leg (RL) lead is placed on the right leg, the right arm (RA) lead is placed on the right arm, and so forth. The electrode cables are then plugged into the electrocardiograph machine for recording the ECG tracings. (From Eubanks DH, Bone RC: *Comprehensive respiratory care,* ed 2, St. Louis, 1990, Mosby–Year Book. Used by permission.)

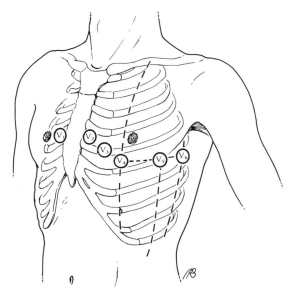

Fig. 10-6 Proper placement of the six precordial leads. (See Table 10-1 for a description of the locations.) (From Eubanks DH, Bone RC: *Comprehensive respiratory care*, ed 2, St. Louis, 1990, Mosby–Year Book. Used by permission.)

b. Get the necessary electrocardiogram machine. (IIA1j1) [R, Ap]

There are three different types of ECG machines. Each is used in different patient situations. First, an electrocardiogram for diagnostic purposes requires a machine capable of receiving electrical input from the four limb leads and six precordial leads. The operator can manually select the combinations needed to get the twelve different combinations for a 12-lead ECG tracing or they can be done automatically. The various electrocardiogram combinations are printed out on ECG paper.

Second, basic bedside rhythm monitoring makes use of a unit that will usually only receive input from the three chest leads. That signal will be sent to an oscilloscope (video display terminal [VDT]) for a real-time display of the patient's rhythm. These ECG machines have several additional features. They will continuously display the patient's heart rate. High and low heart rate alarm settings can be set. If the high or low setting is reached an audible and visual alarm will be triggered. The patient's heart rhythm can be recorded on ECG paper manually by pushing a record button or automatically when an alarm setting is reached. These units are often seen mounted at the patient's bedside in the intensive care unit.

Third, the CPR crash cart will have an ECG machine mounted on it with the additional feature of being connected to the defibrillator. This allows for synchronous defibrillation (cardioversion), which is discussed later. It will have other features that are similar to those seen on bedside monitoring units. Portable versions of these units are used when the patient must be transported. They operate by battery power when unplugged from the wall electrical outlet.

c. Begin electrocardiogram monitoring in an emergency setting. (IIID1) [R, Ap]

Emergency electrocardiogram monitoring is done on any patient with a serious cardiopulmonary problem. If there is a possibility that the patient will experience serious changes in heart rate or rhythm he or she should be continuously monitored. In this case use bedside rhythm monitoring. This unit should have an oscilloscope for viewing the rhythm and additional features for counting the heart rate, setting high and low heart rate alarms, and recording the rhythm on standard ECG paper for a permanent record.

The most common chest electrode pattern used for rhythm monitoring is called lead II. The three chest electrodes are placed as shown in Fig. 10-4, **B.** The negative (right arm, RA) electrode is on the right upper chest. The positive (left leg, LL) electrode is placed on the left lateral chest. The ground (left arm, LA) electrode is placed on the left upper chest. With this electrode configuration, known as Eintho-ven's triangle, the heart's electrical signal is followed as it flows from the right atrium to the left ventricle. This results in the so-called normal ECG tracing with upright P, R, and T waves as shown in Fig. 10-7 and 10-8.

d. Perform an electrocardiogram to find the patient's diagnosis. (IB8j and IC1i) [R, Ap, An]

To determine the patient's diagnosis it is necessary to perform a 12-lead ECG. This test involves the use of an electrocardiograph machine with heat sensitive ECG recording paper, four limb leads, and six precordial leads (see Figs. 10-5 and 10-6). Table 10-1 describes the locations of the precordial leads and the positive and negative electrode combinations that are used to record the heart's electrical signal through the 12 different leads. Each lead individually records the heart's electrical activity but does so from a different position in relation to the heart. These 12 leads give the physician a three-dimensional impression of how the cardiac conduction system and the myocardium are functioning. Abnormal function-ing can be diagnosed. Review the normal anatomy and physiology of the heart and its conduction system if necessary.

Clinical experience is important in performing a diagnostic ECG. Improper placement of the precordial or limb leads can easily result in a misleading ECG tracing and a misdiagnosis. For example, reversing the arm leads will cause the

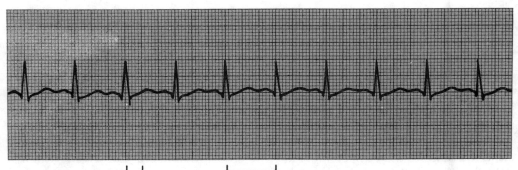

└┘ └──────┘
1 LARGE BLOCK   **3 LARGE BLOCKS BETWEEN EACH QRS COMPLEX**

Fig. 10-7 Example of a normal sinus rhythm. Because there are three large blocks between each R wave, the heart rate is 100 beats per minute. (From Butler HH: How to read an ECG, RN Magazine, 35-45, Jan 1973. Used by permission.)

Table 10-1. Standard Electrocardiogram Leads

		Leads	Positive Electrode		Negative Electrode
Bipolar	1.	I	Left arm	and	Right arm
	2.	II	Left leg	and	Right arm
	3.	III	Left leg	and	Left arm
Unipolar	4.	aV_R	Right arm		
	5.	aV_L	Left arm		Central terminal*
	6.	aV_F	Left leg		
Precordial	7.	V_1	Right of sternum in 4th intercostal space (4th ICS)		
	8.	V_2	Left of sternum in 4th ICS		
	9.	V_3	Midway between V_2 and V_4		
	10.	V_4	Midclavicular line in 5th ICS		Central terminal*
	11.	V_5	Midway between V_4 and V_6		
	12.	V_6	Lateral chest in 5th ICS		

* The *central terminal* is a combination of electrode potentials, producing a summation effect. This serves as the single negative or *indifferent* electrode. The specific combination of electrodes for each lead is automatically determined in the lead selector switch.
From Phillips RE, Feeney MK: *The cardiac rhythms: a systematic approach to interpretation,* ed 3, Philadelphia, 1990, WB Saunders. Used by permission.

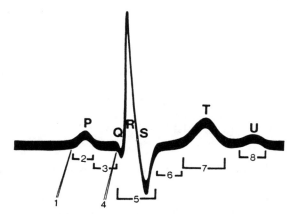

Fig. 10-8 Sequence of electrical events of the cardiac cycle during normal sinus rhythm. (See Table 10-2 for the description of each event.) (From Phillips RE, Feeney MK: *The cardiac rhythms: a systematic approach to interpretation,* ed 3, Philadelphia, 1990, WB Saunders. Used by permission.)

Table 10-2. Electrophysiological Events Represented by the Electrocardiogram

Sequential Electrical Events of the Cardiac Cycle	Electrocardiographic Representation
1. Impulse from the sinus node	Not visible
2. Depolarization of the atria	P wave
3. Depolarization of the A-V node	Isoelectric
4. Repolarization of the atria	Usually obscured by the QRS complex

5. Depolarization of the ventricles
  a. Intraventricular septum
  b. Right and left ventricles
	QRS complex
	  a. Initial portion
	  b. Central and terminal portions

6. Quiescent state of the ventricles immediately after depolarization	ST segment: isoelectric
7. Repolarization of the ventricles	T wave
8. Afterpotentials following repolarization of the ventricles	U wave

From Phillips RE, Feeney MK: *The cardiac rhythms: a systematic approach to interpretation,* ed 3, Philadelphia, 1990, WB Saunders. Used by permission.

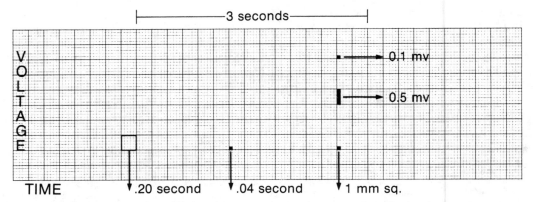

Fig. 10-9 ECG paper with added details on how to interpret time and voltage. (From Patel JM, McGowan SG, Moody LA: *Arrythmias: detection, treatment, and cardiac drugs*, Philadelphia, 1989, WB Saunders. Used by permission.)

QRS to be reversed in lead I. Technical errors in grounding the patient and not keeping the patient still during the ECG will also result in useless tracings because of electrical interference and an unstable baseline.

e.   Interpret the results of the electrocardiogram. (IB8j and IC1i) [R, Ap, An]

It is important to understand how ECG paper is designed so that the heart's electrical signal that is traced on it can be understood. This special paper is heat sensitive and after exiting the ECG machine shows a black line from the heated stylus. Fig. 10-9 shows the grid markings on the paper and how to interpret the ECG tracing for voltage and time. Each large square box is 5 mm in height and represents 0.5 mV (millivolt) of the heart's electrical force. The large square box is divided into five smaller boxes that are 1 mm in height and represent 0.1 mV. Timing of the ECG tracing is determined by the speed with which the paper passes under the heated stylus. Normally this is 25 mm per second. At this speed, each large square box is .20 seconds and each of the five small boxes is .04 seconds. There are 300 large boxes in 1 minute's time (.20 seconds × 300 = 60 seconds).

The following 10 features should be examined in every electrocardiogram:

1. Heart rate
2. Rhythm
3. P wave
4. PR interval
5. QRS interval
6. QRS complex
7. ST segment
8. T wave
9. QT interval
10. U wave

The systematic evaluation of these factors will usually result in a clear understanding of the patient's cardiac function. All these are discussed and illustrated in this section.

The *heart rate* can be most accurately found by counting it for 1 minute; however, this time-consuming method is not always practical. An approximate heart rate can be quickly found. First, find a heartbeat tracing where the R wave is on a heavy vertical line. Then count the number of large boxes between this first R wave and the next R wave (see Fig. 10-7 for an example). Approximate heart rates can be estimated as follows:

Two large boxes = 150 beats per minute (300 divided by 2)
Three large boxes = 100 beats per minute (300 divided by 3)
Four large boxes = 75 beats per minute (300 divided by 4)
Five large boxes = 60 beats per minute (300 divided by 5)
Six large boxes = 50 beats per minute (300 divided by 6)

The *normal cardiac rhythm* must obviously be understood to distinguish it from the abnormal rhythms. The normal adult's cardiac rhythm is usually called normal sinus rhythm (NSR) and has these characteristics:

a. Heart rate between 60 and 100 beats per minute while at rest.
b. Rhythm that varies by no more than ± 10% between QRS complexes.
c. P wave before every QRS complex and upright in lead II.
d. A QRS complex follows every P wave.
e. Proper timing of the components of the ECG rhythm.

The sequential electrical events of the normal cardiac rhythm are detailed in Fig. 10-8 and Table 10-2. Fig. 10-10 shows the normal timing of the components of the ECG tracing.

Abnormal Cardiac Rhythms

The following list of abnormal cardiac rhythms (usually called arrhythmias or dysrhythmias) includes many of those that are commonly encountered in clinical practice. It is beyond the scope of this text to discuss all possible arrhythmias. Instead, those that are either frequently seen and/or dangerous are described. Each of the following cardiac irregularities is: a) defined, b) exemplified, c) described, d) discussed in terms of its clinical significance, and e) accompanied by a treatment (if any) description.

Arrythmias with an SA Node Origin

The following three arrhythmias all originate from the SA node. The electrical signal follows the normal pathway and results in contraction of both atria and ventricles as would be expected. They are distinguished from normal sinus rhythm by the differences in rate and regularity of the impulses. (See the illustrations of pathway and ECG at the left in Fig. 10-11 for an example.)

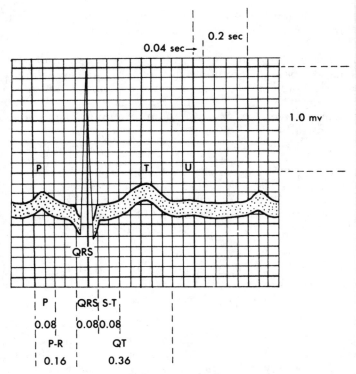

Fig. 10-10 Timing of the electrical events of the cardiac cycle during normal sinus rhythm. (From Spearman CB, Sheldon RL, Egan DF: *Egan's fundamentals of respiratory therapy,* ed 4, St. Louis, 1982, Mosby–Year Book. Used by permission.)

Sinus Arrhythmia

This arrhythmia is characterized by normal complexes but a heart rate that varies with the respiratory cycle (see Fig. 10-12 for an example). Notice how the QRS complexes are closer together on inspiration than on expiration. This is because the increased venous return to the heart during inspiration causes the heart to fill more quickly so that the pulse rate quickens. The opposite rhythm effect is sometimes seen with a patient on a mechanical ventilator. No cardiac treatment is needed. The mechanically ventilated patient should have every attempt made to lower the intrathoracic pressure.

Sinus Tachycardia

Sinus tachycardia in the adult is defined as a heart rate of more than 100 beats per minute while at rest. All complexes are normal and the rate is seldom more than 140 (see Fig. 10-13 for an example). Causes include caffeine, anxiety, fever, pain, or hypotension. Correction of the problem will result in the heart rate decreasing to the normal range. Cardiac drugs are not needed.

Sinus Bradycardia

Sinus bradycardia is defined as a heart rate of less than 60 beats per minute while at rest (see Fig. 10-14). All complexes remain normal. This is commonly seen in well-trained athletes during rest and patients receiving digitalis or morphine. Cardiac drugs are not needed.

If sinus bradycardia is associated with a myocardial infarct, it may result in

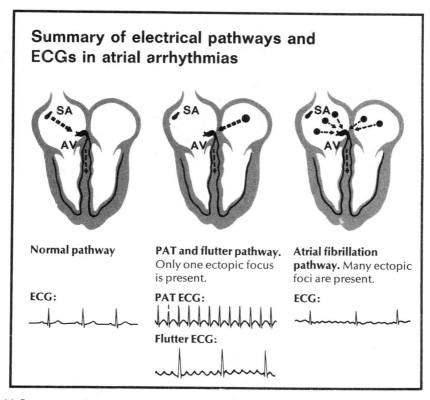

Fig. 10-11 Summary of electrical pathways and ECGs in atrial arrhythmias. (From Butler HH: How to read an ECG, *RN Magazine*, 49-61, Feb 1973. Used by permission.)

fainting or congestive heart failure (pulmonary edema). The patient will need to be treated for the heart attack but also to increase the heart rate. Atropine with or without isoproterenol (Isuprel) is commonly used to speed up the heart rate. A pacemaker will be needed if the patient does not respond to medications and continues to have symptoms.

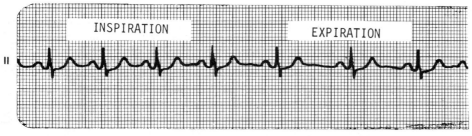

Fig. 10-12 Sinus arrhythmia showing slightly increased heart rate during inspiration and slightly decreased heart rate during exhalation. (From Goldberger AL, Goldberger E: *Clinical electrocardiography,* St. Louis, 1981, Mosby–Year Book. Used by permission.)

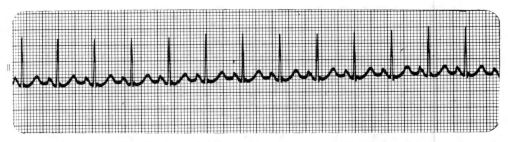

Fig. 10-13 Sinus tachycardia. (From Goldberger AL, Goldberger E: *Clinical electrocardiography,* St. Louis, 1981, Mosby–Year Book. Used by permission.)

Arrhythmias with an Abnormal Atrial Origin

The following three arrhythmias originate in either one or both atria from a source other than the SA node. The electrical signal travels through the atria, which results in their contraction. It then moves on to the AV node and the ventricles, which contract normally. All these arrhythmias result in faster than normal atrial contraction and often in a faster than normal ventricular contraction.

Paroxysmal Atrial Tachycardia (PAT)

PAT (also known as paroxysmal supraventricular tachycardia [PSVT]) is a series of three or more premature atrial contractions. It is characterized by a heart rate between 140 and 250 beats per minute with an average rate of 180. The ECG tracing will show a normal QRS complex after each P wave. See the middle drawings of the conduction and ECG in Fig. 10-11. Notice the abnormal origin of the P wave seen during the PAT episode. The recommended term for any abnormal origin to a heartbeat is focus. The term foci would refer to more than one abnormal site to a heart beat. Fig. 10-15 shows one tracing of the PAT arrhythmia.

Patients with PAT usually complain of a sudden onset of pounding or fluttering in the chest. This is often associated with breathlessness, weakness, and angina pectoris in patients with coronary artery disease. Because of these problems, PAT must be treated. Treatment usually progresses in the following sequence: 1) give a sedative, 2) stimulate the vagus nerve by rubbing the carotid sinus (see Fig. 10-15), 3) give propranolol (Inderol) or a similar medication, and 4) perform synchronized cardioversion. (This last procedure is described in Section 17.) Obviously, if the patient responds to one treatment method there is no need to go on to the next.

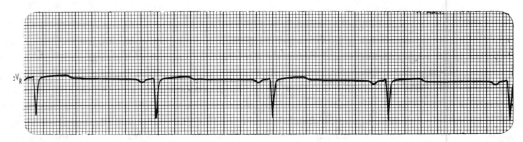

Fig. 10-14 Sinus bradycardia. (From Goldberger AL, Goldberger E: *Clinical electrocardiography,* St. Louis, 1981, Mosby–Year Book. Used by permission.)

PAROXYSMAL ATRIAL TACHYCARDIA (PAT)

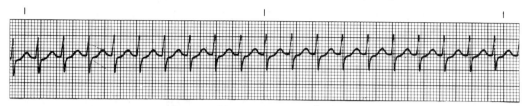

Fig. 10-15 Paroxysmal trial tachycardia (PAT), which is defined as a series of three or more consecutive premature atrial contractions. (From Goldberger AL, Goldberger E: *Clinical electrocardiography*, St. Louis, 1981, Mosby–Year Book. Used by permission.)

Atrial Flutter

Atrial flutter is characterized by a single, fast, abnormal atrial focus that fires at a rate of about 250 to 350 beats per minute. This rate is so fast that the AV node does not pass all of them along to the ventricles. On ECG, it will be noticed that there is a ratio between the fast P waves and the QRS complex. Usually this ratio is 2 : 1, but it may be 3 : 1, 4 : 1, or more. The electrical pathway and ECG tracing are shown in the middle drawings in Fig. 10-11. (See Fig. 10-16 for several example ECG tracings of atrial flutter.) As with PAT, the fast ventricular rate found in atrial flutter is not well tolerated. An attempt must be made to suppress the abnormally fast atrial focus. Digitalis or synchronous cardioversion are the preferred treatments to slow down the heart rate.

Atrial Fibrillation

This condition is identified by the variably shaped P waves and the irregular spacings between the QRS complexes. Each focus is seen on the ECG as a separately shaped P wave. See the electrical pathway and ECG tracing to the right in Fig. 10-11. As with atrial flutter, the AV node does not pass the electrical current from each P wave through to the ventricles. However, with atrial fibrillation, the ratio is not set and there is variable spacing between the QRS complexes and an inconsistent rate (see Fig. 10-17). Patients with atrial fibrillation do not completely empty their ventricles. Often this results in the formation of blood clots that become pulmonary or cerebral emboli. Digitalis and synchronous cardioversion usually are effective treatments. Heparin or coumarin may be added to prolong the blood's clotting time.

Arrhythmias with an AV Node Origin

Both of the following arrhythmias originate in an abnormal atrioventricular (AV) node. The patient may or may not have a normal SA node, atria, and ventricles.

Atrioventricular (AV) Block

AV block is most commonly caused by digitalis toxicity, arteriosclerosis, or myocardial infarction. The latter two may result in scarring, inflammation, or edema. These causes slow down or prevent the transmission of the electrical signal from the SA node through the AV node and to the ventricles. *First degree* AV block is seen with an increased PR interval of at least .20 seconds. Each P wave is followed by a normal QRS complex (see Fig. 10-18). It does not require any treatment. *Second degree* AV block results in some P waves being blocked out completely

ATRIAL FLUTTER

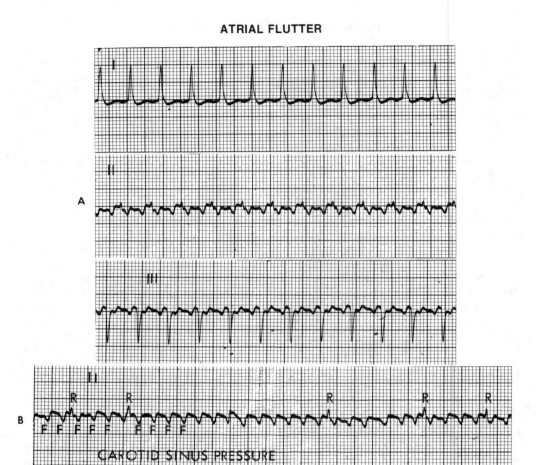

Fig. 10-16 Two examples of atrial flutter. **A,** Note the variable appearance of the flutter waves in different leads. This example shows a 2 : 1 ratio between atrial contractions and ventricular contractions. **B,** This shows how the ventricular rate is decreased after carotid sinus pressure is applied. The "F" letterings show flutter waves made up of rapid P waves from a single foci. The "R" letterings mark R waves when the electrical signal traveled through the AV node to stimulate the ventricles. (From Goldberger AL, Goldberger E: *Clinical electrocardiography,* St. Louis, 1981, Mosby–Year Book. Used by permission.)

with no ventricular response. This more serious condition comes in two different variations. Wenckebach (also known as Mobitz type I) is characterized by a progressively longer PR interval until a P wave is not conducted through at all. Then the cycle starts over again and continues to repeat itself. (See Fig. 10-19 for examples.) Medications such as atropine or isoproterenol may be used to increase the heart rate. Mobitz type II is noticed on the ECG as a rhythm where the PR interval is normal for those that result in a QRS complex but that some P waves are completely blocked (see Fig. 10-20). The ratio between those P waves that conduct and those that are blocked off may be 2 : 1, 3 : 1, or 4 : 1. Mobitz type II is a sign of severe conduction system disease. The usual treatment is to place a cardiac pacemaker into the patient. *Third degree* AV block is also known as complete heart block (see Fig. 10-21). No P waves are conducted through to the ventricles. The ventricles

RAPID ATRIAL FIBRILLATION

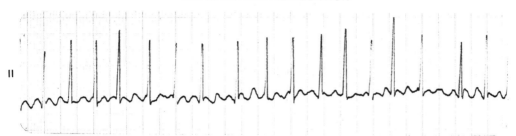

Fig. 10-17 Atrial fibrillation. Note the variable shapes to the P waves indicating their different origins. Also note how the distances between the R waves change considerably. This depends on when an electrical signal from the atria passes through the AV node to the ventricles. (From Goldberger AL, Goldberger E: *Clinical electrocardiography*, St. Louis, 1981, Mosby–Year Book. Used by permission.)

beat about 40 times per minute based on the intrinsic rate of the bundle of His and Purkinje fibers. Obviously, a heart beat this slow is not normal or healthy. Patients have no stamina and frequently faint. A cardiac pacemaker must be placed into these patients.

Junctional Premature Beats

A junctional premature beat is also known as a premature AV nodal contraction (PNC), nodal beat, or junctional beat (see Fig. 10-22). This arrythmia involves the atrioventricular node sending out a premature electrical signal and becoming the primary pacemaker instead of the SA node. The ventricles contract normally with the expected QRS complex.

First degree AV block

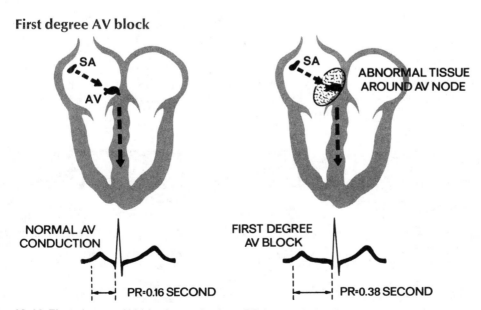

Fig. 10-18 First degree AV block results in a PR interval that is longer than the normal of five small blocks or .20 seconds. (From Butler HH: How to read an ECG, *RN Magazine* 49-61, Feb 1973. Used by permission.)

WENCKEBACH (MOBITZ TYPE I) SECOND-DEGREE AV BLOCK

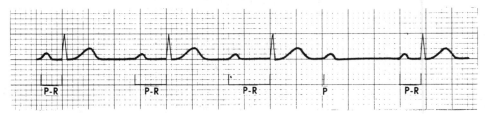

P-R   P-R   P-R   P   P-R

WENCKEBACH (MOBITZ TYPE I) SECOND-DEGREE AV BLOCK

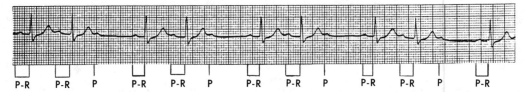

P-R P-R P   P-R P-R P   P-R P-R P   P-R P-R P   P-R

Fig. 10-19 Two examples of Wenckebach (Mobitz type I) second degree AV block. Note how the PR interval progressively lengthens with each beat until one P wave is not conducted through at all. The cycle then repeats itself. (From Goldberger AL, Goldberger E: *Clinical electrocardiography,* St. Louis, 1981, Mosby–Year Book. Used by permission.)

Arrythmias with a Ventricular Origin

Myocardial Infarction (MI)

A myocardial infarction (MI) (also known as a heart attack) is an occlusion of a coronary artery that results in death of some segment of the heart muscle. If large enough, the heart will fail to pump adequately and the patient will die. A smaller infarct will still weaken the heart. In addition, the damaged or dying tissue will act as an abnormal focus for the arrythmias discussed here. The series of ECG changes that occurs during the acute stage of an MI and as the heart heals are shown in Fig. 10-23 and are listed here:

1. The initial ECG may be normal. This happens about 15% of the time. The patient should be admitted for observation and cardiac enzyme studies if symptoms are present.

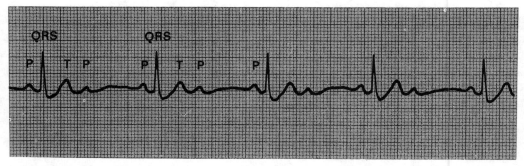

Fig. 10-20 Mobitz type II second degree heart block. Note how the first P wave is conducted through the AV node and the second P wave is not. (From Butler HH: How to read an ECG, *RN Magazine* 49-61, Feb 1973. Used by permission.)

THIRD-DEGREE (COMPLETE) AV BLOCK

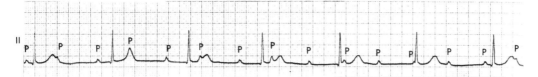

THIRD-DEGREE (COMPLETE) AV BLOCK

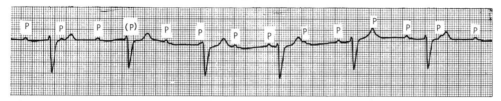

Fig. 10-21 Two examples of third-degree (complete) heart block. Both show P waves that have no relationship with the QRS complexes. The top example has QRS complexes of the normal width indicating that the AV junction is acting as the pacemaker. The bottom example has QRS complexes that are wider than normal because the ventricles are being paced from below the AV junction. Instead, an idioventricular pacemaker is determining the patient's heart rate. (From Goldberger AL, Goldberger E: *Clinical electrocardiography*, St. Louis, 1981, Mosby–Year Book. Used by permission.)

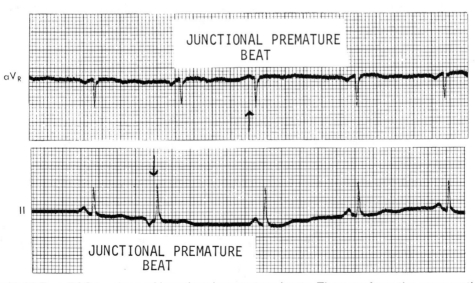

Fig. 10-22 Two ECG tracings of junctional premature beats. They are from the same patient but from different leads. The arrows point out retrograde P waves of opposite polarity from normal. (From Goldberger AL, Goldberger E: *Clinical electrocardiography*, St. Louis, 1981, Mosby–Year Book. Used by permission.)

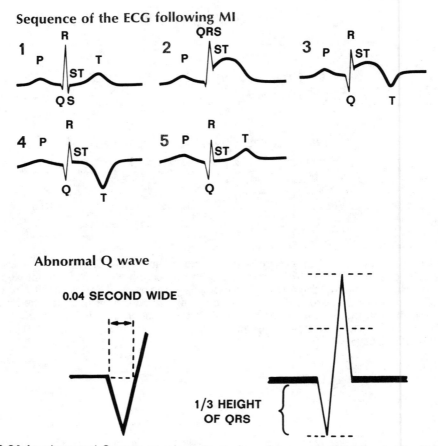

Fig. 10-24 An abnormal Q wave as a long-term sign of a myocardial infarct. The Q wave is considered to be abnormal if it is either more than .04 second wide or more than one third the height of the QRS complex. (From Butler HH: How to read an ECG, *RN Magazine* 50-59, March 1973. Used by permission.)

2. The first sign of an MI is an elevated ST segment. This will occur within a few hours of the injury.
3. Next the T wave will invert. This will happen within hours to days of the infarct.
4. The ST segment returns to the normal baseline position within days to weeks.
5. After a period of weeks to months the T wave becomes upright again. A lasting ECG change will be an enlarged Q wave as shown in Fig. 10-24.

Premature Ventricular Contraction (PVC)

A premature ventricular contraction (PVC) is an abnormal, fast contraction of the ventricles that originates from a focus below the AV node (see Fig. 10-25). This is usually a sign of a diseased or hypoxic ventricle. Pathologic causes include arteriosclerotic heart disease or MI. An example of an isolated PVC is shown in Fig. 10-26 and has these traits:

1. It is premature and happens before the normal heartbeat.
2. There is no P wave.

Normal pathways   PVC pathways

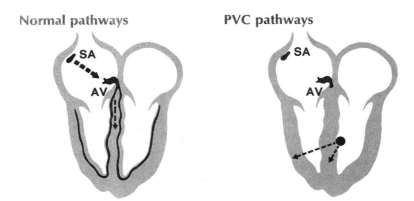

Fig. 10-25 A comparison of the normal electrical pathway and the pathway of a premature ventricular contraction (PVC). This same type of abnormal pathway is seen in ventricular tachycardia and ventricular flutter. (From Butler HH: How to read an ECG, *RN Magazine* 50-59, March 1973. Used by permission.)

3. The QRS complex is bizarre looking and more than .12 seconds wide.
4. The T wave is inverted.
5. Usually there is a fully compensatory pause before the next normal heartbeat (see Fig. 10-27).

A single PVC is not dangerous unless it originates during the T wave when the heart is especially vulnerable to electrical stimulation. Then it could cause ventricular fibrillation. Patients with PVCs should be watched more closely and probably treated when their PVCs are seen more frequently than 1 in 10 beats, seen in groups of two or three, or seen in multiple configurations. For example, two different-looking PVCs mean that there are two different ventricular foci firing prematurely. Bigeminy is when every second beat is a PVC; trigeminy is when every third beat is a PVC. Dangerous PVCs must be rapidly treated. Lidocaine (Xylocaine) is given intravenously if the heart rate is more than 60 beats per minute. If that does not work, procainamide hydrochloride (Pronestyl) is added.

Ventricular Tachycardia

Ventricular tachycardia (VT or V tach) is a serious consequence of untreated premature ventricular contractions (see Fig. 10-28). VT is defined as a series of three or more consecutive PVCs. Runs of VT may be fairly short or prolonged. The

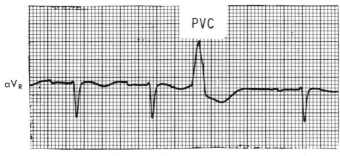

Fig. 10-26 ECG of an isolated premature ventricular contraction (PVC). (From Goldberger AL, Goldberger E: *Clinical electrocardiography,* St. Louis, 1981, Mosby–Year Book. Used by permission.)

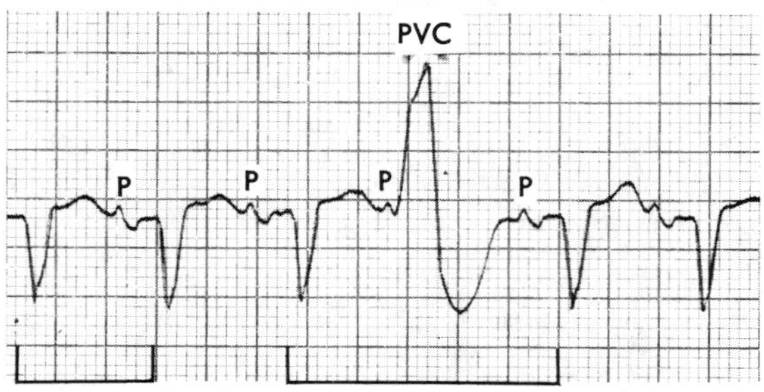

FULLY COMPENSATORY PAUSE

PVC

P   P   P   P

R₁—R₂
520 msec

R₃—R₄
1040 msec

Fig. 10-27 PVCs cause a fully compensatory pause. Note that the interval between the two sinus beats that surround the PVC (R3 and R4 in this case) is exactly two times the normal interval between the sinus beats R1 and R2. Notice that the P waves come on time, except that the third P wave is interrupted by the PVC and therefore does not conduct normally through the AV junction. The next (fourth) P wave also comes on time. The fact that the sinus node continues to pace despite the PVC results in the fully compensatory pause. (From Goldberger AL, Goldberger E: *Clinical electrocardiography*, St. Louis, 1981, Mosby–Year Book. Used by permission.)

rate counted during VT is between 110 and 250 beats per minute. Cardiac output falls dramatically during this arrhythmia. If the patient has a stable blood pressure, VT is treated with lidocaine as an antiarrhythmic. Synchronized cardioversion will be needed if the lidocaine is ineffective. If the VT is sustained and the patient is unresponsive, pulseless, hypotensive, or in pulmonary edema, unsynchronous cardioversion will be necessary. If left untreated, VT will usually progress to either ventricular flutter (see Fig. 10-29) or ventricular fibrillation discussed next. Ventricular flutter looks similar on the ECG as VT except that the rate is usually faster and the rhythm less regular. Its treatment is the same as VT and, if left untreated, will progress to ventricular fibrillation. Both of these arrhythmias originate from a single fast ventricular focus as shown in Fig. 10-25.

Ventricular Fibrillation

Ventricular fibrillation (VF or V fib) is caused when multiple, fast ventricular foci are firing (see Fig. 10-30 for the electrical pathways). When several ventricular foci are firing in an uncoordinated manner the rhythm is chaotic and without any pattern (see Fig. 10-31). There is virtually no cardiac output. The patient is pulseless and without any blood pressure. This is a true medical emergency. If not treated

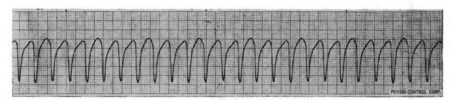

Fig. 10-28 Example of an ECG showing ventricular tachycardia. If this arrhythmia is not treated promptly it will deteriorate into ventricular flutter or ventricular fibrillation. (From Kacmarek RM, Mack CW, Dimas S: *The essentials of respiratory care*, ed 3, St. Louis, 1990, Mosby–Year Book. Used by permission.)

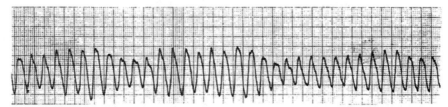

Fig. 10-29 Example of an ECG showing ventricular flutter. If this arrythmia is not treated promptly it will deteriorate into ventricular fibrillation. (From Kacmarek RM, Mack CW, Dimas S: *The essentials of respiratory care,* ed 3, St. Louis, 1990, Mosby–Year Book. Used by permission.)

immediately, brain death will occur within minutes. CPR must be started to provide oxygen to the brain. The treatment of choice for VF is defibrillation as quickly as possible. No attempt is made to synchronize the electrical shock. Fig. 10-32 shows the usual position of the defibrillator paddles. Fig. 10-33 shows an ECG tracing with VF, electrical defibrillation, and the restoration of an effective heartbeat.

Ventricular Asystole

Ventricular asystole (or asystole) is when there is no cardiac electrical signal and no myocardial activity. The ECG tracing will show a flat line indicating that there is no cardiac electrical activity. The presence of this arrythmia is ominous. When seen after the full attempt at CPR, it indicates a nonfunctioning heart. The patient will almost assuredly die. Some physicians may elect to defibrillate the patient in asystole in the attempt to generate some sort of rhythm. Because of the dire consequences of ventricular asystole, it is wise to double check all the equipment. This includes the ECG leads or defibrillator paddles being used to check the rhythm, all electrical connections, and the functioning of the ECG monitor to be sure that there is no technical error.

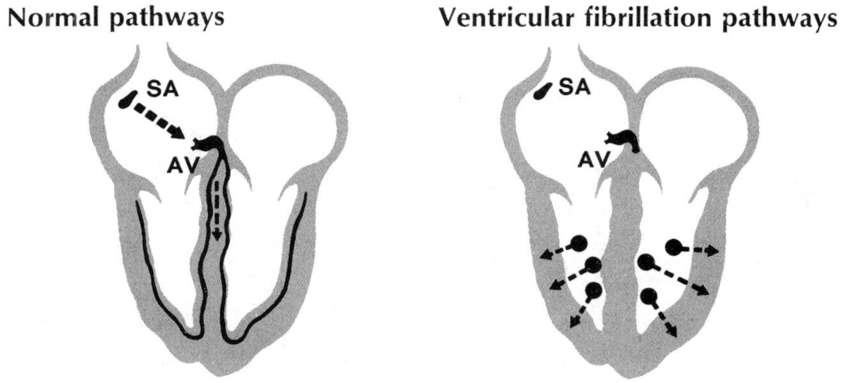

Fig. 10-30 Comparison of the normal electrical pathway and the abnormal electrical pathway seen in ventricular fibrillation. Because there are several electrical foci firing without any coordination, the heart muscle contracts in a chaotic manner and there is no effective pumping action. (From Butler HH: How to read an ECG, *RN Magazine,* 50-59, March 1973. Used by permission.)

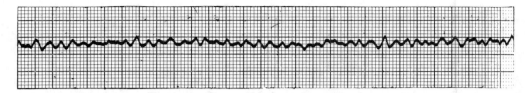

Fig. 10-31 Ventricular fibrillation. Note how no rhythm can be seen on the tracing. (From Goldberger AL, Goldberger E: *Clinical electrocardiography*, St. Louis, 1981, Mosby–Year Book. Used by permission.)

3.   Make the recommendation to defibrillate the patient. (IIID4) [R, Ap, An]

Defibrillation sends a specific amount of direct electrical current (DC) through the patient's chest wall and heart. Its purpose is to stimulate the entire cardiac muscle and electrical system so that the source of an abnormal signal will be suppressed. The SA node usually then takes over as the normal pacemaker. A more complete discussion of the subject is presented in Section 17.

As discussed earlier, synchronized defibrillation (cardioversion) should be performed under the following circumstances: atrial flutter, paroxysmal atrial tachycardia, atrial fibrillation, and ventricular tachycardia unless the patient is pulseless, unresponsive, hypotensive, or in pulmonary edema.

Unsynchronized defibrillation should be performed under the following circumstances: ventricular fibrillation or ventricular tachycardia when the patient is pulseless, unresponsive, hypotensive, or in pulmonary edema. Some physicians may also administer a cardiac shock to a patient in ventricular asystole.

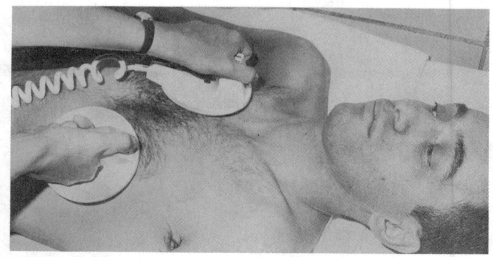

Fig. 10-32 The most commonly used positions for the defibrillation paddles are shown here on the left lateral chest and to the right of the sternum. During a synchronized cardioversion or defibrillation attempt the electrical energy is passed through the chest wall and myocardium. (From Butler HH: *How to read an ECG*, *RN Magazine* 50-59, March 1973. Used by permission.)

| VENTRICULAR FIBRILLATION | ELECTRICAL DEFIBRILLATION | EFFECTIVE HEARTBEAT |

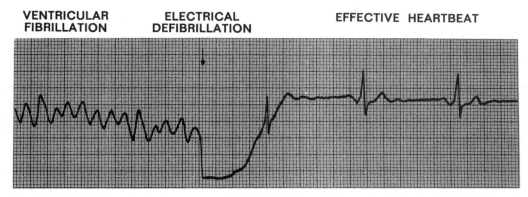

Fig. 10-33 ECG tracing of a successful defibrillation. The more quickly defibrillation is attempted during the resuscitation attempt, the more likely it is to be successful. (From Butler HH: How to read an ECG, *RN Magazine* 50-59, March 1973. Used by permission.)

4. Administer medications during an emergency.
a. Recommend the administration of bicarbonate during an emergency situation. (IIID3) [R, Ap, An]

According to the most recent guidelines, bicarbonate (sodium bicarbonate) should be used, if at all, only after all other CPR procedures have been instituted. Bicarbonate may then used if a diagnosis has been made and the patient has a preexisting metabolic acidosis, hyperkalemia, or tricyclic or phenobarbitol overdose. Bicarbonate may also be beneficial if the patient has been in prolonged arrest or if CPR has been performed for an extended time.

When used, bicarbonate should be given initially at a dose of 1 mEq/kg; a half dose is then given every 10 minutes. If available from arterial blood gases, use the calculated base deficit or bicarbonate concentration as a guideline for giving more bicarbonate. Do not completely correct the base deficit to avoid accidentally making the patient alkalotic.

b. Recommend the instillation of medications through the endotracheal tube during an emergency situation. (IIID8) [R, Ap, An]

Cardiac medications should be instilled down the endotracheal tube when a resuscitation attempt is underway and the patient does not have a functional central or peripheral intravenous (IV) line. The following medications may be instilled into all patients: lidocaine, epinephrine, and atropine. In addition, naloxone may be given to pediatric patients. Adults should be given a dose 2 to 2.5 times the normal intravenous amount. The medication should be diluted by adding 10 ml of normal saline or distilled water. Pediatric patients should be given a dose that is 10 times the normal IV amount. It should be diluted with 1 to 2 ml of normal or half normal saline.

c.   Instill the ordered medication down the endotracheal tube. (IIID9) [R, Ap]

The following steps for instillation are recommended:

1. Disconnect the manual resuscitator from the endotracheal tube and stop the chest compressions.
2. Pass a suction catheter or feeding tube past the distal tip of the endotracheal tube.
3. Quickly inject the drug solution down the catheter.
4. Withdraw the suction catheter.
5. Reconnect the manual resuscitator to the endotracheal tube and give the patient several deep breaths. This helps to force the medication down to the alveolar level or causes aerosolization so that there is faster absorption.
6. Resume chest compressions and ventilation.

5.   Observe the size of the patient's pupils and their reaction to light. (IIID2) [R]

Normally the pupils react to a light being shined into them by constricting. The pupils dilate within 30 to 40 seconds after cardiac arrest and do not constrict normally when the brain is hypoxic. If CPR is being done properly to deliver oxygen to the brain, the pupils should constrict normally. Fixed (nonreactive) and dilated pupils are an ominous sign. Even if the heart can be restarted the brain has probably suffered irreversible damage.

There are several conditions when the pupils will not react as expected. The pupils will remain constricted if the victim has received morphine sulfate or other opiates. The pupils will be dilated if the victim has received atropine, quinidine, or epinephrine. Hypothermia will also cause the pupils to dilate.

6.   Recommend capnography to evaluate the adequacy of resuscitation. (IIID6) [R, Ap, An]

The general discussion of capnography was presented in Section 4; review it if necessary. If quickly available, capnography can be used to help confirm that the endotracheal tube is properly located in the trachea. It is also helpful if the patient is being transported or the endotracheal tube is being repositioned. The presence of exhaled carbon dioxide confirms that the tube is properly positioned in the trachea. In addition, there is clinical evidence that monitoring the exhaled carbon dioxide level during a CPR attempt is helpful in evaluating the patient's response. In general, if chest compressions and assisted ventilation are effective, carbon dioxide will be removed from the tissues and circulated to the lungs for exhalation. If the CPR efforts are ineffective little exhaled carbon dioxide will be measured.

This ends the general discussion on cardiopulmonary resuscitation. The Registry Exams will ask *direct* questions on this material. Patient assessment was covered in detail in Section 1. In addition, some of the information in Sections 2, 4, and 8 relates to performing advanced CPR. More specific information on the role of the respiratory therapist in assisting with a defibrillation attempt is given in Section 17.

Module C.   Patient assessment.

1.   Examine all the data to determine the patient's pathophysiological condition. (IC3a) [R, Ap, An]

Be able to identify the types of arrythmias discussed in this section. Especially important are premature ventricular contactions and ventricular fibrillation.

2.   Take part in the development of the respiratory care plan. (IC3c) [An]

Arterial blood gases should be obtained if possible to check on oxygen, carbon dioxide, and pH values. Bicarbonate administration is also guided by their results. Some reports show that pulse oximetry provides valuable information on the patient's oxygenation during a CPR attempt. It is important that the oximetry site be one that is well perfused to provide useful data. Place an oximetry probe over the earlobe or bridge of the nose rather than a finger or toe.

Be prepared to assist with endotracheal intubation and the insertion of an arterial catheter. Also be prepared to begin mechanical ventilation if the patient is successfully resuscitated. A pulmonary artery catheter may also need to be inserted later.

BIBLIOGRAPHY

AARC Clinical Practice Guideline: Resuscitation in acute care hospitals, *Respir Care* 38(11):1179-1188, 1993.

Abedin Z, Conner RP: *12 lead ECG interpretation: the self-assessment approach*, Philadelphia, 1989, WB Saunders.

Andreoli KG, Fowkes VH, Zipes DP, et al: *Comprehensive cardiac care*, St. Louis, 1979, Mosby—Year Book.

Butler HH: How to read an ECG, *RN Magazine* 35-45, Jan 1973.

Butler HH: How to read an ECG, *RN Magazine* 49-61, Feb 1973.

Butler HH: How to read an ECG, *RN Magazine* 50-59, March 1973.

Davis D: *Differential diagnosis of arrhythmias*, Philadelphia, 1991, WB Saunders.

Emergency Cardiac Care Committee and Subcomittees, American Heart Association: Guidelines for cardiopulmonary resuscitation and emergency cardiac care, *JAMA* 268(16):2184-2281, 1992.

Eubanks DH, Bone RC: *Comprehensive respiratory care*, ed 2, St. Louis, 1990, Mosby—Year Book.

Ferko JG: Airtight advice, *Emergency* 31-36, Jan 1988.

Goldberger AL, Goldberger E: *Clinical electrocardiography*, St. Louis, 1981, Mosby—Year Book.

Hess D, Goff G, Johnson K: The effect of hand size, resuscitator brand, and use of two hands on volumes delivered during adult bag-valve ventilation, *Respir Care* 34(9), 1989.

Hurst JM, Branson RD, Davis K Jr, et al: Cardiopulmonary resuscitation. In Burton GG, Hodgkin JE, Ward JJ: *Respiratory care: a guide to clinical practice*, ed 3, Philadelphia, 1991, JB Lippincott.

Kacmarek RM, Mack CW, Dimas S: *The essentials of respiratory care*, ed 3, St. Louis, 1990, Mosby–Year Book.

Madama VC: Safe mouth-to-mouth resuscitation requires adjunct equipment, caution, *Occupat Health Safety* 60(1):56-64, 1991.

Marriott HJL: *Practical electrocardiography*, ed 7, Baltimore, 1983, Williams & Wilkins.

McPherson SP: *Respiratory therapy equipment*, ed 4, St. Louis, 1990, Mosby–Year Book.

Patel JM, McGowan SG, Moody LA: *Arrythmias: detection, treatment, and cardiac drugs*, Philadelphia, 1989, WB Saunders.

Phillips RE, Feeney MK: *The cardiac rhythms: a systematic approach to interpretation*, ed 3, Philadelphia, 1990, WB Saunders.

Scanlan CL: Emergency life support. In Scanlan CL, Spearman CB, Sheldon RL, editors: *Egan's fundamentals of respiratory therapy*, ed 5, St. Louis, 1990, Mosby–Year Book.

Sills JR: *Respiratory care certification guide: the complete review resource for the entry level exam*, ed 2, St. Louis, 1991, Mosby–Year Book.

Stein E: *Clinical electrocardiography*, Philadelphia, 1987, Lea & Febiger.

Stephenson HE Jr: Cardiopulmonary resuscitation. In Burton GG, Hodgkin JE, editors: *Respiratory care: a guide to clinical practice*, ed 2, Philadelphia, 1984, JB Lippincott.

Sweetwood HM: *Clinical electrocardiography for nurses*, Rockville, Md, 1983, Aspen Systems.

Watson MA: Cardiopulmonary resuscitation. In Barnes TA, editor: *Respiratory care practice*, Chicago, 1988, Year Book Medical.

SELF-STUDY QUESTIONS

1. A completely compensatory pause is seen after which type of heartbeat?
    A. Normal sinus rhythm
    B. Premature ventricular contraction
    C. Paroxysmal atrial tachycardia
    D. Second degree AV block
    E. Ventricular tachycardia

2. A normal sinus rhythm can be identified by:
    I. A resting rate of 60 to 100 beats per minute in an adult
    II. A P wave before every QRS complex
    III. A regular rhythm
    IV. A QRS complex after every P wave
    V. An upright T wave in lead II
    A. I, III
    B. II, IV
    C. II, III, IV
    D. I, II, III, V
    E. I, II, III, IV, V

3. All the following statements are true of a pneumatic (demand valve) resuscitator EXCEPT:
    A. It will fail to cycle off if there is a leak between the face mask and the patient.
    B. The patient cannot trigger it to deliver a tidal volume breath.
    C. The delivered volume will vary if the patient's compliance and resistance change.
    D. It may cycle off earlier than expected during a chest compression.

4. Your ventilator-dependent patient is set up for routine ECG monitoring. Because of refractory hypoxemia, the physician orders 10 cm water of PEEP. Shortly after the PEEP therapy is added, you notice that the patient has developed sinus arrhythmia. Which of the following is the best course of action to follow?
   A. Recommend the administration of atropine.
   B. Defibrillate the patient.
   C. Decrease the PEEP from 10 to 5 cm water and then inform the physician of your decision.
   D. Make a record of the rhythm and inform the nurse and physician of your observation.
   E. Recommend synchronized cardioversion.

5. A patient comes into the emergency room appearing ashen gray and complaining of sudden, severe pain beneath his sternum and shortness of breath. He says that this began after exercising vigorously for 45 minutes. After putting an oxygen mask on the patient what should you do?
   A. Start ECG monitoring.
   B. Recommend that he begin a supervised exercise program at the hospital.
   C. Recommend to the physician that the patient have a complete pulmonary function test.
   D. Perform a peak flow test to check on exercise-induced asthma.
   E. Draw an arterial blood gas sample.

6. The nurse calls you into a patient's room. Looking at the ECG monitor, you notice that the patient is in ventricular tachycardia. You cannot find a carotid pulse and the nurse says that he cannot find a blood pressure. What would you recommend?
   A. Start a nasal cannula at 3 L/min.
   B. Check the other arm for a blood pressure.
   C. Defibrillate the patient.
   D. Intubate the patient and start her on a ventilator.
   E. Synchronized cardioversion of the patient.

7. Counting from the left, the first and sixth rhythms on the ECG strip shown below represent:
   A. Atrial flutter
   B. Second-degree heart block
   C. Unifocal premature ventricular contractions
   D. Premature junctional beats
   E. Multifocal premature ventricular contractions

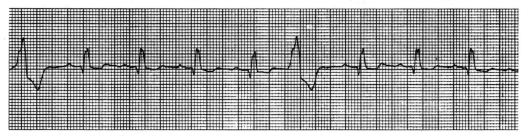

(From Patel JM, McGowan SG, Moody LA: Arrythmias: detection, treatment, and cardiac drugs, Philadelphia, WB Saunders, 1989. Used by permission.)

8. A 65-year-old patient has been successfully resuscitated in the emergency room after suffering a myocardial infarction. He is still unstable with frequent premature ventricular contractions. He needs to be transported to the cardiac care unit for management. Which of the following would be most important for monitoring him during the transportation?
   A. A pulse oximeter
   B. A portable capnography unit
   C. A cardiac care unit ECG machine
   D. A portable ECG machine with defibrillator
   E. A 12-lead ECG unit to record any arrhythmias

9. You are performing chest compressions during a resuscitation attempt while another therapist is manually ventilating the intubated patient. The nurse and physician are both unable to start an IV line to give medications. What would you recommend?
   A. Instill the medications down the endotracheal tube.
   B. Keep trying new sites to start the IV line.
   C. Nebulize the medications.
   D. Give the medications by subcutaneous injection.
   E. Switch with the nurse so that you can try to start the IV line.

10. You are doing oxygen rounds on patients in the coronary care unit. You notice that the patient whose 28% venturi mask you are checking is unresponsive to your questions. Looking up you see the rhythm strip shown below. What would you recommend as a first reaction?

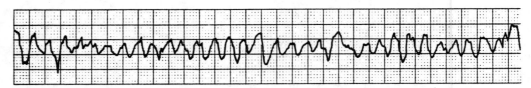

(From Patel JM, McGowan SG, Moody LA: Arrythmias: detection, treatment, and cardiac drugs, Philadelphia, WB Saunders, 1989. Used by permission.)

   A. Remove the oxygen mask because the patient is receiving too much oxygen and is hypoventilating.
   B. Check the calibration on the ECG machine.
   C. Replace the ECG leads.
   D. Increase the oxygen percentage because the patient is hypoxic.
   E. Defibrillate the patient.

11. During a diagnostic ECG, you notice that the QRS complex is inverted on lead II. What would most likely cause this?
   A. The patient has sinus inversus.
   B. The electrodes are attached properly.
   C. The leg electrodes are reversed.
   D. The arm electrodes are reversed.
   E. The unit is out of calibration.

12. Electrocardiogram monitoring would be important with an intensive care unit in all of the following situations EXCEPT:
    A. The patient is hypoxemic.
    B. If it is used to evaluate peripheral perfusion.
    C. The patient has an electrolyte disturbance.
    D. The patient has a history of arrhythmias.
    E. The patient is being given a rapid infusion of potassium.

Answer Key

1. B; 2. E; 3. B; 4. D; 5. A; 6. C; 7. C; 8. D; 9. A; 10. E; 11. D; 12. B.

11

Airway Management

Module A. Perform the following procedures to maintain a patent airway.

1. Recommend the use of an artificial airway. (IIIC10h) [R, Ap, An]

An artificial airway is indicated in any patient who cannot protect his or her airway. The patient could: 1) be at risk of obstructing the upper airway by the tongue falling back, 2) have facial trauma or surgery, 3) be at risk of vomiting and aspirating, and/or 4) need mechanical ventilation for assisted breathing. A number of possible airways are available. Select the best one based on the patient's needs.

An oral pharyngeal airway is used in an unconscious patient who is at risk of obstructing the airway with his or her tongue. It may also be used in an unconscious patient at risk of seizure activity. It will prevent the tongue from being bitten during a seizure. It should not be used in a conscious patient because it may cause gagging.

A nasopharyngeal airway is used to keep the tongue from blocking the airway when an oral pharyngeal airway cannot be used. This would include patients with oral trauma or surgery or patients who are conscious. It is also used as a guide to pass a catheter for tracheal suctioning.

An endotracheal tube is indicated when a patent airway is required for endotracheal suctioning and/or mechanical ventilation. Aspiration is also prevented when the cuff is inflated. An oral endotracheal tube is indicated in most emergency situations because it is faster and easier than placing a nasal endotracheal tube. A nasal endotracheal tube is indicated when the patient has oral trauma or a cervical spine injury prevents the neck from being hyperextended for placing the oral tube.

A tracheostomy tube is indicated for long-term airway management or when facial trauma or surgery prevents an oral or nasal endotracheal tube from being used. This tube also provides a patent airway for suctioning and mechanical ventilation and prevents aspiration. In addition, it is more comfortable than an endotracheal tube and allows the patient to eat and drink. The so-called "talking" tracheostomy tubes permit the patient to vocalize with the aid of an additional source of airflow through the vocal cords.

These types of airways are discussed in more detail in *Respiratory Care Certification Guide* (Sills, 1994) and other standard respiratory care textbooks. There is one additional class of artificial airways—the esophageal obturator airways (EOA). They are not listed as testable by the NBRC and so are not discussed in detail here; however, they are widely used by emergency medical technicians when intubation cannot be performed. It is recommended that the learner become familiar with them because patients coming into the emergency room may have one inserted. There are several versions available and they should not be treated in the same manner as an endotracheal tube. Clinical practice with each type of EOA is recommended.

2.   Perform endotracheal intubation. (IIIB1b) [R, Ap]

Oral endotracheal intubation is the recommended procedure for securing the airway during an emergency. In uncomplicated cases, the patient can be quickly intubated with an apneic period of no more than 20 seconds. This procedure is described in relationship to a "team" of two respiratory therapists doing it. It is difficult, if not impossible, for a single therapist to perform this important task without placing the patient at great risk. Usually the therapist who will intubate is considered the leader and another therapist will act as the assistant. Therapists must feel comfortable in both roles. The steps in an uncomplicated, urgent intubation are described later. This might be seen during a CPR attempt or when respiratory failure is imminent. (See Table 11-1 for a list of indications and contraindications for oral intubation and Table 11-2 for a list of complications.)

The steps of an intubation performed under the controlled environment of an operating room may be quite different. For example, the patient is usually sedated, pharmacologically paralyzed, or both before intubation is tried. It is unlikely that a respiratory therapist will do any intubating in the operating room outside of the initial training sessions.

Steps in an emergency oral endotracheal intubation:

1. Prepare the patient. The assistant should:
   a. Place the head and neck in the sniffer's position.
   b. Ventilate the patient with 100% oxygen by a face mask and manual resuscitator or demand valve.
2. The intubator should put clean gloves on both hands (and possibly a surgical mask and goggles) and perform the following:
3. Prepare the endotracheal tube.
   a. Select the proper endotracheal tube (see Table 11-3 for the recommended tube sizes based on age). If time permits, the next smaller and larger tube size should also be selected.

Table 11-1. Indications and Contraindications for Oral Endotracheal Intubation

General Indications for Endotracheal Intubation
Provide a secure, patent airway.
Provide a route for mechanical ventilation.
Prevent aspiration of stomach or mouth contents.
Provide a route for suctioning the lungs.
Use general anesthesia.

Indications for Oral Intubation
Fastest, easiest method to secure the airway.
Simpler, less invasive method cannot ensure an
  open airway.

Contraindications for Oral Intubation
Cervical spine injury so that the patient's neck
  cannot be hyperextended
Lower facial injury
Oral surgery

Table 11-2. Complications of
Endotracheal Intubation

General Complications
Reflex laryngospasm
Perforation of the esophagus or pharynx
Esophageal intubation
Bronchial intubation
Reflex bradycardia
Tachycardia or other arrhythmias from hypoxemia
Hypotension
Bronchospasm
Aspiration of tooth, blood, gastric contents,
    laryngoscope bulb
Laceration of pharynx or larynx
Nosocomial infection
Vocal cord injury
Laryngeal or tracheal injury from the tube or the
    excessive cuff pressure

Complications of the Oral Route
Cervical spine injury
Tooth trauma from the blade being pulled back
Eye trauma from the handle or the operator's
    hand

Complications after Extubation
Reflex laryngospasm
Aspiration of stomach contents or oral secretions
Sore throat
Hoarseness
Laryngeal edema (postintubation croup)

   b. Inflate the cuff with a 10 or 20 ml syringe. Remove the syringe from
      the one-way valve. Make sure that it will hold the air and then
      deflate the cuff completely.
   c. Lubricate the last few centimeters of the endotracheal tube with a
      water-soluble lubricant.
   d. Lubricate a stylet with the sterile water-soluble lubricant. Place the
      stylet into the tube so that the natural curve of the tube is
      maintained. The tip of the stylet should not go past the end of the
      tube (see Fig. 11-1). Some practitioners may prefer not to use a stylet.
      Many believe that the stylet offers the advantage of being able to
      bend the tube to match the patient's anatomy if a second attempt is
      needed.
3. Prepare the laryngoscope and blade.
   a. Select a laryngoscope handle.
   b. Select a laryngoscope blade. The blades come in several sizes from
      pediatric to adult. There are two main classes of blades—straight and
      curved (see Fig. 11-2). The straight blades (Miller is a common
      brand) are designed to lift the epiglottis to expose the tracheal
      opening. The curved blades (MacIntosh is a common brand) are
      designed to fit into the vallecula (between the base of the tongue and
      the epiglottis). As the blade is lifted, the epiglottis is raised and the
      tracheal opening can be seen. Personal experience and training will
      lead the practitioner to select between the two styles.

Table 11-3. Endotracheal and Tracheostomy Tube Sizes Based on Patient Age

Age	ID in mm	Approximate OD in mm	French Size (OD)
Newborn			
Less than 1000 grams	2.5	4.0	12
1000-2000 grams	3.0	5.0	14
2000-3000 grams	3.5	5.5	16
Greater than 3000 grams to 6 months old	3.5-4.0		16-18
Pediatric			
18 months	4.0	6.0	18
3 years	4.5	6.5	20
5 years	5.0	7.0	22
6 years	5.5	8.0	24
8 years	6.0	9.0	26
Adult			
16 years	7.0	10.0	30
Normal adult female	7.5-8.0	11.0	32-34
Normal adult male	8.0-8.5	12.0	34-36
Large adult	9.0-10.0	13.0-14.0	38-42

It is important to always use the largest tube that can be placed into the patient without causing any harm during the intubation. This is because the larger the internal diameter of the tube is, the less airway resistance it causes. Be prepared to insert a tube that is one size larger or smaller than anticipated based on individual variances.

The approximate mathematical relationship between the outer diameter in mm and French size can be easily calculated. The French size is determined by multiplying the outer diameter in mm by 3. The outer diameter in mm is found by dividing the French size by 3.

    c. Attach the blade to the handle (see Fig. 11-3). Make sure that the light bulb shines brightly.

4. The intubator should tell the assistant to stop ventilating the patient and stand clear so that an intubation can be attempted. The assistant should check his or her watch to silently count off 20 seconds. The intubator should be told when 20 seconds has passed so that the patient can be reventilated if the intubation is proving to be difficult.

5. Open the victim's mouth as widely as possible without using force.

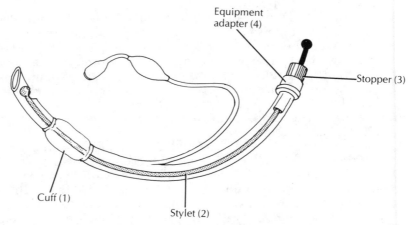

Fig. 11-1 Stylet with stopper properly placed in a standard endotracheal tube to maintain its curved shape. (From Eubanks DH, Bone RC: *Comprehensive respiratory care,* ed 2, St. Louis, 1990, Mosby–Year Book. Used by permission.)

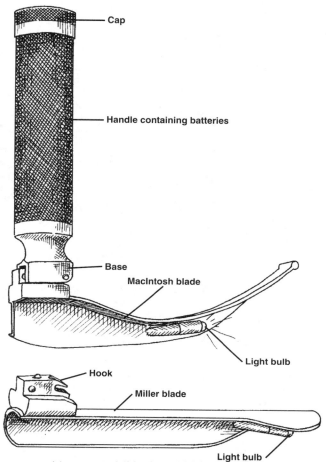

Fig. 11-2 Laryngoscope with a curved (MacIntosh) blade attached. A straight (Miller) blade is below for comparison. Note the component parts and features. (From Sills JR: *Respiratory care certification guide: the complete review resource for the entry level exam*, ed 2, St. Louis, 1994, Mosby–Year Book. Used by permission.)

Remove any dentures or foreign material. Suction out any saliva, blood, or vomitus.

6. Grasp the laryngoscope handle in the left hand. Carefully advance the blade between the teeth or gums along the right side of the mouth. Move the tongue to the left of the mouth to allow a clear view of the oropharynx (see Fig. 11-4). Advance the blade along the base of the tongue until the epiglottis is seen.
7. With a *straight blade:*
   a. Advance the blade so that it barely passes the epilgottis.
   b. Do not advance the blade too far or it will enter the esophagus or trachea.
   With a *curved blade:*
   a. Advance the blade tip into the vallecula.
   b. Lift the blade tip into this space.
8. With either blade, lift the laryngoscope handle and blade toward the patient's chest at a 45° angle (see Fig. 11-5). The straight blade will lift

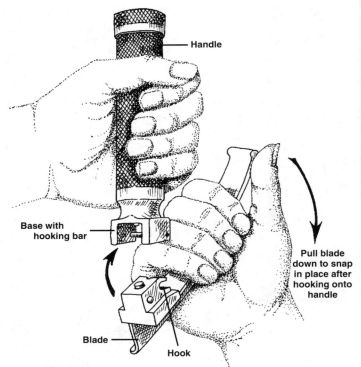

Fig. 11-3 Motions to attach a laryngoscope blade to a handle. (From Sills JR: *Respiratory care certification guide: the complete review resource for the entry level exam,* ed 2, St. Louis, 1994, Mosby–Year Book. Used by permission.)

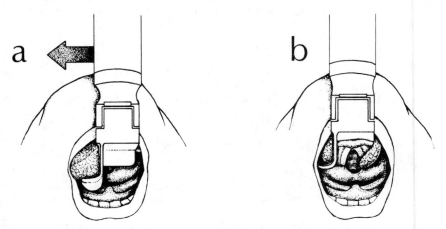

Fig. 11-4 Proper placement of the laryngoscope blade to move the patient's tongue. **A,** The proper placement of the laryngoscope blade to the right of the patient's tongue to move it to the left. This should give a clear view of the glottis. **B,** The tongue partially obstructs the view if it is not moved to the left. (From Shapiro BA, Harrison RA, Kacmarek RM et al: *Clinical application of respiratory care,* ed 4, St. Louis, 1991, Mosby–Year Book. Used by permission.)

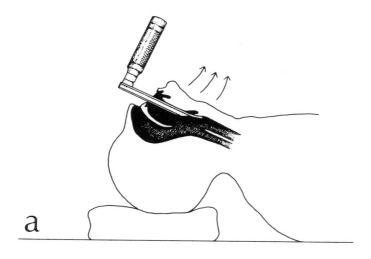

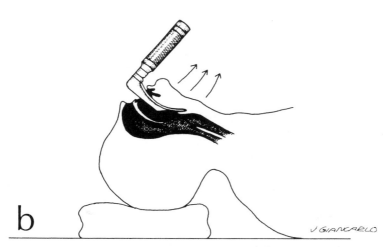

Fig. 11-5 Proper use of the laryngoscope blade to expose the larynx by lifting the glottic structures. Note how the lifting is at a 45° angle toward the patient's chest. *Never* pull back on the blade against the teeth. **A,** A straight blade is used to lift the epiglottis to expose the trachea. **B,** A curved blade is used to lift the soft tissues of the vallecula to expose the trachea. (From Shapiro BA, Harrison RA, Kacmarek RM et al: *Clinical application of respiratory care,* ed 4, St. Louis, 1991, Mosby–Year Book. Used by permission.)

the epiglottis. The curved blade will lift the soft tissues of the vallecula and the epiglottis will lift with them. Do *not* pull back on the patient's upper teeth. If needed, tell the assistant to put downward pressure on the patient's larynx.

9. The vocal cords and glottis should be clearly seen (see Fig. 11-6).
10. Tell the assistant to place the endotracheal tube into your right hand.
11. Place the tube into the patient's mouth and trachea. In the adult, the proximal end of the cuff should be placed 3 to 4 cm past the vocal cords

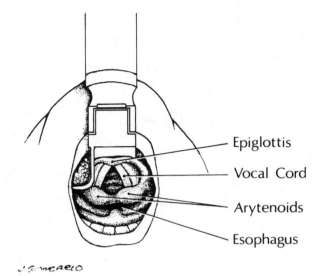

Fig. 11-6 Major anatomic features that will be seen when the epiglottis is lifted. The opening to the trachea can be seen between the vocal cords. (From Shapiro BA, Harrison RA, Kacmarek RM et al: *Clinical application of respiratory care,* ed 4, St. Louis, 1991, Mosby–Year Book. Used by permission.)

    (see Fig. 11-7). In children less than 6 months, with an uncuffed endotracheal tube, place the end of the tube about 1 cm past the vocal cords.

12. Hold the tube in place.
13. Withdraw the laryngoscope blade.
14. Tell the assistant to inflate the cuff. Place about 10 ml of air into the cuff (of an adult's tube) so that some resistance can be felt. The cuff pressure can be measured and adjusted later.
15. Pull out the stylet (if used).
16. The assistant should ventilate the patient with the manual resuscitator bag or a demand valve.
17. The intubator should listen to both lung fields in the upper lobes and bases. Bilateral breath sounds should be heard.
18. If the breath sounds are equal and bilateral, the assistant can secure the tube in place with tape or a tube holder. If the breath sounds are unequal or absent on one side the tube has been placed into a bronchus (usually the right mainstem). The cuff should be deflated and the tube then withdrawn 1 to 2 cm in the adult; less in a child. The cuff should be reinflated and breath sounds listened to again. When the breath sounds are equal the tube can be secured.
19. If no breath sounds are heard, listen over the stomach area. If air is heard bubbling into the stomach, the tube has been placed into the esophagus. Immediately remove the tube. Ventilate the patient and prepare to attempt reintubation with a new endotracheal tube.

    It is especially important to check for bilateral breath sounds after any endotracheal tube has been placed. The right mainstem bronchus is commonly accidentally intubated because it comes off of the trachea at a less acute angle than the left mainstem bronchus. No breath sounds would be heard over the left lung field. The practitioner should only perform those procedures for which he or she has been

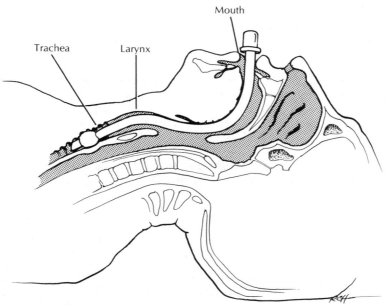

Fig. 11-7 Oral endotracheal tube properly positioned within the trachea. (From Eubanks DH, Bone RC: *Comprehensive respiratory care,* ed 2, St. Louis, 1990, Mosby–Year Book. Used by permission.)

trained. If the patient cannot be intubated with the standard equipment and procedure, an anesthesiologist or trained physician should be called in. Be prepared to assist as necessary.

3. Use an exhaled carbon dioxide detector to confirm the proper placement of the endotracheal tube. (IIID10) [R, Ap, An]

An exhaled carbon dioxide detector can be used to help confirm the proper placement of the endotracheal tube within the trachea. At the time of this writing, Nellcor is the only manufacturer of such a device. Its Easy Cap unit is able to detect exhaled CO_2 and give its approximate concentration.

To use the Easy Cap, removed it from its sealed foil envelope. Its 15-mm ID patient end is then placed on the endotracheal tube adapter. The manual resuscitator or demand valve is then connected to the 15-mm OD equipment end. Each inspiration and exhalation must then pass through the Easy Cap. It has a colored indicator that is CO_2 sensitive. With inspiration (no carbon dioxide) the indicator turns dark purple. As the properly intubated patient exhales CO_2 the indicator turns yellow. The manufacturer recommends that at least six breaths be evaluated to make sure that the reading is accurate. If each exhalation results in the indicator turning yellow you can be certain that the patient's trachea is intubated. If the indicator turns light or deep purple the patient should be evaluated for possible placement of the tube into the esophagus. Listen for bilateral breath sounds. If absent, extubate and reintubate the patient. Use the Easy Cap again to measure the exhaled carbon dioxide level. The unit can be used for up to 2 hours.

Nellcor lists the following as limitations or contraindications to the Easy Cap:

1. The patient must weigh at least 15 kg.
2. The Easy Cap should not be used during mouth-to-tube ventilation.

3. It will not be able to detect right mainstem bronchial intubation.
4. It should not be used to detect hypercarbia.
5. It should not be used to help determine the placement of an esophageal obturator airway.

The Easy Cap could be used in a cardiopulmonary resuscitation attempt to help determine if compressions and ventilations are effective. This is discussed in Section 10 in reference to capnography readings. The same idea applies here. If the CPR efforts are effective the Easy Cap will show a yellow reading indicating that carbon dioxide is being exhaled.

4. Measure and maintain the proper cuff volume and pressure in the endotracheal or tracheostomy tube. (IB9e) [An]

Most brands of modern tubes have cuffs for sealing the trachea that are designed to have a relatively large reservoir volume that fills at a relatively low pressure. The soft, flexible balloon seals the airway by having a large surface area that easily conforms to the shape of the trachea. Because of this, less pressure is needed in the cuff to create a seal. So, less pressure is exerted against the tracheal mucosa. The original esophageal obturator airway (EOA) still has the older low volume, high pressure cuff. The newer esophageal gastric tube airway (EGTA) and other esophageal blocking tubes have low pressure, large volume cuffs.

All manufacturers (except Kamen-Wilkenson) have designed cuffs that must be actively filled with air by way of a one-way valve and syringe. These cuffs have greater than atmospheric pressure in them. The pressure is placed against the wall of the trachea. The greater the pressure on the wall of the trachea, the greater the disruption of normal lymphatic and blood flow. Shapiro, Harrison, Kacmarek et al state that a patient with a normal blood pressure (120/80 mm Hg) will have the following effects at these cuff pressures:

a. Lymphatic flow blockage will occur at pressures greater than 5 mm Hg/8 cm H_2O. Edema of the tracheal mucosa will result.

b. Capillary blood flow blockage will occur at pressures greater than 18 mm Hg/24 cm H_2O. Venous (and lymphatic) drainage will be stopped as a result.

c. Arterial blood flow blockage will occur at pressures greater than 30 mm Hg/42 H_2O. Arterial (and lymphatic and capillary) flow will be stopped as a result.

In general, the clinical goal is to keep the cuff pressure as low as possible to make sure that the circulation through the tracheal wall is normal. It seems reasonable to try to keep the cuff pressure no greater than 15 mm Hg/21 cm H_2O. This would hold true for all normotensive patients. A spontaneously breathing patient must have the cuff inflated to prevent the aspiration of oral secretions into the lungs. It is sometimes necessary to keep a higher cuff pressure in a mechanically ventilated patient. High positive airway pressures can result in an air leak around the cuff if the endotracheal or tracheostomy tube is too small. Ideally, the tube should be replaced with a larger one; however, some patients are too unstable to tolerate reintubation and must simply have the cuff pressure increased temporarily.

Hypertensive patients may be able to tolerate higher cuff pressures before blood flow is stopped. Hypotensive patients will suffer from the loss of blood flow to the tracheal wall at lower cuff pressures than those listed.

It is clear that a cuff pressure greater than the patient's mucosal capillary pressure will prevent the flow of blood through the area covered by the cuff. Tissue ischemia (hypoxemia) will result. If the ischemia is severe enough, tissue necrosis will follow. The higher the cuff pressure and the longer the high cuff pressure is maintained, the greater the likelihood of tissue necrosis. If the necrosis is circumferential (all the way around) to the trachea, tracheal stenosis will likely occur. Tracheal stenosis is found when the diameter of the trachea is narrowed due to scar tissue buildup after the normal mucosa and underlying tissues have died. The patient's airway is permanently narrowed and, if serious, must be surgically corrected. Another severe complication of high cuff pressures and tracheal necrosis is the development of a tracheoesophageal fistula. This is an opening between the trachea and esophagus. A fistula is more likely to develop when the patient also has a nasogastric tube in place. The fistula will permit food to pass into the airway and lungs causing pneumonia. Mechanical ventilation is made more difficult because of the air leak from the lungs to the esophagus. Surgical repair of the fistula is usually required.

There are two slightly different techniques for inflating the cuff to a safe pressure when the patient is on a positive pressure ventilator. They are presented in detail in *Respiratory Care Certification Guide* (Sills, 1994) if they need to be reviewed. Basically, the *minimal leak* technique is used to find the cuff pressure that results in a small leak at the cuff when the patient's airway pressure is greatest. The *minimal occluding volume* technique is used to find the cuff pressure that results in no leak at the cuff when the patient's airway pressure is greatest.

5. Change the endotracheal tube. (IIIC6b) [R, Ap, An]

There are usually only two reasons to have to replace a patient's endotracheal tube. First, the tube should be changed if it is too small and the cuff must be overfilled to seal the airway. Excessive pressure will result in damage to the tracheal wall as previously discussed.

Second, the tube should be replaced if the cuff is leaking or ruptured and the airway cannot be sealed. The patient may be reintubated by the procedure described earlier. Or, a tube changing stylet may be used as shown in Fig. 11-8. The stylet is a hollow, flexible plastic tube that can be bent and can hold its shape. It has a center mark and 1 cm markings counting out to each end. These are to help keep the proper depth for inserting the replacement endotracheal tube. Instrumentation Laboratories makes a unit that they call the JEM 400 Endotracheal Tube Changer (Guide). It can be used on an endotracheal tube that is at least 7-mm interior diameter. The procedure for changing the endotracheal tube with a tube changing stylet includes:

1. Obtain the needed equipment: replacement endotracheal tube and one that is a size smaller, 10-ml syringe to inflate the cuff, sterile gloves, and sterile water-soluble lubricant. Make sure the cuff inflates and deflates properly.
2. Tell the patient what you are going to do. Put on the gloves.
3. Remove the patient's oxygen equipment.
4. Suction the patient's trachea and oral pharynx of secretions.
5. Reoxygenate and ventilate the patient.
6. Place some lubricant on the outside of the stylet.
7. Remove the oxygen equipment and pass the stylet through the endotracheal tube into the patient's trachea.
8. Insert it to about the same depth as marked on the distal end of the endotracheal tube. For example, if the distal end of the endotracheal tube is 22 cm, insert the tube changer to 22 cm.
9. Deflate the cuff on the endotracheal tube.
10. While holding the distal tip of the tube changer in place, pull the defective endotracheal tube over it and out of the patient.
11. Advance the new endotracheal tube over the stylet. Hold the distal end

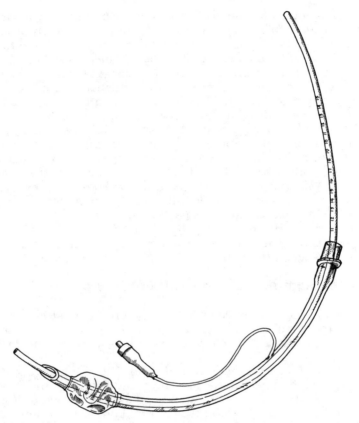

Fig. 11-8 An endotracheal tube changer (guide) inserted through an endotracheal tube. The JEM 400 unit can be inserted through a tube that is 7-mm ID or larger. The tube changer is used to aid in the replacement of an esophageal obturator airway or a defective endotracheal tube with a functional endotracheal tube. See the text for how to use the tube changer instead of traditional intubation equipment. (Modified from Heffner JE: Managing difficult intubations in critically ill patients, *Respir Management* 19:3, 1989.)

      of the stylet and push the new tube into the patient to the same depth mark on the stylet as the old tube.

12. Hold the endotracheal tube in place and remove the stylet.
13. Ensure that the tube has been placed into the trachea to the proper depth by listening for bilateral breath sounds.
14. Inflate the cuff to a safe pressure.
15. Secure the tube in place and note the depth marking at the patient's teeth or gums.
16. Obtain a chest x-ray.

A defective one-way valve or severed cuff inflating tube may not necessarily lead to a reintubation; often it can be bypassed. This is done by slipping a small diameter needle (usually about 21-gauge) into the inflating tube, attaching a three-way stopcock to the hub of the needle, and screwing a 10-cc syringe into one of the stopcock ports (see Fig. 11-9). The cuff pressure can be measured by attaching a pressure manometer to the other port on the stopcock. Air can be added by the 10-cc syringe and the pressure measured simultaneously (see Fig. 11-10). There is

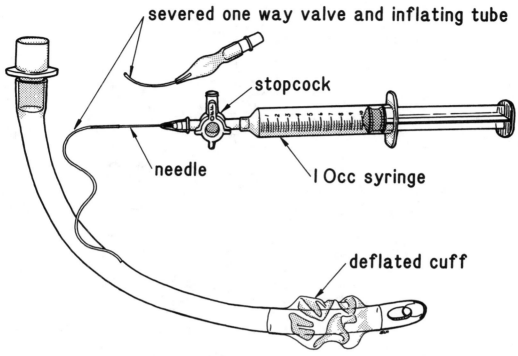

severed one way valve and inflating tube

stopcock

needle

l Occ syringe

deflated cuff

Fig. 11-9 An emergency system for inflating the cuff when the one-way valve and inflating tube are severed. (From Sills JR: An emergency cuff inflation technique, *Respir Care* 31(3):199-201, 1986. Used by permission.)

now a commercially available system to bypass a severed cuff inflating tube. It consists of a blunted needle and a small length of cuff-inflating tube added to a new one-way valve. The unit comes in two needle sizes to fit different size pilot tubes. It is made by Instrumentation Laboratories and is called the Endotracheal/Trach Tube Pilot Tube Repair Kit. Clinical experience has shown that when a patient is too unstable to attempt reintubation, these replacement one-way valve systems can be used to keep the cuff inflated at a safe pressure.

6. Change the tracheostomy tube. (IIIB1d and IIIC6b) [R, Ap, An]

A tracheostomy tube may have to be changed because of a ruptured cuff just as in the endotracheal tube or because of another problem. In addition, patients with a permanent tracheostomy will have the tube changed on a routine schedule as part of the tracheostomy care. These two different situations are discussed separately.

Emergency Tube Change

Let us focus here on the clinical emergency of obstruction when the tracheostomy tube should be replaced. Several things can cause this, such as the cuff being herniated over the end of the tube, a mucus plug blocking the lumen, or the end of the tube being forced into the tracheal tissues. Unfortunately, these problems cannot be seen from the outside. If the patient is in acute respiratory distress and an obstruction is suspected, attempt to pass a suction catheter. Failure to pass it

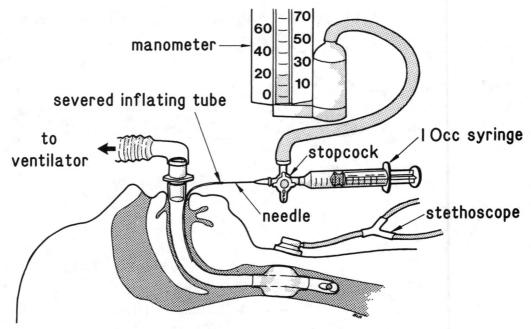

Fig. 11-10 Measuring the intracuff pressure as the cuff is reinflated with an emergency system. The stethoscope is used to listen for the presence of a leak at the larynx. (From Sills JR: An emergency cuff inflation technique, *Respir Care* 31(3):199-201, 1986. Used by permission.)

beyond the end of the tube will confirm the obstruction. A rapid clinical decision will have to be made as to the best action. The tube should be removed if the obstruction is complete and the patient cannot breathe. A spontaneously breathing patient will continue to breathe through the stoma. An apneic patient will have to be temporarily ventilated with mouth-to-stoma breaths. As rapidly and carefully as possible another tracheostomy tube should be inserted. This will usually result in a patent airway. If loose tracheal mucosa is blocking the airway, an endotracheal tube will have to be inserted past the tissue and deeper into the trachea. Call the physician as soon as possible to evaluate the patient's condition.

Routine Tube Change

It is important to avoid, if possible, changing the tube until several days after a fresh tracheostomy procedure. This allows time for the stoma site to form granulomatous tissue as it begins to heal. The site will then be less likely to bleed as the tube is changed. When the tracheostomy tube is changed it is usually part of the tracheostomy wound care. These are typical steps in changing the tracheostomy tube:

1. Gather the necessary equipment: new tracheostomy tube of the same size and the next size smaller, its 15-mm adapter, its obturator, tracheostomy tie strings to secure the tube in the patient (see Fig. 11-11), a sterile 4″ × 4″ gauze pad, sterile scissors, a 10-ml syringe to inflate the cuff, sterile water-soluble lubricant, and sterile gloves. Make sure the cuff inflates and deflates properly.
2. Put the gloves on.

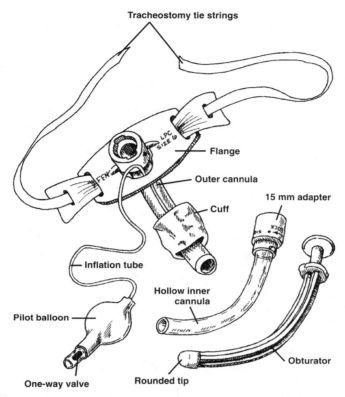

Tracheostomy tie strings

Flange

Outer cannula

15 mm adapter

Cuff

Inflation tube

Hollow inner cannula

Pilot balloon

Obturator

One-way valve

Rounded tip

Fig. 11-11 A typical tracheostomy tube with its component parts and features. (From Sills JR: *Respiratory care certification guide: the complete review resource for the entry level exam,* ed 2, St. Louis, 1994, Mosby–Year Book. Used by permission.)

3. Maintaining sterile technique, make sure the obturator easily fits into and comes out of the tracheostomy tube.
4. Cut a slit into the center of the gauze pad.
5. Apply some lubricant to the tip of the tracheostomy tube.
6. Tell the patient what you are going to do.
7. Remove the oxygen and/or aerosol from the patient.
8. Suction the patient's trachea. Reoxygenate the patient.
9. Untie the tracheostomy strings.
10. Deflate the cuff.
11. Remove the 4″ × 4″ gauze pad.
12. Remove the tracheostomy tube by pulling it in a curved motion toward the patient's chest.
13. Inspect the tracheostomy opening for signs of infection such as redness, pus, or swelling. Report signs of infection to the nurse or physician.
14. Carefully insert the new trachestomy tube with obturator into the stoma. The motion should be opposite that used to remove the original tube. Make sure not to force the tube into the tissues of the trachea.
15. Remove the obturator and insert the 15-mm adapter. Lock it in place.
16. Inflate the cuff to a safe pressure.
17. Listen for bilateral breath sounds.
18. Slide the new 4″ × 4″ gauze pad around the tube such that the slit fits around it.

19. Tie the tracheostomy tie strings behind the patient's neck.
20. Give the patient oxygen and/or aerosol as before.

7. Change the type of humidification equipment. (IIIC6a) [An]

Patients with an oropharyngeal or nasopharyngeal airway may be given supplemental humidity by a simple aerosol mask. This should help to prevent the secretions from becoming too viscous and difficult to cough out.

Patients with an endotracheal or tracheostomy tube in place should ideally be provided 100% relative humidity at body temperature. Typically, an aerosol generator or humidifier warmed to provide 100% of the patient's humidity needs is connected to the endotracheal or tracheostomy tube. This should be provided to any patient with a problem of viscous or large amounts of secretions.

It is acceptable to use a condensing humidifier (heat and moisture exchanger or HME) with an intubated patient who does not have a problem with viscous secretions, pneumonia, or bronchitis. The condensing humidifier makes use of a hygroscopic filter that removes the warmth and natural humidity from the patient's exhaled gas. This moisture evaporates from the filter on the patient's next inspiration. Between 70% and 90% of the patient's body humidity can be met by using this device. Most commonly these are used with a patient who is breathing on a mechanical ventilator.

8. Extubate the patient. (IIIB1d) [R, Ap]

Extubation should only be performed by trained personnel and under the proper conditions to ensure the patient's safety. (See Table 11-4 for a list of complications that can occur after extubation.)

Table 11-4. Complications after Extubation

Endotracheal Tube Removal
Laryngospasm
Regurgitation and aspiration of stomach contents
Aspiration of saliva
Sore throat
Dysphagia
Postintubation laryngeal edema (croup)
Hoarseness from vocal cord edema or paralysis

Tracheostomy Tube Removal
Difficult tube removal from a tight stoma
Granuloma or scar at the stoma
Unhealed, open stoma

Cuff-Related Complications
Granuloma
Tracheomalacia
Tracheal stenosis
Tracheal web formation
Tracheoesophageal fistula
Arterial fistula

a. Endotracheal tube.

The generally recommended steps in extubation include the following:

1. Evaluate the patient's cardiopulmonary status. The reason(s) for the tube being placed should be corrected. The most recent blood gas results should be acceptable. Tracheal secretions should be minimal and not too viscous to be coughed out by the patient. Bedside spirometry results should show an acceptable tidal volume, vital capacity, and maximal inspiratory pressure.
2. Inform the patient about the removal of the tube and the follow-up care that will be needed.
3. The patient's inspired oxygen percentage may be kept the same or increased prior to the extubation. If increased, it should be done at least 5 to 10 minutes before the tube is removed.
4. Suction the trachea until all secretions are removed.
5. Suction the oral pharynx to remove all saliva. Be prepared to suction out additional oral secretions and mucus after extubation.
6. In rapid succession:

    a. Give a deep sigh breath.
    b. Deflate the cuff. Cut the inflation tube to the cuff to ensure its collapse.
    c. Pull out the tube when the lungs are full.

    Alternatively, in rapid succession:

    a. Give a deep sigh breath.
    b. Place a suction catheter through the tube into the trachea. This works best with a self-contained catheter and sheath system.
    c. Deflate the cuff. Cut the inflation tube to the cuff to ensure its collapse.
    d. Pull out the tube when the lungs are full.
    e. Apply suction as the tube is withdrawn.

7. Have the patient cough vigorously to remove any secretions.
8. Apply a cool, bland aerosol by face mask with the previous amount of oxygen.
9. Monitor and evaluate the patient every 30 minutes for several hours. Encourage deep breathing and coughing. Check the vital signs. Measure pulse oximetry or arterial blood gases after 20 minutes. Listen to the breath sounds and larynx. Inspiratory stridor is a sign of laryngeal edema. Be prepared to nebulize racemic epinephrine (Vaponephrine) if needed. Be prepared to reintubate the patient if necessary.

b. Tracheostomy tube.

1. Follow steps 1 to 7 from the previous list.
2. Depending on the physician's order, do one of the following:

    a. Apply a bland aerosol by tracheostomy mask to the stoma site with the previous amount of oxygen.
    b. Cover the stoma site with a sterile 4″ × 4″ dressing. Tape it in place. Apply a bland aerosol by face mask with the previous amount of oxygen.

3. Monitor and evaluate the patient every 30 minutes for several hours. Encourage deep breathing and coughing. Check the vital signs and breath sounds. Measure pulse oximetry or arterial blood gases after 20 minutes. Be prepared to reintubate the patient if necessary.
4. Routine stoma care to ensure healing usually includes the following each shift:

    a. Remove the dressing. Inspect the stoma for signs of infection such as pus, redness, and swelling.
    b. Clean the stoma site with hydrogen peroxide on a sterile gauze pad.
    c. Apply antibiotic ointment to the stoma site.
    d. Reapply a sterile dressing.

Module B.   Airway Equipment.

1.   Oral and nasal endotracheal tubes.
a.   Select the proper tube. (IIIB1a) [R, Ap]

An endotracheal tube is the best emergency device for maintaining a secure airway. It also provides a direct suctioning route to the lungs and prevents aspiration. Mechanical ventilation can easily be provided through it. An endotracheal tube is meant to be a temporary airway; however, it can be kept in patients for weeks if necessary. Virtually all endotracheal tubes used clinically now are made of pliable plastic. Always select a tube that has a large residual volume, low pressure cuff unless there is a specific reason not to. These cuffs have the advantage of easily conforming to the shape of the patient's airway so that a seal can be made without using excessive pressure. For the most part, oral and nasal endotracheal tubes can be used interchangeably. They both serve the same purposes. In a side-by-side comparison, it will be noted that the nasal endotracheal tube is longer and more curved than an oral endotracheal tube. The greater curve of the nasal tube should result in less pressure on the nasal mucosa. An anesthesiologist would request a nasal tube if he or she is going to place it by the nasal route. Oral tubes are used in the majority of patients.

The tubes come in sizes from 4-mm outer diameter (OD) through 4-mm OD so that patients of all ages and sizes can be intubated. The OD size increments are 0.5 mm. The outer wall of the tube varies from 0.5 to 1 mm. This results in the inner diameter (ID) of the tube being reduced by about 1 to 2 mm. It is important to select the tube for the patient that has the largest ID because it will result in the lowest airway resistance. Table 11-3 lists the approximate ID of an endotracheal tube to place into a patient based on his or her age. Once the tube is properly placed into the patient, the excess tube, beyond 3 to 4 cm past the teeth, should be cut off. This will further reduce the airway resistance and mechanical dead space.

Most endotracheal tubes have the standard features shown in Fig. 11-12. There are a number of specialty endotracheal tubes that can be found in limited use. They all share the same characteristics except for some special feature. If available, these tubes are worth looking over.

Pediatric Endotracheal Tubes.—Pediatric endotracheal tubes come in two basic types. One type has a constant diameter. Some manufacturers place a black ring mark on the tube about 2 cm from the tip. During intubation, the tube should be inserted until the mark is at the vocal cords. Manufacturers include Portex and National Catheter. The second type, manufactured by Cole, has a relatively wide proximal part to the body that narrows at the distal end. The design is supposed

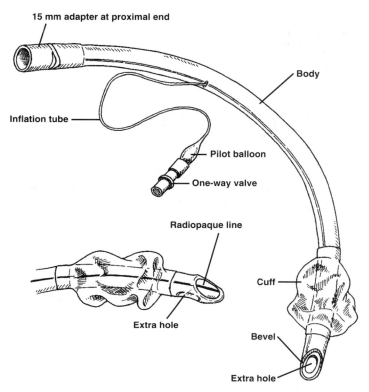

15 mm adapter at proximal end

Body

Inflation tube

Pilot balloon

One-way valve

Radiopaque line

Cuff

Extra hole

Bevel

Extra hole

Fig. 11-12 A typical, modern endotracheal tube with its component parts. The insert shows the important features found at the distal end of the tube. (From Sills JR: *Respiratory care certification guide: the complete review resource for the entry level exam,* ed 2, St. Louis, 1994, Mosby–Year Book. Used by permission.)

to allow the smaller diameter tip to be passed through the vocal cords but prevent the wide "shoulder" from passing into the trachea. Both types of tube end with a single opening with a bevel cut (see Fig. 11-13). Neither type has a cuff on any tube that is 2 to 3 mm ID or smaller.

Armored Tubes.—Armored tubes have a steel spring coiled through them. An advantage of the armored tubes over regular ones is that they will not collapse if the patient should bite down. Furthermore, the tube may be prebent for shape and will not kink like a plastic tube might.

Preformed Tubes.—Preformed tubes have been preshaped for better patient comfort or security. One style has a forward bend so that the tube can be taped to the chin. There is also a pediatric tube with a bend for taping it to the forehead.

Guidable (Trigger) Tubes.—Guidable trigger tubes make it easier to intubate a patient with an anterior larynx or to perform a blind nasal intubation (see Fig. 11-14).

High Frequency Jet Ventilation Tube.—A high frequency jet ventilation tube is made by National Catheter Corporation and called the Hi-Lo Jet Tracheal Tube. It is used only with patients undergoing high frequency jet ventilation (HFJV). It

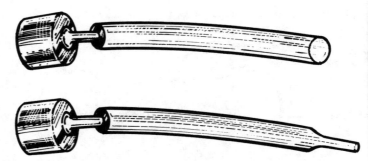

Fig. 11-13 Comparison of the two different types of pediatric endotracheal tubes. The top style of tube is made by several manufacturers and has a uniform diameter. The bottom tube is made by Cole and features a narrowing of the distal tip to pass through the vocal cords. Note that neither has a cuff. (From Burgess WR, Chernick V: *Respiratory therapy in newborn infants and children,* ed 2, New York, 1986, Thieme. Used by permission.)

features four lumens: two for ventilating the patient, one for inflating the cuff, and one for monitoring the proximal airway pressure. See Section 14 for an illustration and more discussion of its clinical use.

There may be other specialty tubes that exist on the marketplace. It would be wise to gain experience with as many different types of endotracheal tubes as possible.

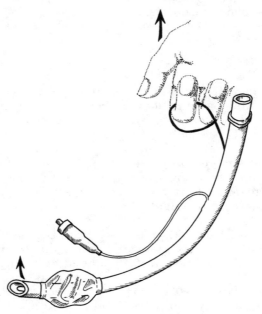

Fig. 11-14 Guidable or "trigger" type endotracheal tube. A wire is imbedded within the wall of the tube. When the ring at the proximal is pulled, the distal tip is flexed up to shorten the radius of the curve. This allows the tube to be directed into an anterior trachea. (Modified from Heffner JE: Managing difficult intubations in critically ill patients, *Respir Management* 19(3), 1989.)

b.   Fix any problems with the tube. (IIB2e4) [An]

Refer to Fig. 11-12 for the components of a standard endotracheal tube. Make sure that the 15-mm adapter is inserted snugly into the proximal end of the tube body. Before intubating the patient, the cuff should be inflated and the syringe disconnected from the one-way valve. This is to make sure that the system works properly. The cuff should hold the air. Do not use any tube with a leaking cuff or one-way valve. Deflate the cuff before placing the tube into a patient.

2.   Double-lumen endotracheal tubes.
a.   Select the proper tube. (IIA1c1) [R, Ap]

Double-lumen endotracheal tubes are used to allow simultaneous independent lung ventilation. A double-lumen tube is also used during special procedures with one lung such as bronchoscopy, bronchoalveolar lavage, lobectomy, and pneumonectomy. The other lung may be mechanically ventilated to maintain the patient's blood gas values (see Fig. 11-15). An adapter can be added to join the two proximal ends of the channels together so that a single ventilator can be used to ventilate both lungs. The Carlens tube is used to preferentially intubate the left bronchus. The White tube is used to preferentially intubate the right bronchus (see Fig. 11-16 for both). Robertshaw makes tubes for either right or left bronchial intubation.

There are several limitations inherent in all double-lumen tubes. First, they can only be used on adults because the smallest size is 8-mm OD. Second, the small internal diameter of the two lumens results in a high airway resistance. Third,

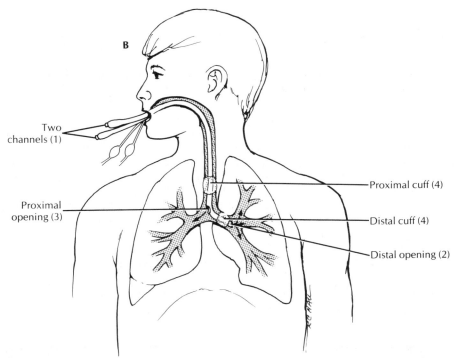

Fig. 11-15 A double-lumen endotracheal tube properly positioned in the patient so that both lungs can be independently ventilated, suctioned, or have special procedures performed. (From Eubanks DH, Bone RC: *Comprehensive respiratory care,* ed 2, St. Louis, 1990. Mosby–Year Book. Used by permission.)

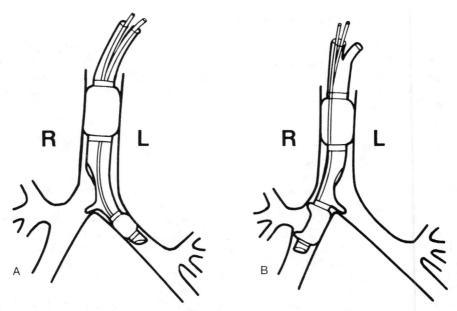

Fig. 11-16 Two types of double-lumen endotracheal tubes. **A,** A Carlens tube; its distal tube enters the left mainstem bronchus. **B,** A White tube; its distal tube enters the right mainstem bronchus. Note how both tubes have a cuff that seals the trachea and a cuff that seals a bronchus. Each has its own inflation tube, pilot balloon, and one-way valve. (From Miller RD, editor: *Anesthesia,* New York, 1981, Churchill Livingston. Used by permission.)

a much smaller than normal suction catheter will have to be used to remove any tracheal secretions.

b. Put the tube together, make sure that it works properly, and identify any problems with it. (IIB1d1) [R, Ap]

Each of the double-lumen endotracheal tubes has its own 15-mm adapter, cuff, one-way valve, pilot balloon, and inflation tube to inflate the cuff. As with traditional endotracheal tubes, both cuffs should be test-inflated. They should hold the air without a leak and then be easily deflated. There is one additional piece of equipment that can be used with a double-lumen tube—a plastic wye that can be used to connect together the proximal ends of both tubes. This is done by removing both 15-mm adapters and inserting one branch of the wye into each of the proximal ends of the tubes. The open end of the wye has a 15-mm adapter so that it can be connected to a ventilator or oxygen source.

c. Fix any problems with the tube. (IIB2e3) [R, Ap, An]

As with a traditional endotracheal tube, do not use a double-lumen tube if the cuffs cannot be inflated and deflated properly. Make sure that both lumens are patent.

3. Fix any problems with intubation equipment: laryngoscope and blades. (IIB2e2) [An]

The laryngoscope is made up of two basic parts: a handle and a blade. The most commonly seen handle is made of stainless steel; some newer units are made of plastic. The handle contains two C-size batteries to power the light source in the blade. They all have a common base with a hooking bar so that the blades can be attached (see Figs. 11-2 and 11-3). The light source will shine when the handle and blade are properly connected because an electrical circuit has been completed. Failure of the light source to shine could be from any of the following problems:

1. The handle and blade are not properly connected and snapped into place. Disconnect them by performing the opposite motions noted earlier. Reconnect them properly.
2. You have cross connected stainless steel and plastic components. As mentioned earlier, only stainless steel handles go with stainless steel blades and plastic handles with plastic blades.
3. The batteries are low as shown by the bulb failing to glow or glowing with a yellow instead of white light. Unscrew the lid from the handle. Replace the old batteries with two new C-size batteries. When reassembled, the bulb should glow with a white light.
4. The batteries are not placed properly. The positive poles (+) must be toward the base of the handle and the negative poles (−) must be toward the cap of the handle. When reassembled, the bulb should glow with a white light.
5. The light bulb in the stainless steel blade is loose or defective. Tighten the light bulb by turning it clockwise. It should light up if it was just loose. Unscrew and throw away a defective light bulb. Replace it with a light bulb of the same size. When reassembled, the bulb should glow with a white light. The newer plastic laryngoscopes use a fiberoptic bundle as the light source; there is no light bulb to tighten or replace.

The discussion on intubation equipment would not be complete without listing all the standard equipment that should be available for both oral and nasal approaches. See Table 11-5 for this list.

Table 11-5. Equipment for Oral and Nasal Intubation

Pediatric and adult laryngoscope handles with batteries
Straight and curved pediatric and adult laryngoscope blades
Variety of nasal and oral endotracheal tubes
Water soluble, sterile lubricant
Metal stylet
Magill forceps for nasal intubation
Hemostat
Tongue depressors
Oropharyngeal airways
Bite block
Nasopharyngeal airways
10-ml syringe with three-way stopcock
Manometer to measure intracuff pressure
Tape or tube restraining device
Yankauer or other oral suction device
Sterile suction catheter for tracheal suctioning
Stethoscope for listening to breath sounds

4.   Fix any problems with a tracheostomy tube. (IIB2e1) [An]

It is important that the various types of tracheostomy tubes be worked with to understand how they operate, what can go wrong with them, and how they should be fixed. Fig. 11-11 shows a standard tracheostomy tube with its components. Fig. 11-17 shows a fenestrated tracheostomy tube and Fig. 11-18 shows a Pitt "speaking" tracheostomy tube.

Most tubes have cuffs that must be inflated before insertion into the patient to make sure that the cuff is sealed and the one-way valve does not leak. Do not use a tube with a leaking cuff or one-way valve. Kamen-Wilkinson endotracheal and tracheostomy tubes are an exception because they have a self-inflating foam cuff. A syringe is used to *deflate* the cuff before placement into the patient. The cuff should stay deflated. A leaking cuff will reinflate and should be discarded. In a properly functioning cuff, removing the syringe and opening the pilot balloon valve to room air pressure results in the cuff inflating.

Make sure that the obturator, inner cannula, and/or plug all fit properly into the outer cannula. They should all easily snap into place and be easily removable. Check this before inserting the tube into the patient. Secretions or foreign matter can plug the lumen of the cannula. Suction to remove any obstruction. If the catheter cannot be inserted beyond the tube and the patient is having respiratory distress, the tube will have to be removed and replaced. A mucus plug or cuff that has herniated or slipped over the end of the tube can cause this.

5.   Fix any problems with a tracheostomy button. (IIB2e1) [An]

Fig. 11-19 shows a standard tracheostomy button and Fig. 11-20 shows a Kistner tracheostomy button. It is recommended that the practitioner be familiar with both types and their component parts.

Make sure that all the component pieces of both types of tracheostomy buttons fit together properly and can be easily disconnected if necessary. The cannula must be kept clear of any secretions, blood, or foreign debris. A suction catheter should be passable through the hollow opening in the cannula. If the button is obstructed and the patient is having trouble breathing through his or her upper airway, the button should be removed and replaced with another or a tracheostomy tube.

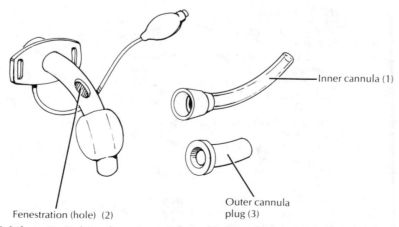

Inner cannula (1)

Outer cannula plug (3)

Fenestration (hole) (2)

Fig. 11-17 A fenestrated tracheostomy tube with its component parts and features. (From Eubanks DH, Bone RC: *Comprehensive respiratory care,* ed 2, St. Louis, 1990, Mosby–Year Book. Used by permission.)

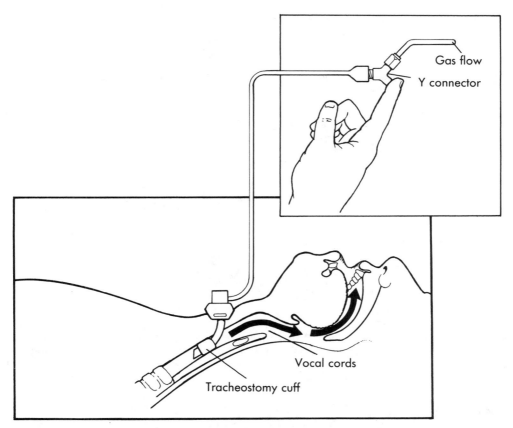

Fig. 11-18 The Pitt tracheostomy tube permits the patient to speak. Note its special feature that directs an outside gas flow past the vocal cords. (From Simmons KF: Airway care. From Scanlan CL, Spearman CB, Sheldon RL, editors: *Egan's fundamentals of respiratory care,* ed 5, St. Louis, 1990, Mosby–Year Book. Used by permission.)

6. Fix any problems with a cuff pressure manometer. (IIB2k2) [Ap]

There are several commercially available cuff pressure manometers. Cufflator is a popular brand. In addition, a blood pressure manometer, three-way stopcock, and 10-ml syringe can be assembled as shown in Fig. 11-10 to measure cuff pressure. With any of these systems it is necessary to keep air-tight connections. An air leak would be indicated if the pressure drops suddenly. Tighten the connections to create a seal so that the pressure is maintained.

7. Exhaled carbon dioxide detector.
a. Get the necessary equipment. (IIA1c2) [R, Ap]

If the clinical goal is to easily and quickly confirm that the endotracheal tube is properly placed there are two choices. A disposable unit such as the Easy Cap end-tidal CO_2 detector made by Nellcor could be selected. Its carbon dioxide indicator changes color from dark purple to yellow when CO_2 is exhaled through it. Another choice is the MiniCAP III CO_2 Detector made by MSA Catalyst Research. It is a reusable item that has a mainstream type of infrared carbon dioxide detector.

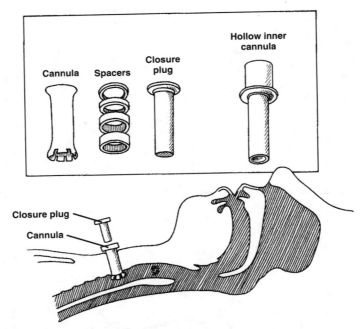

Fig. 11-19 A typical tracheostomy button with its component parts. The airway picture shows the tracheostomy button properly positioned in the patient. (From Sills JR: *Respiratory care certification guide: the complete review resource for the entry level exam,* ed 2, St. Louis, 1991, Mosby–Year Book. Used by permission.)

The unit is powered by a battery pack. Its light-emitting diode (LED) signals the presence of carbon dioxide with each exhalation.

A capnograph should be selected if it is necessary to get a more accurate CO_2 reading. Its general function and the interpretation of capnography tracings was discussed in Section 4. The use of capnography to evaluate the effectiveness of CPR was discussed in Section 10. A possible disadvantage of this system is that it will take more time to set up than the Easy Cap.

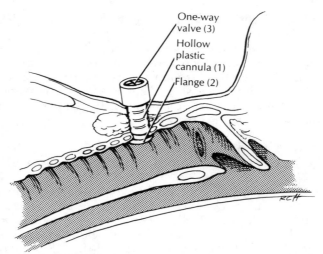

Fig. 11-20 A Kistner tracheostomy button. (From Eubanks DH, Bone RC: *Comprehensive respiratory care,* ed 2, St. Louis, 1990, Mosby–Year Book. Used by permission.)

b. Put the equipment together, make sure that it works properly, and identify any problems with it. (IIB1d2) [R, Ap]

The Easy Cap comes as a single unit within a sealed foil container. Before using it, match the initial purple color of the indicator with the purple color labeled CHECK on the product dome. Do *not* use an Easy Cap unit whose color is not the same or darker than that on the product dome. If the color is correct, the Easy Cap can be used. Remove both caps from the patient and circuit connector ports. The Easy Cap is then attached to the patient's endotracheal tube by its 15-mm ID connector port. The Easy Cap's 15-mm OD circuit end is connected to the manual resuscitator to ventilate the patient. If a heat and moisture exchanger (HME) is used, it should be placed between the patient's endotracheal tube and the Easy Cap and manual resuscitator. The Easy Cap should not be used with a heated humidifier or nebulizer because too much humidity will affect its accuracy. The following items can contaminate the Easy Cap and cause a patchy yellow or white discoloration of the indicator: stomach contents, mucus, pulmonary edema fluid, and intratracheal epinephrine. The color will not change with the breathing cycle. Throw away this Easy Cap unit.

The MiniCAP III has a disposable adapter that connects the mainstream CO_2 detector to the patient's endotracheal tube. The adapter has a 15-mm ID end for attachment to the endotracheal tube and a 15-mm OD end to which the manual resuscitator can be attached. The assembly and operation of a capnograph is discussed in Section 4. Review it if necessary.

c. Fix any problems with the equipment. (IIB2e5) [R, Ap, An]

Because the Easy Cap comes as a self-contained single piece unit there is nothing to repair. Contamination problems with the unit were discussed earlier. If the unit's color changes are not normal, it should be discarded. The caps over the two connector ports must be removed to attach the Easy Cap to the endotracheal tube and manual resuscitator. The 15-mm ID patient connector port will only fit over the endotracheal tube adapter. The 15-mm OD circuit connector port will only fit into the manual resuscitator or demand-valve adapter.

The adapter is the only removable part in the MiniCAP III. It will only fit in one direction into the CO_2 detection unit. As mentioned earlier, only one end of the adapter will fit onto an endotracheal tube and the other end of the adapter will only fit into a manual resuscitator outlet. Troubleshooting with a capnograph was presented in Section 4.

This ends the general discussion on specific airway management procedures and equipment. The Registry Exams may ask questions about this material and the related material presented next. Some information may have to be reviewed from Sections 1, 4, and 10.

Module C. Patient assessment.

1. Examine all the data to determine the patient's pathophysiological condition. (IC3a) [R, Ap, An]

A chest x-ray should always be taken to confirm the location of a newly placed endotracheal or tracheostomy tube. All modern endotracheal and tracheostomy tubes contain a strip of radiopaque material near the distal tip of the tube. This is easily noticed as the white line seen on the chest x-ray and confirms the location of the tip of the tube in the airway (see Fig. 11-12). The chest x-ray should be repeated if there has been a significant change in the patient's condition or if the tube has been pulled back or pushed deeper into the trachea. The chest x-ray will also detect a pneumothorax related to the tracheostomy procedure or other pulmonary conditions.

2. Take part in the development of the respiratory care plan. (IC3c) [An]

In addition to the technical part of the airway, effective communication is important for good patient care. The conscious patient with an endotracheal tube or tracheostomy will be unable to speak. Alternative ways to communicate will have to be provided. Examples include alphabet boards and picture boards for pointing, and pencil and paper for notes. Head nods for yes and no and lip reading are often used. It is important that questions are worded so that they can be answered with a "yes" or "no." Avoid questions that require a lengthy written answer unless the patient seems ready and willing to do so.

It is not possible to predict how a patient will react to the placement of an artificial airway or its prolonged need. Some patients react with relief and relax when the work of breathing is reduced. Others may become angry at the limitations imposed on them. Still others may become depressed. Be prepared to deal with these reactions or changes in the patient's emotional response to this very stressful situation.

BIBLIOGRAPHY

Applebaum EL, Bruce DL: *Tracheal intubation*, Philadelphia, 1976, WB Saunders.

Caldwell SL, Sullivan KN: Artificial airways. In Burton GG, Hodgkin JE, editors: *Respiratory care: a guide to clinical practice*, ed 2, Philadelphia, 1984, JB Lippincott.

Emergency Cardiac Care Committee and Subcommittees, American Heart Association: Guidelines for cardiopulmonary resuscitation and emergency cardiac care: adult advanced cardiac life support, *JAMA* 268(16):2199-2241, 1992.

Eubanks DH, Bone RC: *Comprehensive respiratory care*, ed 2, St. Louis, 1990, Mosby–Year Book.

Fluck RR, Wagner IJ, Wiezalis CP: The esophageal obturator airway: a review, *Respir Care* 27(11):1373-1379, 1982.

Frownfelter DL: Chest physical therapy and airway care. In Barnes TA, editor: *Respiratory care practice*, Chicago, 1988, Year Book Medical.

Heffner JE: Managing difficult intubations in critically ill patients, *Respir Management* 19(3), 1989.

Kovac AL: Dilemmas and controversies in intubation, *Respir Management* 21(4), 1991.

Levitzky MG, Cairo JM, Hall SM: *Introduction to respiratory care*, Philadelphia, 1990, WB Saunders.

McPherson SP: *Respiratory therapy equipment*, ed 4, St. Louis, 1990, Mosby–Year Book.

Plevak DL, Ward JJ: Airway management. In Burton GG, Hodkin JE, Ward JJ, editors: *Respiratory care: a guide to clinical practice*, ed 3, Philadelphia, 1991, JB Lippincott.

Product literature on the Esophageal (Obturator) Airway (EOA) and Esophageal (Gastric Tube) Airway (EGTA), Brunswick Manufacturing Company, Inc, Thacher Lane, Wareham, Mass.

Product literature on the JEM 400 Endotracheal Tube Changer (Guide), Instrumentation Industries Inc, Bethel Park, Penn.

Product literature on the PressureEasy Cuff Pressure Controller, ReviveEasy PtL Airway, and Endotracheal/Trach Tube Pilot Tube Repair Kit, Respironics, Inc, Monroeville, Penn.

Rarey KP, Youtsey JW: *Respiratory patient care*, Englewood Cliffs, NJ, 1981, Prentice Hall.

Roberts JT: *Fundamentals of tracheal intubation*, New York, 1983, Grune & Stratton.

Shapiro BA, Harrison RA, Kacmarek RM et al: *Clinical application of respiratory care*, ed 4, St. Louis, 1991, Mosby–Year Book.

Sills JR: An emergency cuff inflation technique, *Respir Care* 31(3):199-201, 1986.

Sills JR: *Respiratory care certification guide: the complete review resource for the entry level exam*, ed 2, St. Louis, 1994, Mosby–Year Book.

Simmons KF: Airway care. In Scanlan CL, Spearman CB, Sheldon RL, editors: *Egan's fundamentals of respiratory care*, ed 5, St. Louis, 1990, Mosby–Year Book.

Stephenson, HE Jr: Cardiopulmonary resuscitation. In Burton GG, Hodgkin JE, editors: *Respiratory care: a guide to clinical practice*, ed 2, Philadelphia, 1984, JB Lippincott.

Watson MA: Cardiopulmonary resuscitation. In Barnes TA, editor: *Respiratory care practice*, Chicago, 1988, Year Book Medical.

SELF-STUDY QUESTIONS

1. A 45-year-old female patient is brought into the emergency room from an automobile accident. She has facial trauma including a broken nose and jaw. Because of heavy bleeding into her mouth she is having difficulty breathing. Which of the following would you recommend to ensure a safe, effective airway?
   A. Place an oral airway.
   B. Place a tracheostomy tube.
   C. Place a nasopharyngeal airway.
   D. Place a nasal endotracheal tube.

2. The proper endotracheal tube size for a premature newborn is:
   A. 1.5-mm ID
   B. 2.5-mm ID
   C. 3.5-mm ID
   D. 4.0-mm ID
   E. 4.5-mm ID

3. Immediate complications of an oral intubation include all the following EXCEPT:
   A. Tooth trauma
   B. Laceration of the pharynx
   C. Esophageal intubation
   D. Tracheoesophageal fistula
   E. Bronchial intubation

4. You are going to assist in the ambulance transport of a 25-year-old patient. The patient has an oral endotracheal tube and you are going to manually ventilate him during the trip. Which of the following would you choose to help you be sure that the endotracheal tube stays properly situated within the trachea?
   A. Pulse oximetry
   B. Capnography
   C. Easy Cap CO_2 Detector
   D. Electrocardiogram

5.   All the following should be monitored after a patient returns from having a tracheostomy tube placed EXCEPT:
     A.   Cuff pressure
     B.   Bowel sounds
     C.   Bilateral breath sounds
     D.   Excessive bleeding
     E.   Presence of subcutaneous emphysema

6.   Auscultation of a recently intubated patient in respiratory failure reveals diminished breath sounds on the left side of the chest. The most likely cause of this finding is:
     A.   Placement of the endotracheal tube in the right mainstem bronchus
     B.   Placement of the endotracheal tube in the left mainstem bronchus
     C.   Placement of the endotracheal tube in the esophagus
     D.   A pneumothorax on the right side
     E.   A pneumothorax on the left side

7.   All the following are needed for an emergency oral intubation:
     I.   Laryngoscope handle
     II.   Stylet
     III.   Proper laryngoscope blade
     IV.   10-ml syringe
     V.   Magill forceps
     A.   I, II
     B.   I, II, V
     C.   I, II, III, IV
     D.   II, IV, V
     E.   II, III, IV

8.   The proper endotracheal tube size for a 59-kg (130-lb) woman is:
     A.   5.0-mm ID
     B.   6.0-mm ID
     C.   7.0-mm ID
     D.   8.0-mm ID
     E.   9.0-mm ID

9.   You are assisting with the extubation of an adult patient. At what point in the procedure should the tube be removed?
     A.   At the end of a peak inspiratory effort
     B.   At the end of a normal exhalation
     C.   At the start of a tidal volume effort
     D.   At the start of a peak inspiratory effort
     E.   During a forced vital capacity effort

10. Your hospitalized patient rapidly develops ventilatory failure due to an accidental overdose of morphine sulfate for pain control. The preferred method to provide a secure airway would be to:
     A.   Place an oropharyngeal airway.
     B.   Hyperextend the patient's head into the sniffer's position.
     C.   Place an oral endotracheal tube.
     D.   Place an esophageal obturator airway.
     E.   Place a nasal endotracheal tube.

11. Your tracheostomy patient has just returned from a series of x-ray procedures. Suddenly she develops respiratory distress and cannot breathe. Your attempt to pass a suction catheter through the tracheostomy tube does not work. You should proceed to:
    I.   Attempt to pass a smaller suction catheter.
    II.   Remove the tracheostomy tube.
    III. Attempt to ventilate the patient with a manual resuscitator.
    IV.   Replace the tracheostomy tube.
    V.   Call the physician.
    A.   V
    B.   II
    C.   III
    D.   I, III
    E.   IV, V

12. Indications for oral intubation include all the following EXCEPT:
    A.   The patient will require mechanical ventilation.
    B.   The patient has a cervical spine injury.
    C.   The patient will require frequent tracheal suctioning.
    D.   The patient is at risk of vomiting and aspirating.

13. Your patient is an 18-year-old woman who was found unconscious from a drug overdose. She has severe atelectasis of her left lung from lying on that side for 2 days. Her right lung is normal. She is going to require mechanical ventilation to open the atelectatic areas. What endotracheal tube would you suggest so that the abnormal lung may be treated properly?
    A.   Double-lumen
    B.   Standard
    C.   Fenestrated tracheostomy tube
    D.   Armored

14. Your patient has epilepsy and has been having unpredictable seizure activity. What oral endotracheal tube would you suggest be placed into her to provide a secure airway?
    A.   Standard
    B.   Double-lumen
    C.   Preformed
    D.   Armored
    E.   Guidable

Answer Key

1. B; 2. B; 3. D; 4. C; 5. B; 6. A; 7. C; 8. D; 9. A; 10. C; 11. E; 12. B; 13. A; 14. D.

12

Suctioning the Airway

All of the various suctioning techniques (oral, endotracheal, and nasotracheal) should be known by technicians. They are tested exclusively on the Entry Level Exam, but it is still important that therapist students and those taking the Registry Exams be proficient in these procedures.

Module A.   Suctioning devices.

1.   Choose a closed system suctioning catheter. (IIIB3b) [R, Ap]

Closed airway suctioning will be used here to refer to suctioning when the patient remains connected to the original source of oxygen. This may be done through a special aerosol T or, more commonly, with the patient receiving mechanical ventilation. Spontaneously breathing patients are less likely to suffer hypoxemia with sealed airway suctioning because they can continue to inhale the prescribed oxygen percentage. In addition, if the patient is on a ventilator, tidal volume breaths can still be delivered and PEEP levels maintained. If hypoxia does occur it will be less severe and of a shorter duration than with open airway suctioning.

Ballard Medical Products and Concord/Portex have made these units available as a self-contained sterile catheter and protective sheath suctioning system (see Fig. 12-1). In these systems, a flexible, clear plastic sheath covers the catheter to maintain its sterility. Gloves are not needed by the practitioner. The self-contained systems have a financial advantage over the traditional catheter and gloves suctioning method because they can be reused for up to 24 hours. A modified T piece can be attached to the catheter and connected to a patient's endotracheal or tracheostomy tube. Aerosol tubing or a ventilator circuit can be attached to the T piece. This has the clinical benefit of never disconnecting the patient from the source of supplemental oxygen or mechanical ventilation during the suctioning procedure. It must be remembered to completely withdraw the catheter from the endotracheal tube into the sheath or it will act as a partial obstruction. These closed-system suction catheters come with either the traditional straight tip or the Coude tip for selective bronchial suctioning.

Another device to create a sealed system for endotracheal tube suctioning consists of an elbow adapter that has an inner plastic sleeve or diaphragm. As the traditional catheter is inserted into the opening on the elbow adapter, the sleeve or diaphragm conforms to the catheter so that there is no air leak (see Fig. 12-2). This ensures that the ventilator-delivered volumes and pressures are not lost through a leak. Manufacturers include Marquest Medical Products with its Trach Swivel

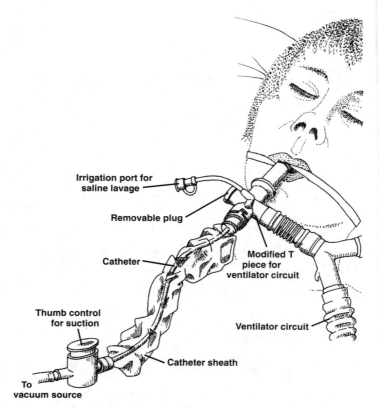

Fig. 12-1 A self-contained catheter and sheath suctioning system. (Based on the Ballard Medical Products suction system and the TRACH-CARE Continuous Suction System. From Sills JR: *Respiratory care certification guide: the complete review resource for the entry level exam,* ed 2, St. Louis, 1994, Mosby–Year Book. Used by permission.)

Adaptor with Port that is used with adults and B + B Medical Technologies with its Neo$_2$Safe adaptor that is used with neonates.

As with traditional catheters, the closed-system suction catheters must be the correct size based on the inner diameter of the endotracheal or tracheostomy tube. Normally a catheter's outer diameter should be no more than one half the inner diameter of the endotracheal tube. See Table 12-1 for the ideal size of the suction catheter based on the different sizes of artificial airways. A larger catheter creates too much obstruction in the tube for the patient to easily breathe around. See Fig. 12-3 for an illustration of the relative sizes of a 12 French suction catheter and an 8-mm ID endotracheal tube.

Module B.   Vacuum regulator systems.

1.   Put the equipment together, make sure that it works properly, and identify any problems with it. (IIB1I1) [R, Ap]

The vacuum regulators come preassembled by the manufacturer. There are two basic types, which are described here. Components must be added to make them fully functional.

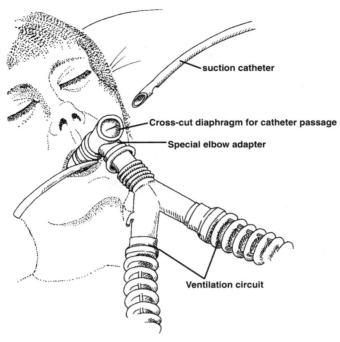

suction catheter

Cross-cut diaphragm for catheter passage

Special elbow adapter

Ventilation circuit

Fig. 12-2 Features and placement of a special elbow adapter that can be suctioned through without losing tidal volume or pressure when the patient is being mechanically ventilated. (From Sills JR: *Respiratory care certification guide: the complete review resource for the entry level exam,* ed 2, St. Louis, 1994, Mosby–Year Book. Used by permission.)

Table 12-1. Recommended Suction Catheter French Sizes for the Various Endotracheal and Tracheostomy Tube Sizes

Age	Inner Diameters of Tube Sizes (mm)	Suction Catheter Size (French)
Newborn		
Less than 1000 grams	2.5	5
1000-2000 grams	3.0	6
2000-3000 grams	3.5	8
Greater than 3000 grams to 6 months old	3.5-4.0	8
Pediatric		
18 months	4.0	8
3 years	4.5	8
5 years	5.0	10
6 years	5.5	10
8 years	6.0	10
Adult		
16 years	7.0	10
Normal adult female	7.5-8.0	12
Normal adult male	8.0-8.5	14
Large adult	9.0-10.0	16

It is recommended to use a suction catheter with an outer diameter that is no more than half of the inner diameter of the endotracheal tube.

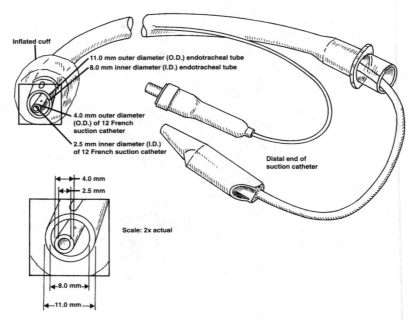

Inflated cuff

11.0 mm outer diameter (O.D.) endotracheal tube
8.0 mm inner diameter (I.D.) endotracheal tube

4.0 mm outer diameter
(O.D.) of 12 French
suction catheter

2.5 mm inner diameter (I.D.)
of 12 French suction catheter

Distal end of
suction catheter

4.0 mm
2.5 mm

Scale: 2x actual

8.0 mm
11.0 mm

Fig. 12-3 The relative sizes of a 12 French suction catheter within an 8 mm ID endotracheal tube. The insert shows them at twice their actual sizes for clarity. Note how when the outer diameter of the catheter is no more than half the inner diameter of the endotracheal tube the patient can still breathe around it.

Portable Vacuum Systems

The portable systems generally include an electrically powered vacuum pump with an on/off switch and a collection jar with lid. Some units have a control valve for adjusting the level of negative pressure. A negative pressure gauge is used to determine how much vacuum is being applied. A length of rubber vacuum tubing is used to pass the negative pressure from the pump to the collection jar. Another length of vacuum tubing is used to pass the vacuum through to the suction catheter. These units come mounted on a wheeled cart so that they may be moved from patient to patient. Portable systems are not as powerful as the central vacuum systems. They will not be very effective at suctioning out large amounts of viscous secretions.

In general, the following steps are needed to make the units operational:

1. Plug the vacuum pump into a working electrical outlet.
2. Place a clean, empty collection jar into its holder on the cart. The jar must be able to hold at least 500 ml of fluid.
3. Slip the rubber lid onto the open top of the collection jar. Both vacuum tubing connectors on the lid must be patent.
4. Slip one end of a short length of vacuum tubing over the connector on the vacuum pump and the other end to one of the tubing connectors on the collection jar lid.
5. Slip one end of a length of vacuum tubing over the other tubing connector on the collection jar lid. The vacuum tubing should be no more

than 3 feet long. The other end of the vacuum tubing is connected to the suction catheter when needed.
6. Determine the negative pressure by:

    a. Pinching closed the long vacuum tubing
    b. Turning on the vacuum pump
    c. Observing the pressure on the negative pressure gauge

7. If the unit has a fixed vacuum level, the observed negative pressure should match that listed by the manufacturer.
8. If the unit has a variable vacuum level, adjust the vacuum control knob to the desired level.

Check the following when trying to determine the cause of a loss of vacuum:

    a. Make sure that the vacuum pump is plugged into a working electrical outlet.
    b. The vacuum pump must be turned on.
    c. Make sure that the vacuum control valve is set at the desired negative pressure.
    d. The lid to the collection jar should be tightly sealed.
    e. The vacuum tubing must tightly connect the pump to the collection jar and the collection jar to the suction catheter.
    f. Make sure that there are no knots or obstructions in the vacuum tubing or catheter.
    g. The collection jar must not be filled above its maximum level.

Correct any potential problems. Do not use a portable vacuum system that will not generate the negative pressure that it is supposed to.

Central Vacuum Systems

Central (wall) vacuum systems are usually available at each patient's bedside in all special care units. Each of the wall outlets is connected through a hospital-wide piping system to a large electrically powered vacuum pump. It is capable of generating a negative pressure of 480 to 635 mm Hg. This is a far greater vacuum pressure than what is needed in most patient care situations. A regulator is used to reduce the vacuum to the desired clinical level (see Fig. 12-4). Either a Quick Connect or Diameter Index Safety System (DISS) connector is used to attach the regulator to the central vacuum system.

Most regulators have a selector knob that allows the user to turn the vacuum off (Off setting) or switch between full vacuum (Full setting) and a regulated level of vacuum (Reg setting). The Full setting opens the unit to the maximum level of vacuum available from the central pump. The Reg setting allows the user to adjust the vacuum level between 0 and 200 mm Hg. A flow of 110 to 150 L/min can be obtained at the maximum negative pressure.

In general, the following steps are needed to make the units operational:

1. Connect the regulator into a working suction outlet.
2. Screw a clean, empty collection jar onto its connector on the regulator. The jar must be able to hold at least 500 ml of fluid.
3. Slip one end of a length of vacuum tubing over the tubing connector on the collection jar. The vacuum tubing should be no more than 3 feet long.

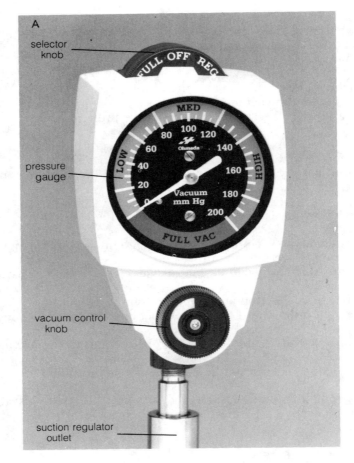

Fig. 12-4 Features of an Ohmeda central vacuum regulator with a three-position selector knob. (Courtesy of Ohmeda, Madison, Wis.)

The other end of the vacuum tubing is connected to the suction catheter when needed.

4. Determine the negative pressure by:

  a. Pinching closed the vacuum tubing (see Fig. 12-5)
  b. Turning the selector knob to Reg
  c. Observing the pressure on the negative pressure gauge

5. Adjust the vacuum control knob to the desired level. In general, the vacuum level is set as low as possible to easily suction out the secretions. Plevak and Ward (1991) and Eubanks and Bone (1990) suggest the following ranges for vacuum:

  a. Adults: 100 to 120 mm Hg
  b. Children: 80 to 100 mm Hg
  c. Neonates: 60 to 80 mm Hg

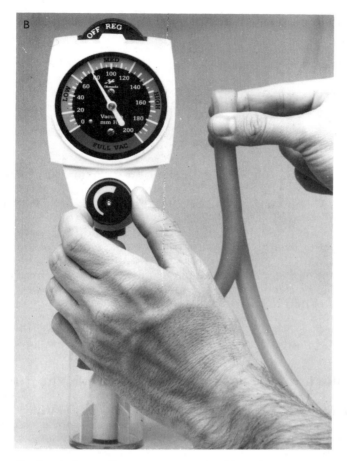

Fig. 12-5 Setting the level of negative pressure on the Ohmeda central vacuum regulator by pinching the vacuum tubing and adjusting the vacuum control knob. The vacuum pressure is seen on the pressure gauge. (Courtesy of Ohmeda, Madison, Wis.)

If the secretions are too viscous to be drawn up the suction catheter, the negative pressure must be increased.

Check the following when trying to determine the cause of a loss of vacuum:

a. Make sure that the regulator is plugged into a working vacuum outlet.

b. Make sure that the vacuum control valve is set at the desired negative pressure.

c. The collection jar should be tightly screwed onto the suction regulator outlet.

d. The vacuum tubing must tightly connect the collection jar to the suction catheter.

e. Make sure that there are no knots or obstructions in the vacuum tubing or catheter.

f. The collection jar must not be filled above its maximum level.

Correct any potential problems. Do not use a central vacuum system outlet that will not generate the negative pressure that it should. Occasionally, there will be less negative pressure than expected when the central vacuum system is being heavily used. There is no problem with the regulator or tubing and the vacuum pressure will increase when fewer people are using it.

C. Modify the suctioning procedure.

1. Make a change in the size and type of suction catheter. (IIIC8a) [An]

As discussed earlier, the outer diameter of the suction catheter should be no more than half the inner diameter of the patient's endotracheal tube. If the secretions are easy to suction out, a smaller catheter may be used. The spontaneously breathing patient is less likely to become hypoxic if the tube is less obstructed.

A catheter with a Coudé tip should be used if the catheter needs to be directed into one or the other mainstem bronchi. Closed-system catheters such as those made by Ballard Medical Products offer two advantages over single use catheters. First, they are more economical if the patient needs frequent suctioning. Second, patients on mechanical ventilators will continue to be ventilated, oxygenated, and have PEEP maintained during the suctioning episode. The newer catheters that offer intermittent or continuous insufflation of oxygen may reduce the hypoxemia that many patients experience during the suctioning procedure; however, they are difficult to use and costly.

2. Change the level of vacuum used when suctioning. (IIIC8c) [An]

In general, the lowest possible vacuum level should be used that adequately removes secretions. Several authors have listed recommended maximum vacuum levels to be applied to adults, children, and neonates. These were listed earlier; however, the AARC Clinical Practice Guidelines on suctioning state that there is a lack of experimental data to support these or any other written maximum pressures.

3. Instill an irrigating solution into the trachea. (IIIC8b) [An]

Sterile normal saline (.9%) is widely accepted as useful to instill into the trachea to dilute and mobilize pulmonary secretions. It should be used whenever secretions are difficult to suction out. Also, by making the secretions easier to remove, a lower vacuum level can be used. In adults, about 5 to 10 ml are instilled into the trachea and then suctioned out with any secretions. Less is used with children, but no universal guidelines are available. Neonates have been reportedly given a few drops to 0.33 ml.

4. Change the frequency of suctioning. (IIIC8d) [An]

Secretions obstruct the airways and should be removed if possible. Often this requires more than one suctioning episode. There is no harm in repeatedly suctioning the patient as long as he or she is reoxygenated in between. Watch for any complications as listed in Tables 12-2 and 12-3. Also, listen to the patient's breath sounds for rhonchi or palpate the chest for secretions in between suctioning efforts. Obviously, stop suctioning when it is no longer needed.

Table 12-2. Hazards/Complications of
Endotracheal Suctioning

Cardiac arrest
Respiratory arrest
Hypoxemia
Cardiac arrhythmias
Bronchospasm
Increased intracranial pressure
Hypertension
Hypotension
Apnea from interruption of mechanical ventilation
Pulmonary hemorrhage
Mechanical trauma to tracheal and bronchial
   mucosa
Infection to and/or from patient and respiratory
   care practitioner
Atelectasis

Table 12-3. Contraindications and
Hazards or Complications of
Nasotracheal Suctioning

Contraindications
Absolute
Epiglottitis
Laryngotracheobronchitis (croup)
Relative
Blocked nasal passages
Nasal bleeding
Acute facial, neck, or head injury
Bleeding disorder
Upper respiratory tract infection
Irritable airway
Laryngospasm

Hazards or Complications
Cardiac arrest
Respiratory arrest
Hypoxemia
Cardiac arrhythmias
Bronchospasm
Increased intracranial pressure
Hypertension
Hypotension
Pulmonary hemorrhage
Infection to and/or from patient and respiratory
   care practitioner
Atelectasis
Pain
Catheter misdirected into esophagus
Gagging and/or vomiting
Uncontrolled cough
Mechanical trauma: nasal turbinates, perforation
   of pharynx, nasal bleeding, bleeding of the
   tracheal and bronchial mucosa

5. Change the duration of the suctioning procedure. (IIIC8e) [An]

Generally speaking, suctioning should take between 5 and 10 seconds; the entire procedure should take between 10 and 15 seconds. Some patients may not be able to tolerate this. Be prepared to suction for a shorter period of time. Suction repeatedly rather than increase the suctioning time.

As listed in Tables 12-2 and 12-3, stop the procedure if the patient becomes hypoxic or has tachycardia, bradycardia, arrhythmias, hypotension, or bronchospasm. Bloody secretions could indicate mucosal damage and would justify stopping the procedure.

Hypoxemia, tachycardia, bradycardia, arrhythmias, hypotension, bronchospasm, pneumothorax, or pulmonary hemorrhage that place the patient's life in danger would indicate the cancellation of the suctioning order. Once the underlying problem has been corrected and safe suctioning can be performed, the order may be resumed.

This ends the general discussion on suctioning the airway. Details on patient assessment that relate to suctioning are found earlier in this section or in Section 1. A few general comments are added here as necessary.

Module D. Patient assessment.

1. Examine all of the data to determine the patient's pathophysiological condition. (IC3a) [R, Ap, An]

Pneumonia and bronchitis result in chest x-ray changes that show areas of infiltrate. Right and/or left lung involvement, individual lobes, and segments with disease can be determined. Suctioning can help to remove secretions so that air is more likely to reach the affected areas. If the left lung is involved, a Coudé catheter should be used to help direct the catheter down the left mainstem bronchus. A mucus trap should be used to obtain a sputum sample to send to the laboratory for culture and sensitivity testing. As the patient's condition improves, the chest x-ray should show clearing of infiltrates.

2. Take part in the development of the respiratory care plan. (IC3c) [An]

Examples of things to consider when making up the respiratory care plan may include but are not limited to:

1. Delivering an aerosolized bronchodilator or mucolytic before suctioning.
2. Performing postural drainage therapy before suctioning.
3. Using a different size catheter.
4. Instilling normal saline into the patient's trachea.
5. Hyperoxygenating the patient before and after tracheal suctioning.
6. Increasing or decreasing the negative pressure based on the viscosity of the secretions.

BIBLIOGRAPHY

AARC Clinical Practice Guideline: Nasotracheal suctioning, *Respir Care* 37(8):898-901, 1992.

AARC Clinical Practice Guideline: Endotracheal suctioning of mechanically ventilated adults and children with artificial airways, *Respir Care* 38(5):500-504, 1993.

Bodai BI, Briggs SW, Goldstein M et al: Evaluation of the ability of the Neo$_2$Safe valve to minimize desaturation in neonates during suctioning. *Respir Care* 34(5):355-359, 1991.

Burton GG: Practical physical diagnosis in respiratory care. In Burton GG, Hodgkin JE, editors: *Respiratory Care*, ed 2, Philadelphia, 1984, JB Lippincott.

Burton GG: Patient assessment procedures. In Barnes TA, editor: *Respiratory care practice*, Chicago, 1988, Year Book Medical.

Caldwell SL, Sullivan KN: Artificial airways. In Burton GG, Hodgkin JE, editors: *Respiratory care*, ed 2, Philadelphia, 1984, JB Lippincott.

Caldwell SL, Sullivan KN: Suctioning protocol. In Burton GG, Hodgkin JE, editors: *Respiratory care*, ed 2, Philadelphia, 1984, JB Lippincott.

Chapman GA, Kim CS, Frankel J et al: Evaluation of the safety and efficiency of a new suction catheter design, *Respir Care* 31(10):889-895, 1986.

Emergency Cardiac Care Committee and Subcommittees, American Heart Association: Guidelines for cardiopulmonary resuscitation and emergency cardiac care, *JAMA* 268(16):2262-2281, 1992.

Eubanks DH, Bone RC: *Comprehensive respiratory care*, ed 2, St. Louis, 1990, Mosby–Year Book.

Frownfelter DL: Chest physical therapy and airway care. In Barnes TA, editor: *Respiratory care practice*, Chicago, 1988, Year Book Medical.

Guidelines for the prevention of nosocomial infections, *AARCTimes* Sep 1983.

Lehre S: *Understanding lung sounds*, Philadelphia, 1984, WB Saunders.

Miller BF, Keane CB: *Encyclopedia and dictionary of medicine, nursing, and allied health*, ed 3, Philadelphia, 1983, WB Saunders.

Nath AR, Capel LH: Lung crackles in bronchiectasis, *Thorax* 35:694, 1980.

Plevak DJ, Ward JJ: Airway management. In Burton GG, Hodgkin JE, Ward JJ, editors: *Respiratory care: a guide to clinical practice*, ed 3, Philadelphia, 1991, JB Lippincott.

Rarey KP, Youtsey JW: *Respiratory patient care*, Englewood Cliffs, NJ, 1981, Prentice Hall.

Scott AA, Koff PB: Airway care and chest physiotherapy. In Koff PB, Eitszmann DV, Neu J, editors: *Neonatal and pediatric respiratory care*, St. Louis, 1988, Mosby–Year Book.

Shapiro BA, Harrison RA, Kacmarek RM et al: *Clinical application of respiratory care*, ed 4, St. Louis, 1985, Mosby–Year Book.

Sills JR: *Respiratory care certification guide: the complete review resource for the entry level exam*, ed 2, St. Louis, 1994, Mosby–Year Book.

Simmon KF: Airway care. In Scanlan CL, Spearman CB, Sheldon RL, editors: *Egan's fundamentals of respiratory care*, ed 5, St. Louis, 1990, Mosby–Year Book.

Smith RM, Benson MS, Schoene RB: The efficacy of oxygen insufflation in preventing arterial oxygen desaturation during endotracheal suctioning of mechanically ventilated patients, *Respir Care* 32(10):865-869, 1987.

Taft AA, Mishoe SC, Dennison FH et al: A comparison of two methods of preoxygenation during endotracheal suctioning, *Respir Care* 36(11):1195-1201, 1991.

White GC: *Equipment theory for respiratory care*, Albany, NY, 1992, Delmar.

Wilkins RL, Hodgkin, JE, Lopez B: *Lung sounds: a practical guide*, St. Louis, 1988, Mosby–Year Book.

Witmer MT, Hess D, Simmons M: An evaluation of the effectiveness of secretion removal with the ballard closed-circuit suction catheter, *Respir Care* 36(8):844-848, 1991.

Wojciechowski WV: Incentive spirometers and secretion evacuation devices. In Barnes TA, editor: *Respiratory care practice*, Chicago, 1988, Year Book Medical.

SELF-STUDY QUESTIONS

1. Steps in making sure that a central vacuum system is working properly include all the following EXCEPT:
    A. Setting the vacuum control at Full.
    B. Screwing a 500-ml collection jar tightly onto the vacuum connector.
    C. Attaching 3 feet of vacuum tubing to the tubing connector on the collection jar.
    D. Pinching closed the vacuum tubing when the vacuum is turned on to measure the vacuum level.

2. Your patient is being mechanically ventilated with 60% oxygen and 8 cm of PEEP. She has twice had her SpO_2 value and blood pressure fall when removed from the ventilator for suctioning. What should be recommended to prevent this from happening again?
    A. Switch to a smaller suction catheter.
    B. Switch to a larger suction catheter.
    C. Increase her PEEP to 10 cm water before and after the suctioning.
    D. Use a closed-system suction catheter.
    E. Remove the PEEP before and after the suctioning.

3. It is difficult to quickly remove the tracheal secretions from your adult patient when using 80 mm Hg of vacuum pressure. What would you do?
    A. Suction for a longer period of time.
    B. Suction more frequently.
    C. Increase the vacuum pressure to 100 mm Hg.
    D. Remove the suction catheter and suction with the larger diameter rubber vacuum tubing.
    E. Replace the central vacuum regulator with a more powerful one.

4. When selecting a catheter's outer diameter for suctioning through an endotracheal tube it is important that it be:
    A. No more than one fourth the inner diameter of the tube
    B. No less than one half the inner diameter of the tube
    C. No less than three fourths the inner diameter of the tube
    D. No more than one half the inner diameter of the tube
    E. No more than three fourths the inner diameter of the tube

5. Your patient has pneumonia in her left lower lobe with a large amount of secretions. What would you recommend to be able to suction her better?
    A. Use the largest diameter suction catheter that is available.
    B. Use a suction catheter with a Coudé tip.
    C. Use the longest suction catheter that is available.
    D. Use a suction catheter with a single opening at the tip.
    E. Increase the length of time that you apply suction.

6. You are suctioning your patient when the vacuum is lost. You should do all the following EXCEPT:
    A. Make sure that the vacuum system is working.
    B. Empty the collection bottle if it is full.
    C. Make sure that there is a tight connection between the suction catheter and the vacuum tubing.
    D. Check the catheter to make sure it is not obstructed.
    E. Get a larger suction catheter.

Answer Key

1. A; 2. D; 3. C; 4. D; 5. B; 6. E.

13 | Intermittent Positive Pressure Breathing (IPPB)

The description of intermittent positive pressure breathing (IPPB) and its indications, contraindications, hazards, and theory of clinical use are presented in *Respiratory Care Certification Guide* (Sills, 1994) and other sources. It is recommended that this information and the functioning of the Bird and Bennett IPPB units be reviewed if necessary. Although it is not specifically listed for testing on the registry exams, at least one equipment-related question has been asked on a recent Written Registry Examination. Furthermore, the information on the functioning of the Bird and Bennett units will also prove essential to understanding their use, and that of other pressure cycled machines, in mechanical ventilation. This topic is discussed in Section 14.

Module A.   IPPB equipment.

1.   Fix any problems with the circuit. (IIB2h1) [An]

Fixing a problem is only possible after the problem is identified. The practitioner should be familiar with both permanent and disposable types of Bird and Bennett circuits. Leaks of any sort in the circuit will prevent the unit from cycling off so that the patient can exhale. Tighten up any friction fit or screw-type connections to stop the leak. A leak at the source gas connection or high pressure hose gas inlet connection will result in a rather loud hissing sound. When tightened properly the hissing and leak will stop.

Debris such as mucus or blood will plug the nebulizer capillary tube and prevent any mist from being formed. Disassemble the nebulizer and rinse it under running water to try to clear the capillary tube. Replace the nebulizer if necessary.

Module B.   Modify IPPB therapy.

1.   Adjust the sensitivity. (IIIC9) [An]

The sensitivity of the IPPB unit refers to how much effort or work the patient will have to perform to turn the unit on for a breath. Commonly the sensitivity is set so that the patient has to generate a negative pressure of only about -1 cm water pressure to begin an inspiration. This can be seen by looking at the needle deflecting into the negative range on the pressure manometer. Ask the patient if the machine can be easily turned on to get a breath. The IPPB unit should not be set so sensitive that it self-cycles.

2.   Adjust the flow. (IIIC9) [An]

The patient should initially feel comfortable with the flow rate and the inspiratory time. Ask the patient a simple question such as, "Is the breath coming too fast or too slow?" He or she will be able to give you a short answer or even a hand gesture in response. As the treatment progresses, the practitioner may be able to adjust the flow to modify the patient's breathing pattern to better achieve the therapeutic goal. For example:

1. Anxious patients may initally need a fast flow. As they are coached to relax and get used to the treatment, the practitioner should try to reduce the flow.
2. Slower flows result in medications being deposited deeper into the lungs. This is important if the patient is having a bronchodilator, mucolytic, or antibiotic nebulized.
3. Faster flows result in the deposition of medications in the upper airways. This is important if the patient is receiving racemic epinephrine for laryngeal edema or xylocaine for a local anesthetic of the upper airway before bronchoscopy.

Turning the inspiratory time/Flow Rate control counterclockwise increases the flow rate on the Bird series. Pulling the Air-Mix knob out from the center body increases the total flow by allowing room air to be entrained along with the source gas. (One question on the second self-assessment Written Registry Exam dealt with this issue.)

Flow rate in the PR-II is determined by the patient's inspiratory effort and how far the Bennett valve is open. Flow can be decreased somewhat by turning the Peak Flow control clockwise. Flow is not affected by the position of the Air Dilution knob.

3.   Adjust the volume and/or pressure. (IIIC9) [An]

A review of the current respiratory care textbooks reveals that all authors agree that the basic goal of IPPB is to deliver a tidal volume that is greater than what the patient does spontaneously. Unfortunately, there is a considerable difference of opinion about what inspiratory volume is being measured or by how much that breath should be increased for therapeutic goals to be achieved. Rather than choose one author over the others, all recommendations are listed here:

1. The AARC Clinical Practice Guideline (1993) on IPPB: The tidal volume delivered during an IPPB assisted breath should be at least 25% greater than the patient's spontaneous breaths.
2. Rarey and Youtsey (1981): IPPB volume should be either a) 3 to 4 ml × ideal body weight in pounds, or b) 10 ml × weight in kilograms.
3. Eubanks and Bone (1990): IPPB volume should be either a) greater than the spontaneous tidal volume, b) at least 10% greater than the spontaneous inspiratory capacity (IC), or c) at least 10% greater than the spontaneous vital capacity (VC).
4. Realey (1990): IPPB volume should be either a) at least 15 ml/kg of ideal body weight, or b) at least one third of the predicted IC.
5. Ziment (1984): IPPB volume should be at least 25% greater than the spontaneous tidal volume.
6. Shapiro, Harrison, Kacmarek et al (1985): IPPB volume should be greater than the spontaneous vital capacity.

7. Respiratory Care Committee of the American Thoracic Society (1980): IPPB volume should be either a) at least 25% greater than the spontaneous tidal volume, or b) at least as great as the spontaneous inspiratory capacity.
8. The AARC Clinical Practice Guideline (1991) on incentive spirometry: IPPB would be indicated to treat atelectasis rather than incentive spirometry if a) the patient's inspiratory capacity (IC) was less than 33% of the preoperative value, or b) the patient's vital capacity (VC) is less than 10 ml/kg of ideal body weight.

If a therapeutic goal is to prevent or treat atelectasis, having the patient inspire a deeper than spontaneous tidal volume breath should help. It seems reasonable to follow the AARC guidelines both as indications and as clinical goals. They can be used as guidelines if an increased tidal volume is used as a substitute for the inspiratory capacity. Based on this assumption, an IPPB delivered tidal volume goal of at least 10 ml/kg of ideal body weight seems reasonable.

Because all of the current IPPB units are pressure cycled, the only way to increase the inspired volume during a passive treatment is to increase the peak pressure. Coaching the patient during an active treatment will result in a larger volume without the need for as great a peak pressure. Decrease the peak pressure if the patient complains of discomfort or cannot hold that much pressure without losing the lip seal.

4. Make a recommendation to add expiratory retard. (IIIC10a) [R, Ap, An]

Expiratory retard is indicated in patients who have small airways disease and are air trapping on exhalation. Patients with emphysema, bronchitis, or asthma tend not to exhale completely their inspired tidal volumes. Over the course of an IPPB treatment this can lead to an increased functional residual volume (FRC) with the increased risk of pulmonary barotrauma. Adding expiratory retard to the treatment has the same effect as pursed lips breathing. The increased back pressure on the smallest airways keeps them open longer so that the more distal air can be exhaled.

It is important to measure the exhaled volumes during the treatment and monitor the patient's response to know how much retard is needed. Too little retard will result in some air trapping and an incompletely exhaled tidal volume. Too much retard will result in an uncomfortably long expiratory time and an increased mean intrathoracic pressure. The proper amount of expiratory retard should result in the patient feeling comfortable with the breathing cycle and being able to completely exhale the tidal volume. Listening to the patient's breath sounds will also be helpful. If wheezing is present, it will be minimized when the proper amount of retard is added. This is because the back pressure is properly adjusted to minimize the small airway collapse.

Bird makes a retard cap that fits over the exhalation valve port on their permanent circuit. The cap has a series of different size holes for exhaled gas to pass through (see Fig. 13-1). By rotating the cap progressively from the largest to the smallest opening, and evaluating the patient at each setting, the proper size opening and amount of retard can be found.

Bennett makes a retard exhalation valve that can be substituted for the regular exhalation valve on their permanent circuit (see Fig. 13-2). The valve consists of a spring attached to a nut and a diaphragm. As the nut is turned counterclockwise the spring pushes the diaphragm closer to the exhalation valve opening. This causes resistance to the exhalation of the tidal volume and a backpressure is created against the airways. If too much pressure is placed against the exhalation valve opening

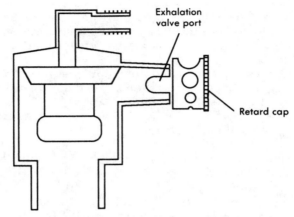

Fig. 13-1 Bird retard cap for providing adjustable expiratory resistance. (From McPherson SP: *Respiratory therapy equipment,* ed 4, St. Louis, 1990, Mosby–Year Book. Used by permission.)

the patient will not be able to exhale back to atmospheric pressure. This is seen on the System Pressure gauge as a pressure of greater than zero. This, in effect, would be IPPB with continuous positive airway pressure (CPAP). This should not be done without an order from the physician. Miller recommends the application of 2.5 to 3 mm or about 5 cm expiratory positive pressure (CPAP). He believes that this amount of pressure will help train the patient to use IPPB properly by making exhalation slower. Remember that the patient's intrathoracic pressure will be increased by this amount.

Be sure to ask the patient's opinion about the use of expiratory retard. The conscious, cooperative patient can tell you if he or she feels like more air is getting out by the use of the retard or if the lungs feel more full because too much retard is being used. Too much retard may also make the expiratory time uncomfortably long.

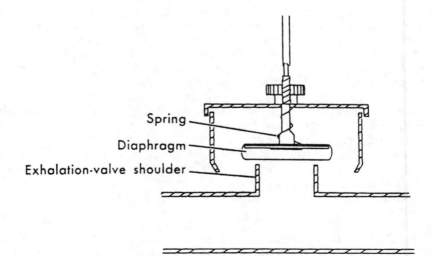

Fig. 13-2 Bennett retard exhalation valve for providing adjustable expiratory resistance. (From McPherson SP: *Respiratory therapy equipment,* ed 3, St. Louis, 1985, Mosby–Year Book. Used by permission.)

Module C. Patient assessment.

1. Examine all the data to determine the patient's pathophysiological condition. (IC3a) [R, Ap, An]

Patients that show signs of hyperinflation, such as those with emphysema or asthma, should have IPPB used at low pressures, if at all. They are at risk for more hyperinflation and the possibility of pneumothorax.

Pulmonary edema has been listed by some authors as an indication for IPPB because it will raise the intrathoracic pressure and reduce blood return to the heart and lungs. In this case, a high pressure would be indicated if tolerated.

2. Take part in the development of the respiratory care plan. (IC3c) [An]

The patient should be fully cooperative to take full advantage of IPPB. It may be counterproductive to try to force an IPPB treatment on a combative or uncooperative patient.

A patient who has a neuromuscular deficit may need assistance in holding the IPPB circuit or keeping a good mouth seal. A mouth seal or face mask treatment may have to be given.

Be prepared to make a recommendation to have a patient use either incentive spirometry, positive expiratory pressure therapy, or IPPB for hyperinflation therapy. Also be prepared to make a recommendation for a patient to use either a metered dose inhaler, small volume nebulizer, or IPPB for the delivery of an aerosolized medication.

BIBLIOGRAPHY

AARC Clinical Practice Guideline: Incentive spirometry, *Respir Care* 30(12):1402-1405, 1991.

AARC Clinical Practice Guideline: Intermittent positive pressure breathing, *Respir Care* 38(11):1189-1195, 1993.

Eubanks DH, Bone RC: *Comprehensive respiratory care*, ed 1, St. Louis, 1985, Mosby–Year Book.

Eubanks DH, Bone RC: *Comprehensive respiratory care*, ed 2, St. Louis, 1990, Mosby–Year Book.

Fluck RJ Jr: Intermittent positive-pressure breathing devices. In Barnes TA, editor: *Respiratory care practice*, Chicago, 1988, Year Book Medical.

Johnson NT, Pierson DJ: The spectrum of pulmonary atelectasis: pathophysiology, diagnosis, and therapy, *Respir Care* 31(11):1107-1120, 1986.

McPherson SP: *Respiratory therapy equipment*, ed 3, St. Louis, 1985, Mosby–Year Book.

McPherson SP: *Respiratory therapy equipment*, ed 4, St. Louis, 1990, Mosby–Year Book.

Miller WF: Intermittent positive pressure breathing (IPPB). In Kacmarek RM, Stoller JK, editors: *Current respiratory care*, Philadelphia, 1988, BC Decker.

Realey AM: Hyperinflation therapy. In Scanlan CL, Spearman CB, Sheldon RL, editors: *Egan's fundamentals of respiratory care*, ed 5, St. Louis, 1990, Mosby–Year Book.

Respiratory Care Committee of the American Thoracic Society: Guidelines for the use of intermittent positive pressure breathing (IPPB), *Respir Care* 25(3), 1980.

Scuderi J, Oslen GN: Respiratory therapy in the management of postoperative complications, *Respir Care* 34(4):281-291, 1989.

Shapiro BA, Harrison RA, Kacmarek RM et al: *Clinical application of respiratory care*, ed 3, Chicago, 1985, Year Book Medical.

Sills JR: *Respiratory care certification guide: the complete review resource for the entry level exam*, ed 2, St. Louis, 1994, Mosby–Year Book.

Weizalis CP: Intermittent positive-pressure breathing. In Barnes TA, editor: *Respiratory care practice*, Chicago, 1988, Year Book Medical.

Welch MA, Shapiro BJ, Mercurio P et al: Methods of intermittent positive pressure breathing, *Chest* 78:3, 1980.

Wilkins RL, Hodgkin JE, Lopez B: *Lung sounds: a practical guide*, St. Louis, 1988, Mosby–Year Book.

Ziment I: Intermittent positive pressure breathing. In Burton GG, Hodgkin JE, editors: *Respiratory care*, ed 2, Philadelphia, 1984, JB Lippincott.

SELF-STUDY QUESTIONS

1. A technician is giving an IPPB treatment with Alupent to an asthmatic patient in the emergency room. During a break in the treatment, the patient complains that his lungs feel too full and he does not feel like all the IPPB volume is getting out. What would you recommend?
   A. Increase the flow.
   B. Add expiratory retard.
   C. Increase the system pressure.
   D. Change to 100% oxygen.
   E. Decrease the sensitivity.

2. A technician calls you to take a look at an IPPB machine and circuit because it cycles off too early. Based on the illustration shown on page 373, what is the most likely problem?
   A. The nebulizer hose is attached to the exhalation valve.
   B. The nebulizer medication jar is loose.
   C. The bacteria filter is missing.
   D. The inspiratory and expiratory hoses are reversed.
   E. The bellows-type spirometer is malfunctioning.

3. A patient with emphysema has been changed from a hand-held nebulizer to IPPB for his bronchodilator therapy. While evaluating the patient during the treatment, you notice that her basilar wheezing has increased and her percussion note indicates hyperinflation with lowered hemidiaphragms. What would you recommend?
   A. Decrease the flow.
   B. Pull out the air-mix knob.
   C. Increase the system pressure.
   D. Add expiratory retard.
   E. Decrease the sensitivity.

4. You are about to give an asthmatic 16-year-old patient her second IPPB treatment. When checking the equipment you notice that it is set with a rather fast inspiratory flow. Her chart had a note that she was very anxious when first admitted. She seems more calm now. How would you start the treatment?
   A. Increase the pressure setting from what it was originally because she will now tolerate a larger breath.

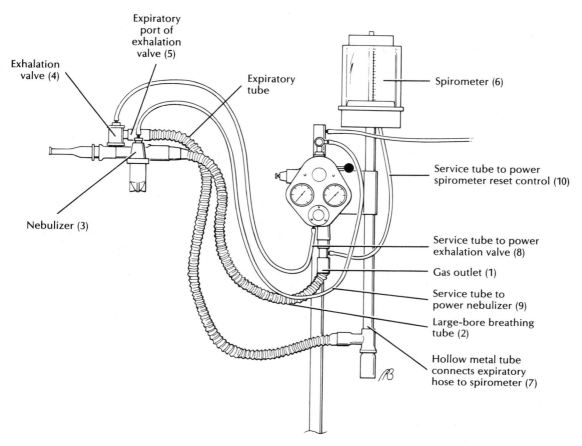

Fig. 13-3 Bennett IPPB unit with permanent circuit and exhaled tidal volume spirometer. (From Eubanks DH, Bone RC: *Comprehensive respiratory care*, St. Louis, 1985, Mosby–Year Book. Used by permission.)

    B.   Keep the flow the same to deliver a larger breath.
    C.   Make the machine as sensitive as possible so that she will not have to work hard to trigger it.
    D.   Tell the patient that you are going to decrease the flow on the machine and want her to tell you if the gas comes fast enough.

5.   Your patient with atelectasis has a spontaneous vital capacity of 600 ml and weighs 180 pounds. Based on this information, what should his IPPB tidal volume be?
    A.   500 ml
    B.   600 ml
    C.   700 ml
    D.   900 ml

6.   Atelectasis has been diagnosed by chest x-ray in a patient whom you are treating by IPPB. To evaluate its effectiveness, which of the following would you evaluate?
    I.   Repeat chest x-ray after the treatments have been given for 2 days.
    II.   Complete blood count.
    III.   Percussion note for the positions of the hemidiaphragms.
    IV.   Breath sounds.
    V.   Maximum voluntary ventilation after the treatments have been given for 2 days.

A.   I, III, IV
B.   I, II
C.   III, V
D.   I, III
E.   III, IV, V

7.   Your patient with COPD has been receiving IPPB treatments on a Bird Mark 7 for 5 days. Expiratory retard was added 4 days ago. Because it has not been evaluated since then, the physician asks you to do so. You proceeded to make the following adjustments in the retard cap settings and make the following observations:

Retard Cap Setting	Exhaled Tidal Volume (ml)	Wheezing	Patient's impression
1 (smallest)	850	None	Exhalation too long
2	825	Some in bases	Exhalation too long
3	800	Some in bases	Comfortable
4	700	All lobes	Lungs feel full
5	675	All lobes	Lungs feel full

Based on this information, which retard cap setting would you recommend?
A.   1
B.   2
C.   3
D.   4
E.   5

Answer Key

1. B; 2. D; 3. D; 4. D; 5. D; 6. A; 7. C.

14

Mechanical Ventilation of the Adult

All publicly available versions of the Written Registry Exam feature mechanical ventilation questions specifically about adults or that could apply to either adult, pediatric, or neonatal patients. There are very few questions that relate specifically to neonatal patients requiring mechanical ventilation. This section is written with the adult patient in mind.

The NBRC is known to ask questions about using specific ventilators and troubleshooting problems with specific ventilators. It is beyond the scope of this book to cover all possible units. That information is available in the manufacturer's literature or equipment books such as McPherson's (1985, 1990) *Respiratory Therapy Equipment*. The NBRC has asked specific questions on the Bennett MA-1 and PR-2, the Bird series, and BEAR series. It would be wise for the learner to become familiar with the workings of the newer ventilators.

Module A. Perform continuous mechanical ventilation to achieve adequate artificial ventilation and/or recommend modifications in ventilatory support based on the patient's response.

1. Recommend changing the type of ventilator to be used on the patient. (IIIC10l) [R, Ap, An]

The decision to place a patient on ventilatory support should not be made without due consideration of the need for ventilatory support. A number of physiologic criteria have been compiled to help the clinician determine when a patient is in respiratory and/or ventilatory failure (see Table 14-1). Remember that the patient may not fail each and every criteria; however, it is likely that the patient will fail one or more of the criteria in each category. Depending on the patient's condition, one particular type of ventilator may be better suited for the patient than another. The main classifications of ventilators are pressure cycled, external negative pressure, volume cycled, and high frequency.

Pressure Cycled Ventilator

Pressure cycled ventilators such as the Bird series or Bennett PR-2 may be acceptable for use with patients who have, and are expected to keep, a normal airway resistance and lung-thoracic compliance. Examples include an unconscious patient from a drug overdose or under anesthesia or a patient with a neuromuscular

Table 14-1. Indications for
Ventilatory Support

Ventilation
Apnea
$PaCO_2 > 55$ mm Hg in a patient who is not
   ordinarily hypercapneic
Dead space : tidal volume ($V_D : V_T$ ratio of greater
   than 0.55-0.6 (55%-60%)
Oxygenation
$PaO_2 < 80$ mm Hg on 50% oxygen or more
$P(A\text{-}a)O_2 > 300\text{-}350$ mm Hg on 100% oxygen
Intrapulmonary shunt > 15%-20%
Pulmonary Mechanics
Spontaneous tidal volume < 3-4 ml/lb or
   7-9 ml/kg of ideal body weight
Vital capacity < 10-15 ml/kg
Maximum inspiratory pressure
   (MIP) < $-20-25$ cm water pressure
Forced expiratory volume in one second (FEV_1) <
   10 ml/kg
Respiratory rate < 12 breaths/min or > 35
   breaths/min in an adult
Miscellaneous
Unconscious patient
Unstable and unacceptable vital signs
Unstable cardiac rhythm due to hypoxemia and/
   or acidosis
Worsening cardiopulmonary or other major organ
   system

disease such as myasthenia gravis or Guillain-Barré syndrome. As long as these patients are stable, the preset pressure will deliver the intended tidal volume. Transport ventilators are usually classified as pressure cycled.

If the patient's airway resistance increases or the patient's lung-thoracic compliance decreases, the tidal volume will decrease. Conversely, if the patient's airway resistance decreases or compliance increases, the delivered tidal volume will increase. In either case, the practitioner has to make frequent adjustments in the preset pressure to hope to keep a stable tidal volume. These units are not practical or safe with unstable patients.

External Negative Pressure Ventilator

An external negative pressure ventilator, such as the Drinker body respirator (iron lung) or chest curaisse, is indicated in similar types of patients. These patients have either a chronic neuromuscular disease, stable COPD, or kyphoscoliosis. They are able to breathe spontaneously through an intact upper airway most of the day. Often these patients are placed in the negative pressure ventilator at night to sleep and rest their respiratory muscles. As long as their compliance and resistance are fairly normal and pulmonary secretions do not require suctioning, these types of ventilators are satisfactory.

Volume Cycled Ventilator

A volume cycled ventilator is indicated whenever the patient's airway resistance or lung-thoracic compliance is expected to change. These types of units will deliver a preset tidal volume to the patient, at whatever pressure is needed, despite changing patient airway and lung conditions. As a result, volume cycled ventilators are recommended in the majority of patients who need ventilatory support. In addition, these types of ventilators come with a built-in alarm system for detecting patient problems. Furthermore, they can be used in a variety of modes, they can deliver therapeutic PEEP, and they can generate more pressure to deliver the tidal volume than the pressure cycled or negative pressure ventilators.

High Frequency Ventilator

A high frequency ventilator is needed whenever the patient's condition calls for a higher respiratory rate or smaller tidal volume than available on a conventional volume cycled ventilator. The Food and Drug Administration (FDA) has approved these units for use during bronchoscopy and laryngoscopy procedures. Patients with a bronchopleural fistula who fail with conventional volume ventilation are also approved for high frequency ventilation. The FDA has limited high frequency jet ventilators to rates of 40 to 150 breaths per minute. Several jet ventilators are available. The Acutronic USA AMS-1000 and Instrument Development Corporation (IDC) Model VS 600 are freestanding units. BEAR Medical Systems has developed the BEAR Jet. It must be used with a volume cycled ventilator that is placed into either the CPAP or IMV mode.

At the time of this writing only one other ventilator has been approved to use higher rates—the Adult Star made by Infrasonics. The Adult Star is classified as an oscillator ventilator and can reach rates of several thousand per minute while delivering very small tidal volumes. It has been used successfully to treat patients with adult respiratory distress syndrome.

2.   Initiate and adjust mechanical ventilation when settings are specified. (IIIB2c) [An]

Typical physician written ventilator orders include the following:

- Mode, such as control, assist/control, IMV, SIMV, pressure support, pressure control, and so forth
- Oxygen percentage
- Respiratory rate
- Tidal volume or minute volume
- Sigh volume and frequency
- Special settings such as mechanical dead space, PEEP, or CPAP

If the order is incomplete the physician should be asked for a clarification unless department protocol allows the therapist to make the decision. Typically the therapist is expected to set the following ventilator controls based on a protocol or the patient's condition and response to the ventilator.

Sensitivity.—Sensitivity is usually set at about -1 to -2 cm water pressure. The patient should not have to work very hard to trigger a machine tidal volume.

Flow.—Flow is adjusted to set the inspiratory time and I : E ratio and/or to meet the patient's needs.

I : E Ratio.—The I : E ratio is adjusted to ensure that the patient can inhale in as physiologically appropriate a manner as possible and completely exhale the inspired tidal volume.

Alarms.—Alarm systems are different for each type of ventilator. Generally speaking, they are set with a safety margin of ±10% from the patient's normal ventilator settings. A variation of greater than 10% results in an audible and/or visual alarm condition.

Gas Temperature.—The goal for most patients is to minimize their humidity deficit by giving gas that is humidified and warmed to near body temperature. It is common to have the gas warmed to 90° to 95°F/35°C. It should be measured in the inspiratory limb of the circuit as close to the patient as possible.

3.   Negative pressure ventilation.
   a.   Initiate external negative pressure ventilation. (IIIB2h) [R, Ap]
   b.   Adjust external negative pressure ventilation. (IIIB2h) [R, Ap]

These ventilators have proven useful in patients with the following characteristics: 1) Normal, intact upper airway; 2) ability to swallow; 3) normal airway resistance; 4) normal lung-thoracic compliance, and 5) ability to ventilate until respiratory muscle fatigue becomes too great.

Patients with the following disease conditions have been successfully ventilated by a negative pressure ventilator: 1) neuromuscular defects such as poliomyelitis, post-polio syndrome, muscular dystrophy, and high spinal cord injury; 2) kyphoscoliosis with resulting restrictive lung disease; and 3) chronic obstructive pulmonary disease during an acute worsening.

Negative pressure ventilators work by creating a negative pressure either around the patient's whole body or over the anterior chest and abdomen. The negative pressure expands the thorax and a tidal volume is inhaled. These devices are not nearly as sophisticated as the other types of ventilators discussed in this or the next section. Typically there is no way to vary the I : E ratio from 1 : 1, the patient cannot trigger any breaths, and alarm systems do not exist. If the patient needs supplemental oxygen it will have to be given by nasal cannula or face mask. There are three basic types of external negative pressure ventilators: drinker body respirator, body wrap, and chest curaisse.

Drinker Body Respirator

The Drinker body respirator (known as the "iron lung") has been in use since 1929. Currently they are made by the J. H. Emerson Company (see Fig. 14-1). More recently, a smaller version called the Portalung has been produced by Life Care, Inc. The patient lies supine with the body inside the closed cylinder; only the head is exposed. Routine nursing care is difficult. Side ports with foam inserts allow some limited contact, but more involved care requires that the patient be removed from the unit. The iron lung is the most powerful of the three types and should be chosen to ventilate the more difficult hospitalized patients. The following steps are used to initiate ventilation:

1. Select a ventilator rate of about 5 to 10 breaths less than the patient's own. The rate can be varied between 14 and 24 per minute.

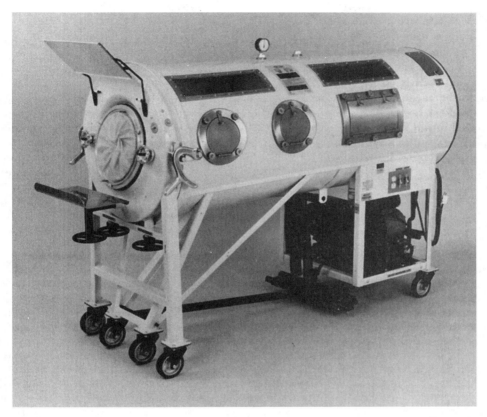

Fig. 14-1 Drinker body respiratory or "iron lung." Note the following features: The patient's head port is at the left end and has a foam rubber seal. The cylinder has two arm ports with seals, a bed pan port, and two glass windows for viewing the patient. The controls and motor for the bellows are below the cylinder at the right end. The bellows covers the right end of the cylinder. A pressure gauge is located at the top of the cylinder. (From LifeCare, Boulder, Colo. Used by permission.)

2. Gradually increase the negative pressure until the patient cannot speak during the inspiratory phase. A pressure of -7 to -15 cm water is enough for most patients. A maximum pressure of -35 cm water can be achieved. It is possible to create a positive pressure during exhalation, if needed, by closing a valve. This is usually limited to times when an assisted cough is called for.
3. Use a hand-held spirometer to measure the patient's tidal volume.
4. After a few minutes ask the patient, "Does the breath feel deep enough, too deep, or not enough? Do you have tingling fingers or feel dizzy (signs of hyperventilation)?"
5. Adjust the negativity and/or rate to meet the patient's needs.
6. Draw an arterial blood gas sample after about 15 minutes. Because the unit must be opened for this, speed is important.

In general, steps 3, 4, 5, and 6 should be used with the body wrap and chest curaisse units as well.

Body Wrap

Body wrap devices have been in use since their development during the polio epidemics of the 1950s. They are also called "pneumowrap," "raincoat," and "poncho." All feature a wind-proof, water-permeable nylon parka. The patient slips into it and lies supine with only the head, hands, and feet exposed. Straps are used to tighten the parka at these sites to prevent air leaks. Ridged plastic anterior and posterior chest pieces are built into the parka (see Fig. 14-2). Negative pressure draws the parka close to the skin and pulls the chest out for a breath to be inhaled. These are not as efficient as the iron lung and become even less so if the posterior chest piece is removed for better patient comfort. Despite the smaller tidal volume generated during passive breathing, these units are popular. Patients find that their portability and ease of entry and exit make them preferable to the iron lung for overnight or intermittent ventilatory assistance. It is recommended that the proper rate and negative pressure settings be determined in the hospital and confirmed by an arterial blood gas analysis before the patient is sent home with the unit.

Chest Curaisse

The chest curaisse has been in existence for more than 60 years. It is also known as the "chest shell" and "tortoise shell." It makes use of a vacuum pump similar to the body wrap device to control the negative pressure. The partial vacuum is applied to the patient by way of a hard plastic shell. It is fitted to cover the chest or preferably the chest and abdomen (see Fig. 14-3). These are the least efficient of all the negative pressure ventilators because less of the patient's body has vacuum applied to it. The patient shell can also cause skin abrasions if it is not carefully fitted to the patient's body contours. Again, it is recommended that the proper rate and negative pressure settings be determined in the hospital and confirmed by an arterial blood gas analysis before the patient is sent home with the unit.

The body wrap and chest curaisse units require an outside source to generate the negative pressure for the tidal volume breath. The simplest units have only a variable rate control and variable negative pressure through an electrically powered vacuum motor. Lifecare International (Lafayette, Colo) has a much more sophisti-

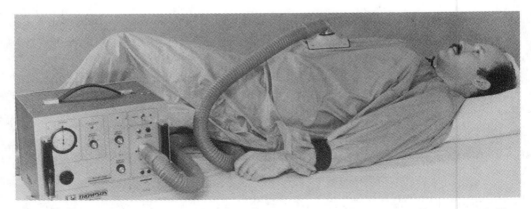

Fig. 14-2 Patient in a body wrap external negative pressure ventilator (Pulmowrap). Note the control box on the left that contains the vacuum motor. A hose connects the vacuum motor to the patient inside the body wrap device. (From Hill NS: Clinical applications of body ventilators, *Chest* 90(6):897-905, 1986. Used by permission.)

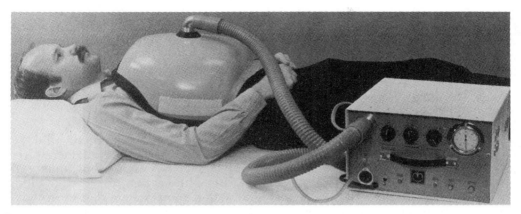

Fig. 14-3 Patient in a chest curaisse (Lifecare). Note the control box on the right that contains the vacuum motor. A hose connects the vacuum motor to the patient inside the chest shell. (From Hill NS: Clinical applications of body ventilators, Chest 90(6):897-905, 1986. Used by permission.)

cated unit. Its NEV-100 is a microprocessor controlled, electrically powered negative pressure ventilator that offers many of the same features available on constant volume ventilators. The modes include control, assist/control, and continuous negative pressure. A sigh can be added to the first two modes. The I : E ratio is variable. It has a low pressure alarm/disconnect alarm. An arterial blood gas analysis should prove that the rate and pressure settings are adequate. The stable patient can then be sent home with the unit.

4. Bilevel (BiPAP) ventilation.
a. Recommend the initiation of bilevel ventilation. (IIIC10r) [R, Ap, An]

Bilevel ventilation is a mode of ventilation where two levels of positive pressure are used to ventilate the patient's lungs. The baseline pressure is greater than zero (similar to PEEP) and the peak pressure is set to deliver a desired tidal volume (similar to IPPB or pressure support ventilation). Both levels can be independently adjusted or not used at all. If only the baseline pressure is elevated, the patient is receiving CPAP. If only the peak pressure is elevated, the patient is receiving pressure support ventilation.

Respironics has developed two devices for bilevel ventilation that can be used in the hospital or home for mask CPAP or mechanical ventilation. They are the BiPAP S-D and newer BiPAP S/T-D Ventilatory Support System. (Note: BiPAP is a registered trade mark of Respironics. Some practitioners mistakenly use the term bilevel ventilation and BiPAP interchangeably.) Both units combine a blower for gas flow with a solenoid system for timed breaths. Supplemental oxygen is not available through the machine; however, it can be added though a side port on the nasal mask to meet clinical goals. It is important to realize that the BiPAP ventilators are not constant volume ventilators with all capabilities and alarm systems.

Bilevel ventilation is indicated in stable, spontaneously breathing patients who present with any of the following clinical situations: elevated carbon dioxide level, hypoxemia despite supplemental oxygen, chronic ventilatory muscle dysfunction, or sleep apnea from upper airway obstruction. It is also used to delay intubation. It is critical only to select patients for bilevel ventilation who are capable of providing some spontaneous ventilation. These patients should also be stable and conscious. Most of the time these patients will be ventilated with the aid of a nasal or face mask (see the next discussion). If the patient is critically ill, unstable, needs to be intubated to secure the airway for secretion removal, and/or needs therapeutic PEEP to maintain the functional residual capacity (FRC), he or she should be placed on a volume cycled ventilator, not a bilevel ventilator.

b. Initiate nasal and mask bilevel ventilation. (IIIB2g and IIIB4b) [R, Ap, An]

The patient must have a properly fitting nasal or face mask to receive bilevel ventilation. These ventilation masks are similar to CPAP masks and will be referred to as such. Remember that mask CPAP is used with hospitalized patients with acute respiratory failure, atelectasis, and other conditions that result in low lung compliance. Mask CPAP in the home is limited to patients with either obstructive sleep apnea or chronic respiratory failure from a neurological disorder. Bilevel ventilation offers patients and clinicians another option in addition to mask CPAP and external negative pressure ventilation.

CPAP masks come in different sizes for children older than 3 years of age and adults. There are two different types of CPAP masks. Nasal masks are designed to cover only the nose. They allow the patient to eat, drink, speak, and use the mouth as a second airway for breathing in case there is a malfunction of the CPAP system. The mouth also acts as a pressure relief route if the CPAP pressure should become too great. Pressures of up to 15 cm water can usually be maintained (see Figs. 14-4 and 14-5). Usually the mask is made of a transparent plastic.

Face masks are designed to cover the nose and mouth. They are similar in design to the masks used during bag-mask ventilation and also made of a transparent plastic. The face mask must be used if the patient has persistent mouth breathing and cannot use a nose mask. With a good seal, pressures of greater than 15 cm water can be maintained.

Both types of CPAP mask have a soft, very compliant seal to closely fit the contours of the face. Straps are needed to hold the mask in place. It is imperative that the mask properly fit the patient's face. Too large a mask will not seal and will allow gas to leak and pressure to drop. This will be seen as a decreased CPAP pressure on the manometer. The patient may show increased snoring or airway obstruction with periods of apnea. Too small or a misfitting mask could cause an uneven distribution of pressure on the face. This could lead to abrasions or pressure sores and ulcers on the face.

The BiPAP S/T-D system can be used for bilevel ventilation or in the CPAP mode. It makes use of a relatively simple circuit and does not have a humidifier, alarm system, or the other attachments seen in a volume cycled ventilator. It is important that only a BiPAP circuit be used with the unit because it has a smooth interior. (A corrugated circuit reduces the delivered gas flow and pressure to the patient.) If other components are needed they must be added on. A bacteria filter should be inserted between the BiPAP unit and the patient circuit. If a humidifier is desired it must be a cascade or wick type of humidifier. A heat and moisture exchanger cannot be used because it creates too much resistance.

The bilevel settings will have to be determined at the bedside by asking for the patient's subjective opinion, listening to breath sounds, checking vital signs, and evaluating arterial blood gas values. See the next discussion for more detail.

If supplemental oxygen is needed it can be added at any of three locations. Adding oxygen to a port on the patient's mask will result in the highest percentage. Oxygen also can be added at the humidifier or the outlet from the BiPAP unit. Up to 15 L/min can be added without affecting the performance of the BiPAP system.

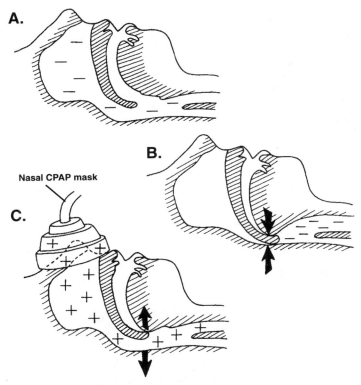

Fig. 14-4 Effect of a nasal CPAP mask. **A,** The normal upper airway remains patent during sleep. **B,** The abnormal upper airway of a patient with obstructive apnea collapses on inspiration during sleep. **C,** The pressure from a nasal CPAP mask keeps the abnormal upper airway patent during sleep. (Modified from Scanlan CL: Respiratory failure and the need for ventilatory support. In Scanlan CL, Spearman CB, Sheldon RL, editors: *Egan's fundamentals of respiratory care,* ed 5, St. Louis, 1990, Mosby–Year Book.)

It is not possible to know the delivered oxygen percentage until after the bilevel ventilation settings are determined. The oxygen flow should be then be gradually increased while the patient's SpO_2 value rises to the desired saturation level.

c. Change either or both levels of positive pressure ventilation. (IIIC7d) [R, Ap, An]

The two levels of ventilation must be independently determined. The baseline level (CPAP or PEEP) must be enough to prevent upper airway obstruction of the soft tissues. The positive expiratory pressure also may be needed to maintain the patient's FRC. The peak pressure must be adequate to deliver an acceptable tidal volume to remove carbon dioxide. If the patient's airway resistance and lung compliance is stable, increasing the peak pressure will deliver a larger tidal volume. Decreasing the peak pressure will obviously decrease the tidal volume.

Ideally, arterial blood gases should be drawn to determine if the machine settings are proper; however, it may be possible to use pulse oximetry values for monitoring patient oxygenation and capnography for monitoring end-tidal carbon dioxide level.

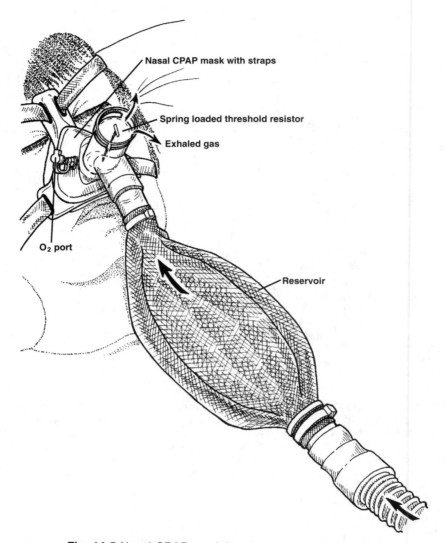

Nasal CPAP mask with straps

Spring loaded threshold resistor

Exhaled gas

O₂ port

Reservoir

Fig. 14-5 Nasal CPAP mask in place on an adult patient.

d. Recommend a change and adjust bilevel ventilation. (IIIB4b and IIIC10r) [R, Ap, An]

There are two advantages of the BiPAP ventilation with mask over intubation and continuous ventilation. First, the patient can talk, eat, and drink because the mask only covers the nose. Second, the unit is capable of delivering enough flow to compensate for a leak around the mask so that the intended ventilator settings are maintained. Mask BiPAP should not be used in a patient who cannot adequately ventilate himself or herself if the mask should come off or if the patient is at risk of aspirating stomach contents.

In 1994 the BiPAP system was approved for use on patients with either an endotracheal tube or tracheostomy tube. Again, only patients who can provide some of their own breathing can be considered for invasive application of the BiPAP system. This is because it does not offer safety systems and a humidifier. To apply a BiPAP system to a patient with an artificial airway the following must be added:

a smooth bore BiPAP ventilator circuit, a cascade-type or wick-type humidifier, and the Respironics Airway Pressure Monitor as an alarm.

Only the function of the BiPAP S/T-D system will be reviewed because it is newer and has more features. The operator can choose between these five modes of operation:

1. Expiratory positive airway pressure (EPAP) from 2 to 20 cm water. This is functionally similar to CPAP.
2. Inspiratory positive airway pressure (IPAP) from 2 to 25 cm water. This is functionally similar to setting the peak pressure on a pressure cycled ventilator. The patient must trigger each IPAP assisted breath.
3. Spontaneous (S) functions such as the pressure support mode where the patient must initiate each assisted breath. The therapist can set IPAP and EPAP levels. This will deliver bilevel ventilation.
4. Spontaneous/timed (S/T) delivers between 6 and 30 ventilator breaths per minute when the patient's respiratory rate drops below the set number. Otherwise, it functions like the spontaneous mode and will deliver bilevel ventilation.
5. Times (T) varies the percent of each cycle in IPAP from 10% to 90%. This allows the therapist to set an I : E ratio. All the first four functions are kept except that the patient cannot trigger an IPAP breath.

With the BiPAP units, the difference between IPAP and EPAP is called pressure boost and delivers the tidal volume. It is important to remember that the delivered tidal volume will vary depending on changes in the patient's airway resistance and lung-thoracic compliance as well as the machine settings. Also, remember that it is not possible to deliver a set inspired oxygen percentage because it can only be added to the port hole on the mask. The patient's tidal volume, vital signs, and arterial blood gases should be monitored for guidance in setting the ventilator's parameters and oxygen flow.

5.   Pressure support ventilation (PSV)
a.   Recommend the initiation of pressure support ventilation. (IIIC10n) [R, Ap, An]

Pressure support ventilation (PSV) is similar to IPPB in that when the patient initiates a ventilator breath a preset pressure is delivered to the airway. That pressure and the patient's cardiopulmonary condition determine the tidal volume. The patient has the flexibility to determine the respiratory rate, minute volume, inspiratory flow through a demand valve, and I : E ratio. PSV can be used as a mode by itself or combined with IMV/SIMV or pressure control ventilation in some current generation ventilators. (See Fig. 14-6 for graphic drawings of breathing in PSV and pressure versus volume tracings.) There are two PSV options depending on the clinical goal: 1) deliver a desired tidal volume, or 2) overcome the patient's calculated airway resistance. Both are discussed next.

b.   Recommend the adjustment of pressure support ventilation. (IIIC10n) [R, Ap, An]

When the pressure support level is adjusted to deliver a tidal volume it is called PSV_{max} (for maximum pressure support ventilation). The clinical guidelines for PSV_{max} are:

a. Use enough pressure to deliver a tidal volume of 10 to 12 ml/kg of ideal body weight.

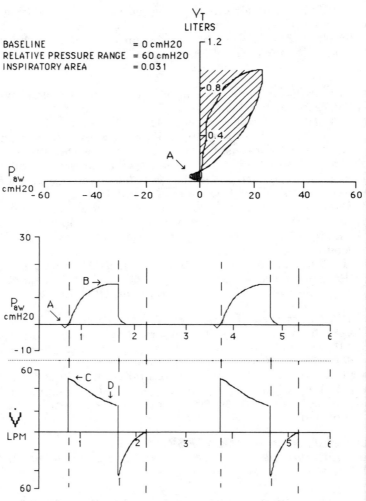

Fig. 14-6 Two graphic tracings of pressure support ventilation. The top graphic shows a pressure-volume loop of a patient triggering a breath. **A,** the amount of work the patient has to provide. The shaded area on the right side indicates how much work was provided by the ventilator.

The bottom graphic shows pressure (Paw) versus time and flow (V) versus time tracings. **A,** where the patient initiated a breath. **B,** where the ventilator cycled off when the pressure support level of 15 cm water was reached. **C,** the high peak flow at the start of the breath. **D,** how the flow rate decreases as the pressure support level is reached. (From Waveforms by Puritan-Bennett. Used by permission.)

b. The patient should not have to assist the ventilator at a rate greater than 20/minute to achieve acceptable arterial blood gas values.

PSV_{max} has been used in patients who have had acute respiratory failure that is resolving. Usually these patients have been maintained on the assist/control mode for several days to minimize their work of breathing while undergoing treatment for their condition. It is felt that PSV_{max} is ideal for reconditioning their diaphragm and other respiratory muscles. Reconditioning occurs when the assist or "trigger" pressure for the breath is kept as low as possible (-1 to -2 cm water pressure) and the tidal volume large. This pattern results in a low respiratory muscle work load. As the patient continues to improve, the PSV level is reduced. The patient's tidal volume will be stable if the patient passively takes in the PSV supported breath. Or the tidal volume can be larger if the patient interacts actively with the pressure that is delivered. (See Fig. 14-7, E, for the pressure-time curve.)

The pressure support level has also been used as a way to overcome the airway resistance caused by the patient's endotracheal tube. It has been felt that too small an endotracheal tube prevents some patients from successfully weaning by the IMV/SIMV mode. The addition of enough pressure support to overcome the additional work of breathing caused by the tube enables the patient to wean successfully and be extubated. The patient's total airway resistance (airways and endotracheal tube) can be determined by this formula:

$$\text{Airway resistance } (R_{aw}) = \frac{\text{peak airway pressure} - \text{plateau pressure}}{\text{flow (in L/sec)}}$$

Flow in liters per second is found by taking the inspiratory flow in liters per minute and dividing it by 60 seconds.

Example

Determine the pressure support level to set to overcome the airway resistance of a mechanically ventilated patient with the following parameters: inspiratory flow of 40 L/min, peak airway pressure of 40 cm water, and plateau pressure of 30 cm water.

$$\text{Flow} = \frac{40 \text{ L/min}}{60 \text{ sec}} = .67 \text{ L/sec}$$

$$\text{Airway resistance } (R_{aw}) = \frac{\text{peak airway pressure} - \text{plateau pressure}}{\text{flow (in L/sec)}}$$

$$R_{aw} = \frac{40 - 30}{.67} = \frac{10}{.67} = 15 \text{ cm water/L/sec}$$

Set the pressure support level at 15 cm water to overcome the resistance of the endotracheal tube. Any greater pressure is delivering some tidal volume. It could be argued that using a pressure to match a resistance is like comparing "apples to oranges"—they are not the same. However, the practice seems to be widely accepted clinically.

The pressure support level is reduced, as tolerated, when the patient's lung-thoracic compliance and/or airway resistance improves. As both return toward normal, the only barrier to extubation is the resistance offered by the endotracheal tube. Some practitioners advocate extubation when the PSV level is 10 cm water or less. This is probably the pressure level needed to overcome the tube's resistance. Therefore the patient should tolerate extubation without any increase in the work of breathing.

6. Pressure control ventilation (PCV).
a. Recommend the initiation of pressure control ventilation. (IIIC10o) [R, Ap, An]

Pressure control ventilation (PCV) involves the delivery of tidal volume breathes that are pressure limited and time cycled. It has been advocated for patients with bilateral low compliance conditions such as seen with adult respiratory distress syndrome (ARDS).

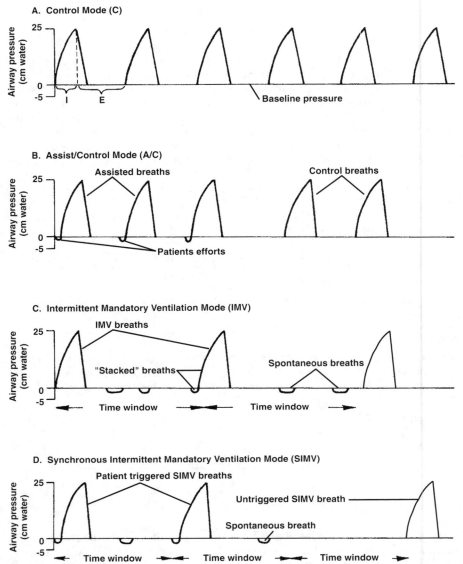

Fig. 14-7 Pressure versus time waveforms for the various modes of mechanical ventilation. **A,** Control mode (C) shows no patient effort and consistent I : E ratios. **B,** Assist/control mode (A/C) shows that the patient's initial effort triggers a machine tidal volume breath. **C,** Intermittent mandatory ventilation mode (IMV) shows spontaneous tidal volume breaths occuring between predetermined machine tidal volume breaths. Note the "stacked" breaths that happen when the patient takes in a breath that is then supplemented by a machine breath. **D,** Synchronous intermittent mandatory ventilation mode (SIMV) shows that a patient effort within a time window results in the delivery of a machine tidal volume. Any other patient efforts within the time window result in a spontaneous tidal volume. If no patient efforts occur within the time window, a machine tidal volume will be automatically delivered. **E,** Pressure support ventilation mode (PSV) shows how the patient must initiate all breaths that are then supported to a predetermined airway pressure. Stable tidal volumes will be seen if the patient inhales passively. Variably larger tidal volumes will result if the patient inhales more actively. **F,** Positive end expiratory pressure (PEEP) therapy can be added to the assist/control mode (as shown) or any other. The elevated baseline pressure prevents alveolar collapse. The sensitivity control must be set at −1 to −2 cm water so that the patient is able to trigger a breath without undue effort. **G,** Continuous positive airway pressure (CPAP) shows that the patient takes spontaneous tidal volumes while exhaling against an elevated baseline pressure.

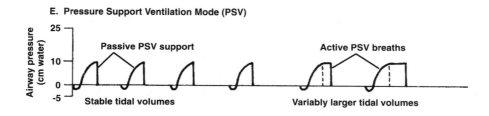

E. Pressure Support Ventilation Mode (PSV)

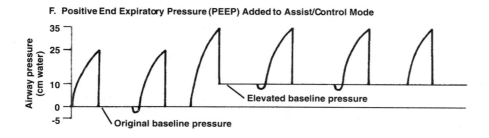

F. Positive End Expiratory Pressure (PEEP) Added to Assist/Control Mode

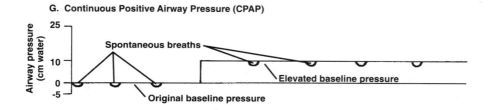

G. Continuous Positive Airway Pressure (CPAP)

Historically these patients have been maintained on a volume cycled ventilator. ARDS patients require very high driving pressures on these machines to deliver the tidal volume. This has resulted in pulmonary barotrauma and/or decreased cardiac output in some patients. If a pulmonary air leak is present, much of the gas will be lost through it and the necessary pleural chest tube. Attempts to increase the tidal volume to make up for the lost gas usually result in an even greater leak. Because of this, the injured tissue cannot heal and seal.

It is hoped that the low pressures used in PCV will prevent the onset of pulmonary barotrauma, or, if barotrauma is present, the lower pressure will help the lung tissues to heal. Another advantage of PCV over volume cycled ventilation is that inspiratory flow decreases toward the end of inspiration. This results in less gas turbulence, which results in a more equal distribution of the tidal volume into low compliance areas.

b. Initiate pressure control ventilation. (IIIB2f) [R, Ap]

Several current generation ventilators have a specific pressure control ventilation mode. Older volume cycled ventilators can be made to function the same way by converting them to a pressure cycled machine. This is done by setting the pressure limit to the desired level and turning the tidal volume up to a higher than desired level. When the ventilator cycles to inspiration a volume is delivered until the pressure limit is reached. The machine then cycles to exhalation and the exhaled tidal volume is measured. However, the I : E ratio cannot be easily adjusted or controlled with these older machines.

Before starting PCV it is important to measure baseline vital signs, arterial blood gases, pulmonary artery catheter values, and so forth on the current ventilator settings. The pressure control level is set as low as possible to achieve an adequate tidal volume for gas exchange. One approach is to set the initial pressure control level at the patient's plateau pressure on the ventilator. Recall that the plateau pressure is found by briefly holding the tidal volume in the lungs. This is the pressure required to overcome the elasticity of the lungs. Whether other ventilator parameters such as rate or oxygen percentage will be changed when pressure control ventilation is started depends on the patient's overall condition. If more than one change is made at a time, it will be difficult to tell which modification caused the resulting blood gases. It is important to monitor the exhaled volume continuously because the tidal volume will decrease if the patient's lung compliance or airway resistance worsens. If either or both improve, the tidal volume will increase. The patient with a pulmonary air leak will lose variable amounts of tidal volume out of the chest tube depending on the same changes in compliance and resistance. It is important to evaluate an arterial blood gas sample with a change in the pressure control level or tidal volume.

The PCV mode is well tolerated by many patients because of the freedom they have to set the rate, inspiratory flow through the demand valve, and minute volume. PCV may also be combined with SIMV and pressure support ventilation as the clinical situation indicates. The following are some suggestions for initial pressure control settings:

- Set the level of PEEP the same as was used on the constant volume ventilator. This is to maintain the patient's FRC.
- Set the pressure control level at the patient's static lung compliance pressure. Be prepared to increase this pressure. The clinical goal is to give a tidal volume close to that delivered previously.
- Set the rate the same as before.
- Set the inspired oxygen the same as before. Some may prefer to set it at 100% until blood gas results show that it can be lowered.
- Set the inspiratory time under pressure control so that the I : E ratio is the same as before.

Check the patient's vital signs for tolerance and get an arterial blood gas sample in about 15 mintues.

c.   Change the pressure control level. (IIIC7c) [R, Ap, An]

As mentioned earlier, the delivered tidal volume varies in the pressure control mode based on the patient's changing airway resistance and lung compliance. Check the blood gases for a rising $PaCO_2$ and dropping tidal volume. If the airway resistance or lung compliance worsens, the pressure control level will have to be increased to maintain or increase the tidal volume. Obviously, as the patient's airway resistance and lung compliance improve (or pulmonary air leak decreases) the pressure control level will have to be decreased to maintain the desired tidal volume.

d.   Recommend a change and adjust pressure control ventilation. (IIIB2f and IIIC10o) [R, ap, An]

In addition to the pressure control level, it is necessary to set and adjust the back-up rate, oxygen percentage, inspiratory gas flow, I : E ratio, alarms, and so forth, as would be done on any mode on any ventilator. Be prepared to make whatever adjustments are necessary based on the patient's condition. (Fig. 14-8 shows two tracings of how the tidal volume can be increased when the inspiratory time is lengthened.) Check the patient's vital signs and blood gases after each change in pressure control ventilation.

7.   Inverse ratio ventilation (IRV).
a.   Recommend the initiation of inverse ratio ventilation. (IIIE10p) [R, Ap, An]

Inverse ratio ventilation (IRV) has been used with success in adults with ARDS who do not respond to pressure control ventilation. The decision to change the I : E ratio is based on the patient's pulmonary condition. The airway resistance and compliance determine how easily air flows into and out of the lungs and how much of the pressure applied to the lungs is transmitted throughout the chest.

Increased inspiratory time and decreased expiratory time should be used in any condition where the patient has a small time constant of ventilation. This would be seen clinically as a normal airway resistance but a low lung-thoracic compliance. Examples of conditions where this is seen include ARDS, pulmonary edema, pneumonia, or an enlarged abdomen.

As a review, the product of the patient's lung-thoracic compliance (C_{LT}) and airway resistance (Raw) is called the time constant of ventilation (T_c) or time constant of the respiratory system (T_{RS}) and is calculated as shown here:

$$\text{Time constant of ventilation (Tc)} = C_{LT} \times \text{Raw}$$

A normal adult has a compliance of 100 ml/cm water pressure (0.1 l/cm water pressure) and an airway resistance of about 2 cm water/L/sec. This person's time constant of ventilation when breathing spontaneously would be calculated as:

$$\text{Time constant of ventilation (Tc)} = C_{LT} \times \text{Raw}$$

$$\text{Tc} = (0.1 \text{ L/cm water pressure}) \times (2 \text{ cm water/L/sec})$$

$$\text{Tc} = .2 \text{ seconds}$$

This brief time constant means that the pressure in the airway is quickly transmitted to the alveoli. If the patient had a condition causing decreased lung compliance, the time constant would become shorter. Conversely, if the patient is intubated or has obstructive airways disease, the airway resistance would increase and the time constant would become longer.

Increasing the inspiratory time to create an inverse I : E ratio keeps the lungs inflated longer to provide more time for oxygen to diffuse. In addition, it keeps the alveoli open longer to help prevent atelectasis and maintain the FRC. Typically, the patient starts out with a normal I : E ratio such as 1 : 2. After other ventilator adjustments prove unsuccessful in maintaining oxygenation, the inspiratory time is increased.

Conversely, a decreased inspiratory time and increased expiratory time should be used in any condition where the patient has a large time constant of ventilation.

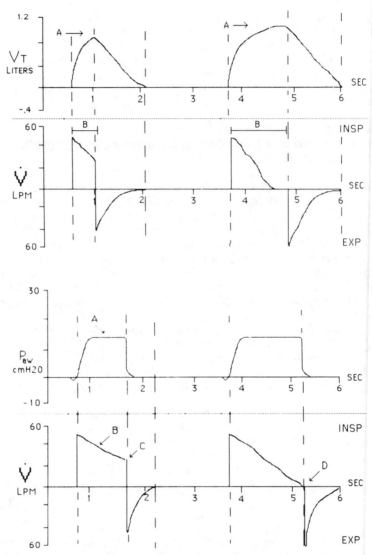

Fig. 14-8 Two sets of graphic tracings of pressure control ventilation. The top two tracings show volume (V_T) versus time and flow (V) versus time. **A,** tidal volume; **B,** inspiratory flow. Note how the tidal volume increases as the inspiratory time is increased. However, as shown in the lower right tracing, as the flow drops to zero no more volume is delivered.

The bottom two tracings show pressure versus time and flow versus time. **A,** the pressure control level being reached with an inspiratory plateau or "square wave" appearance. **B,** a declining inspiratory flow. **C,** the final flow when inspiration is time cycled off and exhalation begins. This graphic can be used to help adjust a longer inspiratory time. If pressure control inverse ratio ventilation (PCIRV) were being optimally adjusted, the inspiration time could be increased until inspiratory flow reached zero. This is indicated by **D.** (From Waveforms by Puritan-Bennett. Used by permission.)

This would be seen clinically as an increased airway resistance but a normal lung-thoracic compliance. Examples of conditions where this is seen include asthma, bronchitis, large amounts of secretions, and airway tumor. The increased expiratory time allows for a complete exhalation of the tidal volume.

Typically, patients being considered for inverse ratio ventilation are already being ventilated in the pressure control mode. Therefore the merging of the two modes is called pressure control inverse ratio ventilation (PCIRV). The following have been listed as specific criteria for starting PCIRV although not all have to be met to justify it:

- Peak pressure greater than 50 cm water
- Static lung compliance less than 40 ml/cm water
- High PEEP level
- More than 60% oxygen is being used
- PaO_2 less than 60 mm Hg
- The minute ventilation greater than 10 L/min
- Shunt fraction greater than 15%
- Bilateral infiltrates seen on chest x-ray film

b.   Initiate inverse ratio ventilation. (IIIB2d) [R, Ap]

Inverse ratio ventilation (IRV) involves either increasing the inspiratory time, decreasing the expiratory time, or both. Furthermore, the ventilator's back-up rate must be monitored for a change unless there are equal adjustments in both the inspiratory and expiratory times. IRV is initiated when the patient fails to respond to pressure control ventilation with a conventional I : E ratio. It is recommended that a set of arterial blood gases be drawn and vital signs recorded before the change is made to PCIRV. The following have been recommended as initial PCIRV settings:

- If the patient is being switched from volume cycled ventilation to PCIRV, set the pressure control level at the patient's static lung compliance pressure. However, if the patient was already on pressure control ventilation at a higher pressure, keep this higher pressure.
- Set the oxygen at 100%.
- Keep the current respiratory rate.
- Keep the I : E ratio at 1 : 1 for now.
- PEEP should be removed if it is currently at less than 8 cm water. Cut the PEEP level in half if it is currently at more than 8 cm water. As the I : E ratio is made inverse, air-trapping will increase the patient's functional residual capacity (FRC).

Draw a set of arterial blood gases after 15 minutes on PCIRV and check the patient's vital signs. Monitor the exhaled tidal volume for a decrease. If the ventilator will give a real-time graph of pressure, volume, and flow these should be monitored for air-trapping (auto-PEEP).

c.   Recommend a change and adjust inverse ratio ventilation. (IIIB2d and IIIC10p) [R, Ap, An]

If the initial set of blood gases on PCIRV does not show adequate oxygenation the inspiratory time will have to be increased. The inspiratory time must be progressively increased and expiratory time decreased if the patient's lung compliance worsens. It is also possible to alternate a 2 to 3 cm water increase in the pressure control level with small increases in the inspiratory time. Blood gases must be analyzed with each increase in inspiratory time, decrease in expiratory time, or increase in pressure control. Once an acceptable PaO_2 is established it is usually not necessary to make further increases in the inspiratory time if the patient's pulmonary condition does not worsen. Look for an increase in $PaCO_2$ or end-tidal CO_2 as a sign of inadequate tidal volume. It may be necessary to increase the pressure control level or decrease the inspiratory time to increase the tidal volume. Also monitor the patient's vital signs and cardiac output, if possible, to look for a decrease in cardiac output. PCIRV ratios as inverse as 3 : 1 or 4 : 1 have been reported. When this happens, the pressure-volume curve takes on a characteristic "square wave" shape as shown in Fig. 14-8.

The advantages of PCIRV over conventional volume ventilation are the lowered peak airway pressure and the longer inspiratory time. The lowered peak pressure is thought to reduce the risk of barotrauma. The longer inspiratory time allows alveoli with long time constants of ventilation to fill and atelectatic areas to reopen. Even if a high peak pressure is developed, the pressure is contained within the stiff lungs and not transmitted to the heart. As the lungs become more compliant, the inspiratory time must be reduced toward normal to prevent the pressure from compressing the heart. Full exhalation of the tidal volume must be assured. This is not usually a problem because the stiff lungs rapidly recoil to the resting level (FRC).

The longer inspiratory time does increase the risk of pulmonary barotrauma, decreased cardiac output, and expiratory air trapping. This last problem is known as auto-PEEP (also called inadvertent PEEP or intrinsic PEEP). Auto-PEEP is end-expiratory pressure in the lungs that cannot be seen on the ventilator's pressure manometer. It is caused by air trapping because of an inadequate expiratory time. It becomes more likely when the inspiratory time is increased, the expiratory time is decreased, or in patients with long time constants of ventilation. Simply put, the next breath is delivered before the patient has exhaled completely. Auto-PEEP is more likely to be found when the I : E ratio becomes 2 : 1 or greater.

It is controversial whether auto-PEEP is desirable or a problem. The key factor seems to be how much total PEEP the patient has. Total PEEP includes therapeutic PEEP and auto-PEEP. The procedure for measuring auto-PEEP is presented later. If auto-PEEP is not desired, care must be taken to measure both the inspired and expired volumes to make sure that they are equal and that the patient is not air trapping. If the patient has auto-PEEP, increase the expiratory time as needed until the tidal volume is completely exhaled. If auto-PEEP is desired it can be measured and adjusted by changing the inspiratory and expiratory times.

The level of auto-PEEP can be determined in two different ways depending on the type of ventilator that is being used. It can be measured on the pressure manometer of most ventilators, such as the Servo 900 B and C and the Puritan-Bennett MA-1 and 7200. Or the trapped expiratory gas can be seen on the graphics display of the BEAR 1000, Bennett 7200, Hamilton Veolar, Respironics Adult Star, and Drager Evita ventilators. The following procedure can be followed for determining the presence or level of auto-PEEP:

1. Note the delivery of a tidal volume.
2. Watch the pressure gauge as it drops to zero (or the level of therapeutic PEEP) at the end of exhalation. Make sure that the patient is exhaling passively to get an accurate reading.
3. Reduce the rate control to delay the next breath.
4. Occlude the expiratory tubing (or push the expiratory-hold button on the Servo 900C or add inflation hold on other ventilators) to prevent any further exhalation for about 3 to 5 seconds.

5. If the pressure gauge is being monitored, see the pressure rise above the baseline pressure. Or if the ventilator has a graphics monitor, seeing the failure of the exhaled tidal volume or expiratory flow to return to baseline confirms the presence and amount of auto-PEEP (see Fig. 14-9).
6. Listen to the patient's breath sounds during a standard breath and during the prolonged exhalation. It is likely that during the standard breath the expiratory sounds will be heard until the inspiratory sounds begin. During the prolonged exhalation the expiratory sounds will continue for a longer time and then end with silence. This silent pause time indicates that there is no more expiratory air flow.

It is important to add any auto-PEEP to the amount of therapeutic PEEP the patient has. This should be recorded as the total level of PEEP. For example, the patient has 5 cm of therapeutic PEEP and 2 cm of auto-PEEP for a total of 7 cm PEEP. It may be felt that the total PEEP level places the patient at risk for barotrauma or decreased venous return and lowered cardiac output. The amount of auto-PEEP can be reduced by decreasing the inspiratory time, increasing the expiratory time, and/or decreasing the tidal volume. Lack of auto-PEEP can be confirmed by the above procedure. If the auto-PEEP cannot be eliminated, therapeutic PEEP can be added to match it. By raising the baseline pressure the patient can more easily trigger an assisted or SIMV breath. It is especially important to decrease the auto-PEEP and therapeutic PEEP levels as the patient's lung compliance improves.

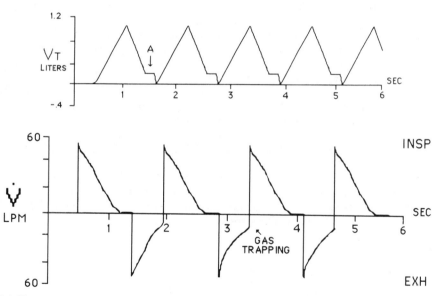

Fig. 14-9 Two graphic tracings of expiratory air trapping. The top graphic shows volume versus time. **A** shows that the exhaled tidal volume tracing does not reach the baseline. The inspiratory tidal volume is greater than the expiratory tidal volume indicating air trapping.

The bottom graphic shows flow versus time. Inspiratory flow is the tracing above the horizontal baseline of zero flow. Expiratory flow is the tracing below the horizontal baseline. It can be seen that the patient's expiratory flow does not return to zero; this indicates air trapping. The higher the flow rate, the more air trapping there is. Air trapping leads to auto-PEEP. It can be minimized by increasing the expiratory time, giving an aerosolized bronchodilator to treat bronchospasm, or suctioning out any secretions. (The top tracing is from Waveforms by Puritan-Bennett. The bottom tracing is from Pressure Control Ventilation Review by Puritan-Bennett. Used by permission.)

It is also very important to return the I : E ratio toward normal as the patient's lung compliance improves. This is done by gradually decreasing the inspiratory time and/or increasing the expiratory time. The patient's blood gas result should be evaluated with each step to be sure that oxygenation is maintained at a safe level.

8. Airway pressure release ventilation (APRV).
a. Recommend the initiation of airway pressure release ventilation. (IIIC10q) [R, Ap, An]

Currently only the Drager Evita (formerly produced as the PPG BioMedical Systems IRISA) ventilator offers airway pressure release ventilation (APRV) or uses this particular terminology for a mode. This unit offers other modes of ventilation as well. In addition, it is microprocessor controlled and includes a monitor for patient data and graphics. The APRV mode has been used with success in ARDS patients who have not responded well to constant volume ventilation. APRV can be described simply as a mode where the patient can breathe spontaneously at two different levels of CPAP. A difference from conventional CPAP is that the two levels are held for set periods of time. The ventilator options for this mode are quite simple. The practitioner sets the low pressure (P_{low}), high pressure (P_{high}), and times that the patient will be at those pressure levels. The low pressure is sometimes refered to as CPAP and high pressure as release pressure. The timing changes from low pressure to high pressure and back to low pressure in effect to deliver a tidal volume. (See Fig. 14-10 for a pressure versus time tracing.)

When comparing APRV to other modes of ventilation there appear to be several similarities between it and pressure control ventilation with PEEP and bilevel ventilation. All have an elevated baseline pressure that allows the patient to breathe spontaneously. All have variable inspiratory times for the higher pressure level. None deliver a set tidal volume to the patient. The only real difference seems to be that the patient can breathe spontaneously at the higher pressure level only with APRV. If the patient does not make any respiratory efforts, APRV would function like pressure control or bilevel ventilation.

b. Initiate airway pressure release ventilation. (IIIB2e) [R, Ap]

A set of blood gases, vital signs, pulmonary artery catheter values, and so forth should be obtained on the current constant volume ventilator settings as a baseline before starting APRV. The following suggestions for initiating APRV are similar to those listed earlier for starting pressure control ventilation.

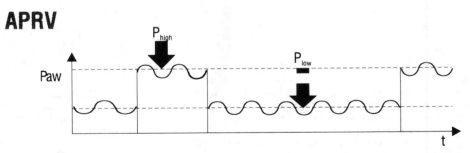

Fig. 14-10 Pressure versus time graphic of airway pressure support ventilation (APRV). The low pressure acts like CPAP, whereas the high pressure delivers a tidal volume. The patient is able to breathe spontaneously at both pressure levels. (From Drager EVITA ventilator technical information. Used by permission.)

- Set the low pressure (CPAP) at the level of PEEP that was used on the constant volume ventilator. This is to maintain the patient's FRC.
- Set the high pressure in a range between the patient's static lung compliance pressure and peak pressure. The clinical goal is to give a tidal volume close to that delivered previously.
- Set the inspired oxygen the same as before. Some may prefer to set it at 100%, as with PCIRV, until blood gas results show that it can be lowered.
- Set the timing of the high pressure and low pressure values so that the I : E ratio and respiratory rate are the same as before. Even if the patient is apneic, as the ventilator switches from high pressure to low pressure the patient exhales a tidal volume.

It will be noticed that these parameters closely match those on the volume cycled ventilator. Monitor the patient's ventilator delivered and spontaneous tidal volumes and rates. Check vital signs. Get an arterial blood gas sample in about 15 minutes.

c. Recommend a change and adjust airway pressure release ventilation. (IIIB2e and IIIC10q) [R, Ap, An]

If the patient's initial blood gas results on APRV show hypoxemia, the following options are available: 1) increase the inspired oxygen percentage if it is not already at 100%, 2) increase the low pressure level (CPAP/PEEP), or 3) increase the high pressure level. Reducing any or all of these options will decrease the patient's PaO$_2$ if it is too high.

If the blood gas results show hypoventilation, the following options are available: 1) increase the high pressure level, or 2) adjust the timing of the low pressure and high pressure values, in effect, to increase the respiratory rate. Do the opposite to increase the PaCO$_2$ if the patient is being hyperventilated.

As with the previous ventilator modalities, the patient should be closely monitored and have an arterial blood gas drawn to evaluate every change.

9. Initiate and adjust different combinations of intermittent mandatory ventilation (IMV), synchronous intermittent mandatory ventilation (SIMV), therapeutic positive end-expiratory pressure (PEEP), pressure support ventilation (PSV), and pressure control ventilation (PCV). (IIIB4a) [R, Ap]

It is presumed that the learner is familiar with the IMV and SIMV modes of ventilation. If not, they can be reviewed in a number of respiratory care textbooks. Fig. 14-7 shows pressure versus time tracings of these and other common modes of ventilation. Table 14-2 lists the signs of IMV/SIMV tolerance or intolerance.

Mandatory Minute Volume Ventilation

Mandatory minute volume (MMV) ventilation is a relatively new variation on the IMV/SIMV mode of ventilation. MMV is a modification of IMV where the patient is assured of a preset minute volume regardless of his or her spontaneous breathing. It has been proposed as an effective way to ventilate and wean patients who can spontaneously breathe but have an unreliable respiratory drive and unstable tidal volume. Examples include patients who have received narcotic, sedative, anesthetic, or neuromuscular blocking medications. Patient conditions for which MMV would be indicated include encephalopathy and cerebral disorders such as

Table 14-2. Indications of
IMV/SIMV Tolerance

Indications that IMV/SIMV is being well tolerated
Stable spontaneous respiratory rate
Stable heart rate
Stable spontaneous tidal volume
Stable vital capacity, MIP, and/or FEV_1
No use or stable use of accessory muscles of
  ventilation
Patient indicates he or she is comfortable
Stable blood gases
Indications that IMV/SIMV is not being well tolerated
Increased spontaneous respiratory rate
Tachycardia or dysrhythmias such as premature
  ventricular contractions
A drop in the spontaneous tidal volume
A drop in the vital capacity, MIP, and/or FEV_1
Beginning or increased use of accessory
  muscles of ventilation
Patient complains of dyspnea
Deterioration of blood gases as seen by a
  falling PaO_2 or SpO_2 and a rapidly falling or
  rising $PaCO_2$

stroke. In addition, MMV may be used during the recovery period of a neuromuscular disease. Ventilators that include the MMV mode are all controlled by a microprocessor and include the Ohmeda CPU-1 and Advent, BEAR 1000, Drager EVITA, and the Hamilton Veolar.

The following parameters have been recommended for the initiation of MMV:

1. Set the ventilator tidal volume according to established guidelines (10 to 15 ml/kg of ideal body weight).
2. The spontaneous breaths may be taken through a demand valve or may be pressure supported. The Hamilton Veolar uses pressure supported breaths to create the desired tidal volume.
3. Determine the minimum minute volume according to the patient's preexisting condition and the clinical goals:

   a. The patient who has been on IMV should have the mandatory minute volume set at 90% of the IMV delivered minute volume. For example, the patient has an IMV rate of 5 breaths/min and tidal volume of 800 ml. Therefore the ventilator is delivering 4 liters of minute volume (5 × 800 ml) and the MMV would be set at 3600 ml (90% of 4 liters).
   b. The patient who has been on assist/control should have the mandatory minute volume set at 80% of the A/C delivered minute volume. For example, the patient has an A/C rate of 10 breaths/min and tidal volume of 1000 ml. Therefore the ventilator is delivering 10 liters of minute volume (10 × 1000 ml) and the MMV would be set at 8 liters (80% of 10 liters).

4. Set the inspired oxygen percent, inspiratory flow, and so forth as the patient's clinical condition requires.

Ideally MMV establishes a minimum safe volume of ventilation. If the patient should inhale less than this volume, the ventilator will deliver as many breaths as necessary at the preestablished tidal volume to make up the difference. Be aware that a patient breathing rapidly with a small tidal volume may move enough gas to exceed the minimum minute volume. Because of this risk, it is important to set a low tidal volume alarm and/or a high respiratory rate alarm to give warning. Do not let the programming of a mandatory minute volume create a false sense of security with these patients.

Determining the Best Therapeutic PEEP Level

PEEP (positive end-expiratory pressure) is generally indicated in any bilateral, generalized pulmonary condition where the functional residual capacity (FRC) is decreased. Examples include generalized atelectasis; pulmonary edema; and conditions where surfactant is diminished or absent, as in ARDS. All these patients show a decreased lung compliance as measured by their static compliance (Cst).

Specific indications for PEEP include:

Intrapulmonary shunt of greater than 15%
Refractory hypoxemia (PaO_2 of less than 60 mm Hg despite an F_IO_2 of up to 0.8 to 1.0)
The patient has had an F_IO_2 of greater than 0.5 for 48 to 72 hours and shows no indication of a rapidly improving PaO_2 so that the F_IO_2 can be lowered to a safer level

Before PEEP is started, the patient should be carefully monitored to establish his or her baseline condition. The same parameters should be monitored after each change in the PEEP level to determine how the patient is tolerating it. The best or optimal level of PEEP is that level which results in the best delivery of oxygen to the tissues (not necessarily the arterial blood). Often a secondary goal is to reduce the inspired oxygen to a safe level. See Table 14-3 for recommendations on what to monitor during the application of PEEP and how to evaluate the data.

The application of PEEP is not without risks; however, these risks are weighed against the potential benefit to the patient. In the profoundly hypoxemic patient, PEEP can be a lifesaver. In the patient whose lungs are recovering, excessive levels of PEEP can result in the problems in the following list. PEEP is *never* indicated in a patient with normal lungs or overly compliant lungs (as in emphysema). The following problems can be fatal if severe enough:

Pulmonary barotrauma
   Pulmonary interstitial emphysema (PIE) seen in a newborn
   Pneumothorax
   Tension pneumothorax
   Subcutaneous emphysema
   Mediastinal emphysema
Decreased venous return to the heart causing a decreased cardiac output and the following
   Tachycardia
   Decreased blood pressure
   Decreased tissue perfusion as measured by a decreased $P\bar{v}O_2$ (mixed venous oxygen level)
   Decreased urine output

Table 14-3. Patient Monitoring During CPAP or PEEP Therapy

Good tolerance of CPAP/PEEP therapy
Increased PaO_2
Increased static lung compliance
Stable cardiac output as shown by:
    Stable heart rate without rhythm disturbances
    Stable blood pressure
    The following, which can only be measured
        through a pulmonary artery/Swan-Ganz
        catheter:
    Stable or increased $P\bar{v}O_2$ (mixed venous
    oxygen)
    Stable cardiac output
    Decreased pulmonary vascular resistance
    Decreased intrapulmonary shunt
Poor Tolerance of CPAP/PEEP Therapy
Increased PaO_2 (This can be deceiving if it is all
    that you look at.)
Decreased static lung compliance
Decreased cardiac output as shown by:
    Increased heart rate and/or rhythm
        disturbances
    Decreased blood pressure
    The following, which can only be measured
        through a pulmonary artery/Swan-Ganz
        catheter:
    Decreased $P\bar{v}O_2$ (mixed venous oxygen)
    Decreased actual cardiac output
    Increased pulmonary vascular resistance
    Increased intrapulmonary shunt

PEEP therapy is usually started at initial levels of 2 to 5 cm water pressure (cm H_2O). The patient is evaluated within 15 to 30 minutes. After the patient's response is determined, 2 to 5 cm more PEEP may be applied. The patient is reevaluated. This process goes on until the best or optimal level of PEEP is determined. (See Fig. 14-11 for a number of physiologic parameters that can be measured.)

There are different approaches to the application of PEEP to find the best level. One approach could be called minimum PEEP. It involves the application of PEEP to the minimum level that allows the inspired oxygen to be lowered to a safer percentage. A clinical goal is to minimize the risk of oxygen toxicity. In this approach, PEEP is raised until the PaO_2 is greater than 60 mm Hg or the SpO_2 is

---

Fig. 14-11 The optimal or best PEEP level is determined by monitoring some or all of the following parameters: PaO_2, effective static compliance (C_{st}), pressure of mixed venous oxygen ($P\bar{v}O_2$), cardiac output (CO), shunt (Qs/Qt), and pulmonary vascular resistance (PVR). Ideally, as the FRC is increased by PEEP, lung compliance is improved and ventilation and perfusion are better matched. Cardiac output should remain stable. It can be measured by the use of the proper pulmonary artery (Swan-Ganz) catheter or indirectly followed by monitoring the patient's heart rate and blood pressure. As can be seen, the optimal PEEP is found at 12 cm water pressure. Excessive PEEP is seen by the resulting drop in static compliance and cardiac output (rising heart rate and falling blood pressure).

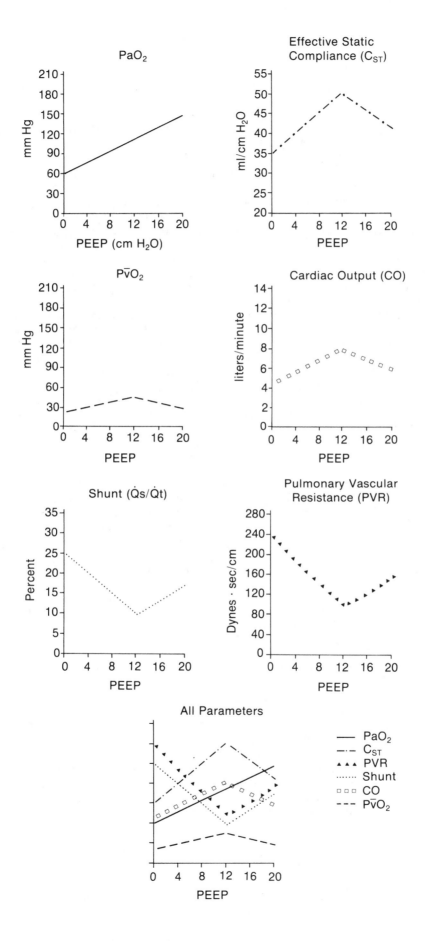

greater than 90% on an F_1O_2 of .60 or less. Usually no more than 10 to 15 cm water of PEEP are needed to achieve this.

Another approach could be called maximum PEEP. This has a clinical goal of reducing the shunt fraction (Qs/Qt) to less than 15%. Commonly this requires much higher levels of PEEP. This much pressure is more likely to have adverse cardiovascular effects on the patient. A pulmonary artery catheter must be placed to monitor the patient's pulmonary wedge pressure, pulmonary vascular resistance, and cardiac output. Often these patients will need additional support to keep the cardiac output clinically acceptable. It may be necessary to give the patient whole blood or balanced electrolyte solutions to support the blood pressure. Dopamine (Intropin) may also be needed to increase the vascular tone to raise the blood pressure. Digitalis (Digoxin) may be needed to increase the heart's pumping ability. The higher PEEP pressures also increase the risk of pulmonary barotrauma. Watch closely for signs of pneumothorax, subcutaneous emphysema, and so forth.

As the patient begins to recover, the PEEP level may be reduced in steps of 2 to 5 cm water pressure. Again, the patient should be evaluated within 15 to 30 minutes after every change in the PEEP level. If the patient's cardiovascular status is normal and there is no evidence of pulmonary barotrauma, the following are recommendations for how to decrease PEEP and oxygen levels:

Decrease PEEP first if the PaO_2 is greater than 60 mm Hg and the F_1O_2 is less than 0.5.
Decrease oxygen first if the PaO_2 is greater than 60 mm Hg and the F_1O_2 is greater than 0.5.

If the patient is showing an adverse reaction to the PEEP level such as decreased cardiac output or barotrauma, the PEEP level should be decreased before the oxygen percentage. Clinical judgment must be used to decide whether a high oxygen level or a high PEEP level is a greater danger to the patient. Minimize or remove whichever puts the patient at greater risk.

Match the mode of ventilation to the patient's problem. It is obvious that the current generation of mechanical ventilators offers the physician and practitioner a number of options for how to best tailor ventilatory support to meet the patient's needs. They must determine which of the following problems the patient must address to best meet his or her needs.

Increased Work of Breathing

Patients who show increased work at breathing may have a very high airway resistance, as in status asthmaticus, or may have a very low lung-thoracic compliance, as in ARDS. Some practitioners believe that the control or assist/control modes, when properly applied to a sedated patient, are best for these problems because the patient's breathing efforts are almost eliminated. Other practitioners believe that IMV or SIMV are physiologically superior modes of ventilation. More recently, pressure support ventilation has been shown to be beneficial to patients with increased efforts at breathing from the high airway resistance caused by a small diameter endotracheal tube.

Hypercapnia

A patient may have hypercapnia (an acute rise in the carbon dioxide level) because of sedation from a morphine or heroin overdose or may have chronic obstructive pulmonary disease with worsening of the chronic hypercapnia. In either case, the patient will become progressively more hypoxemic (unless given supplemental oxygen) as the carbon dioxide level rises. Control or assist/control modes are best for setting a minimum minute volume to determine the maximum carbon dioxide level. As the patient recovers, IMV/SIMV or PSV allow for the gradual reduction of ventilatory support. Mandatory Minute Ventilation has also shown success at setting a minute volume that limits the rise in carbon dioxide as the patient is weaning.

Hypoxemia

If the problem is secondary to a decreased functional residual capacity, as in ARDS or atelectasis, the treatment of choice for hypoxemia is CPAP on a freestanding system or bilevel ventilation or PEEP on a conventional volume cycled ventilator. If the problem is from an increased intrapulmonary shunt, the patient may need PEEP or CPAP as well as up to 100% oxygen. Pressure control inverse ratio ventilation and high frequency jet ventilation have been used with success in hypoxemic patients with a pulmonary air leak who have failed at conventional volume ventilation.

Combining modes of ventilation. All the following were discussed earlier as individual modes of ventilation. When a patient has more than one problem, more than one solution may be needed. The following are combinations of modes from which to choose:

Pressure Control/Pressure Control Inverse Ratio Ventilation, Synchronous Intermittent Mandatory Ventilation and PEEP

Pressure control or, if necessary, pressure control inverse ratio ventilation have been used with success in patients with low compliance and a pulmonary air leak. By limiting the peak pressure, less air seems to leak out and the tissues are more likely to heal. Therapeutic PEEP is applied to increase the patient's FRC to correct hypoxemia. The SIMV feature is added to let the patient breathe spontaneously if desired and stay more synchronized with the ventilator. With lung healing the PEEP level is decreased and the inspiratory time is shortened. SIMV with a constant tidal volume would likely be used during the weaning phase. Fig. 14-8 shows pressure and flow tracings during pressure control ventilation.

IMV/SIMV with Pressure Support and PEEP

IMV or SIMV are used to give the patient a controlled number of deep tidal volume breaths. The patient can breathe as often as desired in between the mandatory breaths. The patient's total minute volume can be determined by adding the combination of IMV/SIMV and pressure supported breaths. A maximum acceptable $PaCO_2$ can be established with the proper combination of IMV/SIMV breaths and pressure support level. A PSV level of more than 10 cm water may be needed. In addition, the pressure support will ensure that the airway resistance of the endotracheal tube is overcome. PEEP therapy is applied to the level necessary to obtain a clinically safe PaO_2 at the lowest possible F_IO_2. (see Fig. 14-12, A, for the pressure-time curve.)

The patients who would benefit from these modes of ventilation have both a ventilation and an oxygenation problem. They have the desire to breathe on their own but a very limited ability to do so. All three modes can be independently

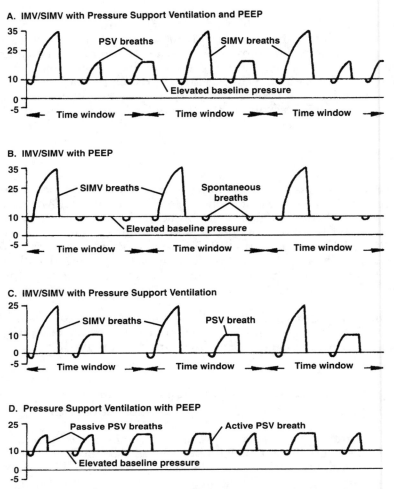

Fig. 14-12 Modification of combinations of IMV/SIMV, pressure support ventilation, and PEEP. **A,** IMV/SIMV with pressure support ventilation and PEEP. **B,** IMV/SIMV with PEEP. **C,** IMV/SIMV with pressure support ventilation. **D,** pressure support ventilation with PEEP. See the text for descriptions of the various combinations and their clinical application.

adjusted for more or less support as indicated by the patient's clinical condition and blood gas results.

IMV/SIMV with PEEP

IMV/SIMV and PEEP therapy are applied as indicated. Pressure support is not needed if the patient is strong enough to overcome the airway resistance of the endotracheal tube and breathe with a clinically acceptable tidal volume. (See Fig. 14-12, B, for the pressure-time curve.)

IMV/SIMV with Pressure Support Ventilation

IMV/SIMV and pressure support levels are increased or decreased based on the factors discussed earlier. This patient has the ability to provide some, but not all, of his or her ventilation. The PaO_2 is clinically acceptable at an oxygen percentage probably no higher than 40%.

A fairly common clinical situation is seen where the recovering patient does well on a gradually decreasing number of IMV/SIMV breaths until he or she can go no lower. The barrier seems to be the airway resistance of the endotracheal tube. The addition of some pressure support overcomes that resistance so that the IMV/SIMV level can be further reduced. When the IMV/SIMV frequency is down to four or less, the patient is providing almost all of his or her minute volume. The greatest barrier to breathing is likely to be the resistance of the endotracheal tube. The decision can then be made to extubate the patient. (See Fig. 14-12, C, for the pressure-time curve.)

Pressure Support Ventilation with PEEP

PSV and PEEP are applied as discussed earlier. This patient has the drive to breathe on his or her own; however, he or she has some limitation in the ability to overcome the resistance of the endotracheal tube or generate a consistently large enough tidal volume. In addition, the patient has a significant oxygenation problem and needs some PEEP therapy. With recovery, both PSV and PEEP can be reduced. They may be reduced individually or simultaneously as the patient's strength and/ or oxygenation improve. (See Fig. 14-12, D, for the pressure-time curve.)

10. Ventilator delivered sigh volume.
a.   Recommend a change in the sigh volume. (IIIC10i) [R, Ap, An]

Most ventilator dependent patients receive a ventilator sigh volume just as they do a tidal volume. A sign volume is typically 1.5 to 2 times the tidal volume if the tidal volume is in the low to middle range of normal. If the patient has a problem of atelectasis or consolidation, a larger sign volume may be indicated. The patient may not need a sigh volume at all if the uncorrected tidal volume is at the 15 ml/ kg upper limit. A patient with bullous emphysema, a pneumothorax, or cardiac status that is sensitive to high peak pressures may be contraindicated for a sigh volume. The patient who is air trapping the tidal volume should have a smaller (possibly no) sigh volume. Compare the inspired and expired volumes to ensure that there is no air trapping.

b.   Recommend a change in the sigh frequency. (IIIC10j) [R, Ap, An]

Most current ventilators allow the clinician to tailor the sigh frequency to best meet the patient's clinical needs. The sigh frequency should be increased in patients with atelectasis or consolidation. The sigh frequency may need to be decreased or eliminated in patients who are air trapping the tidal and/or sigh volumes. The sigh control is usually turned off when a patient is in the IMV/SIMV mode.

11. Recommend a change in the mechanical dead space. (IIIC10g) [R, Ap, An]

Mechanical dead space is added to increase the patient's $PaCO_2$ by making him or her rebreathe some exhaled carbon dioxide. The last part of the tidal volume to be exhaled came from the alveoli and is high in CO_2. This last portion of the tidal volume is exhaled into the dead space tubing. This high CO_2 gas is then inhaled back to the alveolar level and increases the patient's $PaCO_2$. The more dead space tubing there is, the more carbon dioxide is retained. It is important to realize that this same rebreathed volume of gas is lower in oxygen because of its diffusion into the patient's pulmonary circulation. If a large amount of mechanical dead space is added, it will be necessary to increase the F_IO_2 to keep the ordered level. Measure the oxygen percentage between the dead space and the endotracheal/tracheostomy tube adapter.

Mechanical dead space is commonly only used in the control and assist/control modes. It should not be used in IMV/SIMV, pressure support, or CPAP modes unless it adds to the patient's comfort by giving flexibility to the circuit when his or her head is turned.

The following formula can be used to predict what amount of mechanical dead space will produce a desired $PaCO_2$. (Note: The same formula can also be used to calculate the necessary change in either tidal volume or respiratory rate to produce a desired $PaCO_2$.)

$$[(V_T - V_{Danat}) - V_{Dmech}] \times f \times PaCO_2 = [(V_T - V_{Danat}) - V_{Dmech}] \times f \times PaCO_2$$

Where:

V_T = current tidal volume
V_{Danat} = anatomic dead space. This is calculated at 1 ml/lb or 2.2 ml/kg of ideal body weight.
V_{Dmech} = current mechanical dead space
f = ventilator rate
$PaCO_2$ = actual patient $PaCO_2$ value
V_{Dmech} = desired mechanical dead space
$PaCO_2$ = desired patient $PaCO_2$ value

Example

Your patient is a 70-kg/154-lb male who is being ventilated on the control mode (he is apneic). His ventilator settings are: tidal volume of 1000 ml, rate of 12/min, F_IO_2 of 0.3, no added mechanical dead space. His arterial blood gases are: PaO_2 of 90 mm Hg, $PaCO_2$ of 30 mm Hg, pH of 7.48, SaO_2 of 95%, BE 0. The clinical goal is to adjust the patient's mechanical dead space as needed to produce a $PaCO_2$ of 40 mm Hg. In summary:

V_T = 1000 ml current tidal volume
V_{Danat} = 154 ml anatomic dead space. This is calculated at 1 ml/lb or 2.2 ml/kg of ideal body weight.
V_{Dmech} = no added mechanical dead space
f = 12 for ventilator rate
$PaCO_2$ = 30 mm Hg actual patient $PaCO_2$ value
V_{Dmech} = desired amount of mechanical dead space
$PaCO_2$ = 40 mm Hg desired patient $PaCO_2$ value

Placing the data and goal into the formula results in:

$$[(V_T - V_{Danat}) - V_{Dmech}] \times f \times PaCO_2 = [(V_T - V_{Danat}) - V_{Dmech}] \times f \times PaCO_2$$
$$[(1000 - 154) - 0] \times 12 \times 30 = [(1000 - 154) - V_{Dmech}] \times 12 \times 40$$

Simplifying produces:

$$[846] \times 12 \times 30 = [846 - V_{Dmech}] \times 480$$
$$304,560 = (846 \times 480) - (V_{Dmech} \times 480)$$
$$304,560 = 406,080 - 480 \, V_{Dmech}$$
$$-101,520 = -480 \, V_{Dmech}$$
$$211.5 \text{ ml} = V_{Dmech}$$

The solution is to increase the patient's mechanical dead space from zero to 212 ml.

12. Recommend the addition of expiratory retard. (IIIC10a) [R, Ap, An]

Expiratory retard was first discussed in Section 13. It is indicated in any patient who is air trapping and not exhaling completely. It functions like pursed-lip breathing in the spontaneously breathing patient. The backpressure prevents the collapse of the smallest airways (see Fig. 14-13 for the pressure-time waveform). Expiratory retard may be indicated in a patient with asthma, emphysema, or bronchitis. It is important with these types of patients to measure the inspiratory and expiratory tidal volume. Air trapping is confirmed by the expiratory volume being less than the inspiratory volume. When listening to the patient's breath sounds, it will be noted that there is no pause at the end of exhalation before the next inspiration is started. In extreme cases, the pressure manometer will not return to the baseline level. These patients should be checked for the presence and level of auto-PEEP. The proper level of expiratory retard is determined by trial and error. The following parameters should be monitored to find the proper amount:

a. The inspiratory and expiratory tidal volumes should be the same.

b. The patient's breath sounds should reveal wheezing to be absent or minimal and a silent pause at the end of exhalation before the next tidal volume is delivered.

c. There should be no auto-PEEP.

d. The patient should subjectively feel that he or she has exhaled completely before the next breath is given.

It is important to monitor the patient frequently when expiratory retard is being used. As the patient is treated with aerosolized sympathomimetics, corticosteroids, and/or aminophylline, the bronchospasm should diminish. Expiratory retard should not be needed when the airway resistance has returned to normal.

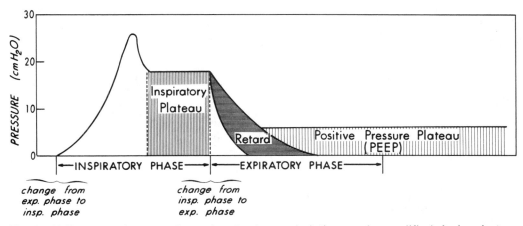

Fig. 14-13 Pressure-time waveform showing how exhalation can be modified. An inspiratory plateau (inflation hold) is seen when the tidal volume is held within the lungs for a period of time. With expiratory retard the gas is more slowly exhaled than during a passive breath. These two modifications of exhalation may or may not be combined with PEEP. (From Kirby RR, Smith RA, Desautels DA: Mechanical ventilation. In Burton GG, Hodgkin JE, editors: *Respiratory care: a guide to clinical practice*, ed 2, Phildelphia, 1984, Lippincott. Used by permission.)

13. Recommend the addition of an inspiratory plateau. (IIIC10b) [R, Ap, An]

Inspiratory plateau (also known as inflation hold) is a technique whereby the patient is temporarily prevented from exhaling the ventilator delivered tidal volume (see Fig. 14-13 for the pressure-time waveform). An inspiratory plateau is added therapeutically to improve the distribution of the tidal volume. Patients with ARDS and pulmonary edema can benefit from it. Oxygenation should improve in direct proportion to the duration of the inspiratory plateau. The duration of inspiratory plateau is measured in different ways depending on the ventilator. For example, the BEAR 5 and Bennett 7200 can have it added in steps of .1 seconds up to several seconds total. The Servo 900 B and C can have it added as a variable percentage of the total duration of the breathing cycle. It is important to reduce the inspiratory plateau as the patient's ventilation and lung compliance improve. Patients with normal ventilation and compliance should not receive any inspiratory plateau.

Notice that the use of an inspiratory plateau increases the inspiratory phase of the breathing cycle. This results in a shorter expiratory time if the rate is kept the same. Or the rate must be reduced to keep the same I : E ratio. Again, as discussed earlier, make sure that the tidal volume is completely exhaled. The patient's condition should be monitored closely to determine if the level of inspiratory plateau is appropriate.

Nontherapeutic inspiratory plateau is added temporarily to determine the plateau pressure on the ventilator. This is considered to be the pressure needed to deliver the tidal volume. With this information, the patient's effective static compliance can be calculated. Its calculation and interpretation are discussed later in this section. An inspiratory plateau of .5 to 1.0 seconds is usually long enough to find the plateau pressure. Remember to turn off the inspiratory plateau afterwards.

14. Initiate and adjust mechanical ventilation when *no* settings are specified. (IIIB2b) [R, Ap]

Typically the therapist is expected to set the following ventilator controls based on a protocol or the patient's condition and response to the ventilator.

Tidal Volume.—The usual goal is to deliver a tidal volume of 10 to 15 ml/kg of ideal body weight. An exception could be a patient who has had a lobectomy or pneumomectomy; he or she would be given a smaller volume.

Sensitivity.—Usually a patient on a volume cycled ventilator should have the sensitivity set at about −1 to −2 cm water pressure. No matter the method by which the ventilator senses the patient's respiratory effort, he or she should not have to work very hard to trigger a machine tidal volume.

Flow.—Flow is adjusted to set the inspiratory time and I : E ratio and/or to meet the patient's needs.

I : E Ratio.—The I : E ratio is adjusted to ensure that the patient can inhale in as physiologically appropriate a manner as possible and completely exhale the inspired tidal volume.

Alarms.—Alarm systems are different for each type of ventilator. Generally speaking, they are set with a safety margin of ± 10% from the patient's normal ventilator settings. A variation of greater than 10% results in an audible and/or visual alarm condition.

Gas Temperature.—The goal for most patients is to minimize their humidity deficit by giving gas that is humidified and warmed to near body temperature. It is common to have the gas warmed to 90° to 95°F/35°C. It should be measured in the inspiratory limb of the circuit as close to the patient as possible.

15. Mean airway pressure.
a. Monitor the mean airway pressure to determine the patient's response to respiratory care. (IIIAld) [R, Ap, An]

Mean airway pressure ($\overline{\text{Paw}}$ or MAP) is the average pressure over an entire breathing cycle. A number of current neonatal and adult ventilators are able to calculate the value (see Fig. 14-14). Mean airway pressure is influenced by the patient's lung-thoracic compliance (C_{LT}), airway resistance (Raw), and ventilator settings. If a volume cycled ventilator is being used, a decrease in compliance or an increase in resistance will result in an increase in the mean airway pressure. This is because it will take more pressure to deliver the tidal volume; a higher peak pressure will be seen. Conversely, if the patient's compliance increases or the resistance decreases, the $\overline{\text{Paw}}$ will decrease. It is important to further evaluate the patient when a change in $\overline{\text{Paw}}$ is noticed. This is because the new pressure, by itself, will not show you whether there has been a change in compliance, resistance, or both. Any treatments that improve lung compliance and reduce airway resistance would be shown by a reduced mean airway pressure. It is important to calculate both dynamic and static compliance (discussed next) when trying to determine how the patient's condition has changed. This can only be done when the patient is on a volume cycled ventilator with a known tidal volume.

b. Recommend a change in the patient's mean airway pressure. (IIIC10c) [R, Ap, An]

In general, an increase in mean airway pressure will increase the patient's oxygenation. This is because the alveoli are kept open longer, allowing more time for diffusion and preventing alveolar collapse. If alveolar ventilation is improved, the $PaCO_2$ may also be reduced. If the mean airway pressure is too high there is an increased risk of pulmonary barotrauma and decreased cardiac output. This is especially true if PEEP is increased to raise the $\overline{\text{Paw}}$. Watch the patient closely

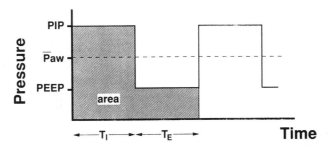

Fig. 14-14 Mathematical derivation of mean airway pressure ($\overline{\text{Paw}}$) and a pressure-time tracing showing where $\overline{\text{Paw}}$ would be found. PIP is the peak inspiratory pressure, PEEP is positive end-expiratory pressure, T_I is inspiratory time, T_E is expiratory time, and K is the waveform constant for the calculation. (From Chatburn RL: Principles and practice of neonatal and pediatric mechanical ventilation, *Respir Care* 36(6):569-595, 1991. Used by permission.)

whenever a ventilator change is made that increases the $\overline{P}$aw. A sudden deterioration in cardiopulmonary function may be caused by a pneumothorax. A reduction in urine output, an increased heart rate, and decreased blood pressure are often seen when the cardiac output is reduced. The mean airway pressure should be reduced if either of these situations is seen. To prevent these complications, it is necessary to reduce the mean airway pressure whenever the patient's pulmonary condition improves. As the compliance increases toward normal it will not be necessary to use as high a mean airway pressure to maintain acceptable blood gases.

There is further discussion on ventilator adjustments that increase or decrease mean airway pressure in Section 15. Because lung compliance cannot be measured on continuous flow IMV mode neonatal ventilators, the monitoring of mean airway pressure is especially important. In general, making the same ventilator adjustments to an adult will result in the same changes in mean airway pressure.

16. Lung compliance and airway resistance.
a. Recommend a lung compliance and airway resistance measurement to get more information about the patient's condition. (IA2r and IA2x) [R, Ap, An]

These calculations are important because they provide valuable information on the patient's pulmonary condition and how the lungs are affected by changes in tidal volume, sigh volume, and therapeutic PEEP.

Static compliance (Cst) is the measurement of work required to overcome the elastic resistance to ventilation. It is a measurement of the compliance of the lungs and thorax (C_{LT}). Static compliance is measured in units of ml/cm water pressure. The normal adult's static compliance is 100 ml/cm water pressure. The procedure for its measurement is given later in this discussion.

Dynamic compliance (Cdyn) is the measurement of the combination of the patient's static compliance and airway resistance (Raw). Dynamic compliance is sometimes called dynamic characteristic. Airway resistance is also known as nonelastic resistance to ventilation. Airway resistance is measured in units of cm water/ L/sec at a standard flow rate of 0.5 L/sec (30 L/min). The normal adult's Raw is 0.6 to 2.4 cm water/L/sec. Do not forget that this procedure is being performed on an intubated patient on a ventilator. The endotracheal tube adds to the patient's total Raw. The smaller the tube is, the greater resistance it offers to gas flowing through it. Altering inspiratory flow also has an influence on the peak pressure measured for the calculation. The lower the flow, the less gas turbulence there is and the lower the peak pressure is. Conversely, a higher flow will create more turbulence and a higher peak pressure will be seen.

b. Determine the lung compliance and airway resistance values to evaluate the patient's response to respiratory care. (IIIA1p) [R, Ap]

The calculation of airway resistance was presented earlier in the discussion of pressure support ventilation. Review it if necessary.

Before the actual calculation of the patient's static and dynamic compliance can be performed, the static compliance of the breathing circuit must be determined. This is because some of the set tidal volume never reaches the patient because it is "lost" as compressed volume in the circuit. The compliance of the breathing circuit is referred to as the compliance factor. It is usually between 2 and 5 ml/cm water pressure. To be as accurate as possible in the calculation of static and dynamic compliance and the calculation of actual tidal and sigh volumes, this lost volume must be subtracted from the exhaled tidal volume. Review the procedure for the calculation of the compliance factor in *Respiratory Care Certification Guide* (Sills, 1994) if necessary.

Several of the microprocessor based ventilators, such as the Puritan-Bennett 7200, will calculate circuit compliance. Furthermore, they can calculate airway resistance and static and dynamic compliance. This information can also be graphed for further interpretation. It is important, however, that the therapist know how to manually perform these calculations and interpret the results.

Procedure for Calculating Static Compliance

1. Determine the compliance factor of the breathing circuit.
2. Reattach the patient to the ventilator. Reset all controls to their ordered or preset positions.
3. Cycle a tidal volume. The patient should be breathing passively; fighting the breath will result in an erroneously high peak pressure and assisting with the breath will result in an erroneously low peak pressure.
4. Briefly prevent the tidal volume from being exhaled. No air should be moving. Note that the pressure manometer shows a peak pressure and then a static or plateau pressure that is stable as long as the tidal volume is held in the lungs. Record the plateau pressure.
5. Calculate the static compliance using this formula:

$$Cst = \frac{\text{exhaled tidal volume} - \text{compressed volume}}{\text{plateau pressure} - \text{PEEP}}$$

where compressed volume = compliance factor × plateau pressure

Procedure for Calculating Dynamic Compliance

1. Determine the compliance factor of the breathing circuit.
2. Reattach the patient to the ventilator. Reset all controls to their ordered or preset positions.
3. Cycle a tidal volume. The patient should be breathing passively; fighting the breath will result in an erroneously high peak pressure and assisting with the breath will result in an erroneously low peak pressure.
4. Note the peak pressure on the manometer. If the pressure at the end of inspiration is less than peak pressure, the pressure at the end of inspiration should be used in the calculation.
5. Calculate the dynamic compliance using this formula:

$$Cdyn = \frac{\text{exhaled tidal volume} - \text{compressed volume}}{\text{peak pressure} - \text{PEEP}}$$

where compressed volume = compliance factor × peak pressure

Example

Calculate the static and dynamic compliance on a ventilated patient without PEEP therapy. The patient has an exhaled tidal volume of 600 ml. The peak pressure is 30 cm water and the static or plateau pressure is 20 cm water (see Fig. 14-15). The compliance factor has been determined to be 4 ml/cm water pressure.

$$\text{Static compliance (Cst)} = \frac{\text{exhaled tidal volume} - \text{compressed volume}}{\text{plateau pressure} - \text{PEEP}}$$

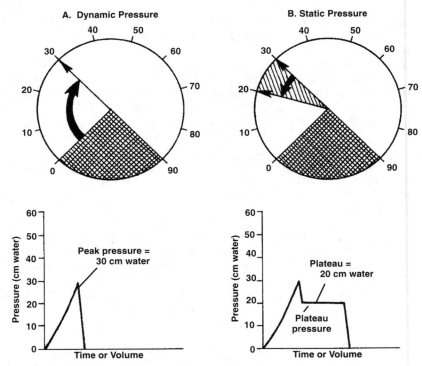

Fig. 14-15 Peak and static pressures without PEEP. **A,** Pressure manometer reading and pressure-volume curve for dynamic pressure. **B,** Pressure manometer reading and pressure-volume curve for static pressure.

where compressed volume = compliance factor × plateau pressure
= 4 ml/cm × 20 cm = 80 ml

$$Cst = \frac{600\,ml - 80\,ml}{20\,cm - 0}$$

$$Cst = \frac{520\,ml}{20\,cm}$$

Cst = 26 ml/cm water pressure

$$\text{Dynamic compliance (Cdyn)} = \frac{\text{exhaled tidal volume} - \text{compressed volume}}{\text{peak pressure} - \text{PEEP}}$$

where compressed volume = compliance factor × peak pressure
= 4 ml/cm × 30 cm = 120 ml

$$Cdyn = \frac{600\,ml - 120\,ml}{30\,cm - 0}$$

$$Cdyn = \frac{480\,ml}{30\,cm}$$

Cdyn = 16 ml/cm water pressure

Example

Calculate the static and dynamic compliance on a ventilated patient with PEEP therapy. The same patient has an exhaled tidal volume of 600 ml. Due to refractory hypoxemia 10 cm of PEEP therapy is started. The peak pressure is now 36 cm water and the static or plateau pressure is now 25 cm water (see Fig. 14-16). The compliance factor has been determined to be 4 ml/cm water pressure.

$$\text{Cst} = \frac{\text{exhaled tidal volume} - \text{compressed volume}}{\text{plateau pressure} - \text{PEEP}}$$

where compressed volume = compliance factor × plateau pressure
$$= 4 \text{ ml/cm} \times (25 \text{ cm} - 10 \text{ cm of PEEP})$$
$$= 4 \text{ ml/cm} \times 15 \text{ cm} = 60 \text{ ml}$$

$$\text{Cst} = \frac{600 \text{ ml} - 60 \text{ ml}}{25 \text{ cm} - 10 \text{ cm}}$$

$$\text{Cst} = \frac{540 \text{ ml}}{15 \text{ cm}}$$

Cst = 36 ml/cm water pressure

$$\text{Cdyn} = \frac{\text{exhaled tidal volume} - \text{compressed volume}}{\text{peak pressure} - \text{PEEP}}$$

where compressed volume = compliance factor × peak pressure
$$= 4 \text{ ml/cm} \times (36 - 10 \text{ cm of PEEP})$$
$$= 4 \text{ ml/cm} \times 26$$
$$= 104 \text{ ml}$$

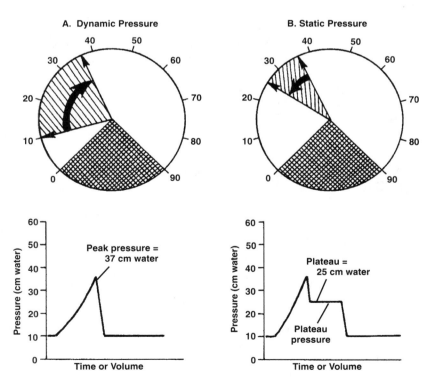

Fig. 14-16 Peak and static pressures with PEEP. **A,** Pressure manometer reading and pressure-volume curve for dynamic pressure. **B,** Pressure manometer reading and pressure-volume curve for static pressure.

$$Cdyn = \frac{600\,ml - 104\,ml}{36\,cm - 10\,cm}$$

$$Cdyn = \frac{496\,ml}{26\,cm}$$

Cdyn = 19 ml/cm water pressure

c. Interpret the lung compliance values to evaluate the patient's response to respiratory care. (IIIA1r6) [R, Ap, An]

There are six possible combinations of increasing or decreasing static and/or dynamic lung compliances. Each has its own possible causes, which will be covered in turn. The example discussed earlier and illustrated in Fig. 14-15 is used as a starting point for these variations.

It must be remembered that the patient must be passive on the ventilator for the measured values to be accurate. If the patient is assisting with the breath, the peak and plateau pressures will be too low. If the patient is fighting the breath, the pressures will be too high. Check two or three breaths for increased accuracy. Let the patient have a normal breath or two between each of the peak and plateau pressure measurement breaths.

Decreased Dynamic Compliance (Cdyn) with a Stable Static Compliance (Cst)

This is noticed as an *increase* in the peak pressure with an unchanged plateau pressure (see Fig. 14-17). Causes include bronchospasm, coughing, secretions in the airways, water or kinking in the inspiratory limb of the circuit, or biting the endotracheal tube. Correcting the underlying problem by aerosolizing a bronchodilator, suctioning, and so forth results in the peak pressure returing to the original level.

Note that the inspiratory resistance has doubled from the original 10 cm to 20 cm while the plateau pressure has not changed. This confirms that the problem originates in the airway or breathing circuit. The patient's lung compliance has not changed.

Increased Dynamic Compliance (Cdyn) with a Stable Static Compliance (Cst)

This is noticed as a *decrease* in the peak pressure with an unchanged plateau pressure (see Fig. 14-18). This represents an improvement in the patient's airway resistance from the original condition. Secretions could be diminished, mucus plugs cleared, or bronchospasm corrected.

Note that the inspiratory resistance has decreased from the original level of 20 cm to just 5 cm. This confirms that the patient's airway resistance has decreased. The patient's lung compliance has not changed.

False Decreased Dynamic Compliance (Cdyn) with True Decreased Static Compliance (Cst)

This is noticed as an *increase* in *both* the peak and plateau pressures (see Fig. 14-19). This is seen when the patient's lung-thoracic compliance worsens. The plateau pressure is elevated and the Cst is decreased. Pulmonary conditions that

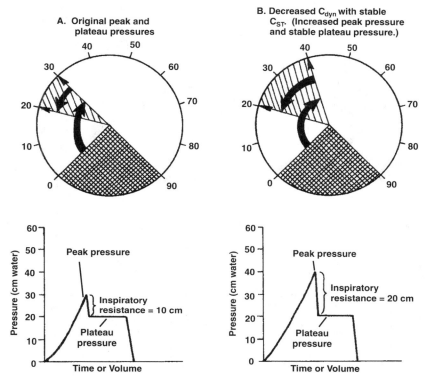

Fig. 14-17 Decreased dynamic compliance (Cdyn) with a stable static compliance (Cst). **A,** Original pressure manometer reading and pressure-volume curve. **B,** Altered pressure manometer reading and pressure-volume curve.

result in a lowered compliance include ARDS and IRDS, pneumonia, pulmonary edema, atelectasis, consolidation, hemothorax, pleural effusion, air trapping, pneumomediastinum, and pneumothorax. Examples of chest wall and abdominal conditions that lower compliance include the various chest wall deformities, circumferential chest or abdominal burns, enlarged liver, pneumoperitoneum, peritonitis, abdominal bleeding, and herniation. Advanced pregnancy may also lower compliance.

As an artifact of the stiffer lungs, the peak pressure is also elevated and the Cdyn is decreased; however, the difference between the peak and plateau pressures remains 10 cm water. This demonstrates that there is no real increase in the patient's airway resistance.

True Decreased Dynamic Compliance (Cdyn) with True Decreased Static Compliance (Cst)

This is also noticed as an *increase* in *both* the peak and plateau pressures (see Fig. 14-20). This is seen with the combination of a decreased lung compliance and an increased airway resistance. Causes of both of these problems were discussed earlier.

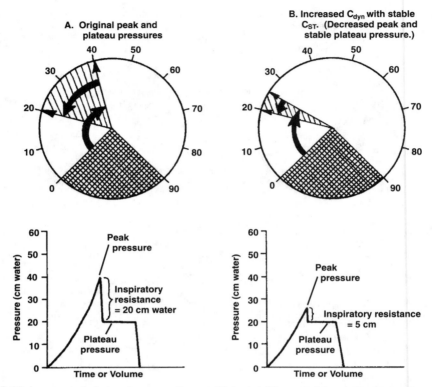

Fig. 14-18 Increased dynamic compliance (Cdyn) with a stable static compliance (Cst). **A,** Original pressure manometer reading and pressure-volume curve. **B,** Altered pressure manometer reading and pressure-volume curve.

False Increased Dynamic Compliance (Cdyn) with True Increased Static Compliance (Cst)

This is noticed as a *decrease* in *both* the peak and plateau pressures (see Fig. 14-21). This will be seen when the patient's lung-thoracic compliance improves. The plateau pressure decreases and, as an artifact, the peak pressure also decreases.

Notice that the difference between the peak and plateau pressures remains 10 cm water. This indicates that the patient's airway resistance is unchanged.

True Increased Dynamic Compliance (Cdyn) with True Increased Static Compliance (Cst)

This is also noticed as a *decrease* in *both* the peak and plateau pressures (see Fig. 14-22). This is seen when the patient's airway resistance and lung-thoracic compliance improve.

Notice that the plateau pressure has decreased indicating more compliant lungs. Also notice that the difference between the peak and plateau pressures has decreased from 20 to 10 cm water. This demonstrates that the airway resistance has also decreased.

All six examples of increasing or decreasing static and/or dynamic lung compliance make use of a single tidal volume that is analyzed for peak and plateau pressures. Some practitioners advocate using several different tidal volumes when

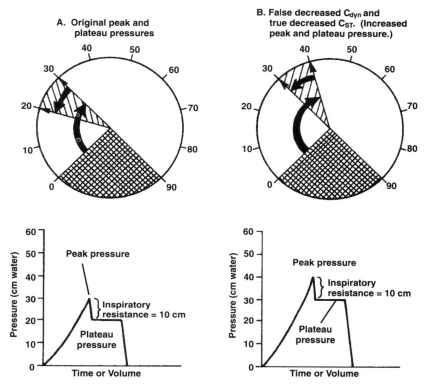

Fig. 14-19 False decreased dynamic compliance (Cdyn) with true decreased static compliance (Cst). **A,** Original pressure manometer reading and pressure-volume curve. **B,** Altered pressure manometer reading and pressure-volume curve.

measuring dynamic and static pressures. The procedure involves delivering a series of tidal volumes, determining the static and dynamic pressures at each volume, and then dividing the tidal volumes by the respective pressures. The various values are plotted on a graph to find the patient's optimal tidal volume that results in the highest static compliance value. Fig. 14-23 shows a series of these graphs. As can be seen, the curves for diseased lungs and airways are quite different from the normal person or a patient with pulmonary emboli. A pulmonary embolism should be considered if the patient's condition deteriorates rapidly and there is no change in the dynamic and static compliance values.

17. Perform and/or interpret pressure-volume and flow-volume loops. (IC1n) [R, Ap, An]

All the currently available microprocessor ventilators are capable of plotting pressure-volume and flow-volume loops and displaying them on the units's video display. These ventilators include the Puritan-Bennett 7200, BEAR 5 and 1000, Hamilton Veolar, Infrasonic's Adult Star, and Drager EVITA. These units contain software programs that allow the practitioner to measure and graph a variety of data. Pressure-volume tracings and flow-volume loop tracings were presented in Section 3. Review that information if necessary for the interpretation of the results. In addition, a number of tracings are included in this section. Fig. 14-6 has tracings of pressure support ventilation, Fig. 14-8 has tracings of pressure control ventilation, and Fig. 14-9 has tracings of air trapping and auto-PEEP.

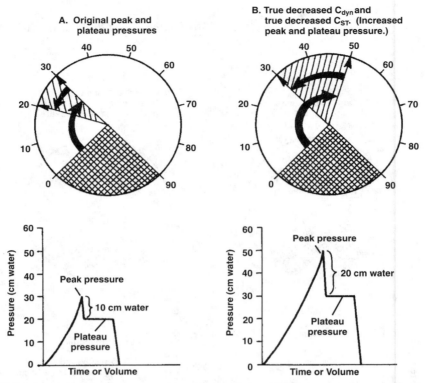

Fig. 14-20 True decreased dynamic compliance (Cdyn) with true decreased static compliance (Cst). **A,** Original pressure manometer reading and pressure-volume curve. **B,** Altered pressure manometer reading and pressure-volume curve.

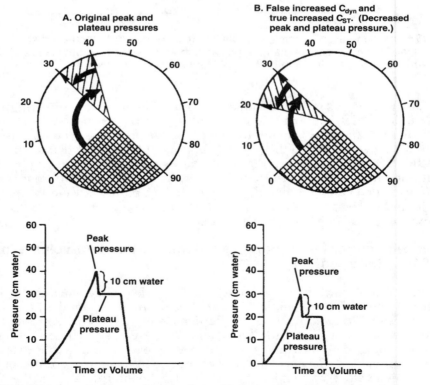

Fig. 14-21 False increased dynamic compliance (Cdyn) with true increased static compliance (Cst). **A,** Original pressure manometer reading and pressure-volume curve. **B,** Altered pressure manometer reading and pressure-volume curve.

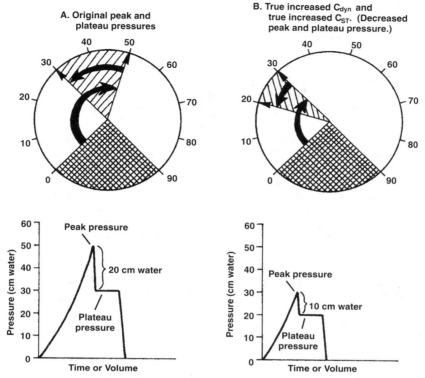

Fig. 14-22 True increased dynamic compliance (Cdyn) with true increased static compliance (Cst). **A,** Original pressure manometer reading and pressure-volume curve. **B,** Altered pressure manometer reading and pressure-volume curve.

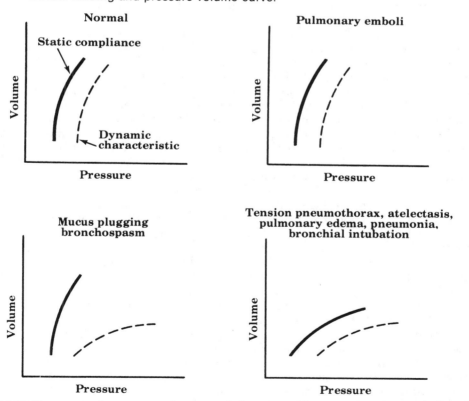

Fig. 14-23 Pressure-volume curves for normal airways and lungs, pulmonary embolism (no change in airway resistance or lung compliance), increased airway resistance, and decreased lung compliance. (From Pilbeam SP: *Mechanical ventilation: physiological and clinical applications,* St. Louis, 1986, Multi-Media Publishing. Used by permission.)

18. Sedate or paralyze the patient.
a. Recommend the use of sedatives or muscle relaxants (paralyzing agents) as needed. (IIIC10d) [R, Ap, An]

An adult who is attempting to inhale or exhale out of sequence with the ventilator is said to be "bucking" or "fighting" the ventilator. This problem is most commonly seen in the control and assist/control modes. If the asynchrony between the patient's efforts and the ventilator is too great, there is an increased risk of hypoxemia, air trapping, and pneumothorax. Carefully evaluate the patient to determine if he or she is breathing rapidly because of pain, anxiety, or improper adjustment of the ventilator. Make sure that the gas flow, rate, pressure limit, and so forth are correctly set for the patient's condition. Sedation or paralysis should be considered only after all other causes of asynchrony have been ruled out.

b. Recommend specific sedating or muscle relaxing agents for use on patients. (IIIC10e) [R, Ap, An]

It is important to consider the following patient conditions before making a medication choice for controlling the patient's breathing efforts:

a. Is the patient in pain? If so, an opiate analgesic such as morphine sulfate is commonly given. It can be given as a single dose by intramuscular injection but most often it is given intravenously for faster onset. Morphine will have the additional effects of reducing anxiety and inducing sleep. Because like all opiates it is a central nervous system depressant, make sure that the ventilator alarm systems are functioning properly in case the patient becomes disconnected. The relatively new opiate analgesic alfentanil (Alfenta) has also gained acceptance. It can be given intravenously as a single dose or dripped in continuously. Unlike morphine, it does not cause histamine to be released. Watch for chest-wall rigidity with its use.

b. Is the patient agitated? Try to communicate with a conscious, cooperative patient to find out what the problem is. If the patient's problem can be corrected, he or she will probably relax and breathe in synchrony with the ventilator. It may be impossible to evaluate an uncooperative patient for mental state; however, asynchrony with the ventilator for no known reason can often be attributed to anxiety or fear. The benzodiazepines are the drug of choice for treatment of agitation. They include diazepam (Valium) and midazolam (Versed). When given intravenously they have a sedating effect within minutes.

It should be noted that it is widely accepted to give patients in pain and/or patients who are agitated a combination of morphine and Valium. They have a synergistic effect so both can be given in smaller doses than if only one drug were given. Watch for apnea or a possible drop in heart rate and blood pressure when the patient becomes suddenly relaxed.

c. Does the patient need to be paralyzed? If it is necessary to cause total muscular relaxation along with apnea, a skeletal muscle paralyzing agent should be used. Usually a short-term, depolarizing neuromuscular blocker such as succinylcholine (Anectine) is used during a difficult intubation. A single intravenous dose will paralyze a combative patient for about 10 minutes. For paralysis during mechanical ventilation, one of the following long-term, nondepolarizing neuromuscular blocking agents is commonly used: pancuronium (Pavulon), atracurium (Tracrium), and vencuronium (Norcuron). These are all given intravenously and will cause paralysis lasting 2 to 4 hours.

Remember that these paralyzing agents have no effect on the patient's ability to feel pain or to be afraid of what is happening. Pain medications, such as morphine, must be given as necessary. A sedating agent, such as Valium, is always given to counteract the emotional stress of being awake but unable to move.

19. Make a recommendation to extubate the patient. (IIIC10k) [R, Ap, An]

Extubation can usually be safely accomplished when the patient has met the criteria listed in Table 14-4, has demonstrated the ability to breathe effectively for a prolonged period of time as measured by the listed criteria, has acceptable arterial blood gas results, is alert enough to protect his or her airway, and can effectively cough out any secretions. It may be found that some patients need the endotracheal tube even though they no longer need ventilatory support. The tube provides a suctioning route if the patient is unable to cough out large amounts of secretions. The tube also protects the airway from the risk of aspiration in a comatose patient who may vomit.

Module B. Mechanical ventilation equipment.

Note: The literature produced by the manufacturers and the descriptions used in many standard texts break down the various ventilators into more catagories than used by the NBRC. To avoid confusion, this text uses the NBRC's more simplified terminology. A pneumatically powered ventilator is defined here as powered by compressed gas. It may be electrically controlled with electrical alarm systems.

Fluidic ventilators are defined here as being pneumatically powered and partially or completely controlled by fluidic methods. Fluidic controls make use of compressed gas for cycling and other ventilator functions.

An electrically powered ventilator is defined here as being electrically powered and controlled. Almost all currently used volume cycled ventilators, external negative pressure ventilators, high frequency jet ventilators, and high frequency oscillator ventilators are electrically powered.

A microprocessor ventilator is defined here as being controlled by a microprocessor (minicomputer). Most are electrically powered but may be pneumatically powered.

Table 14-4. Indications that the Patient can Probably Be Weaned from the Ventilator

Oxygenation
PaO_2 of 80 mm Hg or greater or $SpO_2 > 90\%$ on 50% oxygen or less
$P(A-a)O_2 < 300\text{-}350$ mm Hg on 100% oxygen
Intrapulmonary shunt of less than 15%
Ventilation
$PaCO_2 < 55$ mm Hg in a patient who is not ordinarily hypercapneic
Dead space : tidal volume ($V_D : V_T$) ratio $< 0.55\text{-}0.6$ (55%-60%)
Pulmonary Mechanics
Spontaneous tidal volume of 3-4 ml/lb or 7-9 ml/kg of ideal body weight
Vital capacity of at least 10-15 ml/kg
Maximum inspiratory pressure (MIP) $> -20-25$ cm water pressure
Forced expiratory volume in one second (FEV_1) > 10 ml/kg
Respiratory rate of 12-35/minute (adult) (It is common to see an increase in the respiratory rate.)
Micellaneous
Conscious and cooperative patient who wants to breathe spontaneously
Stable and acceptable normal blood pressure and temperature
Stable cardiac rhythm; heart rate should not increase by more than 15% to 20%
Corrected underlying problem that led to ventilatory support
Normal fluid balance and electrolyte values
Proper nutritional status

1. Ventilators.
a. Fix any problems with a pneumatic ventilator. (IIB2d1) [An]

Make sure that all connections are tight; there are more connections with the addition of the humidification system and expiratory limb to the bellows spirometer. A major leak commonly causes a prolonged inspiratory time or failure to cycle to exhalation. Tightening of the leak results in a return to the normal I : E ratio and delivery of the desired tidal volume.

A defective exhalation valve or one in which the small bore tubing has popped off will send gas through the circuit and not to the patient. If a bellows spirometer is being used, you will notice that it fills during inspiration instead of during expiration as normal.

b. Fluidic ventilators.
i. Get the necessary equipment for the procedure. (IIA1b1) [R, Ap]

Currently the only widely used adult fluidic ventilator is the Monaghan 225.

ii. Put the equipment together, make sure that it works properly, and identify any problems with it. (IIB1c1) [R, Ap]
iii. Fix any problems with the equipment. (IIB2d3) [R, Ap, An]

All versions of fluidic ventilators are pneumatically powered and have fluidic controls. Make sure that the oxygen source is up to the required pressure of 50 psig. Fluidic controls are very sensitive to any obstruction. Also make sure that inlet and outlet filters are kept clear.

c. Fix any problems with an electric ventilator. (IIIB2d2) [An]

A low volume could be from a leak; check all connections and tighten them as needed. The volume can be measured directly as it leaves the ventilator to see if it is accurate or if the unit is delivering the wrong volume. If the unit shows a volume entering the spirometer instead of the test lung during inspiration, the exhalation valve is broken or the high pressure line to a Bennett MA-1 has popped off. The valve must be replaced if broken. All alarms must be working properly. Some are powered by batteries that need to be replaced when discharged.

d. Fix any problems with a microprocessor ventilator. (IIB2d4) [An]

Microprocessor ventilators usually have self-diagnosing software built into them. If a problem with the unit is detected it will be displayed on the monitor. There is usually little to repair on the ventilator except to change a defective computer chip.

e. High frequency jet ventilators (HFJV).
i. Get the necessary equipment for the procedure. (IIA1b2) [R, Ap]

Examples of freestanding jet ventilators include the Acutronic USA AMS-1000 and Instrument Development Corporation (IDC) Model VS 600. Bear Medical Systems developed the BEAR Jet that must be used with a volume cycled ventilator that may be placed in the CPAP or IMV mode during use of the jet. The FDA has limited the rate of all jet ventilators to between 40 and 150 breaths per minute.

The proper endotracheal tube must be used before the patient can be ventilated. Ideally, the patient must be intubated with a HiLo Jet tube from National Catheter Corporation (see Fig. 14-24). This tube is designed with a catheter through which the jetted gas is sent to the main lumen. Based on the physical principles that govern jets, additional gas is entrained through the main lumen. This entrained gas should be humidified if the jet gas is dry. All exhaled gas passes out through this main lumen. If the jet ventilator is used with a conventional volume cycled ventilator, the exhaled tidal volume can be measured through the ventilator's spirometry system. The ventilator's alarm systems can also be used and IMV breaths and PEEP can be added if needed. If the patient is too unstable to be extubated and reintubated, a special endotracheal tube adapter can be added (see Fig. 14-25). Jet gas enters through the cannula and additional inspiratory and all expiratory gas go through the main lumen of the adapter.

Humidification was a problem with earlier HFJV systems. The Acutronic USA AMS-1000 has its own humidification system. The IDC Model VS 600 does not. With it, a standard intravenous pump is used to drip water or normal saline at a rate of 5 to 7 ml/hour through the endotracheal tube adapter. The IV system must have a back-check valve to prevent the inspiratory pressure from forcing the fluid back up the IV tubing. The fluid is nebulized by the jet gas during inspiration. The BEAR Jet does not have a humidification system of its own. It is used with a

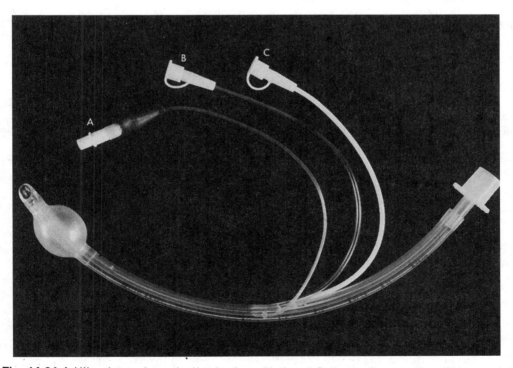

Fig. 14-24 A HiLo Jet endotracheal tube from National Catheter Corporation. This special purpose endotracheal tube features four lumens. *A,* pilot line to the cuff. *B,* for measuring the proximal airway pressure within the endotracheal tube above the cuff. *C,* the jet catheter used for delivering small bursts of tidal volume gas from a high frequency jet ventilator (HFJV). It opens within the endotracheal tube below the cuff. The main lumen of the endotracheal tube is used for suctioning and adding entrained, humidified gas from a conventional volume cycled ventilator. (From McPherson SR: *Respiratory therapy equipment,* ed 4, St. Louis, 1990, Mosby–Year Book. Used by permission.)

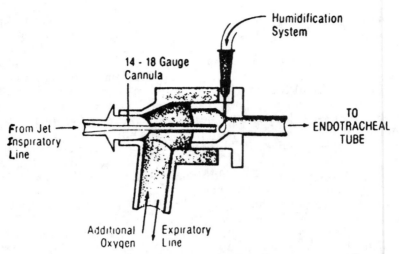

Fig. 14-25 A schematic drawing of a tracheostomy/endotracheal tube adapter and endotracheal tube adapter that have been modified for use with a high frequency jet ventilator (HFJV). A jet injector cannula has been added to the tracheostomy/endotracheal tube adapter. A needle has been pushed through the endotracheal tube adapter to drip saline into it for humidity. This system would be used if a patient could not be intubated with a HiLo Jet endotracheal tube. (From Carlon GC, Miodownik S, Ray C Jr et al: Technical aspects and clinical implications of high frequency jet ventilation with a solenoid valve, *Crit Care Med* 9(1):45-50, 1981. Used by permission.)

conventional volume ventilator and the entrained gas is humidified through the cascade humidifier on it.

> **ii. Put the equipment together, make sure that it works properly, and identify any problems with it. (IIB1c2) [R, Ap]**
> **iii. Fix any problems with the equipment. (IIB2d5) [R, Ap, An]**

Fig. 14-26 shows a schematic drawing of a high frequency jet ventilator. Although the three currently available ventilators have basic differences in how they are designed, they share these common features:

1. 50 psig source gas(es) of oxygen or oxygen and air are needed to generate a driving pressure.
2. A drive pressure control lets the operator set the peak pressure of the jet.
3. An inspiratory time control sets the I : E ratio.
4. Rate can be varied between 40 and 150 per minute.
5. The inspired oxygen percentage can be dialed either on the unit itself or on an external air-oxygen blender before going into the unit.
6. Humidification must be provided by either a dedicated cascade system or one joined to a volume cycled ventilator.

As with any ventilator, make sure that all connections are tight. Leaks are a particular problem because of the high pressures leaving the unit and the small tidal volumes that are delivered.

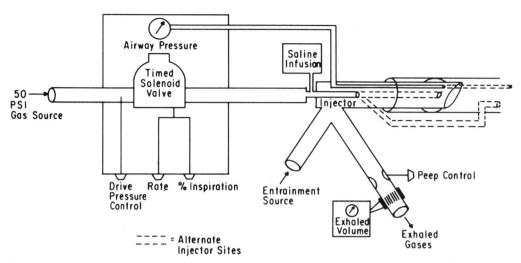

Fig. 14-26 Schematic diagram of the jet ventilator concept. (From MacIntyre NR: *Jet ventilation in the adult with breathing rates up to 150 BPM*, Riverside, Calif, 1985, Bear Medical Systems. Used by permission.)

f.   High frequency oscillator ventilators.
  i.   Obtain the necessary equipment for the procedure. (IIA1b3) [R, Ap]

At the time of this writing, the Infrasonics Adult Star is the only high frequency oscillator ventilator available for adults. It is a self-contained unit with a humidifier. The Adult Star does require a special circuit made just for it.

  ii.   Put the equipment together, make sure that it works properly, and identify any problems with it. (IIB1c3) [R, Ap]
  iii.   Fix any problems with the equipment. (IIB2d6) [R, Ap, An]

Experience with the equipment is recommended. The circuit is designed to combine two separate flows of gas for the patient's tidal volume. As with any circuit, make sure that all connections are tight. The ventilator is controlled by a microprocessor that can help to diagnose any problems with the equipment.

g.   Bilevel ventilator.
  i.   Obtain the necessary equipment for the procedure. (IIA1b4) [R, Ap]

At the time of this writing, the Respironics BiPAP system is the only bilevel ventilator. There are two different special circuits that may be used with it; both have a smooth bore. One circuit is used if the patient is being ventilated by a nasal or face mask. The other circuit is used if the patient has an endotracheal or tracheostomy tube. If the patient requires additional humidification, a cascade unit is required. A heat and moisture exchanger should not be used because it causes too much resistance.

    ii.   **Put the equipment together, make sure that it works properly, and identify any problems with it. (IIB1c4) [R, Ap]**

    iii. **Fix any problems with the equipment. (IIB2d7) [R, Ap, An]**

Follow the manufacturer's guidelines for putting the circuit on the unit and adding the cascade humidifier. As with any ventilator be wary of leaks in the circuit or humidifier. In addition, if the nasal or face mask does not fit properly there will be a leak at the patient's face. The mask may have to be adjusted or replaced with one that fits better.

  h. **Transport ventilators.**
    i.   **Obtain the necessary equipment for the procedure. (IIA1b5) [R, Ap]**

Examples of adult transport ventilators include the Bio-Med IC-2A, Ohmeda Logic 7, Omni-Vent D/MRI, Life Support Products AutoVent 2000/3000, and Newport E 100i. All are pneumatically powered by a high pressure oxygen source such as a cylinder. They may be electrically, pneumatically, or fluidically controlled. See the manufacturer's guidelines for details. The Omni-Vent D/MRI is made specifically for taking a patient for a magnetic resonance image because it will not be affected adversely by the strong magnetic field. Additional equipment includes:

- A full oxygen cylinder to power the ventilator.
- A circuit suited for the unit.
- If humidification is needed, get an appropriate heat and moisture exchanger.

It is important that if the patient is to be transported by helicopter or airplane that the ventilator not be sensitive to the drop in barometric pressure. If the ventilator can be used in the IMV/SIMV mode, the patient should inhale through a demand valve. An H-valve and reservoir balloon IMV system should not be used. The ventilator should have solid state electronics that can stand up to being bumped around.

    ii.   **Put the equipment together, make sure that it works properly, and identify any problems with it. (IIB1c5) [R, Ap]**

Make sure that all the equipment and circuits are working properly before leaving with the patient. Calculate the duration of the cylinder so that you will not run out of gas. Make sure the battery is fully charged.

    iii. **Fix any problems with the equipment. (IIB2d8) [R, Ap, An]**

Problems with a circuit disconnection or leak or heat and moisture exchanger obstruction are usually easy to identify and correct. Replace an empty cylinder with a new full one.

  i. **Home care ventilators.**
    i.   **Get the necessary equipment for the procedure. (IIA1b6) [R, Ap]**

Examples of home care ventilators include Life Products LP5 and LP6, LifeCare PLV-100 and PLV-102, Puritan-Bennett Companion 2800, and BEAR 33. All are electrically powered and can have oxygen added if needed by the patient. They are either electrically controlled or microprocessor controlled and offer a variety of breathing modes. Obviously, they require an appropriate breathing circuit. None offer a built-in humidifier; therefore a cascade humidifier or heat and moisture exchanger needs to be added on.

ii. Put the equipment together, make sure that it works properly, and identify any problems with it. (IIB1c6) [R, Ap]

Make sure that the unit is plugged into a working electrical outlet. Depending on the manufacturer's requirements and the patient's needs, oxygen will have to be added. This could be done with a bank of oxygen cylinders or an oxygen concentrator. Make sure that the circuit and humidifier are put together properly. Keep the air inlet filter clear of debris.

iii. Fix any problems with the equipment. (IIB2d9) [R, Ap, An]

Be prepared to tighten any loose connections, clean out the air intake filter, replace empty oxygen cylinders, add water to the humidifier, and take care of any other routine care issues. Make sure the patient's family has a working manual resuscitation bag. They need to know how to use it if the ventilator should fail.

2. Ventilator breathing circuits.
a. Fix any problems with a continuous mechanical ventilation (CMV) circuit. (IIB2h2) [An]

A number of companies produce circuits for the various types of ventilators including the ventilator manufacturers. There is considerable variation based on the manufacturer and the type of ventilator it is designed for. Common, but not universal, features of the inspiratory limb of the circuit include water trap, humidification system, nebulizer, thermometer or temperature probe, pressure monitoring port, and oxygen monitoring port.

Common, but not universal, features of the expiratory limb of the circuit include exhalation valve and water trap. A wye connects the inspiratory and expiratory limbs of the circuit and attachs the circuit to the patient (see Fig. 14-27 for a generic CMV ventilator circuit). It is generally recommended that the circuit and humidification system be changed every 24 hours to minimize the chance of pathogens growing in it; however, pathology studies have shown that circuits can be used for longer periods of time without endangering the patient. Make sure that the water level is properly maintained in the humidifier.

Check the circuit and connections for leaks if the volume is low. Check the volume leaving the ventilator if it does not match the set and returned volume. The volume control or spirometer may be out of calibration. If, during inspiration, the unit shows a volume entering the spirometer instead of the test lung or patient, the exhalation valve is broken or the high pressure line to it has popped off. Replace them as needed.

b. H-valve assembly for intermittent mandatory ventilation (IMV).
i. Obtain the necessary equipment for the procedure. (IIA1e) [R, Ap]

Hudson RCI is a manufacturer of an H-valve and related components depicted in Fig. 14-28, which is an example of a closed- or positive-pressure type of IMV system. The same H-valve can be added into the ventilator circuit as shown in Fig.

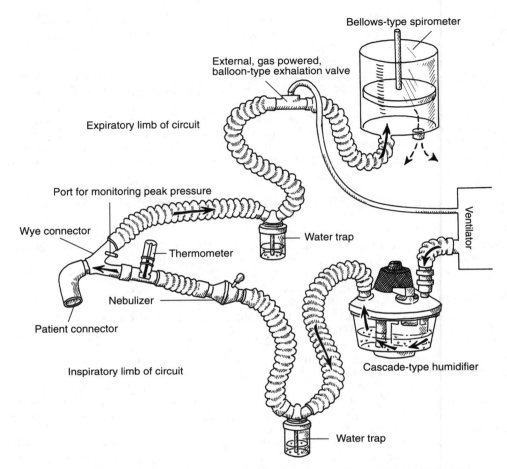

Fig. 14-27 Patient breathing circuit for continuous mechanical ventilation.

14-29, which is an example of an open- or ambient-pressure IMV system. These older IMV systems were first added on to ventilators such as the Bennett MA-1.

ii. Put the equipment together, make sure that it works properly, and identify any problems with it. (IIB1f) [R, Ap]

Closed- or Positive-Pressure IMV System

See Fig. 14-28 for the typical set-up of this Hudson RCI system. Gases from both the ventilator and IMV system flow through the cascade humidifier. IMV flow must be great enough to keep the bag inflated so that the excess gas flows through the humidifier to the patient or is vented out past the partially clamped orifice on the anesthesia bag. IMV flow should never be so great that the pressure manometer on the ventilator shows a constant positive pressure (unless therapeutic PEEP is being applied).

Placing the one-way valve backwards prevents any flow from passing through to the patient. If the flow through the IMV system is too great, the bag will overfill

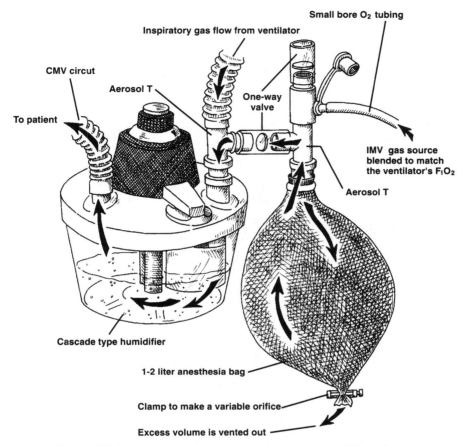

Fig. 14-28 Detail of a closed- or positive-pressure IMV system.

and pressure will build up in the circuit. The patient may complain of it being hard to exhale and a positive pressure will be seen on the manometer. The flow must be decreased to the IMV system. The opposite problem is inadequate flow through the IMV system. This is seen as the reservoir bag collapsing on inspiration, the patient complaining of not getting enough air, or the pressure gauge registering a negative pressure on inspiration. Obviously, the flow to the system must be increased.

Open- or Ambient-Pressure IMV System

See Fig. 14-29 for the typical set-up of an open- or ambient-pressure IMV system. A length of aerosol tubing is added for a reservoir instead of the anesthesia bag. The IMV gas is humidified by either a heated, large volume nebulizer (as shown) or a second cascade humidifier. Gas from the ventilator flows through the original cascade humidifier.

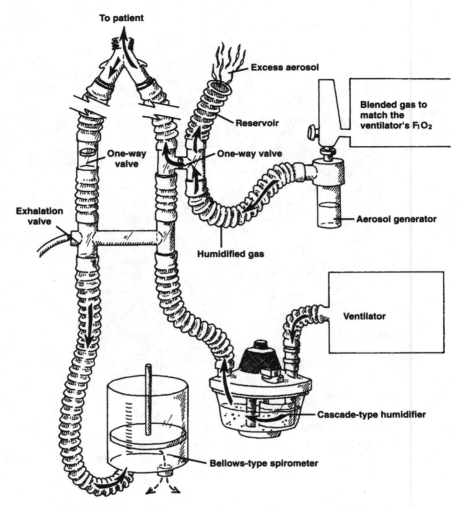

To patient

Excess aerosol

Blended gas to match the ventilator's F$_I$O$_2$

Reservoir

One-way valve

One-way valve

Exhalation valve

Aerosol generator

Humidified gas

Ventilator

Cascade-type humidifier

Bellows-type spirometer

Fig. 14-29 Detail of an open- or ambient-pressure IMV system.

Typically, 100 to 200 ml of aerosol tubing is added as a reservoir. Flow through a nebulizer must be great enough that excess mist can be seen escaping from the reservoir during a patient's spontaneous inspiration. Gas flow through a cascade humidifier must great enough that it can be felt coming out of the end of the reservoir during a spontaneous inspiration. Increase the flow if it cannot.

Placing the one-way valve backwards prevents any added flow from passing through to the patient. Indeed, placing the valve in the reversed position will result in the IMV breath being vented out into room air. Placing the valve properly allows gas to pass through to the patient as intended.

Both IMV system configurations must have a thermometer placed into the inspiratory limb of the circuit near the patient to ensure that the desired temperature is maintained. Make sure in both configurations that the oxygen percentage is the same through both the IMV system and the ventilator. Ventilator alarms for low exhaled volume and/or patient disconnection must be functional.

c. Change the patient's ventilator circuit as needed. (IIIC7b) [An]

Either a permanent or a disposable circuit may be selected based on the type of ventilator on which it must be placed. A circuit with an external exhalation valve must be used with ventilators such as the Bennett MA-1 and MA-2 and BEAR 3. The Puritan-Bennett 7200, BEAR 1000, and Servo 900 B and C feature internal exhalation valves and therefore do not need a circuit with one. If the patient needs to receive aerosolized medications, the circuit should either include a nebulizer or be able to accept one. If not included, the nebulizer or metered dose inhaler adapter will have to be added into the inspiratory limb of the circuit.

The compression factor and internal resistance of the circuit should also be considered. The compression factor is a main determinant of how much compressed volume is lost. Remember that the compressed volume is subtracted from the set tidal volume to determine the actual delivered tidal volume. The compression factor varies with the material used to construct the circuit, the temperature of the inhaled gas, and the peak inspiratory pressure placed against the circuit. Commonly, permanent circuits have a slightly lower compression factor than disposable circuits. Some circuits have a smooth rather than a corrugated interior surface. The smooth surface has less resistance resulting in less turbulence and less back pressure. Therefore more of the peak pressure is directed to deliver the tidal volume. A smooth bore circuit is required with the BiPAP Ventilatory Support System by Respironics. It is recommended that a low compressed volume and low resistance circuit be used whenever high pressures are required to deliver low tidal volumes. This is usually the case during high frequency ventilation.

Heated wire circuits have been used to maintain a constant temperature throughout the circuit and minimize condensation. They have been used for some time with neonatal ventilators. Because they are not typically used with adult patients, further discussion on this is included in Section 15.

3. Continuous positive airway pressure (CPAP) systems.
a. Fix any problems with a CPAP breathing circuit. (IIB2h3) [An]

Freestanding CPAP breathing circuits vary considerably. Most commonly, each respiratory care department develops its own breathing circuit to meet its needs. Several manufacturers have developed CPAP systems for home use. Examples include Vital Signs, which produces the Downs CPAP mask and the Downs Flow Generator, and Respironics, which produces the BiPAP S/T-D Ventilatory Support System. Traditionally the complete circuit of any system is changed after 24–48 hours of use to minimize the risk of infection. Fig. 14-30 shows the typical components used in a CPAP breathing circuit. The components of the system include some or all of the following depending on the patient's needs: air/oxygen blender; pediatric or adult flowmeter on the blender; cascade humidifier; inspiratory circuit of large bore/aerosol tubing with water trap and one-way valve, wye to connect the inspiratory and expiratory limbs of the circuit, and patient connector (elbow adapter) to endotracheal/tracheostomy tube; CPAP prongs or CPAP mask; expiratory circuit of large bore/aerosol tubing with water trap, one-way valve, pressure manometer for measuring the CPAP level, low pressure/disconnection audible alarm, CPAP device, anesthesia bag as reservoir, variable resistance clamp on the

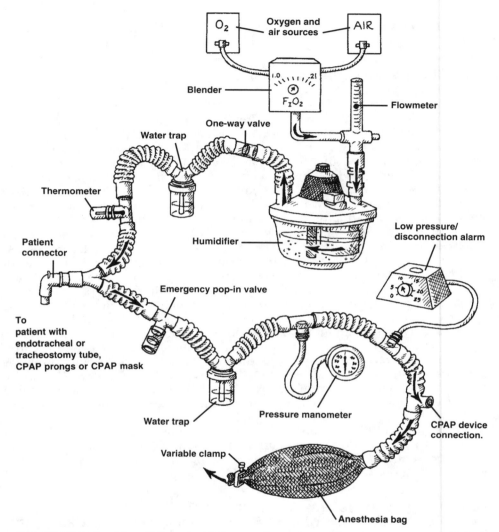

Fig. 14-30 Patient breathing circuit for continuous positive airway pressure (CPAP).

tail of the anesthesia bag, Brigg's/T-adapters for connecting the various features, and an emergency pop-in valve in case gas flow is stopped.

The CPAP level is adjusted by means of a variety of threshold resistors. These range from a variable clamp on an anesthesia bag, a column of water with a length of expiratory tubing inserted below the surface, a vertically mounted ball bearing, and a spring-loaded resistor. Illustrations and further discussion of all of these systems are included in *Respiratory Care Certification Guide* (Sills, 1994).

All CPAP systems must be adjusted by checking the pressure level on the manometer. Set the low pressure/disconnection audible alarm to sound at a few centimeters below the CPAP level. For example, if 10 cm CPAP is ordered, set the alarm to sound if the pressure drops below 8 cm CPAP.

Flow through the CPAP breathing circuit must be sufficient to meet the patient's needs. A flow of 2 to 3 times the patient's minute volume is usually enough;

however, the minute volume often cannot be accurately measured. In this case set the flow so that the pressure manometer drops no more than 2 cm water below the CPAP pressure during a peak inspiration. Flow is also inadequate if the patient shows an increased use of accessory muscles of respiration or complains of increased work of breathing. Too high a flow is seen by an inadvertently high level of CPAP and/or the patient complaining of it being difficult to exhale. Adjust the flowmeter setting and clamp on the anesthesia bag so that it is somewhat inflated with excess air escaping out past the clamp. With all of the devices, gas will escape through the path of least resistance. All or some may escape through the anesthesia bag or CPAP device or both. The bag should collapse somewhat during the patient's inspiration and expand somewhat during the expiration.

A sudden drop in the CPAP level to zero indicates a disconnection at the patient or somewhere in the breathing circuit. Check all connections and reassemble the break. The patient may need to be manually ventilated while the problem is corrected. Make sure that the water level is properly maintained in the humidifier. Fill it with sterile, distilled water as often as necessary. In addition, the water column systems must be frequently monitored because of water loss due to evaporation.

b. Fix any problems with a CPAP nasal or face mask. (IIB2a4) [An]

As discussed earlier, it is imperative that the mask properly fit the patient's face. Too large a mask will not seal and will allow gas to leak and pressure to drop. This will be seen as a decreased CPAP pressure on the manometer. The patient may show increased snoring or airway obstruction with periods of apnea. Too small or a misfitting mask could cause an uneven distribution of pressure on the face. This could lead to abrasions or pressure sores and ulcers on the face.

A sudden drop in the CPAP level to zero indicates a disconnection at the patient or somewhere in the breathing circuit. Check all connections and reassemble the break. If the CPAP level drops more than 2 cm of water pressure during an inspiration, the flow is inadequate and should be increased. Flow is also inadequate if the patient shows an increased use of accessory muscles of respiration or complains of increased work of breathing. Too high a flow is seen by an inadvertently high level of CPAP and/or the patient complaining of it being difficult to exhale.

4. Perform volume, flow, and pressure calibration on a ventilator for quality control. (IIB3f) [R, Ap, An]

Follow the manufacturer's guidelines for quality control procedures on mechanical ventilators. The microprocessor ventilators usually have a software package that performs self-diagnostic tests on the unit. If a problem is found it is printed on the monitor. Obviously, the ventilator should deliver the volume, flow, and pressure that is set on the control. Do not use a ventilator that fails a quality control check.

5. Change the type of humidification equipment. (IIIC6b) [An]

Heated Humidifier

Heated humidifiers are used when long-term ventilation (greater than 96 hours) is needed or when a heat and moisture exchanger (HME) is contraindicated. The humidifier should be capable of providing close to 100% relative humidity. Passover systems are preferred with neonates.

The temperature is usually maintained so that gas delivered to the patient is at $33 \pm 2°C$ (about 91°F). At this temperature it should deliver 30 mg/L of water vapor. Exceptions, when ordered by the physician, would be running at a cooler than body temperature when the patient has a fever or running at a warmer than body temperature (about 110°F or 44°C) when the patient is hypothermic. A temperature probe should be set into the inspiratory limb of the circuit near the wye.

Always follow the manufacturer's guidelines for assembly. All connections must be air tight to avoid loss of tidal volume to the patient. Make sure that the water level is kept in the recommended range to properly humidify the gas. If temperature alarms come with the system, set the high at no more than 37°C and the low at no less than 30°C.

Heat and Moisture Exchanger

A heat and moisture exchanger (HME) is commonly used when the patient will be ventilated for less than 96 hours or when the patient is being transported and does not have a secretion problem. HMEs are designed to be warmed by the patient's exhaled breath and absorb the water vapor from the gas. The next inspired volume is then warmed and humidified by evaporation. Do not use an HME that cannot deliver at least 30 mg/L of water vapor to the patient.

Most of these units are preassembled by the manufacturer; there is nothing to add. An exception is the Siemens unit that has a replaceable filter. It may be necessary to attach a length of large bore/aerosol tubing or an elbow adapter to make the unit fit onto the wye or endotracheal tube. All come with standard 15-mm or 22-mm connector ends; air should flow easily through them with little resistance. Any disconnections can be easily noticed and reconnected. Replace any unit that has a mucus plug or other debris obstructing the channel. This might be demonstrated by the patient's peak airway pressure suddenly rising. Typically, these units are replaced every 24 to 48 hours when the breathing circuit is replaced.

This ends the general discussion on the application of mechanical ventilation to adult patients. Refer to Sections 1, 2, 3, and 4 or earlier in this section for most of the necessary details on patient assessment. Some additional comments are added as needed.

Module C.   Patient assessment.

1.   Examine all the data to determine the patient's pathophysiological condition. (IC3a) [R, Ap, An]

Remember to get an ABG after every ventilator change that could result in a different PaO_2 (pulse oximetry may be substituted) and/or $PaCO_2$ (end-tidal CO_2 may be substituted).

Physical responses to mechanical ventilation, as measured by the vital signs, can vary considerably. A patient who is anxious, angry, or in pain will have an increase in the vital signs. A patient who is relaxed, has reduced work of breathing, and whose blood gas values are now normal will have a return to normal vital signs.

Watch carefully for the patient whose drop in blood pressure coincides with a tachycardia. This patient may be having decreased venous return to the heart from an increased intrathoracic pressure.

2. Take part in the development of the respiratory care plan. (IC3c) [An]

Because an intubated patient cannot speak, it is necessary to communicate by asking simple questions that can be answered in a "yes" nod or "no" shake of the head. Other methods of communication are a pad of paper and pencil or picture boards.

It is not possible to predict how a patient will react to the initiation of mechanical ventilation or its prolonged need. Some patients react with relief and relax when the work of breathing is reduced. Others may become angry at the limitations imposed on them. Still others may become depressed.

Be prepared to make recommendations on changing ventilator parameters based on the patient's condition, blood gas values, chest x-ray, and vital signs.

3. Make a recommendation to insert a chest tube into the patient. (IIIC8f) [R, Ap, An]

A chest x-ray and physical exam of the patient will reveal if air or fluid is abnormally found around the lung(s) or heart. If a patient has a tension pneumothorax, a pleural chest tube must be inserted to remove the air and relieve the pressure within the chest. A nontension pneumothorax of greater than 10% is often also treated by inserting a pleural chest tube. A pleural chest tube is also placed to remove blood or other fluid from the pleural space.

A pneumomedistinum, pneumopericardium, or pneumoperitoneum that puts the patient at risk must also be treated. A chest tube is then inserted into the area where the abnormal air is found. The same chest tube would also remove any abnormal collection of fluid. A chest tube is usually placed behind the heart to remove any blood that should leak out after open heart surgery.

4. Measure the volume of air lost through a patient's pleural chest tube. (IIIC7a) [R, Ap, An]

If the patient is being ventilated on a constant volume ventilator, the amount of air that is lost through the pleural chest tube can be calculated. This is done by subtracting the measured exhaled volume from the measured inhaled volume (the set tidal volume). For example:

Inspired tidal volume = 500 ml
Exhaled tidal volume = − 400 ml

100 ml of tidal volume is lost through the pleural chest tube

It is not always possible to measure a consistent tidal volume when pressure control ventilation or a similar mode is used. In a case like this it is only possible to make a qualitative judgment on pleural air leak. In other words, if air is seen to bubble out through the pleural drainage system, an air leak is present. When the air stops bubbling the pleural tear has healed. See Section 17 for a complete discussion on pleural drainage systems.

BIBLIOGRAPHY

AARC Clinical Practice Guideline: Humidification during mechanical ventilation, *Respir Care* 37(8):887-890, 1992.

AARC Clinical Practice Guideline: Patient-ventilator system checks, *Respir Care* 37(8):882-886, 1992.

AARC Clinical Practice Guideline: Ventilator circuit changes, *Respir Care* 39(8):797-802, 1994.

American Association for Respiratory Care: Consensus statement on the essentials of mechanical ventilation, *Respir Care* 37(9):1000-1008, 1992.

Banner MJ, Lampotang S: Clinical use of inspiratory and expiratory waveforms. In Kacmarek RM, Stoller JK, editors: *Current respiratory care*, Philadelphia, 1988, BC Decker.

Barnes TA: Mechanical ventilation. In Barnes TA, editor: *Respiratory care practice*, Chicago, 1988, Year Book Medical.

Bone RC: Pressure-volume measurements in detection of bronchospasm and mucous plugging in acute respiratory failure, *Respir Care* 21(7), 1976.

Bone RC: Monitoring ventilatory mechanics in acute respiratory failure, *Respir Care* 28(5), 1983.

Bone RC: Acute respiratory failure: classification, differential diagnosis and introduction to management. In Burton GG, Hodgkin JE, editors: *Respiratory care*, ed 2, Philadelphia, 1984, JB Lippincott.

Boysen PG, McGough E: Pressure-control and pressure-support ventilation: flow patterns, inspiratory time, and gas distribution, *Respir Care* 33(2), 1988.

Branson RD, Campbell RS, Davis K Jr et al: Altering flowrate during maximum pressure support ventilation (PSV$_{max}$): effects on cardiorespiratory function, *Respir Care* 35(11):1056-1064, 1990.

Branson RD, Chatburn RL: Technical description and classification of modes of ventilator operation, *Respir Care* 37(9):1026-1044, 1992.

Branson RD, Hurst JM: Laboratory evaluation of moisture output of seven airway heat and moisture exchangers, *Respir Care* 32(9):741-747, 1987.

Branson RD, Hurst JM, DeHaven CB Jr: Synchronous independent lung ventilation in the treatment of unilateral pulmonary contusion: a report of two cases, *Respir Care* 29(4):361-367, 1984.

Branson RD, Hurst JM, DeHaven CB Jr: Mask CPAP: state of the art, *Respir Care* 30(10):846-857, 1985.

Chatburn RL: High frequency ventilation: a report on a state of the art symposium, *Respir Care* 29(8):839-849, 1984.

Chatburn RL: Estimating appropriate pressure support levels (letter), *Respir Care* 30(10):925-926, 1985.

Chatburn RL: A new system for understanding mechanical ventilation, *Respir Care* 36(10):1123-1155, 1991.

Chatburn RL: Classification of mechanical ventilators, *Respir Care* 37(9):1009-1025, Sept 1992.

Corbridge T, Hall JB: Status asthmaticus in the adult: assessment, drug therapy, and mechanical ventilation, *Respir Management* 21(5):119-126.

Craig KC, Pierson DJ, Carrico CJ: The clinical application of positive end-expiratory pressure (PEEP) in the adult respiratory distress syndrome (ARDS), *Respir Care* 30(3):184-201, 1985.

DesJardins TR: *Cardiopulmonary anatomy and physiology: essentials for respiratory care*, Albany, NY, 1988, Delmar Publishers.

Drinker PA, McKhann CF III: The iron lung: first practical means of respiratory support, *JAMA* 256(11):1476-1480, 1986.

Earl J: Should we support pressure support? *Respir Care* 34(2):125-128, 1989.

Earl J: Full ventilatory support: a point of view, *Respir Care* 34(8):741-744, 1989.

East TD, Elkhuizen PHM, Pace NL: Pressure support with mandatory minute ventilation supplied by the Ohmeda CPU-1 prevents hypoventilation due to respiratory depression in a canine model, *Respir Care* 34(9):795-800, 1989.

Ershowsky P, Kreiger B: Changes in breathing pattern during pressure support ventilation, *Respir Care* 32(11):1011-1016, 1987.

Eubanks DH, Bone RC: *Comprehensive respiratory care: a learning system*, ed 2, St. Louis, 1990, Mosby—Year Book.

Failing T, Van Way CW: Ventilatory support in chest trauma, *Respir Management* 20(3):61-65.

Felix WR, MacDonnell KF, Jacobs L: Resuscitation from drowning in cold water, *The New England Journal of Medicine*, April 2, 1981.

Flasch M: Negative-pressure ventilatory support in the home, *Respir Ther* 16(5):21-25, Sept/Oct 1986.

Greer K: Hypothermia: a quiet killer, *Advance for Respiratory Therapists*, Jan 15, 1990.

Guidelines for invasive applications with BiPAP systems, Respironics: Monroeville, Penn.

Gurevitch MJ: Selection of the inspiratory : expiratory ratio. In Kacmarek RM, Stoller JK, editors: *Current respiratory care*, Philadelphia, 1988, BC Decker.

Hess D: Perspectives on weaning from mechanical ventilation, with a note on extubation, *Respir Care* 32(3):167-171, 1987.

Hess D, McCurdy S, Simmons M: Compression volume in adult ventilator circuits: a comparison of five disposable circuits and a nondisposable circuit, *Respir Care* 36(10):1113-1118, 1991.

Hill NS: Clinical application of body ventilators, *Chest* 90(6):897-905, 1986.

Hill NS, Eveloff SE, Carlisle CC et al: Efficacy of nocturnal nasal ventilation in patients with restrictive thoracic disease, *Am Rev Respir Dis* 145(2):365-371, 1992.

Hirsch C, Kacmarek RM, Stanek K: Work of breathing during CPAP and PSV imposed by the new generation mechanical ventilators: a lung model study, *Respir Care* 36(8):815-828, 1991.

Hodgkin JE, Gray LS, Burton GG: Techniques in ventilatory weaning. In Burton GG, Hodgkin JE, editors: *Respiratory care*, ed 2, Philadelphia, 1984, JB Lippincott.

Kacmarek RM: The role of pressure support ventilation in reducing work of breathing, *Respir Care* 33(2):99-120, 1988.

Kacmarek RM: Systematic modification of ventilatory support. In Barnes TA, editor: *Respiratory care practice*, Chicago, 1988, Year Book Medical.

Kacmarek RM: Essential gas delivery features of mechanical ventilators, *Respir Care* 37(9):1045-1055, 1992.

Kacmarek RM, Foley K, Cheever P et al: Determination of ventilatory reserve in mechanically ventilated patients: a comparison of techniques, *Respir Care* 36(10):1085-1092, 1991.

Kacmarek RM, Hess D: Pressure-controlled inverse-ratio ventilation: panacea or auto-PEEP? *Respir Care* 35(10):945-948, 1990.

Kacmarek RM, Mack CW, Dimas S: The essentials of respiratory care, ed 3, St. Louis, 1990, Mosby—Year Book.

Kirby RR: Modes of mechanical ventilation. In Kacmarek RM, Stoller JK, editors: *Current respiratory care*, Philadelphia, 1988, BC Decker.

Kirby RR, Smith RA, Desautels DA: Mechanical ventilation. In Burton GG, Hodgkin JE, editors: *Respiratory care*, ed 2, Philadelphia, 1984, JB Lippincott.

Levizky MG, Cairo JM, Hall SM: *Introduction to respiratory care*, Philadelphia, 1990, WB Saunders.

MacIntyre NR: *Pressure support ventilation: potential clinical application*, Winter 1986, pp 1-7, Mead Johnson Pharmaceutical Division.

MacIntyre NR: *Jet ventilation in the adult with breathing rates up to 150 BPM*, Riverside, Calif, 1985, Bear Medical Systems.

MacIntyre NR: Respiratory function during pressure support ventilation, *Chest* 89(5):677-683, 1986.

MacIntyre NR: Pressure support: inspiratory assist. In Kacmarek RM, Stoller JK, editors: *Current respiratory care*, Philadelphia, 1988, BC Decker.

MacIntyre NR: Weaning from mechanical ventilatory support: volume-assisting intermittent breaths versus pressure-supporting every breath, *Respir Care* 33(2):121-125, 1988.

Make BJ, Gilmartin ME: Care of ventilator-assisted individuals in the home and alternative community sites. In Burton GG, Hodgkin JE, Ward JJ, editors: *Respiratory care: a guide to clinical practice*, ed 3, Philadelphia, 1991, JB Lippincott.

Marini JJ: Mechanical ventilation: taking the work out of breathing? *Respir Care* 31(8):695-702, 1986.

Marini JJ: What derived variables should be monitored during mechanical ventilation? *Respir Care* 37(9):1097-1107, 1992.

Martz KV, Joiner JW, Rodger MS: *Management of the patient-ventilator system: a team approach*, ed 2, St. Louis, 1984, Mosby–Year Book.

McPherson SP: *Respiratory therapy equipment*, ed 3, St. Louis, 1985, Mosby–Year Book.

McPherson SP: *Respiratory therapy equipment*, ed 4, St. Louis, 1990, Mosby–Year Book.

Morganroth ML, Morganroth JL, Nett LM, et al: Criteria for weaning from prolonged mechanical ventilation, *Arch Intern Med* 144:1012-1016, 1984.

Pennock BE, Kaplan PD, Carlin BW et al: Pressure support ventilation with a simplified ventilatory support system administered with a nasal mask in patients with respiratory failure, *Chest* 100(5):1371-1376, 1991.

Pilbeam SP: *Mechanical ventilation: physiological and clinical applications*, St. Louis, 1986, Multi-Media Publishing.

Product literature, High frequency jet ventilation: applications for laryngoscopies and bronchoscopies, Instrument Development, Pittsburgh, Penn.

Product literature on the NEV-100 ventilator, Puritan-Bennett, LIFECARE, LaFayette, Colo.

Product literature on Pressure Control Ventilation, Puritan-Bennett.

Product literature on the suggested protocol for initiation of the BiPAP S/T or BiPAP S/T-D Ventilatory Support System, Respironics.

Quan SF, Parides GC, Knoper SR: Mandatory minute volume (MVV) ventilation: an overview, *Respir Care* 35(9):898-905, 1990.

Rarey KP, Youtsey JW: *Respiratory patient care*, Englewood Cliffs, NJ, 1981, Prentice Hall.

Register SD, Downs JB: F_1O_2 and PEEP. In Kacmarek RM, Stoller JK, editors: *Current respiratory care*, Philadelphia, 1988, BC Decker.

Scanlan CL: Physics and physiology of ventilatory support. In Scanlan CL, Spearman CB, Sheldon RL, editors: *Egan's fundamentals of respiratory care*, ed 5, St. Louis, 1990, Mosby–Year Book.

Scanlan CL: Respiratory failure and the need for ventilatory support. In Scanlan CL, Spearman CB, Sheldon RL, editors: *Egan's fundamentals of respiratory care*, ed 5, St. Louis, 1990, Mosby–Year Book.

Scanlan CL: Selection and application of ventilatory support devices. In Scanlan CL, Spearman CB, Sheldon RL, editors: *Egan's fundamentals of respiratory care*, ed 5, St. Louis, 1990, Mosby—Year Book.

Shapiro BA, Harrison RA, Kacmarek RM et al: *Clinical application of respiratory care*, ed 3, Chicago, 1985, Year Book Medical.

Shelledy DC, Mikles SP: Newer modes of mechanical ventilation. I. Pressure support. *Respir Management* July/Aug 1988, 14-20, 1988.

Shelledy DC, Mikles SP: Newer modes of mechanical ventilation. II. Mandatory minute volume ventilation, *Respir Management* July/Aug 1988, 21-28, 1988.

Sills JR: *Respiratory care certification guide: the complete review resource for the entry level exam*, ed 2, St. Louis, 1994, Mosby—Year Book.

Spearman CB: Appropriate ventilator selection. In Kacmarek RM, Stoller JK, editors: *Current respiratory care*, Philadelphia, 1988, BC Decker.

Spearman CB, Sheldon RL, Egan DE, editors: *Egan's fundamentals of respiratory care*, ed 4, St. Louis, 1982, Mosby—Year Book.

Stoller JK: Establishing clinical unweanability, *Respir Care* 36(3):186-198, 1991.

Strumpf DA, Carlisle CC, Millman RP et al: An evaluation of the respironics BiPAP Bi-Level CPAP device for delivery of assisted ventilation, *Respir Care* 35(5):415-422, 1990.

Tobin MJ: Monitoring of pressure, flow, and volume during mechanical ventilation, *Respir Care* 37(9):1081-1096, 1992.

Tobin MJ, Lodato RF: PEEP, Auto-PEEP, and Waterfalls, *Chest* 96(3):449-451, 1989.

Vandine JD: Mechanical ventilators. In Barnes TA, editor: *Respiratory care practice*, Chicago, 1988, Year Book Medical.

Waldhorn RE: Nocturnal nasal intermittent positive pressure ventilation with bi-level positive airway pressure (BiPAP) in respiratory failure, *Chest* 101(2):516-521, 1992.

Wright J, Gong H: "Auto-PEEP": Incidence, magnitude, and contributing factors, *Heart Lung* 19(4):352-357, 1990.

SELF-STUDY QUESTIONS

1. Your patient is being ventilated in the assist/control mode on a Bennett MA-1 ventilator. The nurse calls you to evaluate the patient because "the bellows alarm is going off." When you arrive you notice that the patient's chest is barely moving during a control breath, the peak pressure does not rise above 3 cm water, and the bellows rises when the control breath is delivered. The most likely cause of these findings is:
   A. The machine is self-cycling.
   B. The inspiratory and expiratory limbs of the circuit are reversed at the Cascade humidifier.
   C. The tubing to the exhalation valve is disconnected.
   D. The spirometer is out of calibration.
   E. The endotracheal tube is misplaced into the esophagus.

2. Pressure control inverse ratio ventilation (PCIRV) is indicated in the following condition:
   A. Emphysema
   B. Asthma
   C. Chronic bronchitis
   D. Pulmonary contusion
   E. ARDS

3. Mean airway pressure is:
    A. Pmax divided by flow
    B. Pmax minus the plateau pressure
    C. Pmax divided by inspiratory time
    D. The average pressure throughout the breathing cycle
    E. Tidal volume divided by peak pressure

4. Factors causing a decreased lung compliance include:
    I.   Pulmonary edema
    II.   Pulmonary fibrosis
    III. Emphysema
    IV.   ARDS
    A. I, II
    B. II, III
    C. I, II, IV
    D. I, II, III, IV
    E. III

5. Expiratory retard would be indicated in a patient with:
    A. Pulmonary edema
    B. Air trapping on exhalation
    C. Pleural effusion
    D. Pneumothorax

6. Mandatory minute volume (MMV) ventilation is:
    I.   Similar to assist/control ventilation
    II.   Indicated when weaning a patient with an unstable respiratory drive
    III. Designed to make sure that at least a minimum minute volume is delivered
    IV.   A substitute for CPAP
    A. II, III
    B. I
    C. III
    D. IV
    E. I, IV

7. The maximum rate that the Food and Drug Administration (FDA) has approved for a high frequency jet ventilator is:
    A. 60
    B. 100
    C. 125
    D. 150
    E. 175

8. Weaning should be terminated when:
    I.   The patient becomes restless and agitated.
    II.   Cardiac dysrhythmias occur.
    III. The patient complains of fatigue.
    IV.   The patient's PaO_2 is 90 on 40% oxygen.
    A. II
    B. I, III
    C. I, II
    D. I, II, III, IV
    E. I, II, III

9. If a patient has just returned from surgery for a left pneumonectomy, the ventilator delivered tidal volume should be:
    A. Less than normal based on ideal body weight
    B. The same as normal based on ideal body weight
    C. Larger than normal based on ideal body weight

10. All the following parameters indicate the need for intubation and mechanical ventilation EXCEPT:
    A. Respiratory rate greater than 35/minute
    B. Vital capacity of less than 15 ml/kg of ideal body weight
    C. Maximum inspiratory pressure of less than 25 cm water
    D. $P(A-a)O_2$ on 100% oxygen of 40 mm Hg
    E. V_D/V_T is 0.7

11. The "Iron lung" is indicated for all the following types of patients EXCEPT:
    A. ARDS
    B. Neuromuscular defects
    C. Kyphoscoliosis
    D. COPD in acute failure

12. The parameters found with an ideal optimal PEEP study are:
    I.   Pulmonary compliance improves
    II. PaO_2 rises
    III. Percent shunt decreases
    IV.   Pulmonary vascular resistance increases
    V.   Pulmonary vascular resistance decreases
    VI.   Blood pressure falls and heart rate increases
    A. II, IV, VI
    B. I, II, III, V
    C. II, III, V, VI
    D. II, V, VI
    E. I, II, III, IV

13. Your polio patient is being ventilated with a chest cuirass. She complains of being short of breath. You check her tidal volume and find that it has dropped by about one half. The most likely reason for this would be:
    A. Someone has changed the I : E ratio.
    B. Someone has changed the rate.
    C. Air is leaking between her chest and the cuirass shell.
    D. The patient is closing her glottis.

14. You are working with an obstructive sleep apnea patient receiving bilevel ventilation on the BiPAP ventilator via a nasal mask. During a sleep period you notice that he is snoring. You would recommend the following ventilator adjustment:
    A. Increase the respiratory rate.
    B. Increase the upper level pressure.
    C. Increase the lower level pressure.
    D. Switch the patient to a face mask.

15. What is the effective static compliance if the corrected tidal volume is 700 ml, the ventilator's peak pressure is 56 cm water, the plateau pressure is 48 cm water, and there is 12 cm water of PEEP?
    A. 16 ml/cm water

B.   15 ml/cm water
C.   19 ml/cm water
D.   12.5 ml/cm water
E.   58 ml/cm water

16.   You are working with an 80 Kg (176 lb) patient who is apneic after suffering a stroke. He is being ventilated on the control mode with the following settings:

Minute volume	8 liters
Rate	10
I : E ratio	1 : 3
Inspired oxygen	40%
Mechanical dead space	200 ml

The arterial blood gas results show:

PaO_2	90 torr
$PaCO_2$	50 torr
pH	7.30
HCO_3^-	24 mEq/L

You would recommend which of the following:
A.   Decrease the mechanical dead space.
B.   Decrease the patient's minute volume.
C.   Change the I : E ratio to 1 : 2.
D.   Increase the inspiratory flow.
E.   Add 5 cm water PEEP.

17.   Factors causing an increased peak pressure without changing static pressure include:
   I.   Retained secretions
   II.   Pleural effusion
   III.   Bronchospasm
   IV.   Pulmonary edema
   A.   II, IV
   B.   I, II
   C.   I, III
   D.   III, IV
   E.   I, II, III, IV

18.   Which of the following will have the greatest impact on the mean airway pressure?
   A.   Increasing the inspiratory flow
   B.   Adding 5 cm PEEP
   C.   Adding .5 seconds of inflation hold
   D.   Increasing the inspiratory time by .25 seconds
   E.   Decreasing the sensitivity

Answer Key

1. C; 2. E; 3. D; 4. C; 5. B; 6. A; 7. D; 8. E; 9. A; 10. D; 11. A; 12. B; 13. C; 14. C; 15. C; 16. A; 17. C; 18. B.

15

Mechanical Ventilation of the Neonate

Module A.   Perform continuous mechanical ventilation to achieve adequate artificial ventilation and/or recommend modifications in ventilatory support based on the patient's response.

A critique of the most recent versions of the Written Registry Exam reveals that only about 2% of the questions deal with the application of continuous positive airway pressure (CPAP) and mechanical ventilation to the neonate. The NBRC tests much more heavily on the application of these techniques on adult patients. Of the 10 scenarios presented in the recent versions of the Clinical Simulation Exam, only two to three concerned neonatal or pediatric patients. CPAP and/or mechanical ventilation may be involved in these situations. As in all other sections, the alphanumeric codes and difficulty levels in this section are based on the Detailed Examination Outline for the Written Registry Examination. This section is also written to include material that has been tested on previous Clinical Simulation Examinations.

1.   Continuous positive pressure breathing (CPAP).
a.   Physiologic effects.

CPAP (and PEEP) increase the patient's functional residual capacity (FRC). In neonates, the most common cause of a decreased FRC is infant respiratory distress syndrome (IRDS). This condition is caused by the lack of surfactant in the lungs of the premature neonate. The neonate with IRDS has relatively airless lungs that are prone to atelectasis. This results in hypoxemia. In addition, each tidal volume breath requires a greater than normal inspiratory effort (see Fig. 15-1). The restoration of FRC in the neonate will increase its PaO_2, decrease the percentage of shunt, narrow the alveolar to arterial difference in oxygen, and reduce its work of tidal volume breathing. CPAP must be used with caution in neonates with persistent pulmonary hypertension of the newborn (PPHN). An excessive amount of pressure in the alveoli will compress the capillary bed. This will decrease pulmonary blood flow, which will in turn increase blood flow through the patent ductus arteriosus and worsen the problem.

b.   Indications, contraindications, and hazards.

CPAP is indication for any condition that results in an unacceptably low PaO_2 secondary to a decreased FRC. Some neonates respond so well to CPAP that mechanical ventilation is not needed. In general, contraindications include any

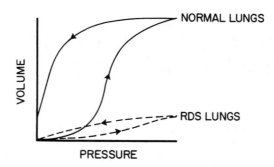

Fig. 15-1 Pressure-volume curves for a normal neonate and for one with infant respiratory distress syndrome (IRDS). The normal neonate's lungs inhale a relatively large tidal volume at a low pressure. Note how when the same pressure is placed against the lungs of the infant with RDS the tidal volume is much smaller. To get a normal tidal volume the RDS infant must generate a much greater negative pressure. (From Carlo WA, Martin RJ: Principles of neonatal assisted ventilation, *Pediatr Clin North Am* 33(1):221-237, 1986. Used by permission.)

CPAP related condition that results in a worsening of the patient's original status. Some neonates cannot tolerate CPAP and progressively hypoventilate as the pressure level is increased. Clinical judgment is needed to decide how high the PaCO$_2$ will be allowed to rise before discontinuing the CPAP and beginning mechanical ventilation. In general, the PaCO$_2$ should not be greater than 50 to 55 mm Hg as long as the pH is at least 7.25. An absolute contraindication is apnea resulting in hypoxemia and hypotension. These infants should be mechanically ventilated. See Table 15-1 for a complete listing of indications, contraindications, and hazards.

c. Initiation.

Before starting CPAP, a set of baseline arterial blood gases should be taken. Transcutaneous oxygen monitoring or pulse oximetry may be substituted in some clinical situations if oxygenation is the only parameter that needs to be measured. The neonate's vital signs should also be recorded. Assemble the CPAP circuit and pressure device. The decision must be made whether to apply the CPAP above the epiglottis (see Figs. 15-2 and 15-3) or to intubate the infant and apply the CPAP within the trachea. Among the factors to be considered are the neonate's gestational age and weight, amount of secretions needing suctioning, pulmonary problem, and the likelihood of mechanical ventilation eventually being needed. More mature and larger infants with few secretions and relatively stable pulmonary conditions will most likely have CPAP applied above the epiglottis by nasal prongs or nasopharyngeal tube. In contrast, less mature and smaller infants (less than 1000 to 1200 grams) who will need suctioning and have relatively unstable pulmonary conditions will probably be intubated. Mechanical ventilation can then be easily started if needed.

CPAP is usually started at about 2 to 3 cm water pressure. Some practitioners believe that if CPAP is initiated through an endotracheal tube, the starting point should be 4 to 5 cm water pressure. The reason for the difference is the effect of the epiglottis on the airway pressure. The spontaneously breathing infant with respiratory distress will close its epiglottis at the end of exhalation to apply about 2 cm water pressure against the lower airway. This so-called "epiglottal PEEP" is often heard as an expiratory grunt. When the trachea is intubated the epiglottis cannot close and the epiglottal PEEP is lost. Therefore some believe that it must be "added" to the CPAP level through the endotracheal tube.

Table 15-1. Indications, Contraindications, and Hazards of CPAP Therapy

Indications
Infant respiratory distress syndrome (IRDS)
Bronchiolitis with pneumonia
Pulmonary edema
Apnea of prematurity or obstructive sleep apnea
Physical exam shows some, if not all, of the
 following:
 Respiratory rate 30%-40% greater than normal
 Substernal and suprasternal retractions
 Expiratory grunting
 Cyanosis
 Chest x-ray shows atelectasis or pulmonary
  edema
Arterial blood gases showing:
 PaO_2 less than 50-60 mm Hg on 50%-70%
  oxygen
 $PaCO_2$ less than 50-55 mm Hg
 pH greater than 7.25
Weaning from mechanical ventilation when the
 IMV rate is about 4-12/minute, the pulmonary
 condition is improved, blood gases show
 acceptable $PaCO_2$, and there is acceptable
 PaO_2 on PEEP. The CPAP level is set to match
 the level of PEEP used on the ventilator.
Contraindications
Prolonged apnea leading to hypoxemia and
 hypotension
Untreated pneumothorax or other evidence of a
 pulmonary gas leak
Unstable cardiovascular status such as
 bradycardia and hypotension
Elevated $PaCO_2$ with unacceptable respiratory
 acidosis
Unilateral pulmonary problem
Hazards
Persistent pulmonary hypertension of the
 newborn (PPHN)
Increased intracranial pressure that can cause
 intraventricular hemorrhage
Decreased cardiac output
CPAP may be ineffective if the neonate weighs
 less than 1000-1200 grams

It should be noted that the inspired oxygen percentage is usually kept at the previously set level. It is important to make only one change at a time so that each adjustment in care can be evaluated for its own effect. For example, if you simultaneously increased the oxygen percentage by 10% and started 5 cm water of CPAP, it would not be known whether the increase in PaO_2 was from the additional oxygen, the CPAP, or both. Often the long-term inspired oxygen is limited to 40% to 50% because of concern of the possibility of pulmonary oxygen toxicity.

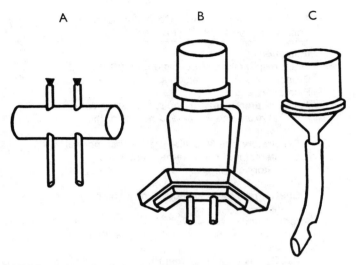

Fig. 15-2 Nasal CPAP devices for infants. **A,** Jackson-Reese tubes. **B,** Argyle nasal cannula (prongs). **C,** Endotracheal tube cut shorter for nasopharyngeal insertion (NP tube). (From Blodgett D: *Manual of pediatric respiratory care procedures,* Philadelphia, 1982, JB Lippincott. Used by permission.)

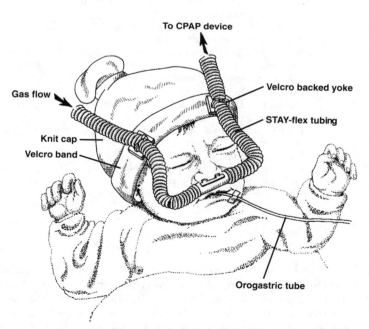

Fig. 15-3 An assembly for supporting nasal CPAP prongs in an infant. (Modified from an advertisement of the Stayflex tubing system from Ackrad.) (From Sills JR: *Respiratory care certification guide: the complete review resource for the entry level exam,* ed 2, St. Louis, 1994, Mosby–Year Book. Used by permission.)

d. Adjustment and weaning.

Blood gases and vital signs must be evaluated at the starting CPAP level. The heart rate, blood pressure, and respiratory rate should be stable or improved. Blood gases should be measured in about 15 to 20 minutes. See Table 15-2 for the recommended blood gas limits. In general, the PaO_2 should be kept between 60 and 70 mm Hg, $PaCO_2$ less than 50 to 55 mm Hg, and pH at least 7.25. If the PaO_2 is too low and the patient's vital signs are acceptable, the CPAP may be increased in a step of 2 to 3 cm water. The vital signs and blood gases should then be reevaluated. If necessary, the process of adding CPAP and reassessing the patient can be continued. It is rare to find that more than 10 cm water CPAP is necessary. Mechanical ventilation is indicated if more than 12 cm water pressure are needed. Depending on the patient, even less may not be well tolerated. The infant may become exhausted from exhaling against the back pressure. That would be seen clinically as decreased chest movement from the smaller tidal volume. The $PaCO_2$ would probably increase. It may be necessary to place the infant on mechanical ventilation to decrease the work of breathing and than add PEEP to maintain the FRC. When nasal prongs or a nasopharyngeal tube are used, CPAP pressures of greater than 8 cm water may cause the infant's mouth to open. This results in the loss of CPAP. A crying infant will also open its mouth and lose the CPAP. In either case, the CPAP pressure gauge will drop to zero or fluctuate below the set pressure.

As the patient improves, it is necessary to reduce the CPAP level so as not to cause pulmonary barotrauma. The pressure level can be reduced in steps of about 2 to 3 cm water. The vital signs and blood gases should be reassessed after each step. The apparatus is usually removed when the CPAP level is down to 2 to 3 cm water. The infant is then placed into an oxyhood at the same oxygen percentage as before or 5% to 15% higher. If the infant has an endotracheal tube that is needed for suctioning or a secure airway, the pressure is usually left at 2 to 3 cm water. After extubation, the infant is placed into an oxyhood as before.

If the infant was breathing more than 50% oxygen while on the CPAP it may be more important to lower the oxygen before decreasing the CPAP level. The following guidelines may prove helpful when decided whether to first lower the oxygen percentage or the CPAP level:

a. If the patient has been breathing more than 50% oxygen for more than 48 hours and has stable vital signs without any pulmonary barotrauma, decrease the oxygen first. Lower the inspired oxygen in 5% to 15% steps and check the oxygen-

Table 15-2. Commonly Recommended Blood Gas Goals for CPAP and Mechanical Ventilator Therapy

	Age of Neonate	
	Less than 72 hours	Greater than 72 hours
PaO_2 (mm Hg)	60-70	50-70
$PtcO_2$ (mm Hg)	Greater than 50,* less than 90*	Greater than 40,* less than 90*
SpO_2	92%-96%	92%-96%
$PaCO_2$ (mm Hg)	35-45†	45-55
$PtcCO_2$ (mm Hg)	May be used after correlation with $PaCO_2$ as discussed in Section 2.	
pH	7.25-7.45	7.25-7.45

* $PtcO_2$ values may be used after they have been shown to correlate within 15% of the PaO_2 from an arterial blood gas.
† With CPAP this value may be increased to 50-55 mm Hg as long as the pH is at least 7.25.

ation level after each reduction. Attempt to get the oxygen down to 40%, if possible. Then decrease the CPAP level.

b. If the patient is breathing 50% oxygen or less and has unstable vital signs or pulmonary barotrauma, decrease the CPAP first. After the CPAP is reduced (or removed entirely) and the patient is stable, reduce the inspired oxygen.

2. Mechanical ventilation.
a. Recommend changing the type of ventilator to be used on the patient. (IIIC10l) [R, Ap, An]

Most neonatal mechanical ventilators are pneumatically powered with electrical controls and alarm systems. They are used in the IMV mode and feature a continuous flow of gas. They are usually time cycled and pressure limited to prevent an excessive peak airway pressure. They can have PEEP added. Furthermore, they are capable of reaching the FDA limited rate of 150 breaths/minute. Examples include the BEAR Cub, Sechrist IV-100B and IV-200, Babybird 2A, Healthdyne 105, and Infrasonics Infant Star ventilators. It is recommended that the general function of these and the following ventilators be reviewed. It is beyond the scope of this textbook to offer any details; the reader is referred to McPherson's (1990) *Respiratory Therapy Equipment* or manufacturer's literature for more information.

High frequency ventilation (HVF) has been approved by the Food and Drug Administration (FDA) for use in the rescue of neonates with IRDS and a bronchopulmonary fistula or pulmonary interstitial emphysema (PIE) who fail under conventional ventilation. HFV has also been used, with parental permission, in the short-term support of neonates with a congenital diaphragmatic hernia until corrective surgery can be performed. The Bunnell Life Pulse High Frequency Ventilator is an example of a high frequency jet ventilator (HFJV) and can have the frequency adjusted to several hundred breaths per minute. The Infrasonics High Frequency Ventilator is built in tandem with the Infrasonics Infant Star Neonatal ventilator. It features a technology called high frequency flow interruption (HFFI) and is capable of a rate of more than 1000 breaths per minute. Finally, the SensorMedics 3100 Oscillatory Ventilator is classified as a high frequency oscillator (HFO). It is able to deliver several thousand breaths per minute by actively forcing the tidal volume both into and out of the patient by use of a piston pump. All these machines deliver very small tidal volumes at very high rates. Because of this the peak and mean airway pressures are lower than with conventional ventilation. This helps to prevent pulmonary barotrauma or allow damaged lung tissue to heal.

A volume cycled ventilator can be used on a neonate or infant who weighs more than 10 kilograms. Any conventional volume cycled ventilator can be used if it can be set to deliver a small enough tidal volume. Volume oriented ventilation can also be performed with a pneumatically powered neonatal ventilator if the patient is apneic. This technique is discussed later.

b. Initiate and adjust mechanical ventilation when settings are specified. (IIIB2c) [An]

As presented in Section 14, typical physician written ventilator orders include the following:

- Mode such as CPAP, IMV, high frequency ventilation, and so forth
- Oxygen percentage
- Respiratory rate
- Flow in liters per minute
- I : E ratio

- Tidal volume or minute volume (only on a volume cycled ventilator)
- Sigh volume and frequency (only on a volume cycled ventilator)
- Special settings such as PEEP or CPAP level

If the order is incomplete the physician should be asked for a clarification unless department protocol allows the therapist to make the decision.

c. Initiate and adjust mechanical ventilation when *no* settings are specified. (IIIB2b) [R, Ap]

Typically the therapist is expected to set the following ventilator controls based on a protocol or the patient's condition and response to the ventilator: sensitivity, flow, I : E ratio, alarms, and gas temperature.

Sensitivity.—There is no sensitivity control on traditional continuous flow neonatal ventilators. The IMV mode is used with these units. Some of the newer ventilators have the ability to sense a neonate's respiratory effort and trigger a machine delivered breath. The BEAR Cub does this with an add-on feature that senses a change in flow when the neonate inspires. The Drager Babylog 8000 has this flow sensing feature built into the unit. The Sechrist IV-200 uses two electrocardiogram leads on the neonate's chest to sense a change in electrical impedence (skin resistance) as a sign of respiratory effort. An older child on a volume cycled ventilator should have the sensitivity set at about −1 to −2 cm water pressure. No matter the method by which the ventilator senses the patient's respiratory effort, the neonate or child should not have to work very hard to trigger a machine tidal volume.

Flow.—Flow is adjusted to set the inspiratory time and I : E ratio and/or to meet the patient's needs.

I : E Ratio.—The I : E ratio is adjusted to ensure that the patient can inhale in as physiologically appropriate a manner as possible and completely exhale the inspired tidal volume.

Alarms.—Alarm systems are different for each type of ventilator. Generally speaking, they are set with a safety margin of ± 10% from the patient's normal ventilator settings. A variation of greater than 10% results in an audible and/or visual alarm condition.

Gas Temperature.—The goal for most patients is to minimize their humidity deficit by giving gas that is humidified and warmed to near body temperature. It is common to have the gas warmed to 90° to 95°F/35°C. It should be measured in the inspiratory limb of the circuit as close to the patient as possible.

d. Initiate and adjust different combinations of intermittent mandatory ventilation (IMV), synchronous intermittent mandatory ventilation (SIMV), and therapeutic PEEP. (IIIB4a) [R, Ap]

A review of the literature dealing with neonatal critical care shows that there are few universally accepted strategies for the use and modification of CPAP/PEEP and mechanical ventilation. In fact, a number of authors specifically contradict the recommendations of other authors. What is presented here is an attempt to describe what are widely accepted approaches to mechanical ventilation and related therapy.

The approach used in this discussion focuses on adjusting the ventilator and treating a neonate based on its pathological problem.

i. Indications for mechanical ventilation.

All authors agree that apnea is an absolute indication for mechanical ventilation. A general indication would be any condition that causes respiratory failure. This is usually documented by unacceptable arterial blood gases. Table 15-3 lists indications for mechanical ventilation.

ii. Time constants of ventilation.

It is important in any patient requiring mechanical ventilation to consider both the patient's lung-thoracic compliance and airway resistance when setting inspiratory and expiratory times. It is especially important in neonates because in comparison to adults they are less compliant and have greater resistance. In addition, they are usually ventilated at faster rates. As a review, the respective lung-thoracic compliances (C_{LT}) and airway resistances (Raw) of normal adults and infants are shown here:

Adult lung-thoracic compliance: 100 ml/cm water pressure (0.1 L/cm water pressure)
Neonatal lung-thoracic compliance: 5 ml/cm water pressure (.005 L/cm water pressure; about 20 times stiffer than an adult)
Adult airway resistance: 2 cm water/L/sec
Neonatal airway resistance: 20 to 40 cm water/L/sec (about 10 to 20 times more resistance to airflow than an adult)

Table 15-3. Common Indications for the Initiation of Mechanical Ventilation

Respiratory Failure
PaO_2 less than 50 mm Hg despite maximal CPAP therapy (12 cm water) and greater than 50% inspired oxygen
$PaCO_2$ greater than 55 mm Hg
Neurological
Complete apnea
Apneic periods leading to hypoxemia and bradycardia
Intracranial hemorrhage
Drug depression
Pulmonary Conditions
Infant respiratory distress syndrome (IRDS)
Diffuse pneumonia
Pulmonary edema
Meconium aspiration
Diaphragmatic hernia
Prophylactic use
Cyanotic congenital cardiac defect
Persistent pulmonary hypertension of the newborn (PPHN)
Postoperatively after major thoracic or abdominal surgery

In addition, the placement of an endotracheal tube to facilitate mechanical ventilation will result in a total pulmonary resistance ranging from 50 to 150 cm water/L/sec. The time constant of ventilation (T_c or time constant of the respiratory system—T_{RS}) is calculated as the product of compliance and resistance:

Time constant in seconds = compliance (L/cm water) × resistance (cm water/L/sec)

For example, using these values for a spontaneously breathing normal neonate, its time constant would be calculated as:

$$T_c = \text{compliance (.005 L/cm water)} \times \text{resistance (30 cm water/L/sec)}$$
$$= .005 \times 30$$
$$= .15 \text{ seconds}$$

While technically impractical to measure the time constant of ventilation at the bedside, the concept is important because it relates to two important clinical considerations during mechanical ventilation. First, it relates to the pressure that develops at the alveolar level as the tidal volume is delivered. For each time constant, progressively more of the peak inspiratory pressure (PIP) is applied within the alveoli (see Fig. 15-4). As can be seen, at three time constants 95% of the PIP is applied to the alveoli. At five time constants, virtually the entire PIP is applied at the alveolar level. Second, the time constant relates to how rapidly the lung recoils to baseline (FRC) during an exhalation. As shown in Fig. 15-4, at one time constant 63% of the tidal volume has been exhaled. It will take three time constants to exhale 95% and five time constants to completely exhale.

The clinical significance of this relates directly to the pulmonary condition of the patient. Infants with stiff lungs and normal resistance, as found in IRDS, will have a short time constant. Alveolar pressure will quickly increase to match the peak inspiratory pressure. The lungs will then rapidly recoil during exhalation so that there is little chance of air trapping. Infants with normal compliance and increased resistance, as found in meconium aspiration, will have a long time con-

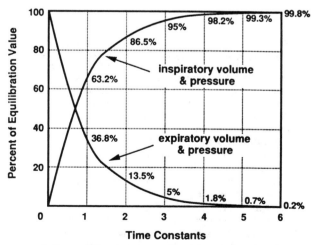

Fig. 15-4 Graphic presentation of the percentage of inspiratory and expiratory volume and pressure in comparison to time constants of ventilation. (From Chatburn RL: Principles and practice of neonatal and pediatric mechanical ventilation, *Respir Care* 36(6): 569-595, 1991. Used by permission.)

stant. It will take a relatively long time for the alveolar pressure to reach the PIP. Also, a relatively long time will be needed for the exhalation to be complete. Because of this, these infants are at risk for air trapping and auto-PEEP.

iii. Initiation and adjustments based on the patient's condition.
a. Patients with normal cardiopulmonary function.

Patients with normal cardiopulmonary function could need mechanical ventilation because of apnea from anesthesia, paralysis, or a neurological condition. The initial ventilator parameters for this type of patient are listed in Table 15-4. Because this patient is apneic and neither assisting nor fighting against the ventilator-delivered breath, it is possible to calculate an approximate tidal volume (volume-oriented ventilation). The following formula would be used:

$$\text{Calculated tidal volume} = (T_I \times \dot{V}) - Vc$$

Where:

T_I = inspiratory time provided that the pressure limit is not reached
(If the pressure limit is reached before the inspiratory time limit is reached, part of the inspiratory time is spent as an inflation hold and no additional tidal volume is delivered.)
$\dot{V}$ = inspiratory flow rate on the ventilator in ml/sec
Vc = volume compressed in the circuit and ventilator
(This is found by multiplying the peak inspiratory pressure by the manufacturer's stated compliance factors for the circuit and ventilator.)

For example, estimate the delivered tidal volume for an apneic 5 kg infant. The ventilator parameters are: inspiratory flow 5.5 L/min, frequency of 20/min, I : E ratio of 1 : 3, inspiratory time of .75 seconds, and expiratory time of 2.25 seconds. Peak inspiratory pressure (PIP) is 15 cm water. The internal compliance of the ventilator is 0.4 ml/cm water and the circuit compliance factor is 1.6 ml/cm water.

Table 15-4. Common Mechanical Ventilator
Parameters for Neonates with Normal Lungs

Delivered tidal volume: 6-8 ml/kg (This may be
    estimated by calculation if the neonate is
    apneic and the pressure limit is not reached.)
Pressure limit: 12-18 cm water
Frequency: 20/minute
I : E ratio: 1 : 2 to 1 : 10
Inspiratory time (T_I): At least .4 seconds
Expiratory time (T_E): At least .5 seconds
PEEP: None unless 2-3 cm water is added to
    replace "epiglottal PEEP"
Inspiratory flow: Sufficient to see the chest move
    and hear bilateral breath sounds during the
    inspiration. Start with at least twice the infant's
    estimated minute volume (respiratory
    rate × estimated tidal volume of 7 ml/kg).
    Check the blood gases for the $PaCO_2$.
Oxygen percentage: 40%

$$\text{Calculated tidal volume} = (T_I \times \dot{V}) - V_C$$

Where:

T_I = .75 seconds
$\dot{V}$ = 5.5 L/min. This is converted to ml/sec by dividing the flow in L/min by 60 seconds. So 5.5 L/min = .092 L/sec or 92 ml/sec
V_C = 0.4 + 1.6 ml/cm water = 2 ml/cm water
    = 2 ml/cm water × 15 cm water PIP
    = 30 ml

Therefore:

Calculated tidal volume = (.75 × 92) − 30
                    = (69) − 30
                    = 39 ml. This is within the ideal tidal volume range of 30 to 40 ml (based on 5 kg weight × 6 to 8 ml/kg).

It must be emphasized that this is only a calculated tidal volume. Leaks in the system, a decrease in the patient's compliance, or an increase in the patient's resistance will decrease the true tidal volume. Conversely, an increase in the patient's compliance or a decrease in the patient's resistance will increase the true tidal volume. Also, if the pressure limit is reached before the inspiratory time is completed, less volume than expected will be delivered. This is because part of the inspiratory time is spent as an inflation hold and no additional tidal volume is delivered (see Fig. 15-5). Finally, the infant must be completely passive during the delivery of the breath.

It is important to evaluate the patient's blood gases, vital signs, breath sounds, and any other pertinent clinical information before changing any ventilator parameters. As the patient recovers and begins to breathe spontaneously, it will probably be necessary to reduce the ventilator-delivered minute volume. It will encourage the child to breathe more because the final goal is to completely wean and extubate

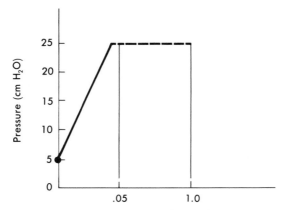

Fig. 15-5 Pressure-time curve seen with the pressure limit set at 25 cm water and the inspiratory time being increased from .5 to 1 second. The pressure limit is reached when the inspiratory time is about .5 second. As the inspiratory time is increased to 1 second (or greater) the pressure limit is held at 25 cm water resulting in a "square wave" pressure curve. (From Betis P, Thompson JE: Mechanical ventilation. In Koff PB, Eitzman DV, Neu J: *Neonatal and pediatric respiratory care*, St. Louis, 1988, Mosby–Year Book. Used by permission.)

the patient. The most accepted way to reduce the ventilator-delivered minute volume is to reduce the ventilator rate. A reduction of about 10% is a good starting place but will have to be tailored to meet the patient's needs. The tidal volume will be maintained as originally set. Obtain a set of blood gases in 20 minutes (or follow the transcutaneous or pulse oximetry values) and check the patient's vital signs to see how well the adjustment is tolerated.

If the blood gases show an elevated $PaCO_2$, the ventilator-delivered minute volume will have to be raised. This can be done by increasing either the alveolar ventilation or respiratory rate. Alveolar ventilation can be increased by either increasing the inspiratory flow or pressure limit (if it has been reached) to increase the tidal volume. The ventilator rate may be increased if the flow and pressure limit cannot be increased. An increase of about 10% is a good starting place but will have to tailored to meet the patient's needs. As before, blood gases and vital signs should be monitored after every change to see if the increase is well tolerated and accomplishing what was intended.

If the blood gases show that the $PaCO_2$ is lower than desired, the ventilator-delivered minute volume will have to be decreased. The first parameter to adjust is usually the rate. Try decreasing it about 10% and check another set of blood gas values. If other parameters need to be reduced, try decreasing the inspiratory flow or inspiratory time about 10% to decrease the tidal volume. Again, check the blood gas values after every adjustment.

If the blood gases show that the PaO_2 is higher or lower than necessary, the oxygen percentage will have to be adjusted. An increase or decrease of about 5% is a good starting place but will have to be adjusted as needed. If the patient does not respond to the increased oxygen as expected, the patient should be reevaluated. It may be necessary to reclassify him or her into one of the following categories.

b.   Patients with decreased lung compliance and normal airway resistance such as Infant Respiratory Distress Syndrome (IRDS).

While IRDS is the most common cause of decreased lung compliance and normal airway resistance, it will be seen in other lung conditions including pneumonia and pulmonary edema (see Fig. 15-6). The greatest challenge presented in the care of these infants is to oxygenate them without causing oxygen toxicity or pulmonary barotrauma. Common recommendations for the initial ventilator settings are listed in Table 15-5. As discussed earlier, blood gases, vital signs, and so forth must be monitored after the infant is placed on the ventilator. Any further adjustments can then be determined and evaluated by another set of blood gases and vital signs.

The issue of time constants of ventilation help to better understand the various options available for adjusting the ventilator. As presented earlier, the time constant of ventilation (T_c or time constant of the respiratory system—T_{RS}) is calculated as the product of compliance and resistance. For example, using the following values for a mechanically ventilated neonate with IRDS, its time constant would be calculated as:

T_c = compliance (.001 L/cm water because the lungs are less
     compliant) × resistance (100 cm water/L/sec because the infant is intubated)
     = .001 × 100
     = .1 seconds (Compare this with a T_c of .15 for a normal, spontaneously breathing neonate.)

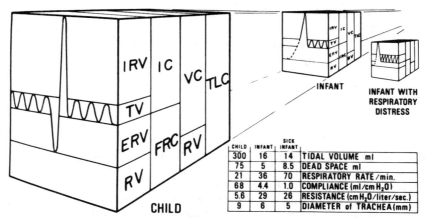

CHILD	INFANT	SICK INFANT	
300	16	14	TIDAL VOLUME ml
75	5	8.5	DEAD SPACE ml
21	36	70	RESPIRATORY RATE /min.
68	4.4	1.0	COMPLIANCE (ml/cm H₂O)
5.6	29	26	RESISTANCE (cmH₂O/liter/sec.)
9	6	5	DIAMETER of TRACHEA(mm)

Fig. 15-6 Comparison of the lung volumes and capacities of a 6-year-old child, normal infant, and infant with IRDS. Note the relatively low compliance and high resistance of the normal infant to the child, and the infant with IRDS to the normal infant. (From Chatburn RL, Lough MD: Mechanical ventilation. In Lough MD, Doershuk CF, Stern RC, editors; *Pediatric respiratory therapy,* ed 3, Chicago, 1985, Year Book Medical. Used by permission.)

Neonates with IRDS have a relatively short time constant; therefore the tidal volume and ventilating pressure are delivered rather quickly to the lungs. However, because the lungs are so stiff there is usually no problem with the tidal volume being fully exhaled as long as 5 time constants are allowed. An expiratory time of at least .5 seconds is usually set initially. The various options available for increasing oxygenation are discussed on the following pages.

Increased Inspired Oxygen

Up to 100% oxygen can be given to the neonate in the short term. Hypoxemia cannot be tolerated and supplemental oxygen is usually the best way to correct it; however, there are several limiting factors. First, it is commonly held that giving more than 50% oxygen for more than 48 to 72 hours increases the risk of pulmonary oxygen toxicity. Second, if more than 80% oxygen is given, some poorly ventilated alveoli will have all of the oxygen absorbed from them leading to denitrogenation

Table 15-5. Common Mechanical Ventilator Parameters for Neonates with Low Compliance and Normal Resistance

Delivered tidal volume: 6-8 ml/kg
Pressure limit: 20-25 cm water
Frequency: 30-40/min (This may need to be raised significantly.)
I : E ratio: 1 : 1 to 1 : 3 (This may eventually need to be altered to an inverse I : E ratio.)
Inspiratory time (T_I): Between .4 and .7 seconds (This may need to be increased.)
Expiratory time (T_E): At least .5 seconds (This may need to be decreased.)
PEEP: 2-3 cm water (This may need to be increased.)
Inspiratory flow: Sufficient to see the chest move and hear bilateral breath sounds during the inspiration. As a general rule, the faster the rate is, the higher the flow must be to deliver an adequate tidal volume. Check the blood gases for the $PaCO_2$.
Oxygen percentage: 40% (This may need to be increased.)

absorption atelectasis. Third, if the hypoxemia is caused by a decreased FRC because of the lack of surfactant and small lung volumes, increasing the oxygen will not markedly increase the PaO_2. Other solutions, such as those discussed here, will have to be used.

Increased Inspiratory Flow

Increasing the flow will increase the tidal volume until the pressure limit is reached. Increasing the tidal volume should result in an increased PaO_2 and is likely to reduce the $PaCO_2$. If the pressure limit is reached, the delivered tidal volume is held in the lungs for the duration of the inspiratory time. This acts as an inflation hold and should also increase the PaO_2. The mean airway pressure would be raised by increasing the flow. (See Fig. 15-7 for the pressure waveforms seen during low flow and high flow conditions.) Under high flow conditions the pressure waveform takes on a characteristic square shape (square wave) because the pressure limit is reached. This pattern of ventilation is currently widely used with these types of patients.

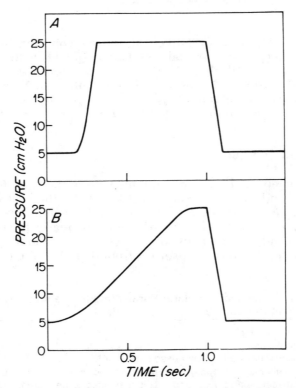

Fig. 15-7 Comparison of pressure-time curves showing the influence of inspiratory flow when the pressure limit is set at 25 cm water pressure. **A,** the curve at a high flow rate. The pressure limit is reached very early in the inspiratory time with a resulting "square wave" flow pattern. **B,** The curve at a low flow rate. The pressure limit is not reached until the inspiratory time is almost 1 second. (From Chatburn RL, Lough MD: Mechanical ventilation. In Lough MD, Doershuk CF, Stern RC, editors: *Pediatric respiratory therapy,* ed 3, Chicago, 1985, Year Book Medical. Used by permission.)

Increased Inspiratory Time Leading to Inverse Ratio Ventilation

i.   Recommend the initiation of inverse ratio ventilation. (IIIC10p) [R, Ap, An]

ii.   Initiate inverse ratio ventilation. (IIIB2d) [R, Ap]

iii. Recommend a change and adjust inverse ratio ventilation. (IIIB2d and IIIC10p) [R, Ap, An]

As with increasing the flow, increasing the inspiratory time will increase the tidal volume until the pressure limit is reached. If the pressure limit is reached, any increased inspiratory time will act as inflation hold. This will also raise the mean airway pressure and should result in an increased PaO_2. (See Fig. 15-5 for the pressure waveform change as the inspiratory time is increased.)

Some authors have advocated an increased inspiratory time as an important way to improve oxygenation. This has led to the use of inverse I : E ratios of up to 3 : 1 (.33) or 4 : 1 (.25) to produce an adequate PaO_2. The inspiratory time should be increased in small time increments and followed in 20 minutes with a blood gas to determine if the desired improvement in oxygenation was achieved. Inspiratory time is increased only as long as necessary to result in a satisfactory PaO_2. Great care must be taken to adjust expiratory time, respiratory rate, or both when a prolonged inspiratory time is used. Obviously expiratory time will have to be reduced to keep the same rate as the inspiratory time is increased, or the rate will have to be reduced as the inspiratory time is increased if the expiratory time cannot be reduced. Care must be taken to ensure that the tidal volume is fully exhaled to avoid auto-PEEP.

As the neonate's lung compliance improves, the inspiratory time must be decreased for two reasons. First, the alveolar pressure will be more readily transmitted throughout the lungs and could decrease venous return to the heart. That would result in a decreased cardiac output. Second, the more normal lungs would be more prone to barotrauma. The inspiratory time should be decreased in small time increments and followed with a set of blood gases to be sure that the neonate is not hypoxemic.

Increased Positive End-Expiratory Pressure (PEEP)

This has the greatest effect on improving the patient's FRC and will probably be the most effective at increasing the PaO_2. As discussed with CPAP therapy, the pressure is usually started out at 2 to 3 cm water. A blood gas is then checked and, if necessary, PEEP is added in 2 to 3 cm water increments. Commonly between 4 and 7 cm are needed; it is rare for more than 8 to 10 cm of PEEP to be needed. Another blood gas should be checked for PaO_2 after every addition of pressure. PEEP will have the greatest impact on raising the mean airway pressure of all the options presented here. Excessive PEEP could cause a decreased venous return to the heart and decreased cardiac output. It also could cause barotrauma resulting in pulmonary interstitial emphysema (PIE), pneumothorax, or pneumomediastinum. Care must be taken to carefully evaluate the patient after each increase in PEEP. Watch for a sudden deterioration in the patient's condition as a sign of a pulmonary air leak. As the patient's PaO_2 improves, the PEEP level should be reduced in steps of about 2 to 3 cm water. As always, recheck the blood gases with each adjustment.

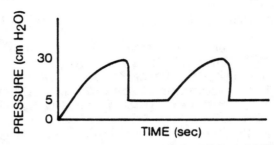

Fig. 15-8 Pressure-time curve showing the effect of the addition of PEEP on the tidal volume. Initially, the tidal volume is delivered by the pressure difference of 30 cm water (difference between 0 and 30 cm water pressure). With the addition of 5 cm water PEEP, the pressure difference is reduced to 25 cm water (difference between 5 and 30 cm water pressure). This results in less tidal volume being delivered. (From Burgess WR, Chernik V: *Respiratory therapy in newborn infants and children*, ed 2, New York, 1986, Thieme. Used by permission.)

Increased Pressure Limit

It may become necessary to increase the pressure limit when it is reached by the peak inspiratory pressure to deliver a larger tidal volume. It may also be necessary to raise the pressure limit to restore the original tidal volume after the addition of PEEP. This is because the original tidal volume is reduced when PEEP is added and the peak inspiratory pressure reaches the pressure limit. This is shown in Fig. 15-8. To restore the original tidal volume the pressure limit (and peak inspiratory pressure) would have to be increased by the same amount as the added PEEP. It is important to remember that as PEEP is reduced, the pressure limit must also be reduced by the same amount. This will maintain the original tidal volume.

Increased Respiratory Rate

Increasing the ventilator respiratory rate will increase the minute volume and probably raise the PaO_2 and lower the $PaCO_2$. Patients with stiff lungs and short time constants of ventilation often respond well to an increased respiratory rate. Some authors advocate using rates of up to 150/minute on conventional ventilators if necessary. (Note: The FDA has set the rate limit of 150/minute on conventional IMV mode ventilators.)

Even though rates greater than this are considered to be experimental, some authors report success at rates of between 150 and 600/minute on high frequency jet ventilators and up to 3000/minute on high frequency oscillator ventilators. Reported benefits of these high rates are lower peak inspiratory pressure and mean airway pressure. This has been reported to reduce the frequency of barotrauma and decrease cardiac output while maintaining acceptable blood gases. Other authors report no significant difference in complications or survival rate between conventional pressure-limited IMV ventilation and high frequency ventilation. Currently, it can only be concluded that high frequency ventilation may prove beneficial to some neonates who fail with conventional ventilation. Unfortunately, there are no universally accepted guidelines on when to switch an infant from conventional ventilation to high frequency ventilation.

Instillation of Exogenous Surfactant

In 1991 the FDA approved the use of exogenous surfactant that can be directly instilled into the trachea of IRDS neonates. Exosurf Neonatal (a synthetic product) and Survanta (a bovine lung extract) have been successfully used clinically. These drugs have proven very beneficial to premature neonates with inadequate natural surfactant. After the drug is administered, the patient's lung compliance improves dramatically. Usually there can then be rapid reductions in the ventilator-delivered oxygen percentage, rate, pressure limit, and PEEP. It can be hoped that as more neonatologists learn how to administer these drugs and adjust the ventilator parameters accordingly, fewer ventilator related complications will be seen.

Each of the options discussed in this section has its advocates; however, it would seem logical that the best possible care would come from the proper application of each option when it is best suited to the patient's condition. To that end, Chatburn, Waldemar, and Lough (1983) have developed a rather comprehensive approach to the adjustment of the various ventilator parameters to optimize the care of the IRDS infant. They use the initial and subsequent blood gas results to direct the various ventilator changes that have been discussed. Due to the complexity of the logic in the algorithm, it is recommended that their articles, listed in the bibliography, be read to appreciate fully its use.

c.   **Patients with increased airway resistance and normal lung compliance such as meconium aspiration syndrome (MAS).**

Although meconium aspiration is a commonly seen cause of increased airway resistance and normal lung compliance, it is also seen in infants with excessive airway secretions or bronchospasm. Their problem is one of getting airflow into and out of the lungs. This uneven airflow results in hypoxemia, air trapping, auto-PEEP, and an increased risk of barotrauma. Because of these issues there are two key clinical goals. The first is to minimize turbulence during inspiration by reducing the inspiratory flow as much as possible. The second is to give a long enough expiratory time to prevent air trapping. Common recommendations for the ventilator settings are listed in Table 15-6. As discussed earlier, blood gases, vital signs, and so forth must be monitored after the infant is placed on the ventilator. Listen to the breath sounds to detect the end of exhalation and a pause before the start of the next inspiration. This is to ensure that the exhalation has been complete and there is no air trapping that would lead to auto-PEEP. Any further adjustments can then be determined and evaluated by another set of blood gases and vital signs.

Table 15-6. Common Mechanical Ventilator Parameters for Neonates with Increased Airway Resistance and Normal Lung Compliance

Delivered tidal volume: 6-8 ml/kg
Pressure limit: 12-18 cm water
Frequency: 10-20/minute
I : E ratio: 1 : 3 to 1 : 10
Inspiratory time (T_I): Between .4 and .7 seconds (This may need to be increased.)
Expiratory time (T_E): At least .5 seconds (This may need to be increased.)
PEEP: 2-3 cm water if needed
Inspiratory flow: Sufficient to see the chest move and hear bilateral breath sounds during the inspiration.
Oxygen percentage: 40%

Let us look again at the issue of time constants of ventilation to better understand the various options for adjusting the ventilator. Using the following values for a mechanically ventilated neonate with meconium aspiration, its time constant would be calculated as:

T_c = Compliance (.005 L/cm water) × resistance (150 cm water/L/sec because the infant is intubated and has an obstuctive problem)
= .005 × 150
= .75 seconds (Compare this with a T_c of 0.15 for a normal, spontaneously breathing neonate and a T_c of 0.1 for a ventilated infant with IRDS.)

This relatively long time constant means that the tidal volume and peak inspiratory pressure are rather slowly delivered to the alveoli. There is little chance of causing barotrauma from high ventilating pressures; however, it will take a fairly long inspiratory time to deliver an adequate tidal volume. Care must be taken to provide enough expiratory time for the tidal volume to be exhaled completely. Briefly then, the challenge is to deliver an adequate tidal volume to maintain acceptable blood gases at a rate slow enough to prevent air trapping on exhalation.

In general, the inspiratory flow and rate are kept low, inspiratory and expiratory times are kept relatively long, and the I : E ratio should favor a long time for complete exhalation. Furthermore, it is important to frequently suction the airway to remove meconium or secretions. Postural drainage and percussion are also provided to mobilize the secretions so that they can be suctioned out. Usually these procedures and the natural breakdown of meconium result in reduced airway resistance within a few days. Ventilatory support can then be lessened.

d. Patients with persistent pulmonary hypertension of the newborn (PPHN).

Persistent pulmonary hypertension of the newborn (PPHN) is also referred to as persistent pulmonary hypertension (PPH), persistent fetal circulation (PFC), or persistence of the fetal circulation. Infants with PPHN present clinically with an elevated pulmonary artery pressure and a right-to-left shunt through a patent ductus arteriosus and/or the foramen ovale. Because of this their oxygenation fluctuates greatly. The problem may be seen right after birth or up to 24 hours later. PPHN seems to result from fetal hypoxemia and acidosis. These, in turn, are caused by or associated with maternal drug addiction, infection, preeclampsia, abruptio placenta, postterm gestation, oligohydramnios, and meconium staining or aspiration. The following four tests are done to help confirm the diagnosis:

1. Hyperoxia test: This is the first test and is done after an arterial blood gas has shown a low PaO_2. The test involves having the patient inspire 100% oxygen for about 10 minutes and obtaining a second arterial blood gas. If the PaO_2 does not improve to more than 50 mm Hg, a fixed right-to-left shunt is proven. The shunt could be from PPHN or a cyanotic heart defect. If the PaO_2 does go over 100 mm Hg, the neonate probably has parenchymal lung disease and should be treated accordingly.

2. Preductal and postductal arterial blood sampling: Simultaneously draw a blood gas from the right radial or brachial artery to check the preductal PaO_2, and from the left brachial, left radial, either femoral artery, or the umbilical artery catheter to check the postductal PaO_2. A drop in saturation from preductal to postductal blood of greater than 10% or a drop in PaO_2 of greater than 15 to 20 mm Hg indicates shunting. For example, a preductal PaO_2 of 70 mm Hg and a postductal PaO_2 of 45 mm Hg would indicate significant shunting. This same test could be

performed noninvasively with either transcutaneous oxygen monitoring or pulse oximetry monitoring. The $PtcO_2$ monitors should be placed over the right upper chest for preductal blood and left upper chest, abdomen, or either thigh for postductal blood. Pulse oximetry monitors should be placed on the right hand for preductal blood and left hand or either foot for postductal blood. Again, a greater than 15 to 20 mm Hg drop in preductal to postductal $PtcO_2$ or a greater than 10% drop in saturation in preductal to postductal SpO_2 would confirm a significant shunt.

It is important to note that if the neonate has a shunt through the foramen ovale instead of the ductus arteriosus, this test will be negative. The preductal and postductal oxygen levels will be the same. Shunting through the foramen ovale is seen in as many as 50% of PPHN babies.

3. Hyperoxia-hyperventilation test: The infant is manually ventilated with 100% oxygen at a rate and pressure adequate to significantly reduce the carbon dioxide level. When this "critical $PaCO_2$" (usually between 20 and 30 mm Hg) is reached, the pulmonary artery pressure will drop, the lungs will be better perfused, and the PaO_2 will improve. Although the patient's color will likely change from cyanotic to pink and the $PtcO_2$ and SpO_2 values will improve, the test is confirmed by a postductal PaO_2 of greater than 80 mm Hg. The critical $PaCO_2$ value, ventilation rate, and manometer pressure on the manual ventilator should be recorded. These values can be used later to set the mechanical ventilator parameters.

4. Echocardiography: This procedure can be used to identify an intracardiac shunt through the foramen ovale or evidence of increased right ventricular pressure as a sign of pulmonary hypertension.

Any infant who shows signs of PPHN, such as positive results to any of the earlier tests or the need for more than 70% oxygen to prevent hypoxemia, should be considered for hyperventilation therapy. The goal is to reduce pulmonary artery hypertension and thus reduce shunting and improve the PaO_2. This is accomplished by hyperventilating the patient to his or her critical $PaCO_2$. Table 15-7 lists common ventilator parameters used to treat persistent pulmonary hypertension. Once the proper ventilator settings are found and the blood gas goals are met, the patient is maintained at this level for one or more days. It is often necessary to pharmacologically paralyze the infant with pancuronium bromide (Pavulon) or a similar drug to ensure that the patient's breathing is synchronized with the ventilator. This is

Table 15-7. Common Mechanical Ventilator Parameters to Treat a Neonate with Persistent Pulmonary Hypertension

Delivered tidal volume: 6-8 ml/kg or greater to hyperventilate the neonate

Pressure limit: As low as possible but be prepared to raise to more than 45 cm water to deliver an adequate tidal volume

Frequency: It is rapid enough to decrease the $PaCO_2$ to the critical level of probably between 20 and 30 mm Hg. Rates of up to 150/minute have been used.

I : E ratio: 1 : 2 (This will depend on the respiratory rate needed to decrease the carbon dioxide level.)

Inspiratory time (T_I): Between .4 and .7 seconds (This will need to be decreased at higher respiratory rates.)

Expiratory time (T_E): At least .5 seconds (This will need to be decreased at higher respiratory rates.)

PEEP: None if possible to lower the mean airway pressure and prevent crushing of the pulmonary capillary bed

Inspiratory flow: It is sufficient to see the chest move and hear bilateral breath sounds during the inspiration. Flow will have to be increased at higher respiratory rates.

Oxygen percentage: 70%–100% to keep the PaO_2 greater than 55 mm Hg and ideally between 115 and 120 mm Hg especially important when high ventilator rates are needed. After about 24 hours the ventilator is adjusted to increase the $PaCO_2$ by 1 to 2 mm Hg. If the peak inspiratory pressure is greater than 45 cm water it should be reduced first. A blood gas is drawn to see if the PaO_2 is stable and if the $PaCO_2$ increased the desired small amount. If this first reduction in support is tolerated, it may be slowly followed by further reductions. Each step back from hyperventilation should be small so that the $PaCO_2$ only increases by 1 to 2 mm Hg each time.

As this is going on, the patient should be supported in every other way. The medication tolazoline (Priscoline) is a pulmonary vasodilator that has proven to be successful in about 1 of 6 neonates with PPHN that receive it. Watch for signs of pulmonary barotrauma or bronchopulmonary dysplasia from the high peak pressures and oxygen percentages required with these patients.

At the time of this writing the gas nitric oxide (NO) is being tried as a pulmonary artery vasodilator. Early investigations indicate that when a small amount of nitric oxide is inhaled the neonate with PPHN shows clinical improvement. If this becomes an accepted treatment modality, it might become an NBRC testable item.

e.   Patients with bronchopulmonary dysplasia (BPD).

The neonate with BPD was usually born prematurely with a low birth weight. He or she is a survivor of IRDS but has suffered serious lung damage in the process. It is controversial whether high peak pressures, high mean airway pressures, high inspired oxygen percentages, or a combination of these factors is the main cause of BPD. It is important to try to minimize all of them so that new lung tissues can grow to replace what has been damaged. It is important to try to wean these infants as quickly as possible to avoid further ventilator-induced damage. If acceptable blood gases can be maintained with a ventilator rate of less than 15/minute, the infant may be extubated. Nasal CPAP may be used to help maintain the PaO_2. See Table 15-8 for the commonly recommended ventilator settings for a BPD patient.

A number of medications are used to help optimize the patient's pulmonary function. Methylxanthines such as aminophylline or caffeine are beneficial as respiratory stimulants. There is further evidence that they help to strengthen the diaphragm and decrease muscle fatigue. The diuretic furosemide (Lasix) has been widely reported to improve lung compliance and airway resistance by decreasing any pulmonary edema fluid. Remember that patients receiving Lasix must be given a potassium-chloride supplement to replace what is lost through the kidneys. Some

Table 15-8. Common Mechanical Ventilator Parameters for Neonates with Bronchopulmonary Dysplasia

---

Delivered tidal volume: 6-8 ml/kg

Pressure limit: As low as possible and not to exceed 25 cm water

Frequency: It is as low as possible to maintain the $PaCO_2$ between 35 and 45 mm Hg. Some authors report accepting a $PaCO_2$ as high as 55 to 65 mm Hg to minimize the need to increase peak and mean pressures.

I : E ratio: 1 : 2 to 1 : 10

Inspiratory time (T_I): Between .3 and .7 seconds

Expiratory time (T_E): At least .5 seconds to allow for a complete exhalation

PEEP: No more than 2-4 cm water

Inspiratory flow: It is sufficient to see the chest move and hear bilateral breath sounds during the inspiration.

Oxygen percentage: It is as low as possible to keep the PaO_2 between 55 and 65 mm Hg. Some authors report accepting a PaO_2 as low as 35 mm Hg to minimize the need to increase peak and mean pressures. It must be noted that a PaO_2 below 55 mm Hg increases the risk of pulmonary hypertension.

authors have reported the use of corticosteroids to be helpful in weaning because of increased pulmonary compliance. This possible advantage must be balanced against the known problems associated with the prolonged use of the medication. Finally, a dietary supplement of vitamin E may increase lung healing. Hopefully the current and future use of synthetic surfactants early in the treatment of the IRDS neonate will reduce the incidence of BPD.

3. Mean airway pressure.
a. Monitor the mean airway pressure to evaluate the patient's response to respiratory care. (IIIA1d) [R, Ap]

Mean airway pressure is the average pressure over an entire breathing cycle. A number of current neonatal and adult ventilators are able to calculate the value. Review Fig. 14-14 for how the $\overline{P}aw$ is measured and the mathematical equation is derived. $\overline{P}aw$ is influenced by both the patient's lung thoracic compliance (C_{LT}) and airway resistance (Raw). If the ventilator settings are unchanged, a decrease in compliance or an increase in resistance will result in an increase in the mean airway pressure. This is because in a neonatal ventilator the pressure limit will be reached earlier and held for the duration of the inspiratory time. Conversely, if the patient's compliance increases or the resistance decreases, the $\overline{P}aw$ will decrease. It is important to further evaluate the patient when a change in $\overline{P}aw$ is noticed. This is because the new pressure by itself will not show you whether there has been a change in compliance, resistance, or both. Any treatments that improve lung compliance and reduce airway resistance would be shown by a reduced mean airway pressure.

b. Recommend a change in the patient's mean airway pressure. (IIIC10c) [R, Ap, An]

In general, an increase in mean airway pressure will increase the patient's oxygenation. This is because the alveoli are kept open longer allowing more time for diffusion and preventing alveolar collapse. If alveolar ventilation is improved, the $PaCO_2$ will also be reduced.

If the mean airway pressure is too high there is an increased risk of pulmonary barotrauma and decreased cardiac output. This is especially true if PEEP is increased to raise the $\overline{P}aw$. Watch the patient closely whenever a ventilator change is made that increases the $\overline{P}aw$. A sudden deterioration in cardiopulmonary function may be caused by a pneumothorax. A reduction in urine output, an increased heart rate, and decreased blood pressure are often seen when the cardiac output is reduced. The mean airway pressure should be reduced if either of these situations is seen. To prevent these complications, it is necessary to reduce the mean airway pressure whenever the patient's compliance improves.

Usually the mean airway pressure is the result of the patient's lung compliance, airway resistance, and the various ventilator settings. The initial mean airway pressure should be considered along with the ventilator settings when interpreting the first set of arterial blood gases. Based on the blood gas results, ventilator adjustments may be needed. Note the $\overline{P}aw$ at each adjustment.

A number of ventilator control adjustments will influence the patient's mean airway pressure. (See Fig. 15-9 for several examples of airway pressure tracings based on ventilator control changes.) If the patient's compliance and resistance are stable, the $\overline{P}aw$ will be *increased* by the following: 1) an increased inspiratory flow, 2) an increased pressure limit (assuming the pressure limit had been previously reached), 3) an increase in PEEP, 4) an increased inspiratory time (assuming no change in ventilator rate and a decreased expiratory time), and 5) a decreased expiratory time (assuming an increased ventilator rate). These ventilator adjust-

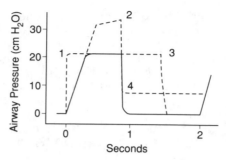

Fig. 15-9 Pressure-time tracings showing four different ventilator settings that can be used to increase the mean airway pressure. *1,* the inspiratory flow is increased. *2,* the pressure limit is increased. *3,* the inspiratory time is increased. This also changes the I : E ratio by reducing the expiratory time if the rate is kept the same. *4,* PEEP is added. (From Harris TR: Physiological principles. In Goldsmith JP, Karotkin EH, editors: *Assisted ventilation of the neonate,* Philadelphia, 1981, WB Saunders. Used by permission.)

ments should result in an increased PaO_2 and possibly a decreased $PaCO_2$. Measure blood gases to be sure of the patient's response.

If the patient's compliance and resistance are stable, the $\overline{P}aw$ will be *decreased* by the following: 1) a decreased inspiratory flow, 2) a decreased pressure limit (assuming the pressure limit had been previously reached), 3) a decrease in PEEP, 4) a decreased inspiratory time (assuming no change in ventilator rate and an increased expiratory time), and 5) an increased expiratory time (assuming a decreased ventilator rate). These ventilator adjustments may result in a decreased PaO_2 and possibly an increased $PaCO_2$. Measure blood gases to be sure of the patient's response.

It should be noted that of all the various controls that have an influence on the mean airway pressure, PEEP has the greatest impact. There is usually a one-for-one relationship between the addition or removal of PEEP and the resulting $\overline{P}aw$. For example, the $\overline{P}aw$ is 10 cm water when 5 cm water of PEEP is added. The resulting $\overline{P}aw$ is seen to become 15 cm water. If 2 cm of PEEP is removed the $\overline{P}aw$ will drop to 13 cm water.

4. Perform and/or interpret pressure-volume and flow-volume loops. (IC1n) [R, Ap, An]

This subject was presented in some detail in Section 14 because several adult microprocessor ventilators give a graphic display of the patient's tidal volume, peak pressure, and inspiratory and expiratory flows. At the time of this writing only the Drager Babylog 8000 is capable of giving similar graphic information. This information is clinically useful because expiratory flow can be monitored to look for air trapping and auto-PEEP. As discussed earlier, this is a concern if the neonate has obstructive airways disease or if a high respiratory rate is being used.

5. Sedate or paralyze the patient.
a. Recommend the use of sedatives or muscle relaxants (paralyzing agents) as needed. (IIIC10d) [R, Ap, An]

An infant who is attempting to exhale when the IMV breath is being delivered is said to be "bucking" or "fighting" the ventilator. This problem is almost unavoidable because the IMV breaths cannot be synchronized on the majority of neonatal ventilators. If the asynchrony between the infant's efforts and the ventilator are too great, there is an increased risk of hypoxemia and pneumothorax. Carefully evaluate the patient to determine if the patient is breathing rapidly because of pain or improper adjustment of the ventilator. Make sure that the flow, rate, pressure limit, and so forth are correctly set for the patient's condition. Sedation or paralysis should be considered only after all other causes of asynchrony have been ruled out.

b. Recommend specific pain relieving or muscle relaxing agents for use on patients. (IIIC10e) [R, Ap, An]

Refer to Section 14 for the general considerations on the use of pain relieving or muscle relaxing agents. Antianxiety agents are not typically used with neonates. Morphine sulfate or other opiates are typically used for pain but other less powerful medications may also be tried. If the patient needs to be paralyzed, pancuronium (Pavulon), atracurium (Tracrium), and vencuronium (Norcuron) are commonly used. Remember that these paralyzing agents have no affect on the patient's ability to feel pain or to be afraid of what is happening. Pain medications must be given as necessary.

6. Make a recommendation to extubate the patient. (IIIC10k) [R, Ap, An]

Specific steps in weaning were discussed earlier with each of the types of common pathological conditions and the various modes of ventilation. Remember to evaluate your patient's blood gases and vital signs before and after making a change in the ventilator parameters. If the patient deteriorates, the ventilator setting(s) should be placed as before.

The decision to extubate with CPAP therapy and ventilator management based on the neonate's pathological condition was discussed earlier. As a review, if the patient's blood gases and vital signs are acceptable at minimal ventilator support and the endotracheal tube is not needed for a suctioning route, the tube can be removed. Follow-up on blood gases and frequent monitoring of vital signs and breath sounds should be done after extubation. Be prepared to reintubate if the patient deteriorates or a suctioning route is needed.

Module B.   Mechanical ventilation equipment.

1.   Ventilators.

As discussed in Section 14, the literature produced by the manufacturers and the descriptions used in many standard texts break the various ventilators into more catagories than used by the NBRC. To avoid confusion, this text uses the NBRC's more simplified terminology. A pneumatically powered ventilator is defined here as powered by compressed gas. It may be electrically controlled with electrical alarm systems. Fluidic ventilators are defined here as being pneumatically powered and partially or completely controlled by fluidic methods. Fluidic controls make use of compressed gas for cycling and other ventilator functions. Both of these types of neonatal ventilators use compressed air and oxygen that go to an air-oxygen mixer (blender) to determine the inspired oxygen. The gas then goes to a flowmeter where the continuous flow per minute through the ventilator circuit is set. Depending on the ventilator, either compressed air or oxygen are used to drive the other control functions in fluidic ventilators such as the Sechrist.

An electrically powered ventilator is defined here as being electrically powered and controlled. Compressed air and oxygen go to a blender where the inspired oxygen is set. A microprocessor ventilator is defined here as being controlled by a microprocessor; it may be pneumatically or electrically powered.

a.   Fix any problems with a pneumatic ventilator. (IIB2d1) [An]

It is beyond the scope of this text to discuss in detail the functions of pneumatic ventilators and the following types of ventilators. Refer to the manufacturer's literature or McPherson's (1990) *Respiratory Therapy Equipment* for specific information. Examples of neonatal pneumatic ventilators include the Babybird, BEAR BP200, BEAR Cub, and Healthdyne 105. Personal experience with the units is recommended.

Make sure that the air and oxygen high pressure hoses are screwed tightly into the air-oxygen blender. A gas leak will be heard as a whistling or hissing sound. If either gas source is cut off to the blender its alarm will sound.

b.   Fluidic ventilators.
i.   Obtain the necessary equipment for the procedure. (IIB2d1) [R, Ap]

The Sechrist IV-100B and IV-200 ventilators are pneumatically powered and electrically and fluidically controlled.

ii.   Put the equipment together, make sure that it works properly, and identify any problems with it. (IIB1c1) [R, Ap]
iii.   Fix any problems with the equipment. (IIB2d2) [R, Ap, An]

Fluidic ventilators are prone to the same kind of problems with leaking high pressure air and oxygen hoses as pneumatic ventilators. In addition, they are very sensitive to obstructions. Make sure that all inlet filters are intact and free of debris.

c.   Fix any problems with an electric ventilator. (IIB2d2) [An]

At the time of this writing, there are no exclusively neonatal units that fit the earlier definition of an electric ventilator; however, some adult ventilators can deliver tidal volumes small enough for a pediatric patient. Make sure that the electrical power source is secure. Do not use a unit that will not power up or operate properly.

d.   Fix any problems with a microprocessor ventilator. (IIB2d4) [An]

The Infrasonics Infant Star and Drager Babylog 8000 are electrically and pneumatically powered and controlled by a microprocessor. Some of the current generation of primarily adult ventilators are capable of delivering tidal volumes and rates appropriate for infants. Examples include the Puritan-Bennett 7200 and BEAR 1000 ventilators. Microprocessor ventilators typically come with self-diagnostic software. If a problem is detected the unit will display it on the monitor. There is little to repair with these units at the bedside. Occasionally a computer chip will have to be replaced in the department.

e. High frequency jet ventilators.
  #### i. Obtain the necessary equipment for the procedure. (IIA1b2) [R, Ap]

The Bunnell Life Pulse High Frequency Ventilator and Infrasonics Infant Star HFV (high frequency ventilator) are examples of high frequency jet ventilators.

  #### ii. Put the equipment together, make sure that it works properly, and identify any problems with it. (IIB1c2) [R, Ap]
  #### iii. Fix any problems with the equipment. (IIB2d5) [R, Ap, An]

Hands-on experience with these ventilators is recommended. The following are needed for proper assembly: 1) a pressurized oxygen source, 2) a pressurized air source, 3) an air-oxygen proportioner (blender), 4) a pressure regulator for controlling the patient's peak pressure, 5) an injector line to add the jet volume to the endotracheal tube, and 6) an intravenous infusion pump to supply a steady drip of water to the jet ventilator injector line for nebulization.

f. High frequency oscillator ventilators.
  #### i. Obtain the necessary equipment for the procedure. (IIA1b3) [R, Ap]

The SensorMedics 3100 High-Frequency Oscillatory Ventilator is an example of a high frequency oscillator ventilator.

  #### ii. Put the equipment together, make sure that it works properly, and identify any problems with it. (IIB1c3) [R, Ap]
  #### iii. Fix any problems with the equipment. (IIB2d6) [R, Ap, An]

Hands-on experience is recommended with high frequency oscillator ventilators. They need the following basic accessories for assembly: 1) a pressurized oxygen source, 2) a pressurized air source, 3) an air-oxygen proportioner (blender), and 4) a passover or cascade humidifier.

g. Transport ventilators.
  #### i. Obtain the necessary equipment for the procedure. (IIA1b5) [R, Ap]

The Bio-Med Devices MVP-10 is an example of a pediatric transport ventilator.

  #### ii. Put the equipment together, make sure that it works properly, and identify any problems with it. (IIB1c5) [R, Ap]
  #### iii. Fix any problems with the equipment. (IIB2d8) [R, Ap, An]

The MVP-10 is pneumatically powered and pneumatically and fluidically controlled. It must have high pressure air and oxygen sources to function. It operates like many other pneumatic ventilators and is prone to the same operational problems.

    h.   **Home care ventilators.**
        i.   **Obtain the necessary equipment for the procedure.**
           (IIA1b6) [R, Ap]

The LifeCare PLV-102 and Puritan-Bennett Companion 2800 are two examples of home care ventilators that can deliver small enough tidal volumes for pediatric patients. Both will deliver a volume as small as 50 ml.

        ii. **Put the equipment together, make sure that it works properly, and identify any problems with it. (IIB1c6) [R, Ap]**
        iii. **Fix any problems with the equipment. (IIB2d9) [R, Ap, An]**

Both the LifeCare PLV-102 and the Puritan-Bennett Companion 2800 are microprocessor controlled and electrically powered. They must have a stable electrical supply. They also must have an oxygen source for adding to the tidal volume if more than room air is required by the patient. An oxygen analyzer should also be put in-line to monitor the oxygen percentage because it will vary with a changing respiratory rate or tidal volume.

2.   **Ventilator breathing circuits.**
    a.   **Fix any problems with continuous mechanical ventilation (CMV) circuits. (IIB2h2) [An]**

Neonatal ventilator circuits are basically the same as adult circuits with an inspiratory limb and an expiratory limb. Water traps are usually added. An obvious difference is the smaller diameter so that there is less compressible volume. Some are smooth bore to minimize gas turbulence and some have a heated wire running through them to keep a constant temperature and eliminate condensation. It is important that a heated wire circuit be used only with the servo-controlled humidifier for which it is designed. Mixing circuits and humidifiers can lead to either overheating or underheating problems. Furthermore, do not cover a heated wire circuit with a blanket. The circuit should not be allowed to touch the patient to avoid burns. If the patient is inside of an incubator, the circuit's temperature probe must be kept outside.

An added feature is a third small-bore tubing for measuring the proximal airway pressure. The tube runs from the patient wye to the proximal airway pressure nipple on the ventilator. Make sure that all the connections are tight to prevent gas leaks.

    b.   **Change the patient's ventilator circuit. (IIIC7b) [An]**

Commonly, disposable single patient use corrugated plastic circuits are utilized. They are inexpensive and meet the needs of most patients. Condensation is drained out into water traps that are placed at low points in the natural draping of the inspiratory and expiratory limbs of the circuit. If excessive moisture is a problem or if the gas temperature must be maintained within a narrow range, a heated wire circuit may be used. These types of circuits are built with a heated wire either loosely threaded through the lumen or coiled within the tubing itself. They are integrated with the humidification system and a servo unit for automatic temperature regulation. As would be expected, these circuits are considerably more expensive than the disposable types and may be sterilized and reused between patients.

Another possible concern with disposable, corrugated circuits is their relatively high internal resistance and compressible volume. The corrugations lead to gas turbulence that increases as the flow is raised. When the tubing is warmed it becomes more stretchable. This results in more tidal volume lost to the circuit instead of being delivered to the patient. It is recommended when high flow rates and ventilating pressures are needed, as in high frequency ventilation, that a smooth bore and low compressible volume circuit be used instead of the standard disposable type.

3. Continuous positive airway pressure (CPAP) systems.
a. Fix any problems with a CPAP breathing circuit. (IIB2h3) [An]

The general discussion and an illustration related to CPAP systems was presented in Section 14. Freestanding neonatal systems are similar to those used with adults. All currently available neonatal ventilators offer a CPAP mode. This allows the practitioner to easily switch the neonate from IMV to CPAP without the need to set up new equipment.

b. Fix any problems with a nasal CPAP device. (IIB2a4) [An]

Nasal CPAP devices are widely used with neonates. These babies commonly are born prematurely and have IRDS. Their immature lungs lack sufficient surfactant and need the CPAP pressure to keep the alveoli open. Often nasal CPAP will meet the patient's needs so that endotracheal intubation and mechanical ventilation can be avoided. Nasal CPAP works with neonates because they are obligate nose breathers.

Nasal CPAP is associated with the hazards of gastric distension and reflux aspiration. These occur when the airway pressure forces air into the stomach. A gastric tube is usually inserted to vent the air out. There are two different devices for administering nasal CPAP. A nasopharyngeal tube is actually an endotracheal tube that has been cut shorter (see Fig. 15-2, **C**). Select a tube that is the largest that can be easily inserted into the patient. Nasal prongs come in short and long versions (see Fig. 15-2, **A** and **B**); both types involve prongs that fit into both nostrils. The prongs come in different diameters so that the proper size can be found to fit the internal diameter of the infant's nares.

A sudden drop in the CPAP level to zero indicates a disconnection at the patient or somewhere in the breathing circuit. Check all connections and reassemble the break. The patient may need to be manually ventilated while the problem is corrected.

If the CPAP level drops more than 2 cm of water pressure during an inspiration, the flow is inadequate and should be increased. Flow is also inadequate if the patient shows an increased use of accessory muscles of respiration or appears to have an increased work of breathing. Too high a flow is seen by an inadvertently high level of CPAP and/or it appearing that the patient is having a difficult time exhaling. A common problem with small diameter tubes like these is mucus plugging. A plugged tube may result in a back-up of gas and could increase CPAP; however, depending on the CPAP system, there may be no change in pressure. Careful patient monitoring is important. Watch for a decrease in a drop in oxygenation, an increase in the respiratory rate, and/or retractions as signs of airway obstruction. Suction to clear out the mucus plug or remove the tube and place a new one.

4. Perform volume, flow, and pressure calibration on a ventilator for quality control. (IIB3f) [R, Ap, An]

Follow the manufacturer's guidelines for quality control procedures on mechanical ventilators. The microprocessor ventilators usually have a software package that performs self-diagnostic tests on the unit. If a problem is found it is printed on the monitor. Obviously the ventilator should deliver the volume, flow, and pressure that is set on the control. Do not use a ventilator that fails a quality control check.

5.   Change the type of humidification equipment. (IIIC6b) [An]

The general discussion of humidification equipment was presented in Sections 7 and 14. See the figures there and the general discussion for set-ups in ventilator and CPAP breathing circuits. Both types are capable of providing 100% relative humidity. Passover systems are preferred with neonates. The gas temperature is usually maintained close to the neonate's body temperature to maintain a neutral thermal environment. Make sure that the water level is kept in the recommended range to properly humidify the gas.

Module C.   Neonatal assessment.

Refer to Sections 1 and 2 or earlier in this section for a detailed discussion on neonatal assessment. Some additional discussion is presented here.

1.   Examine all the data to determine the patient's pathophysiological condition. (IC3a) [R, Ap, An]

Some discussion on pathology is presented in the earlier discussion. It is recommended that the most common neonatal and pediatric cardiopulmonary diseases and conditions be reviewed.

2.   Take part in the development of the respiratory care plan. (IC3c) [An]

Be prepared to make recommendations on changing ventilator parameters based on the patient's condition, blood gas values, chest x-ray, and vital signs.

3.   Make a recommendation to insert a chest tube into the patient. (IIIC8f) [R, Ap, An]

A chest x-ray and physical exam of the neonate will reveal if air or fluid is abnormally found around the lung(s) or heart. If a patient has a tension pneumothorax a pleural chest tube must be inserted to remove the air and relieve the pressure within the chest. A nontension pneumothorax of greater than 10% is often also treated by inserting a pleural chest tube. A pleural chest tube is also placed to remove blood or other fluid from the pleural space.

A pneumomedistinum, pneumopericardium, or pneumoperitoneum that puts the patient at risk must also be treated. A chest tube is then inserted into the area where the abnormal air is found. The same chest tube would also remove any abnormal collection of fluid. A chest tube is usually placed behind the heart to remove any blood that should leak out after open heart surgery.

4.   Measure the volume of air lost through a patient's pleural chest tube. (IIIC7a) [R, Ap, An]

If a neonate is being ventilated on a constant volume ventilator the amount of air that is lost through the pleural chest tube can be calculated. This is done by subtracting the measured exhaled volume from the measured inhaled volume. For example:

Inspired tidal volume =   40 ml
Exhaled tidal volume = −30 ml
                          10 ml of tidal volume is lost through the pleural chest
                          tube

    It is not possible to measure tidal volume when the neonate is ventilated by any other means. In a case like this it is only possible to make a qualitative judgment on pleural air leak. In other words, if air is seen to bubble out through the pleural drainage system an air leak is present. When the air stops bubbling the pleural tear has healed. See Section 17 for a complete discussion on pleural drainage systems.

BIBLIOGRAPHY

AARC Clinical Practice Guideline: Application of continuous positive airway pressure to neonates via nasal prongs or nasopharyngeal tube, *Respir Care* 39(8):817-823, 1994.

AARC Clinical Practice Guideline: Neonatal time-triggered, pressure-limited, time-cycled, mechanical ventilation, *Respir Care* 39(8):808-816, 1994.

AARC Clinical Practice Guideline: Surfactant replacement therapy, *Respir Care* 39(8):824-829, 1994.

Aloan C: *Respiratory care of the newborn*, Philadelphia, 1987, JB Lippincott.

Avery ME et al: Is chronic lung disease in low birth weight infants preventable? A survey of eight centers, *Pediatrics* 79(1):26-30, 1987.

Betis P, Thompson JE: Mechanical ventilation. In Koff PB, Eitzman DV, Neu J: *Neonatal and pediatric respiratory care*, St. Louis, 1988, Mosby—Year Book.

Boros SJ, Matalon SV, Ewald R et al: The effect of independent variations in inspiratory-expiratory ratio and end expiratory pressure during mechanical ventilation in hyaline membrane disease: the significance of mean airway pressure, *J Pediatrics* 91(5):794-798, 1981.

Burgess WR, Chernick V: Respiratory therapy in newborn infants and children, ed 2, New York, 1986, Thieme.

Carlo WA, Martin RJ: Principles of neonatal assisted ventilation, *Pediatr Clin North Am* 33(1):221-237, 1986.

Cavanagh K: High frequency ventilation of infants: an analysis of the literature, *Respir Care* 35(8):815-830, 1990.

Chatburn RL: High frequency ventilation: a report on a state of the art symposium, *Respir Care* 29(8):839-849, 1984.

Chatburn RL: Principles and practice of neonatal and pediatric mechanical ventilation, *Respir Care* 36(6):569-595, 1991

Chatburn RL, Lough MD: Mechanical ventilation. In Lough MD, Doershuk CF, Stern RC, editors: *Pediatric respiratory therapy*, ed 3, Chicago, 1985, Year Book Medical.

Chatburn RL, Waldemar AC, Lough MD: Clinical algorithm for pressure-limited ventilation of neonates with respiratory distress syndrome, *Respir Care* 28(12)1579-1586, 1983.

Coghill CH, Haywood JL, Chatburn RL et al: Neonatal and pediatric high-frequency ventilation: principles and practice, *Respir Care* 36(6):596-612, 1991.

Finer NN, Kelly MA: Optimal ventilation for the neonate. 1. Continuous positive airway pressure, *Respir Ther* 43-47, Jan/Feb 1983.

Finer NN, Kelly MA: Optimal ventilation for the neonate. 2. Mechanical ventilation, *Respir Ther* 73-78, March/April 1983.

Gagnon C, Simoes J: The management of the mechanically ventilated infant receiving pancuronium bromide (Pavulon), *Neonatal Network,* pp 20-24, Dec 1985.

Goldberg RN, Bancalari E: Bronchopulmonary dysplasia: clincial presentation and the role of mechanical ventilation, *Respir Care* 31(7):591-598, 1986.

Goldberg RN, Bancalari E: Therapeutic approaches to the infant with bronchopulmonary dysplasia, *Respir Care* 36(6):613-621, 1991.

HIFI Study Group: High-frequency oscillatory ventilation compared with conventional mechanical ventilation in the treatment of respiratory failure in preterm infants, *New England Journal of Medicine* 320(2):88-93, 1989.

Jobe A: Surfactant treatment for respiratory distress syndrome, *Respir Care* 31(6):467-475, 1986.

Koff PB, Eitzman DV, Neu J: Neonatal and pediatric respiratory care, ed 2, St. Louis, 1993, Mosby—Year Book.

MacDonald KD: *Operation and clinical application of the BEAR NVM-1 neonatal volume monitor,* BEAR Medical Systems product literature.

McPherson SP: Respiratory therapy equipment, ed 4, St. Louis, 1990, Mosby—Year Book.

Milner AD, Hoskyns EW: High frequency positive pressure ventilation in neonates, *Archives of Disease in Childhood* 64:1-3, 1989.

Miyagawa CI: Sedation of the mechanically ventilated patient in the intensive care unit, *Respir Care* 32(9):792-805, 1987.

Nicks JJ, Becker MA: High-frequency ventilation of the newborn: past, present, and future, *RT* 4(4), 1991.

Pilbeam SP: *Mechanical ventilation: physiological and clinical applications,* St. Louis, 1986, Multi-Media Publishing.

Pirie GE, Cain DL: Options for ventilating the pediatric patient. 2. Choosing the right technique, *Respir Ther* 60-68, July/Aug 1983.

Pirie GE, Cain DL: Options for ventilating the pediatric patient. 3. Circuits and humidification systems, *Respir Ther* 73-84, Sept/Oct 1983.

Product literature on Infrasonics Infant Star HFV, Infrasonics, Inc., San Diego, California.

Ramsden CA, Reynolds EOR: Ventilator settings for newborn infants, *Arch Dis Child* 62:529-538, 1987.

Schmidt JM: Nitric oxide therapy in neonates; adding to the arsenal, *Respir Ther* 7(5):37-42, 1994.

Smith I: The impact of surfactant on neonatal intensive care unit management, *RT* 4(4):22-26, 1991.

Spear ML, Spitzer AR, Fox WW: Hyperventilation therapy for persistent pulmonary hypertension of the newborn, *Perinatology/Neonatology* 9(5):27-34, 1985.

Tobin MJ: What should the clinician do when a patient "fights the ventilator"? *Respir Care* 36(5):395-406, 1991.

SELF-STUDY QUESTIONS

1. The neonate less than 72 hours old with pulmonary problems should have its PaO_2 kept in the _____ range on the lowest inspired oxygen level.
   A.   40-45 torr
   B.   45-50 torr
   C.   60-70 torr
   D.   80-90 torr
   E.   90-100 torr

2. If CPAP is administered through an endotracheal tube the child should be extubated when the CPAP pressure is:
    A. 0 cm water
    B. 2 cm water
    C. 4 cm water
    D. 6 cm water
    E. 8 cm water

3. Apneic spell leading to bradycardia indicates:
    A. Starting CPAP
    B. Starting mechanical ventilation
    C. Starting an aerosolized bronchodilator
    D. Ending CPAP

4. Switching from CPAP to IMV mode is indicated by:
    I.   CPAP of 8 to 10 cm water with a resulting PaO_2 of less than 50 torr
    II. F_IO_2 of 0.8 or more resulting in a PaO_2 of less than 50 torr
    III. $PaCO_2$ of greater than 60 torr
    A. I
    B. II
    C. I, II
    D. I, II, III

5. Identify the rationale for the use of pressure limiting or "square wave ventilation."
    I.   It increases the $PaCO_2$.
    II.   It reduces the peak pressure.
    III. It decreases the $PaCO_2$.
    IV.   It increases the patient's oxygenation.
    V.   There is no change in the patient's $PaCO_2$.
    A. I, II, III
    B. I, III
    C. I, II, IV
    D. II, IV, V
    E. I, II, IV, V

6. Given the following choices, which would you select to decrease $PaCO_2$ in a neonate on the Sechrist ventilator?
    I.   Increase the inspired oxygen.
    II.   Decrease the pressure limit if it has been reached.
    III. Increase the respiratory rate.
    IV.   Increase the flow if the pressure limit has not been reached.
    V.   Increase the pressure limit if it has been reached.
    A. I
    B. II
    C. III, IV, V
    D. II, III
    E. V

7. Hyperventilation is recommended in which of the following types of patients?
    A. Meconium aspiration
    B. Persistent pulmonary hypertension of the newborn
    C. Infant respiratory distress syndrome
    D. Infant with normal lung compliance

8. Increasing the pressure limit on the ventilator increases the patient's risk of:
    A. Retrolental fibroplasia form hyperoxia
    B. Oxygen toxicity
    C. Pneumothorax
    D. Tracheo-esophageal fistula

9. You are taking care of a newborn who has aspirated meconium. You would recommend which of the following ventilator settings:
    A. I : E of 1 : 2
    B. I : E of 2 : 1
    C. I : E of 1 : 4
    D. I : E of 1 : 1
    E. The I : E ratio is unimportant.

10. Given the following choices, which would you select to increase PaO_2 in a neonate on the Sechrist ventilator?
     I.   Increase inspiratory time.
     II.   Increase the pressure limit if it is reached during an inspiration.
     III. Decrease flow.
     IV.   Increase PEEP.
     V.   Decrease the IMV rate.
     A. III
     B. II, III
     C. V
     D. III, IV
     E. I, II, IV

11. If you increase PEEP without increasing the pressure limit by the same amount the patient's
     A. Minute volume will increase.
     B. Tidal volume will decrease.
     C. Minute volume will remain unchanged.
     D. $PaCO_2$ will decrease.
     E. Tidal volume will increase.

12. You are working with a neonate who has persistent pulmonary hypertension of the newborn (PPHN). He has right upper chest and left thigh transcutaneous oxygen monitors in place. His PaO_2 by umbilical artery catheter is 60 torr on 40% oxygen on the ventilator. His $PtcO_2$ at both sites is 55 torr. The nurse suctions his endotracheal tube and calls you over when the thigh $PtcO_2$ alarm sounds. You notice that even though he is back on the ventilator his thigh reading remains at 30 torr while his shoulder $PtcO_2$ has returned to 55 torr. The most likely problem is:
     A. The thigh monitor should be placed on the right thigh.
     B. The shoulder monitor needs recalibrating.
     C. The inspired oxygen is wrong on the ventilator.
     D. His ductus arteriosus has opened.
     E. His coarctation of the aorta has spasmed closed.

Answer Key

1. C; 2. B; 3. B; 4. D; 5. D; 6. C; 7. B; 8. C; 9. C; 10. E; 11. B; 12. D.

16 | Home Care and Pulmonary Rehabilitation

Module A.   Home care.

1.   Interview the patient.
a.   What is the patient's home environment like? (IB5c) [R]

Ideally, what a patient's home environment is like is determined by visiting the patient's home; however, the following questions can also be asked in the hospital. The home environment is an important consideration in discharge planning with the patient and family. Barriers to the patient's mobility and/or complete recovery must be identified so that they can be eliminated or minimized. The following questions will help the practitioner learn about the home the patient will return to:

"How many floors does your home have?"
"Do you have to go up a set of stairs to get into your home?"
"Is your bedroom on the main floor?"
"If your bedroom is upstairs, can it be relocated to a room on the main floor?"
"If your bedroom was relocated to the main floor, would it be easy for you to get to a bathroom and the kitchen?"
"Does anyone who lives with you smoke?"
"Is there anything else in or around your home that puts smoke or dust into the air?"

The answers to these types of questions may lead you to think of other questions about the patient's home environment. Think of the patient's disease or condition and the answers that are given to determine a discharge plan that will minimize any inconveniences or barriers.

b.   What is the patient's family and social life like? (IB5c) [R]

The patient's family and social life is an important consideration in discharge planning with the patient and family. Whether the patient is an adult or a child, it is important to know about his or her home life. Probably no one knows more about the patient or cares more about his or her well being than the immediate family. Very close friends can assist the family or even replace a nonexistent one.

The following questions can be asked of an adult patient and family:

"Is your spouse able to help you at home?"
"Do you have other family members who can help you at home?"

"Are there neighbors or family friends who can help you at home?"
"Do you belong to any clubs or church? Can you get to them?"
"Do you garden, have a pet, or have any hobbies at your home?"

The following questions can be asked of the family of a minor child:

"Do both parents live at home? If not, with whom does the child live? Do both parents care for the child?"
"Are there any siblings who can help in caring for the child?"
"Do you have other family members who can help you care for the child at home?"
"Are there neighbors or family friends who can help you care for the child at home?"
"Does the child belong to any clubs or church? Can you get the child to them? Can they help you care for the child at home?"
"Can you get the child to and from school?"

The answers to these types of questions may lead you to think of other questions about the patient's family and social life. Think of the patient's disease or condition and the answers that are given to determine a discharge plan that will minimize any disturbances in family life.

c.   What is the patient's nutritional status? (IB5c) [R]

The patient's nutritional status is an important part of the patient's background. Patients who have been ill for more than a few days should be suspected of suffering, to some degree, from malnutrition and/or dehydration. The longer they have been ill and not eating and drinking the more they will be malnourished and dehydrated. Ask the following questions of the patient or family:

"How long have you been sick?"
"Were you able to eat and drink normally before you became sick?"
"How long has it been since you were able to drink normally? Do you feel thirsty now?"
"How long has it been since you were able to eat normally? Do you feel hungry now?"
"Is it more difficult to cough out your secretions now than before you became sick?"

2.   Determine the patient's ideal therapeutic goals. (IIIE2a) [R, Ap, An]

Determining the patient's ideal therapeutic goals is best done in a team approach. The patient's physician, nurse, and respiratory therapist should work together. The first consideration should be the patient's diagnosis. Next, determine if the patient's condition is permanent, improving, or worsening. Objective information such as arterial blood gas results, pulmonary function testing results, chest x-ray findings, sputum production, and vital signs must be evaluated. The patient cannot be expected to do more than he or she is physically capable. It is also important to evaluate the patient's mental state. Is he or she emotionally ready to go home and be taught about self-care? Each patient's therapeutic goals must be individualized. If the patient is not physically or emotionally ready to take care of himself or herself, the family or a paid care provider is needed. The following are common therapeutic goals:

1. The primary goal is to increase the patient's functional ability as much as possible. This can best be determined by finding out what the patient wants to be able to do in his or her life. From this, a list of attainable short- and long-term goals can be developed. One of the primary short-term goals should be that the patient feels better. He or she should be able to control or reduce any symptoms.

    Make sure that the patient's goals are realistic and can be reached. The family needs to be involved with any major decision making. Often it is helpful to break a large goal down into several smaller tasks. That way the patient and family receive frequent positive feedback.

2. Improve the patient's self-image. This should follow when goal number 1 is reached.

3. Increase the patient's ability to exercise. This may depend on the level of the patient's disability. In general, the worse the patient's lung disease, the less able the patient is to increase his or her exercise level.

4. Decrease the frequency and length of any hospitalizations.

5. Prolong the patient's life by the proper use of oxygen and other respiratory care modalities.

3. Discharge planning.

a. Describe and teach the planned therapeutic goals to the patient and his or her family. (IIIE2f) [R, Ap]

Effective teaching methods include the following:

1. Speak at the patient's and family's level of understanding. Medical language usually reserved for peer discussions will not be understandable by people without a medical background. Yet, using overly simple explanations can be insulting to someone who is intelligent and/or well educated. In either case, the important information will not get across as intended. Give the patient written instructions as needed.

2. Frequently ask the patient and family whether they have any questions and then answer them.

3. Have the patient and family explain back to you in their own words how they understand what you just described.

4. Have the patient and family demonstrate back to you all procedures and techniques.

5. Reteach anything that is misunderstood.

6. Retest the patient and family as needed.

7. Document in the patient's chart what has been instructed.

b. Communicate important information to the patient and family. (IIIA2b) [R, Ap]

For important legal and medical reasons the following should be communicated:

1. The physician writes the discharge order. If the patient decides to leave against medical advice he or she must sign a form that releases the physician and hospital from any responsibility for ill effects from the decision.

2. Make sure that arrangements have been made to pay for the medical stay.

3. Tell the patient and family of physician orders for home-care procedures, medications, treatments, and so forth.

4. Gather all necessary equipment and supplies that the patient is to take home. Instruct the patient and family in their use. Document in the chart that this was done.
5. Help the patient in dressing, if needed, and organizing personal belongings.
6. Escort the patient and belongings to a car and make sure that the patient and belongings are safely loaded into it.

c.   Council the patient and family about smoking cessation and smoking cessation programs. (IIIA2c) [R, Ap]

Despite denials by the cigarette manufacturers, there is absolute proof that smoking causes emphysema, chronic bronchitis, lung cancer, and heart disease. These conditions occur in the smoker as well as a nonsmoking spouse and children. Asthmatics often find that their bronchospasm is worsened when they inhale tobacco smoke. Obviously it is important that any patient with a smoking-related cardiopulmonary disease cease smoking. The patient's family must also stop smoking. Continued exposure to tobacco smoke will harm the patient.

Because the nicotine found in tobacco is highly addictive, many patients find that they cannot stop smoking without suffering from withdrawal symptoms. To aid in stopping smoking it is often helpful to meet with a group of people who are also trying to stop. This group support helps the patient feel less alone in his or her efforts to stop smoking. Psychological support is very important in helping many patients quit. The American Lung Association and American Cancer Society as well as many hospitals offer smoking cessation clinics at a modest cost. The patient's physician also needs to be involved in this process. The physician can offer support and prescribe a nicotine replacement system, as described next.

d.   Recommend the use of a nicotine patch or nicotine gum. (IIIC11h) [R, Ap, An]

If the patient has been unable to stop smoking due to withdrawal symptoms it is likely that he or she is addicted to nicotine. In these cases it is very difficult for the patient to quit by willpower alone. The physician can order a nicotine replacement system that will greatly aid in smoking cessation. Although no smoking cessation plan works in every case, the highest percentage of patients are able to stop smoking if they have a combination of psychological support and gradual reduction in nicotine.

At the current time there are two well-established nicotine replacement and reduction systems. Nicotine polacrilex (Nicorette) is a gum that is chewed by the patient to release a dose of nictone. The patient can give himself or herself the desired amount of nicotine by varying the number of sticks of gum and the rate of chewing. The plan is for the patient to gradually reduce the number of sticks of Nicorette gum and be weaned off of nicotine. Drawbacks of the gum are its unusual taste and that some patients have developed mouth sores.

Nicotine transdermal patches are the second nicotine reduction system. Prostep, Nicoderm, and Habitrol are three brands of patch that, when placed onto the skin, allow a set amount of nicotine to be absorbed. With these systems, the patient starts with a relatively high dose of the drug and over a period of weeks goes through a series of patches with less and less nicotine. The patches should not be worn over areas of damaged or irritated skin and should be taken off at night to sleep. If a skin irritation develops, the physician should be informed.

The patient should be under a physician's care when either of these nicotine replacement and reduction systems is being used. Also, it is critical that the patient not smoke while using one of these systems. Patients who continue to smoke run the risk of a nicotine overdose, which increases the risk of a myocardial infarction.

4. Examine the patient's home and recommend how it can be modified to ensure safety and meet infection control standards. (IIIE2d) [R, Ap]

Evaluate the following aspects of the patient's home environment:

1. Does the patient live alone or have a spouse or companion to help provide care? Make sure that telephone numbers to relatives, helpful neighbors, the patient's physician, ambulance service, local hospital, pharmacy, and any other support services are posted by each telephone.
2. Make sure that all respiratory care equipment is cleaned and functioning properly.
3. Check that home oxygen systems are working properly. If the patient has an oxygen concentrator, make sure that the filters are cleaned and that the alarms are set and working. Make sure that an oxygen cylinder, regulator, and oxygen delivery system are working properly as a back-up system if the oxygen concentrator fails.
4. Have the patient centrally locate all necessary items for daily living. The patient should avoid unnecessary stair climbing. It might be recommended that the patient convert the living room, if it is located near the kitchen and bathroom, into a bedroom. Clothing can be modified with velcro fasteners, snaps, and/or zippers if the patient cannot use buttons easily. Shoes can be more easily put on with a long-handled shoehorn. Avoid shoes with laces. A long-handled comb or brush will make grooming easier.
5. The kitchen should be modified so that all commonly used equipment is on the counter. Everyday dishes, utensils, and foods should be placed so that they can be easily reached in cabinets and drawers within an arm's reach. The patient should not have to bend over, stoop down, or climb onto a footstool to get anything that is needed.
6. The bathroom may need to have handholds added to the walls by the toilet and shower or tub for extra security when using these facilities. A shower chair can be added so that the patient can sit while bathing. A hand-held shower head might make bathing easier.
7. Check the home for airborn irritants. Smoking by the patient or anyone else in the home must be stopped. The patient should avoid contact with other forms of indoor pollution such as aerosol sprays, paints, varnishes, dust, and so forth. A HEPA (high efficiency particulate air) filtration system is best for removing indoor airborn pollutants and irritants. Indoor kerosene fueled space heaters should not be used because of their release of carbon monoxide.
8. The patient should avoid contact with any known allergens, people who smoke, or substances to which he or she has a bad reaction.

5. Home respiratory care procedures.
   a. Change, as necessary, any respiratory care treatments or procedures used in the home. (IIIE2e) [R, Ap, An]

See next discussion.

b. Monitor and maintain any respiratory care equipment used in the patient's home. (IIIE2c) [R, Ap]

Home care equipment is essentially the same as that found in any hospital. The same types of equipment problems can occur in the patient's home as in the hospital. Those who wish to learn more about specific brands of home care equipment are referred to McPherson's (1988) *Respiratory Home Care Equipment* or the manufacturer's literature. The examinee should review, if necessary, any or all respiratory care procedures because they can be performed in the home care setting as well as in the hospital.

Past Written Registry Exams have included questions on the maintenance of oxygen concentrators and the use of back-up sources of oxygen when an oxygen concentrator fails. In addition, questions have been asked about how to deal with a home care patient whose nasal cannula has no flow through it. Telephone instructions include having the patient place the cannula under water to check for bubbling, tightening all tubing connections, confirming that gas is flowing from the oxygen concentrator, cleaning its filters, replacing a defective cannula, or switching to an oxygen cylinder if the concentrator has malfunctioned.

c. Apnea monitoring.
i. Perform apnea monitoring. (IB8k) [R, Ap, An]

Apnea monitoring is indicated in an infant who has documented periods of apnea of prematurity due to an immature central nervous system. This condition is seen in infants less than 35 weeks gestational age. The usual guidelines for monitoring include that the apnea lasts longer than 20 seconds and is associated with bradycardia with a heart rate of less than 100 beats per minute. Hypoxemia is often demonstrated by cyanosis, pallor, or documented desaturation through pulse oximetry. In addition, the infant may show marked limpness, choking, or gagging. Other conditions such as intracranial hemorrhage, patent ductus arteriosus, upper airway obstruction, hypermagnesemia, infection, maternal narcotic agents, and so forth should be ruled out before apnea of prematurity is confirmed. If this is the infant's problem, it is usually outgrown by the time the infant is 40 weeks postconceptional age. Home apnea monitoring is *not* indicated in normal infants, preterm infants without symptoms of apnea, or to test for sudden infant death syndrome (SIDS). See Table 16-1 for guidelines on starting and stopping home apnea monitoring.

Apnea monitors currently in use sense respiratory efforts through the changing electrical impedence measured through the chest wall as the infant breathes. Impedence is resistance to the flow of electricity through the skin and other organs. The monitor sends out a small, constant electrical current that results in a voltage

Table 16-1. Guidelines for Starting and Stopping Home Apnea Monitoring

Indications to start home apnea monitoring
Infant has had one or more apparent life-threatening apnea events.
Infant is preterm and symptomatic of apnea.
Infant is a sibling of two or more SIDS victims.
Infant has central nervous system based hypoventilation.
Indications to stop home apnea monitoring
Two to three months have passed without a significant number of alarms.
Two to three months have passed without an apnea episode.
Infant can tolerate stress of illnesses (e.g., nasopharyngitis) or immunizations (e.g., diptheria-tetanus-pertussis [DPT]) without apnea episodes.

across the two electrodes on the infant's chest. As the infant breathes and the chest wall expands and contracts there is a resulting change in voltage. This fluctuation is measured and interpreted as inhalation and exhalation. Similarly, smaller voltage changes are measured with each heartbeat. This is measured and interpreted as the heart rate.

The following are desirable features on a home apnea monitor: 1) ability to store and display events for later analysis, 2) identification of breathing patterns and apnea periods, 3) identification of heart rate patterns, 4) estimation of tidal volume, and 5) identification of hypoxemia by pulse oximetry. An example of such a unit is the Aequitron Medical 9550 Respiration and Heart Rate Monitor. Setting up a home apnea monitor involves placing the electrodes properly on the infant's chest, turning on the monitor, and setting the proper high and low limits for the alarms.

Two electrodes are usually placed where there is the greatest amount of movement during breathing. Most of the time this is on the infant's upper chest between the nipples and armpits (see Fig. 16-1). With older infants the electrodes might have to be placed on the sides over the lower ribs. Occasionally one electrode is placed on the chest and the other on the infant's abdomen. Some monitoring systems require that a Velcro belt be placed around the infant over the electrodes to keep them in place. (Obviously this will only work if both electrodes are on the chest.) Other systems make use of electrodes with an adhesive. In either case, for best results the infant's chest should be washed with mild soap and water and dried before the electrodes are placed. This will result in the best electrical conduction. Do not use baby oils, lotions, or powders over the electrode sites. Attach the lead wires to the electrodes. These connect to the patient cable that is then connected to the monitor. Occasionally static electricity will cause some interference with the signal. A third chest electrode is then added to act as a ground wire.

The monitor should be plugged into a working electrical outlet and turned on. Set the unit to charge the internal battery so that it can be made portable for later use. See that the infant's respiratory and heart rates are being sensed and displayed.

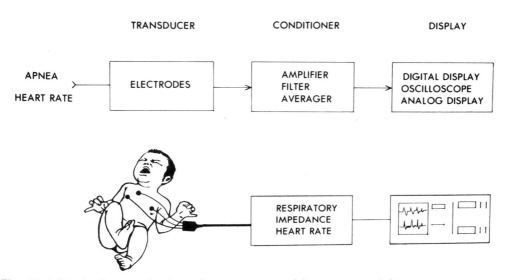

Fig. 16-1 Block diagram for impedence apnea and heart rate monitor. (From Lough MD: *Newborn respiratory care procedures.* In Lough MD, Williams TJ, Rawson JE, editors: *Newborn respiratory care,* Chicago, 1979, Year Book Medical. Used by permission.)

If pulse oximetry is a feature on the unit, the probe should be properly placed on the infant and an SpO$_2$ value should be displayed. Set the high and low alarm values according to the physician's orders or established protocols. For example:

1. Set the apnea alarm to trigger after 20 seconds.
2. Set the low heart rate alarm to trigger if the heart rate is less than 100 beats per minute.
3. If available, set the pulse oximeter alarm to trigger if the SpO$_2$ drops below 90%.
4. If available, set the high heart rate alarm to trigger if the heart rate is greater than 150 beats per minute.

Multiple alarms provide for a greater margin of patient safety. They also indicate what physiologically deteriorates first in the infant. These back-up alarm systems are important because the apnea monitor senses chest wall movement not air movement. It is possible for the infant to have an upper airway obstruction and continue to make breathing attempts; therefore the apnea monitor would not alarm because the chest wall is moving. The bradycardia or desaturation alarms would signal that the infant is in trouble.

It is critically important that the parent(s) know about the infant's medical condition. They need to understand how the monitor functions and what to do if the alarms go off. They should demonstrate their knowledge of the monitor's functions and be given written instructions on it. The parents should not be more than 10 seconds away from the infant at any time, which would mean that the infant would not be apneic for more than 30 seconds (20 seconds alarm delay and 10 seconds for the parents to respond). The parents must know how to give tactile stimulation to the infant, use the manual resuscitator, call for emergency help, and perform infant cardiopulmonary resuscitation.

ii. Interpret apnea monitoring results. (IB8k) [R, Ap, An]

Alarm situations fall into two basic categories: patient alarms and equipment alarms. Patient alarms mean that the infant is either apneic, has a heart rate below or above an acceptable level, or is desaturated. One, any two, or all three alarms could be triggered. Other than the audible alarm a visual alarm flashes to show the problem(s), and the recording device keeps track of the events. The parents should be instructed to first care for the infant, then, when the infant is back to normal, the alarms can be reset.

There are three types of equipment alarms: electrode or lead problem, low battery, or monitor failure. The unit should have different visual and audible alarms for equipment failure so that the family will not mistakenly think that the infant is in trouble. An electrode or lead problem alarm usually occurs because the electrode came off of the infant or the lead disconnected. The family should be taught how to fix these types of problems. A low battery alarm indicates that there is not much time left for the monitor to function on battery power. The family should be instructed to plug the monitor into a functioning electrical outlet and the unit should be set to recharge the battery. A monitor failure alarm indicates a serious internal problem with the monitor. It is not functioning properly and should not be used. The family should be instructed to continuously observe the infant and call the home care company for a replacement monitor.

Apnea monitors in current use record and store the above alarm situations. The information can usually be downloaded into a computer for a visual display of breathing and heart rate patterns, equipment problems, and the dates and times of their occurences. The therapist or physician should review all this data to determine what kind of problems the patient was having.

iii. Maintain apnea monitors. (IIIE2h) [R, Ap]

There is little to maintain on an apnea monitor. Make sure that the battery is recharging properly, test that the audible and visual alarms go off when an alarm limit is reached, and confirm that the high and low alarm limits are set properly.

The monitor is usually cleaned by wiping it off with a soft cloth that has been dampened. A mild detergent may be added. Do *not* use water, alcohol, or solvents to clean the unit as the electronic components may be damaged. Use another soft cloth to dry off the monitor. The lead wires and patient cable are cleaned in the same way. Follow the manufacturer's guidelines for caring for or replacing the skin electrodes. Typically, permanent electrodes are washed in mild soap and water daily and then rinsed and dried. Alcohol should not be used on them. Disposable electrodes are usually discarded after 2 or 3 days. If an electrode belt is used to hold the electrodes on the infant's chest, it should be washed and dried according to the manufacturer's guidelines.

6. Evaluate the patient's progress. (IIIE2g) [R, Ap, An]

The therapist must have a thorough understanding of the patient's condition and individual goals to evaluate his or her progress toward meeting them. Objectively consider the patient's physical, emotional, and social condition. The therapist must also listen to the patient's subjective opinion about his or her situation. Be prepared to make recommendations to the patient and attending physician for modifying the goals depending on the patient's changing condition.

Module B.   Pulmonary rehabilitation.

1.   How much exercise can the patient tolerate and how active is the patient on a daily basis? (IB5b) [R]

The following subject areas and questions will help you to further determine the patient's exercise tolerance and activities of daily living:

Personal grooming
  "Do you get short of breath when dressing?"
  "What is the most difficult part of dressing?"
  "Are you able to wash your hair regularly?"
  "Are you (men) able to shave regularly?"
  "Does using extra oxygen help you to do these things without getting as short of breath?"
In-home activities
  "Can you go up and down stairs without getting short of breath?"
  "Can you walk through your home without getting short of breath?"
  "Can you cook or prepare nutritious meals?"
  "Does using extra oxygen help you to do these things without getting as short of breath?"
Out-of-home activities
  "Can you go shopping without getting short of breath?"
  "What clubs, church, and so forth do you attend regularly?"
  "Can you do yard or garden work?"
  "Do you have a pet dog that you walk through the neighborhood?"
  "Does using extra oxygen help you to do these things without getting as short of breath?"

The patient with chronic and severe cardiopulmonary disease will tell you of a very restricted and limited lifestyle. Extra oxygen may have only a limited benefit. The patient with chronic, but moderate, cardiopulmonary disease will be able to live a somewhat limited but full lifestyle. Extra oxygen may help greatly at times when the patient becomes short of breath. The otherwise healthy patient who has an acute cardiopulmonary disease should tell of a previously full and enjoyable lifestyle. Extra oxygen may be needed now but hopefully not on recovery.

2. Determine the patient's ideal therapeutic goals. (IIIE2a) [R, Ap, An]

The patient's physical condition must be evaluated before designing an exercise program. Besides COPD, the patient may have other conditions that would further limit his or her ability to safely participate in a rehabilitation program. See Table 16-2 for the suggested parameters to assess. If the patient is too ill or too limited in ability, he or she should not be placed into a rehabilitation program.

While the patient's physical condition is the most important thing to evaluate from a safety point of view, other aspects of his or her life must also be looked into. These include a nutritional evaluation, a psychosocial evaluation, and a vocational evaluation. Because these areas are beyond the scope of practice of most respiratory therapists, other experts must be called in by the physician to do this. In addition, any patient who is still smoking must be enrolled in a smoking cessation program.

Table 16-2. Patient Evaluation Before Starting a Pulmonary Rehabilitation Program

History
Complete physical exam
Chest x-ray
Resting diagnostic electrocardiogram
Complete blood count
Serum electrolytes
Urinalysis
Arterial blood gases
Theophylline level
Sputum analysis
Pulmonary function tests
  Spirometry
  Lung volume study
  Diffusion capacity
  Before and after bronchodilator study
Pulmonary stress test including:
  Electrocardiogram
  Blood pressure
  Heart rate
  Respiratory rate
  Pulse oximetry
  Maximum ventilation
  Oxygen consumption
  Carbon dioxide production
  Respiratory quotient
(See Section 3 for information on pulmonary
  function testing and Section 17 for
  information on cardiopulmonary stress
  testing.)

Similar to preparing a patient for home care, all the patient's physical condition information must be evaluated. Each patient must have an individualized program and be physically and emotionally prepared to begin the rehabilitation program. As discussed next, the patient will be placed into either an open- or closed-end program format. The starting and ending points of the program will be determined based on the patient's physical condition, heart rate target, and stress test results.

3. Begin a graded exercise program and monitor the patients' progress. (IIIE2b) [R, Ap]

A graded exercise program is an individually structured sequence of events that is designed to safely increase the patient's exercise tolerance. It is a critical component of any pulmonary rehabilitation program.

In 1942, the Council of Rehabilitation defined rehabilitation "as the restoration of the individual to the fullest medical, mental, emotional, social, and vocational potential of which he/she is capable." In 1974, The American College of Chest Physicians' Committee on Pulmonary Rehabilitation adopted the following:

> Pulmonary rehabilitation may be defined as an art of medical practice wherein an individually tailored, multidisciplinary program is formulated which through accurate diagnosis, therapy, emotional support, and education, stabilizes or reverses both the physio- and psychopathology of pulmonary diseases and attempts to return the patient the *highest possible functional capacity* (italics added) allowed by his pulmonary handicap and overall life situation.

It further states: "In the broadest sense, pulmonary rehabilitation means providing good, comprehensive respiratory care for patients with pulmonary disease."

The patient with pulmonary disease who is inactive because of his or her condition will experience a slow deterioration in overall body function. It is well known that physical activity is important for general health. Table 16-3 lists the effects of inactivity.

The remainder of this discussion focuses on how to start a patient in a graded exercise program and monitor his or her progress through it. (Note that the education of the patient about normal and abnormal lung function, respiratory care procedures,

---

Table 16-3. Effects of Inactivity

Metabolism
Decreased metabolic rate, decreased protein catabolism, negative nitrogen balance, decubitus ulcers, imbalance of cellular electrolytes, and gastrointestinal hypomotility

Psychosocial
Decreased learning ability, decreased motivation to learn, decreased retention of new material, decreased problem-solving ability, exaggerated or inappropriate emotional reactions, perceptual and motor changes, and increased somatic concerns

Respiratory system
Decreased movement of secretions, decreased use of respiratory muscles, and development of microatelectasis and infection

Muscular system
Loss of normal muscle tone, decreased muscle efficiency, increased local muscle Vo_2, rapid onset of fatigue, and contracture

Cardiopulmonary system
Decreased cardiac output, venous stasis, thromboembolism, and pulmonary emboli

Skeletal system
Osteoporosis, reabsorption of calcium from the bone, and increased incidence of compression fractures

From May DF: *Rehabilitation and continuity of care in pulmonary disease*, St. Louis, 1991, Mosby–Year Book.

medications, and so forth is addressed in earlier sections of this book or other textbooks dedicated solely to pulmonary rehabilitation.)

Benefits of an Exercise Program

The benefits of the exercise program must be stressed to the patient to gain his or her acceptance of it. If the patient does not believe that the program will make his or her life better, it will not be followed. In 1981 the American Thoracic Society Executive Committee adopted the following as principle objectives of pulmonary rehabilitation:

1. To control and alleviate as much as possible the symptoms and pathologic complications of respiratory ailments.
2. To teach the patient how to achieve optimal capability for carrying out his or her activities of daily living.

Most authors agree with the following general therapeutic goals:

1. The primary goal is to increase the patient's functional ability as much as possible. This can best be determined by finding out what the patient wants to be able to do with his or her life on a daily basis. From this list of activities of daily living (ADL), a series of short- and long-term goals can be developed. One of the primary short-term goals should be that the patient feels better. He or she should be able to control or reduce any symptoms. This alone will improve the patient's quality of life. Make sure that the patient's goals are realistic and can be reached. The family needs to be involved with any major decision making. Often it is helpful to break a large goal down into several smaller tasks so that the patient and family receive frequent positive feedback.
2. Improve the patient's self-image. This should follow when goal number 1 is reached. The patient should experience less anxiety and depression and also feel better about himself or herself.
3. Increase the patient's ability to exercise. This may depend on the level of the patient's disability. In general, the worse the patient's lung disease is, the less able the patient is to increase his or her exercise level.
4. Decrease the frequency and length of any hospitalizations.
5. Prolong the patient's life by the proper use of oxygen and other respiratory care modalities.

Note that the benefits did not list an improvement in the patient's cardiopulmonary condition. Numerous studies have documented that pathologic changes seen in chronic obstructive pulmonary disease (COPD) do *not* improve despite the patient being in a rehabilitation program. It is important that the therapist correct any misunderstanding of this.

Individualized Graded Exercise Program

The program format and features may vary considerably. Minimally the patient's physician should specify four parts to the exercise prescription: mode, intensity, duration, and frequency. The following program formats and suggestions are typical of what might be ordered.

Program Format

There are two basic types of formats. Each has its own advantages and disadvantages depending on what the patient's limitations and preferences may be. The **open-end format** allows the patient to enter and progress through the program at his or her own pace. Because each patient's goals are individualized, the time of their accomplishment is relatively unimportant as long as progress is being made. The program facilitator (often a respiratory therapist) acts as a coordinator. This may include making sure that educational materials are available for the patient, exercise equipment is available, and the patient's questions are answered. The patient may stay in the program until the last goal is achieved. The advantages of this program are that it is self-directed and can be adjusted if the patient has a schedule conflict. The disadvantage of this program is that there is no group support or involvement with other people who have COPD.

The **closed-end format** involves the program facilitator setting up a formal schedule of educational topics and exercise sessions. These group events commonly last from 1 to 3 hours and may occur from one to three times per week. The whole program can vary in length from 8 to 16 weeks depending on the content. These events are attended by a group of patients who share a common problem and have common goals to cope with it. One major advantage of this program is that most patients do better when they have peers to call on for emotional support. The facilitator will probably find that it is easier to schedule speakers when a sure time frame can be set. The disadvantages of this program relate to the loss of individual goals and attention. If a patient misses a session he or she will have to wait for the topic to be repeated at the next program. If the group is too large, the facilitator may not have time to help a patient with an individual goal.

Strength Training

Many patients are so weak from years of relative inactivity that they must regain muscle strength before working on increased endurance. The specific muscle groups that need strengthening can be determined by physical examination. In general, the large muscle groups of the legs and arms and inspiratory muscles must be strengthened.

Before beginning strength training, the patient must perform calisthenics for about 10 minutes as a "warm up." It is important to stretch the muscles and joints and increase circulation before starting more vigorous activity. See Fig. 16-2, groups 1 to 7, for a series of progressively more demanding calisthenic exercises. All patients should at least be able to perform the calisthenics shown in groups 1 and 2 for a warm up. The patient must focus on breath control (pursed-lips breathing) during the warm-up period to avoid dyspnea.

Arm and leg strengthening can be done in a variety of ways for about 10 minutes. Typically, a 1- or 2-lb weight is used. Barbell weights can be held as the arms are moved to the back, front, sides, and overhead to strengthen the arms, shoulders, and chest and back muscles. Ankle weights can be strapped on. The legs are then moved to the back, front, sides, and the legs lifted with knees bent. Or, the initial calisthenics can be repeated with added weight. The abdominal muscles can be strengthened by having the patient lie on his or her back and placing a 2-lb weight on the abdomen. The patient then concentrates on maintaining breath control against the added weight.

Inspiratory muscle strengthening is done in two ways. First, the patient is told to take in a deep sigh and hold it for a brief time. This both stretches the rib cage and increases the work load of the primary and secondary inspiratory muscles. The

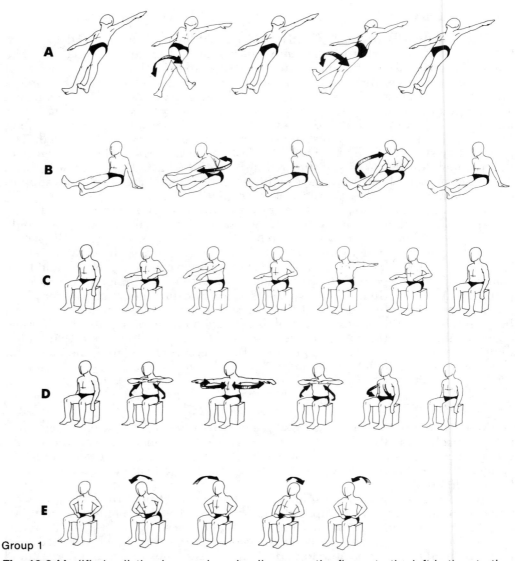

Group 1

Fig. 16-2 Modified calisthenic exercises. In all groups, the figure to the left is the starting point. The figures to the right show the sequence of steps in the exercise. The patient can adjust the pace of the exercises to either increase or decrease the energy that is spent. In general, 10 to 15 repetitions per minute are chosen by most patients. The exercises shown in groups 1 and 2 are useful during the warm-up period of either a strength or endurance program. The exercises shown in groups 3 and 4 are more demanding and can be used for muscle reconditioning by many patients in an endurance program. The most demanding exercises are those shown in groups 5, 6, and 7. Patients with only moderate disability may be able to progress to this level for further muscle conditioning. (From May DF: *Rehabilitation and continuity of care in pulmonary disease,* St. Louis, 1991, Mosby–Year Book. Used by permission.)

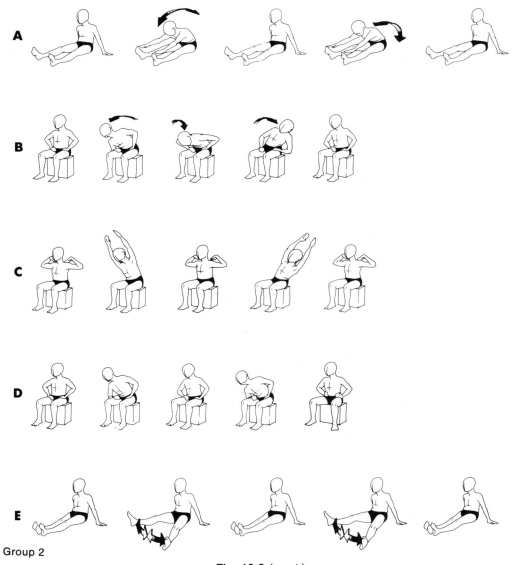

Group 2

Fig. 16-2 *(cont.)*

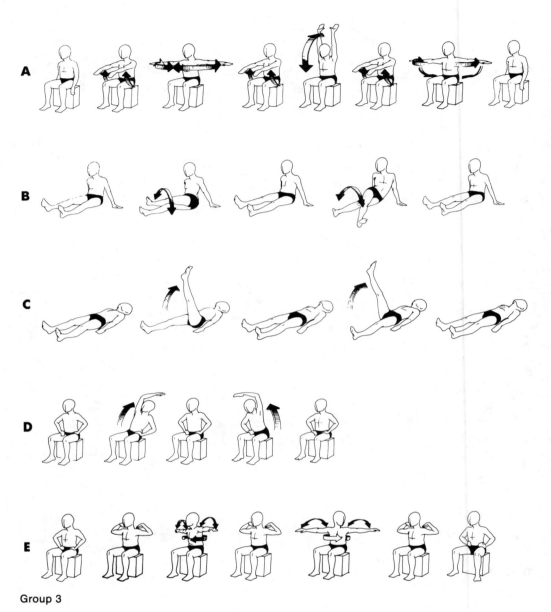

Group 3

Fig. 16-2 (*cont.*)

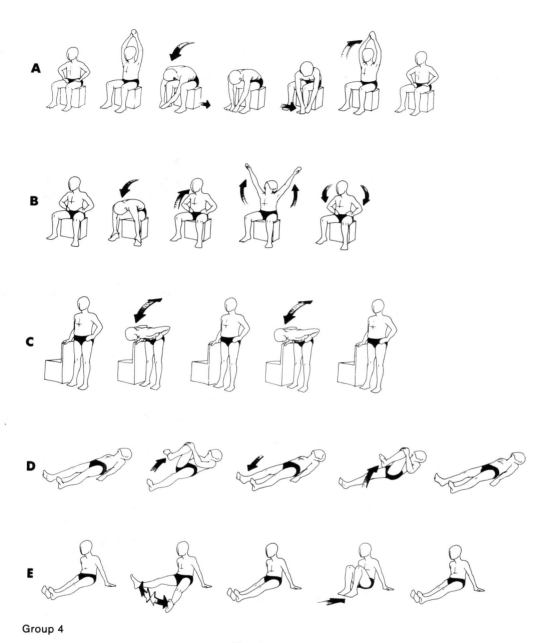

Group 4

Fig. 16-2 *(cont.)*

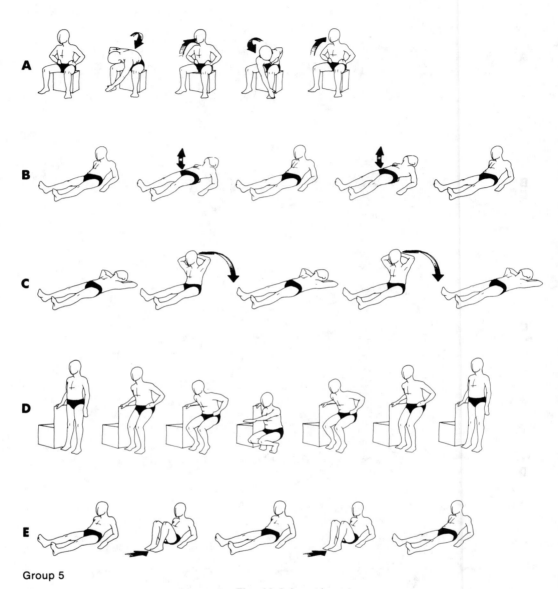

Group 5

Fig. 16-2 *(cont.)*

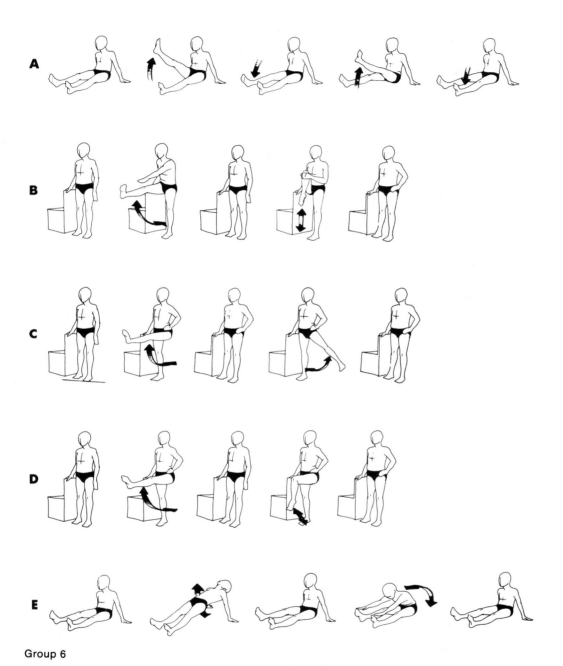

Group 6

Fig. 16-2 *(cont.)*

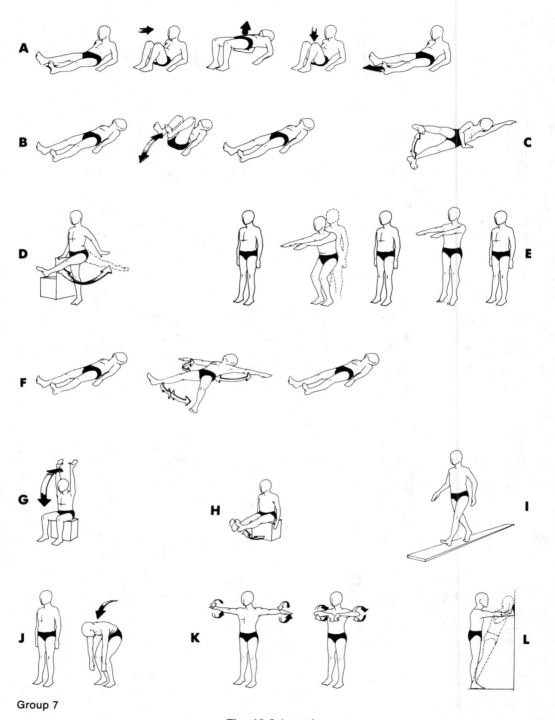

Group 7

Fig. 16-2 *(cont.)*

deep sigh should be repeated several times. Second, the patient uses a specific inspiratory muscle training device. The PFLEX device is popular because it is inexpensive and can be gradually adjusted to increase the work load as the patient improves. See Section 6 for a complete discussion of its use.

Finally, the patient should spend about 10 minutes in "cool-down" activities. This could involve more light calisthenics or slow walking. The cool-down period allows the body to return to a slower metabolic rate while still maintaining good circulation to the arms and legs. This will help to eliminate any lactic acid that might have built up in the muscles during the more vigorous exercise. Increased lactic acid may cause some of the muscle aches after exercise. Inform the patient that there may be some muscle soreness the next day. It can be relieved by taking an antiinflammatory medication such as aspirin if the physician approves. See Table 16-4 for specific guidelines for a strength training program.

It is helpful, but not necessary, for the patient to have access to professional body building equipment found in many gymnasiums. In addition, a physical therapist is helpful in designing a training program.

Endurance Training

Endurance training is designed to build up the patient's stamina to perform activities of daily living (ADL). It does this by improving the functioning of the patient's cardiopulmonary and cardiovascular systems. When these systems are functioning better they can meet the patient's need for increased oxygen delivery to and carbon dioxide removal from exercising muscles.

Endurance training must be preceded by the patient performing calisthenics for about 10 minutes as a "warm up." Just as in strength training, it is important

Table 16-4. Guidelines for Strength and Endurance Training

Strength Training
This involves a low number of repetitions of a high intensity activity, such as lifting weights.
  Warm-up period involving calisthenics for about 10 minutes.
  The following strengthening program should last about 10 minutes:
    a. Three sets of 10 to 15 repetitions of an activity.
    b. Each set is followed by a rest period of a few minutes.
    c. The patient should work at 85% to 90% of the maximum capacity of the muscles being exercised.
  Cool-down period involving calisthenics for about 10 minutes.
  The patient should exercise every other day; there should be a rest day between the exercise days.
  This program may precede or be done simultaneously with an endurance program.
  It will take 4 to 8 weeks for improved strength to be realized.
Endurance Training
This involves a high number of repetitions of a relatively low intensity activity, such as walking.
  Warm-up period involving calisthenics for about 10 minutes.
  The patient should do the following:
    a. Exercise continuously for about 20 to 30 minutes.
    b. Exercise at a level that results in the target heart rate being maintained.
  Cool-down period involving calisthenics for about 10 minutes.
  The patient should exercise every other day; there should be a rest day between the exercise days.
  This program may follow or be done simultaneously with a strength program.
  It will take 4 to 8 weeks for improved endurance to be realized.

Modified from May DF: *Rehabilitation and continuity of care in pulmonary disease*, St. Louis, 1991, Mosby–Year Book.

to stretch the muscles and joints and increase circulation before starting more vigorous activity. See Figure 16-2, groups 1 to 7, for a series of progressively more demanding calisthenic exercises. All patients should be able to at least perform the calisthenics shown in groups 1 and 2 for a warm up. Patients who can perform the activities shown in groups 3 and 4 will gain some endurance training as well. Some very debilitated patients may not be able to perform at this higher level. Some less debilitated patients will eventually be able to advance to the highest levels. The patient must focus on breath control (pursed-lips breathing) during the warm-up period to avoid dyspnea.

The actual endurance exercise that is selected must meet the patient's needs. He or she can walk, use a treadmill, ride a bicycle ergometer, swim, or do a combination of these. The method that is selected must be both practical and fun for the patient. For this reason, walking is usually the main activity; however, the upper body should not be ignored. An arm ergometer, rowing machine, or barbell weights can be used for upper body endurance.

A key concept of the endurance program is that the patient must exercise at a level great enough to raise the heart rate to a predetermined level. The increased heart rate reflects the increased metabolic rate and work being performed by the patient. The target heart rate must be maintained for 20 to 30 minutes to have any muscle training effect. Exercising at a lower heart (and metabolic) rate will not be as beneficial. Exercising at a higher heart rate may be dangerous to the patient. Karvonen's formula is used to determine the target heart rate for endurance training:

Target heart rate (HR) = [% intensity (maximum HR − resting HR)] + resting HR

Where:

    Target HR = the target heart rate for the exercise period
    % intensity = 60% to 80%
    Maximum HR = maximum HR determined by either of the following formulas:
        a) Maximum HR = 220 − age of the patient
        b) Maximum HR = 210 − (age of the patient × .65)
    Resting HR = the patient's resting heart rate

Example

Determine the target heart rate for a 50-year-old patient (of either sex) who is enrolled in an endurance training program. The patient has a resting heart rate of 80 beats per minute. The patient's maximum heart rate is 170 (220 − 50 for the patient's age = 170).

Target HR = [% intensity (maximum HR − resting HR)] + resting HR

Lowest target HR = [.60 (170 − 80)] + 80
         = [.60 (90)] + 80
         = [54] + 80
         = 134 beats per minute

Highest target HR = [.80 (170 − 80)] + 80
         = [.80 (90)] + 80
         = [72] + 80
         = 152 beats per minute

The range of target heart rates for this patient is 134 to 152 beats per minute. The patient must monitor his or her heart rate during the exercise period to make sure that it stays within this range. This is most easily accomplished by feeling the radial or carotid pulse and counting heartbeats for a 15-second period, then multiplying by four to find the heart rate for 1 minute.

Finally, as in strength training, the patient should spend about 10 minutes in "cool-down" activities. This could involve light calisthenics or slow walking. As discussed earlier, the cool-down period allows the body to return to a slower metabolic rate while still maintaining good circulation to the arms and legs. This will help to eliminate any lactic acid that may have built up in the muscles during the endurance exercise. See Table 16-4 for specific guidelines for an endurance training program.

Assessment of the Patient's Progress in the Program

The following indicate that the patient is making progress:

1. The patient subjectively feels that he or she is doing as well as can be expected. The patient is motivated to try new things.
2. Symptoms are reduced or at least under control.
3. Cardiopulmonary function tests and blood gases show improvement. Even a slowing in the patient's former rapid rate of decline is a good sign.
4. The patient reports an increase in the distance that can be walked at his or her own pace.
5. The patient reports an increase in the 6-minute or 12-minute walk distance. The 6-minute or 12-minute walk is a measurement of how far a person can maximally walk in the given time period.

The following would indicate that the patient's health is deteriorating:

1. He or she subjectively feels worse. The patient is afraid to try new things.
2. Symptoms are worse. The patient feels dyspneic at less exertion than before.
3. The sputum has changed. It could be viscid and harder to cough out or have changed color to yellow or green. The patient may be coughing out more than before or less if it cannot be brought up.
4. Cardiopulmonary function tests and blood gases are worse. The patient may need more oxygen, an aerosolized bronchodilator, or other cardiopulmonary medications.
5. The patient cannot walk or perform as much work as before without having the symptoms worsen.

Module C.   Patient assessment.

1.   Examine all the data to determine the patient's pathophysiological condition. (IC3a) [R, Ap, An]

The therapist should be familiar with the home care or rehabilitation patient's cardiopulmonary status. It is important to have a solid understanding of pathophysiology to determine what could be causing a sudden change in the patient's condition.

2.   Take part in the development of the respiratory care plan. (IC3c) [An]

As mentioned earlier, the respiratory therapist should be a member of the patient's home care or rehabilitation team. Be prepared to evaluate the patient's condition and make suggestions for changing goals, methods, and so forth.

BIBLIOGRAPHY

AARC Clinical Practice Guideline: Oxygen therapy in the home or extended care facility, *Respir Care* 37(8):918-922, 1992.

Aloan C: *Respiratory care of the newborn,* Philadelphia, 1987, JB Lippincott.

Bell CW, Blodgett D, Goike C et al: *Home care and rehabilitation in respiratory medicine,* Philadelphia, 1984, JB Lippincott.

Belman MJ, Wasserman K: Exercise training and testing in patients with chronic obstructive pulmonary disease, *Basics of Respiratory Disease* 10(2), 1981.

Burgess WR, Chernick V: *Respiratory therapy in newborn infants and children,* ed 2, New York, 1986, Thieme.

Christopher KL: At-home administration of oxygen. In Kacmarek RM, Stoller JK, editors: *Current respiratory care,* Toronto, 1988, BC Decker.

Connors G, Hilling L, editors: *American Association of Cardiovascular and Pulmonary Rehabilitation: guidelines for pulmonary rehabilitation programs,* Champaign, Ill, 1993, Human Kinetics.

Connors GA, Hodgkin JE: Pulmonary rehabilitation. In Burton GG, Hodgkin JE, Ward JJ, editors: *Respiratory care: a guide to clinical practice,* ed 3, Philadelphia, 1991, JB Lippincott.

Cruver N, Solliday N: Fundamentals of exercise stress testing for lung disease, *Respir Care* 27(9):1050-1057, 1982.

Edge RS: Infection control. In Barnes TA, editor: *Respiratory care practice,* Chicago, 1988, Year Book Medical.

Eichenwald EC, Stark AR: Apnea of prematurity. In Koff P, Eitzman D, Neu J, editors: *Neonatal and pediatric respiratory care,* ed 2, St. Louis, 1993, Mosby–Year Book.

Eubanks DH, Bone RC: *Comprehensive respiratory care,* ed 2, St. Louis, 1990, Mosby–Year Book.

Gilmartin M: Transition from the intensive care unit to home: patient selection and discharge planning, *Respir Care* 39(5):456-480, 1994.

Hodgkin JE: Home care and pulmonary rehabilitation. In Kacmarek RM, Stoller JK, editors: *Current respiratory care,* Toronto, 1988, BC Decker.

Holden DA, Stelmach KD, Curtis PS et al: The impact of a rehabilitation program on functional status of patients with chronic lung disease, *Respir Care* 35(4):332-341, 1990.

Homedco Home Infant Monitoring Guidelines, Homedco, Fountain View, California.

Lough MD: Newborn respiratory care procedures. In Lough MD, Williams TJ, Rawson JE, editors: *Newborn respiratory care,* Chicago, 1979, Year Book Medical.

Lucas J, Golish JA, Sleeper G et al: *Home respiratory care,* Norwalk, 1988, Appleton & Lange.

May DF: *Rehabilitation and continuity of care in pulmonary disease,* St. Louis, 1991, Mosby–Year Book.

McPherson SP: *Respiratory home care equipment,* Dubuque, Iowa, 1988, Kendall/Hunt.

McPherson SP: *Respiratory therapy equipment,* ed 4, St. Louis, 1990, Mosby–Year Book.

Mulligan SC, Masterson JG, Devane JG et al: Clinical and pharmacokinetic properties of a transdermal nicotine patch, *Clin Pharmacol Ther* 47(3):331-337, 1990.

Nett LM: The physician's role in smoking cessation, *Chest Suppl* 97(2):28s-32s, 1990.

Petty TL: Pulmonary rehabilitation: better living with new technology, *Respir Care* 30(2):98-107, 1985.

Petty TL, Nett LM: *Enjoying life with emphysema,* Philadelphia, 1987, Lea & Febiger.

Product literature on the Model 9200 Respiration/Heart Rate Monitor, Aequitron Medical, Minneapolis, Minn.

Pulmonary rehabilitation: official American Thoracic Society statement. *Am Rev Respir Dis* 124:663-666, 1981.

Rennard SI, Daughton D: Transdermal nicotine for smoking cessation, *Respir Care* 38(3):290-293, 1993.

Sills JR: *Respiratory care certification guide: the complete review resource for the entry level exam,* ed 2, St. Louis, 1994, Mosby–Year Book.

Sobush D, Dunning M, McDonald K: Exercise prescription components for respiratory muscle training: past, present, and future, *Respir Care* 30(1):34-42, 1985.

Taylor C, Lillis C, LeMond P: *Fundamentals of nursing: the art and science of nursing care,* ed 2, Philadelphia, 1993, JB Lippincott.

Whitaker K: *Comprehensive perinatal and pediatric respiratory care,* Albany, NY, 1992, Delmar Publishers.

Wyka KA: Cardiopulmonary rehabilitation. In Scanlan CL, Spearman CB, Sheldon RL, editors: *Egan's fundamentals of respiratory care,* ed 5, St. Louis, 1990, Mosby–Year Book.

Wyka KA: Respiratory home care. In Scanlan CL, Spearman CB, Sheldon RL, editors: *Egan's fundamentals of respiratory care,* ed 5, St. Louis, 1990, Mosby–Year Book.

Yee AR, Hodgkin JE, Zorn EG et al: Pulmonary rehabilitation. In Burton GG, Hodgkin JE, editors: *Respiratory care,* ed 2, Philadelphia, 1984, JB Lippincott.

SELF-STUDY QUESTIONS

1. The theraputic goals of a rehabilitation program include all the following EXCEPT:
   A. Decreased hospitalizations
   B. Reversal of lung disease
   C. Increase the patient's energy level
   D. Increase the patient's ability to perform activities of daily living
   E. Improve the patient's self-image

2. Your patient with COPD had been coughing out about 20 ml of white colored mucus per day until 3 days ago. Since then she has only been coughing out 5 ml. She tells you that the mucus is more difficult to cough out and she is getting more short of breath. What is the most likely cause of these recent changes?
   A. Her lung disease is improving.
   B. She is overhydrated.
   C. She has an infection or mucus plugging.
   D. The secretions are being unconsciously swallowed.
   E. The treatments have decreased the amount of mucus she is producing.

3. When visiting a home care patient she tells you that she cannot feel any oxygen coming to her nasal cannula from the oxygen concentrator. You would do all the following EXCEPT:
   A. Refill the humidifier bottle with sterile water.
   B. Place the cannula prongs under water to see if any gas is coming out.
   C. Tighten all the equipment connections.
   D. Switch the patient over to her tank of oxygen.
   E. Replace the cannula if it is defective.

4. Upon surveying a patient's home you notice that it has four steps leading into the front door. The patient's bedroom is upstairs and his wife smokes about one pack of cigarettes a day. You would recommend all the following EXCEPT:
   A. The patient's wife should stop smoking.

B.   He should use a cane when climbing stairs.

C.   The patient's bedroom should be moved downstairs.

D.   A ramp should be added to ease entering the front door.

5.   The components of a strength training program include:
   I.   Cool-down period
   II.   Strengthening exercises performed daily
   III.   Warm-up period
   IV.   Strengthening exercises performed every other day
   V.   Exercises performed for 20 to 30 minutes continuously
   A.   I, II
   B.   III, IV, V
   C.   II, III, V
   D.   I, III, IV
   E.   I, III, V

6.   You are supervising a patient who is participating in an endurance training rehabilitation program. Her target heart rate is between 130 and 150 beats per minute. She is exercising on a bicycle ergometer and her heart rate is 167 beats per minute. What would you advise her to do?
   A.   Stop exercising immediately and sit down.
   B.   Only exercise until she begins to perspire.
   C.   Continue exercising if she feels that she can handle the work load.
   D.   Exercise a maximum of 10 minutes each day.
   E.   Slow down on the ergometer until her heart rate drops to the target level.

7.   Home apnea monitoring can usually be stopped when all the following conditions exist EXCEPT:
   A.   The infant has gone 30 days without an apnea episode.
   B.   The infant has had a DPT immunization without any consequences.
   C.   Three months have passed without any alarms sounding.
   D.   Two months have passed without an apnea episode.

8.   Your patient and her husband are both smokers. She is about to be discharged after treatment for bronchitis. Which of the following would you recommend?
   I.   She should stop smoking.
   II.   She should see her physician about help to stop smoking.
   III.   Her husband should stop smoking.
   IV.   She should go to a store and purchase some Nicorette gum to chew to help her stop smoking.
   A.   I, II
   B.   I, IV
   C.   I, II, III
   D.   I, II, III, IV

Answer Key

1. B; 2. C; 3. A; 4. B; 5. D; 6. E; 7. A; 8. C.

17

Special Procedures

Module A. Participate in air or land patient transportation. (IIID7) [R, Ap]

Be prepared to perform, during transport, all the respiratory care practices and procedures that have been described in this text as well as in *Respiratory Care Certification Guide* (Sills, 1994) or other books that describe the duties of a technician or therapist. It is extremely important that all equipment and supplies be accounted for before leaving the hospital. Obviously, once under way, there is no way to obtain something that was forgotten. To help ensure that this does not happen, it is wise to have a checklist of everything that could be needed. In addition, all equipment must be checked for proper function. Calculate the duration of the oxygen cylinders at expected liter flows. Make sure that batteries and light bulbs work and have spare bulbs.

If mechanical ventilation will be needed, bring a unit that is lightweight, portable, has solid state circuitry, and can be powered by both alternating current (AC) and direct current (DC) from batteries. If the ventilator will be used for helicopter or nonpressurized cabin fixed-wing aircraft, it must be able to deliver an IMV/SIMV mode through a demand valve rather than through a reservoir system. The function of the ventilator should not be affected by high altitude dramatic changes in atmospheric pressure. An example of such a unit is the Uni-Vent by IMPACT Instrumentation.

Module B. Assist the physician who is performing the following procedures.

1. Cardioversion. (IIIE1h) [R, Ap]

Cardioversion (also called countershock) refers to deliberately sending a direct current (DC) electrical shock through the patient's heart. Its purpose is to suppress an abnormal heartbeat so that the normal pacemaker at the sino-atrial (SA) node will take over. This is accomplished if a great enough electrical current is sent through the chest wall to cause the depolarization of a critical mass of myocardial cells. After this, the SA node should take over as the pacemaker, provided that the heart muscle is oxygenated and not too acidotic. There are two different types of cardioversion: defibrillation (also called unsynchronized cardioversion) and synchronized cardioversion. Both were introduced in Section 10 for the treatment of specific arrythmias.

Defibrillation is performed in an emergency situation. Patients who need to be defibrillated include those in ventricular fibrillation or ventricular tachycardia when they are pulseless, unresponsive, hypotensive, or in pulmonary edema. Because the fastest possible action is needed, no attempt is made to synchronize the defibrillation shock with the heart's rhythm. While CPR is being performed, the defibrillator unit is prepared. The defibrillating paddles (large positive and negative electrodes) are placed on the patient's anterior and left lateral chest wall. The physician or other qualified person (respiratory therapist, registered nurse, or paramedic) performing the defibrillation should call out, "Stand clear." All other medical personnel should stand back from the patient and the bed and not touch anything that is electrically grounded. When the buttons on the paddles are pushed, the shock is administered. If successful, the patient's normal heartbeat will return to normal sinus rhythm. If the initial shock is unsuccessful, CPR is continued. The defibrillator is then recharged for another attempt as quickly as possible. See Table 17-1 for the sequence of increasingly more powerful countershocks that can be given.

Synchronized cardioversion is similar in some ways to defibrillation. An electrical shock is sent through the heart to suppress paroxysmal atrial tachycardia, atrial flutter, atrial fibrillation, or hemodynamically stable ventricular tachycardia so that the SA node will take over. Its major difference from defibrillation is that the electrical shock is administered automatically by the defibrillator after an R wave

---

Table 17-1. Wattage Used in Synchronous Cardioversion and Defibrillation

---

Synchronized Cardioversion of an Infant
0.5-1.0 joules (watt-seconds) per kilogram
Stepwise increases in energy should be used if
   the initial shock fails to convert the rhythm.
Synchronized Cardioversion of an Adult
Atrial flutter and paroxysmal atrial tachycardia:
   50 joules
   Stepwise increases in energy should be used if
      the initial shock fails to convert the rhythm.
Atrial fibrillation:
   100 joules
   Stepwise increases in energy should be used if
      the initial shock fails to convert the rhythm.
Ventricular tachycardia with a regular form and
   rate with or without a pulse:
   100 joules
   Stepwise increases in energy should be used if
      the initial shock fails to convert the rhythm.
Ventricular tachycardia with an irregular form and
   rate:
   200 joules
   Stepwise increases in energy should be used if
      the initial shock fails to convert the rhythm.
Defibrillation
Infant:
   2 joules per kilogram
   4 joules per kilogram for second and
      succeeding attempts
Adult:
   200 joules on first attempt
   200-300 joules on second attempt
   Up to 360 joules on third and succeeding
      attempts

is recognized by the ECG monitor. The ECG electrodes must be in place and the best lead (often lead II) selected to show a clear, strong, upright R wave. The defibrillator unit is set for synchronized cardioversion. The physician holds the paddles on the patient's anterior and left lateral chest wall. When the discharge buttons are pushed on the paddles, the shock is sent after the next R wave is identified by the ECG monitor.

This procedure is not considered to be an emergency; however, it is performed as quickly as possible so that the patient does not stay in the abnormal rhythm any longer than necessary. Synchronized cardioversion is performed only if medical treatment with antiarrhythmia drugs or carotid artery massage have no affect. Because these patients are usually conscious, they should be sedated with Valium or a similar medication. Patients who are hypotensive or already unconscious should not be sedated.

The respiratory therapist's role in either type of cardioversion could include:

a. Making sure that the ECG electrodes are properly positioned for either monitoring or diagnosing the rhythm, as the physician requires.

b. Making sure that the ECG monitor and electrocardiograph are working properly.

c. Making sure that the ECG lead is selected that results in a strong R wave; usually the R wave will be upright in lead II.

d. Charging the defibrillator to the power level ordered by the physician.

e. Adding the electrode cream to the electrode paddles to decrease the skin's resistance to electricity.

f. Being prepared to keep a patent airway, manually ventilate the patient, and/or begin chest compressions, if necessary.

2. Bronchoscopy.
a. Recommend a bronchoscopy procedure to get additional information on the patient's condition. (IA2u) [R, Ap, An]

Bronchoscopy is a procedure that involves looking directly into the patient's tracheobronchial airways. The physician can perform a number of diagnostic and therapeutic tasks under direct vision. (See Table 17-2 for uses, limitations, and risks of both types of bronchoscopy.)

Rigid tube bronchoscopy has been performed for more than 50 years. The rigid bronchoscope is a straight, hollow stainless steel tube (see Fig. 17-1). It has a distal light source so that the airway can be seen and a side port for providing oxygen or mechanical ventilation to the patient. The right and left mainstem bronchi can be observed by passing a mirror through the main channel. A hook or net can be passed through the main channel into the trachea or either brochus to remove a foreign body. The rigid bronchoscope is preferred for the treatment of massive hemoptysis or to remove a foreign body.

Flexible fiberoptic bronchoscopy (FFB) has been used clinically since the mid 1960s. It has gained wide popularity because it is better tolerated by the patient and allows for better visualization and collection of specimens from smaller bronchi (see Figs. 17-2 and 17-3).

b. Select a fiberoptic bronchoscope for the planned procedure. (IIA1l) [R, Ap]

The adult bronchoscopy tube is about 5 to 6 mm OD and the pediatric tube is about 3-mm OD. The small diameters and ability to guide the catheter allow the operator to look into the bronchus to each lung segment (segmental bronchi). The

Table 17-2. Uses, Limitations, and Risks of Bronchoscopy

Rigid bronchoscopy

Diagnostic use:

Biopsy of tumors within the main airway

Therapeutic uses:

Treatment of massive hemoptysis by cold-saline lavage or placement of a Fogarty catheter to occlude the airway

Removal of foreign body in infants and small children

Aspiration of inspissated secretions and mucus plugs

Limitations:

Cannot be used for observing or treating problems beyond the left or right mainstem bronchus

Cannot be used with patients with disease or trauma of the cervical spine who cannot hyperextend their neck

Cannot be used with patients with disease or trauma of the jaw who cannot open their mouth widely enough to pass the tube

Fiberoptic bronchoscopy

Diagnostic uses:

Search for the origin of a positive sputum cytology

Evaluate lung lesions and perform transbronchial biopsy of lung tissue (should only be done under fluoroscopic control)

Stage lung cancer preoperatively

Investigate unexplained hemoptysis, unexplained cough, localized wheeze, or stridor

Search for the etiology of unexplained paralysis of a vocal cord or hemidiaphragm

Search for the etiology of superior vena cava syndrome, chylothorax, or unexplained pleural effusion

Assessment of airway patency and investigate suspected bronchial tear or other injury after thoracic trauma

Investigate a suspected tracheoesophageal fistula

Investigate problems related to an endotracheal tube such as tracheal damage, airway obstruction, or tube placement

Obtain mucus for identification of pathogens

Investigate suspected injury secondary to inhaled superheated gas and smoke from an enclosed fire

Investigate suspected injury secondary to the aspiration of gastric contents

Perform bronchoalveolar lavage

Therapeutic uses:

Remove secretions or mucus plugs that cannot be cleared by other methods

Remove small foreign bodies

Table 17-2. (cont.)

Remove abnormal endobronchial tissue or
foreign material by forceps or laser
techniques

**Increased risks related to rigid or fiberoptic
bronchoscopy**

Recent myocardial infarction or unstable
angina

Unstable cardiac arrhythmia

Partial tracheal obstruction

Unstable bronchial asthma

Severe hypoxemia

Hypercarbia

Pulmonary hypertension (risk of hemorrhage
after biopsy)

Bleeding disorder (risk of hemorrhage after
biopsy)

Lung abscess (airway could be flooded with
purulent material)

Pulmonary infection from contaminated
equipment

Pneumothorax from transbronchial biopsy

Respiratory failure requiring mechanical
ventilation of the patient

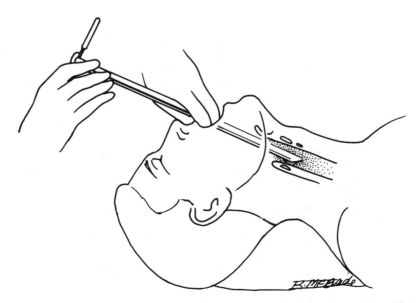

Fig. 17-1 A rigid tube bronchoscope being inserted into a patient's trachea. Note how the head and neck must be hyperextended. (From Simmons KF: Airway care. In Scanlan CL, Spearman CB, Sheldon RL, editors: *Egan's fundamentals of respiratory care,* ed 5, St. Louis, 1990, Mosby–Year Book. Used by permission.)

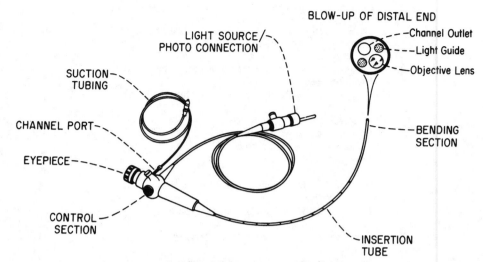

Fig. 17-2 A flexible fiberoptic bronchoscope with its components and special features. (From Simmons KF: Airway care. In Scanlan CL, Spearman CB, Sheldon RL, editors: *Egan's fundamentals of respiratory care,* ed 5, St. Louis, 1990, Mosby–Year Book. Used by permission.)

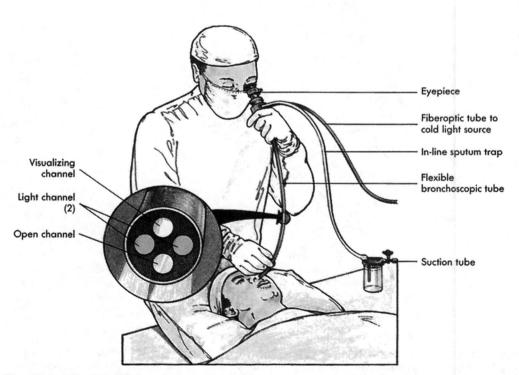

Fig. 17-3 A flexible fiberoptic bronchoscopy being performed on a patient. (From Williams SF, Thompson JM: *Respiratory disorders,* St. Louis, 1990, Mosby–Year Book. Used by permission.)

fiberoptic bronchoscope is preferred over the rigid one when the patient is being mechanically ventilated or has disease or trauma to the skull, jaw, or cervical spine. As shown in Fig. 17-2, a photo connection allows the assistant to either take still photographs of pulmonary anatomy or videotape the entire procedure.

A limitation of the pediatric unit is that there is no channel outlet for suctioning purposes. This is because of its small size. If a patient has an obstructing bronchial tumor, a special laser fiberoptic bronchoscope is used to burn away part of it. This enables the patient to breathe easier but is not a cure for the cancer.

c. Put the fiberoptic bronchoscope together, make sure that it works properly, and identify any problems with it. (IIB1m) [R, Ap]

The fiberoptic bronchoscope comes preassembled (see Fig. 17-2 for its primary features). If photographing or videotaping is planned, the camera must be attached at the photo connection. Have a central or portable suctioning system set up with suctioning tubing. In addition, the following must be checked for proper functioning:

1. Make sure the light source shines through to the distal end of the bronchoscope.
2. Look through the eyepiece. Point the distal end of the bronchoscope at a close object and adjust the lens to bring it into focus.
3. Adjust the thumb control to bend the distal tip.
4. Pass biopsy forceps or brush through the channel port to the outlet.
5. Make sure the suctioning tubing will connect to the channel port.

d. Fix any problems with the equipment. (IIB2n) [R, Ap]

If the light source does not work you will have to check with the manufacturer's equipment manual to help you determine if it could be something simple such as a burned out light bulb or a more serious problem. Similarly, problems with the camera equipment can be resolved by checking the manufacturer's equipment manual.

Failure to pass a biopsy forceps or brush through the channel port probably means that there is an obstruction such as dried blood or tissue. Try applying suction through the channel port to clear out the debris. It may also be helpful to squirt sterile distilled water from a syringe through the channel. Try suctioning again or pushing the biopsy forceps through the channel. If alternating suction, instilling water, and pushing the forceps through the channel does not dislodge the debris, the unit cannot be used. Try soaking the bronchoscope in water to soften the debris before repeating the above processes. If the channel cannot be cleared the unit must be sent back to the manufacturer for repairs.

e. Assist with the procedure. (IIIE1a) [R, Ap]

Typical duties of the respiratory therapist during bronchoscopy may include the following:

1. Inform the patient of the procedure and have him or her sign the medical release form.
2. Have a sedative or pain relieving agent administered if needed.
3. Nebulize a topical anesthetic, such as 4% lidocaine, to the airway.
4. Check the fiberoptic unit for proper function: working light source,

working thumb control to flexible tip, eyepiece focus can be adjusted, patency of the suction/biopsy channel.

5. Check the functioning of the biopsy brush and forceps.
6. Set up and monitor the patient's electrocardiogram.
7. Monitor the patient's vital signs.
8. Place and monitor the pulse oximeter on the patient.
9. Administer oxygen via a nasal catheter or the suction/biopsy channel on the unit.
10. Collect all suctioned or other specimens for culture and sensitivity.
11. Perform biopsies and brushings for cytology.
12. Operate any photographic equipment.
13. If the patient is being mechanically ventilated during fiberoptic bronchoscopy, perform the following:

   a. Place a bronchoscopy adapter between the endotracheal tube and wye of the circuit. This will keep a seal around the bronchoscopy tube to minimize any drop in tidal volume.

   b. Watch for an increase in the peak pressure from the increased resistance caused by the bronchoscopy tube.

   c. Be prepared to make adjustments in inspired oxygen, rate, flow, and tidal volume.

   d. Be prepared to switch from conventional volume ventilation to high frequency jet ventilation if needed.

14. Tend to the patient's comfort.
15. Disinfect the equipment between patients.

3. Thoracentesis.
a. Recommend the insertion of a chest tube. (IIIC10f) [R, Ap, An]

A chest tube (also called tube thoracostomy) may be inserted into either one or both pleural spaces around the lungs, the mediastinal space, or pericardial space around the heart. This procedure is indicated when air and/or fluid in any of these spaces interferes with normal lung or heart function. Table 17-3 lists the indications for the insertion of a chest tube.

b. Put a pleural drainage system together, make sure that it works properly, and identify any problems with it. (IIB1l2) [R, Ap]

Modern drainage systems consist of either three or four chambers or sections designed to regulate the vacuum level, hold any drained fluids, prevent any outside air from entering the patient's thorax, and act as a pressure relief valve in case the vacuum regulator should fail. Argyle and Pleurovac are two well-known manufacturers. The systems for draining the pleural space are discussed here, but the principles are the same for draining the mediastinal and pericardial spaces. Refer to Fig. 17-6 for the assembly and operation of the three-chamber drainage system. The four-chamber drainage system is shown in Fig. 17-7 and is discussed concurrently.

Table 17-3. Indications for the Insertion of a
Chest Tube

Pleural Space (See Fig. 17-4, **D.**)
Tension pneumothorax
Greater than a 10% to 20% simple pneumothorax
Hemothorax
Empyema
Pleural effusion
Chylothorax
Mediastinal Space
Free air
Free blood or other fluid
Pericardial Space (See Fig. 17-5.)
Cardiac tamponade
Pneumopericardium

Vacuum Level

The operation of the wall/central vacuum systems was discussed in Section 12. It is common practice to set a partial vacuum of -15 to -20 cm water pressure to the pleural space.

Suction Control

The suction control chamber is dry when the unit is unpacked. Follow the manufacturer's instructions for adding the correct amount of water to it. The proper water level is generally 15 to 20 cm high and results in that level of vacuum being applied to the patient's pleural space.

It is normal to have room air drawn into the opening on top and bubbling through the water column. This corresponds to bottle/chamber C in Fig. 17-7. The constant air bubbling will cause the water level to gradually drop from evaporation. Water will have to be added occasionally.

Water Seal

The water-seal chamber is a safety feature. It is dry when unpacked. Follow the manufacturer's directions as to the amount of water to add. Typically, the water-seal tube should have about 2 cm of water in it for any patient air to bubble through. As indicated by the arrows, it is designed to permit air to leave the patient's chest cavity. (Air will also be seen bubbling through when fluid enters the drainage collection chamber and displaces some of its air.) However, room air cannot be drawn "backwards" through the water to enter the chest if the vaccum fails or is disconnected. The water-seal chamber corresponds to bottle/chamber B in Fig. 17-7.

It is important to check the water-seal chamber regularly to see if there is any air bubbling through from the patient's chest. If so, the patient has an active air leak. If the chest tube has been placed into the pleural space, it shows that the patient has an unhealed pneumothorax or bronchopleural fistula. If the chest tube has been placed into the mediastinum or pericardium, it indicates that air is leaking

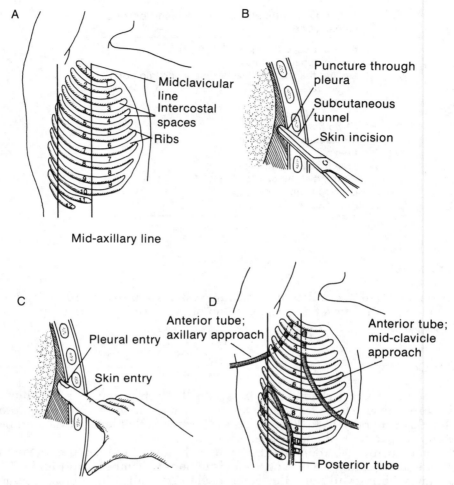

Fig. 17-4 Technique for inserting a pleural chest tube. **A,** Anatomical landmarks. **B,** Dissecting through the tissues with a hemostat. **C,** Using a finger to widen the opening and ensure that the lung has not been punctured. **D,** Proper tube placement. Air is removed by a tube that is placed toward the apex of the lung. Fluid is removed by a tube placed toward the posterior base of the lung. (Modified from Anderson HL, Bartlett RH: Respiratory care of the surgical patient. In Burton GG, Hodgkin JE, Ward JJ, editors: *Respiratory care: a guide to clinical practice,* ed 3, Philadelphia, 1991, JB Lippincott.)

through a tear in the lung structures to these areas. When the air leak stops, it indicates that the tissues have healed over the tear. Any air leakage will cause the water level to gradually drop from evaporation; therefore some water will have to be added occasionally.

Drainage Collection

The drainage collection chamber is designed to hold any fluid that is removed from the pleural space. It is divided into several sections that are marked off for volume measurement. The volume that has accumulated in the chamber should

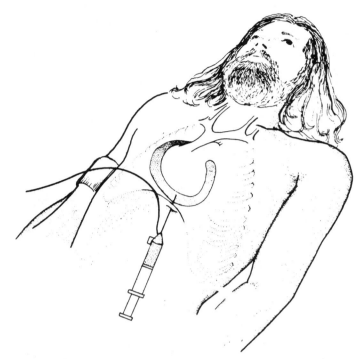

Fig. 17-5 Pericardiocentesis with a needle and syringe. A pericardial or mediastinal chest tube is also inserted by a substernal approach. (From Sproul CW, Mullanney PJ, editors: *Emergency care: assessment and interventions,* St. Louis, 1974, Mosby–Year Book. Used by permission.)

be recorded each hour. A sudden, significant increase in the amount of drainage should be called to the physician's attention. This is especially important if the patient is losing blood. Note the color of the drainage. Blood would obviously be red, chyle would be white, and pus from an empyema would be yellow or green.

This chamber corresponds to bottle/chamber A in Fig. 17-7. The whole drainage system will have to be replaced when the drainage collection chamber becomes filled.

Pressure Relief Valve on the Four-Chamber System

This additional chamber is a safety feature and is seen on four-chamber systems such as those shown in Fig. 17-7. Its purpose is to act as a escape route for any gas leaking from the patient if the vacuum system is accidentally turned off or disconnected. Without the relief valve, air pressure from a pneumothorax could increase to a dangerous level. Instead, the air and pressure are released. In three-chamber systems, the pressure has to build up to the point that water in the suction control chamber "geysers" out before the pressure is relieved.

c.   Fix any problems with the pleural drainage system. (IIB2m) [R, Ap, An]

A number of problems can occur with chest drainage systems. The practitioner must understand how the systems are designed to work and how to recognize and correct the situation. See Table 17-4 for examples of problems. Fig. 17-8 lists important considerations when assessing the patient on chest drainage.

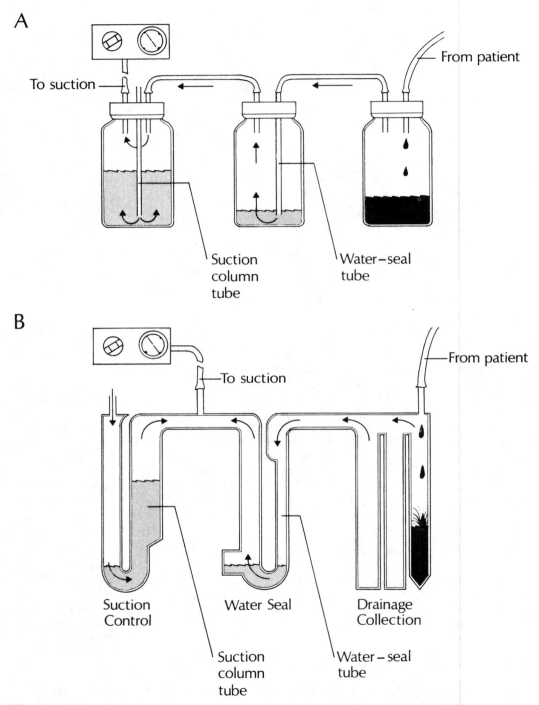

Fig. 17-6 Three-chamber pleural drainage systems. **A,** Homemade three-chamber drainage system. The depth that the suction column tube is placed under water determines the level of vacuum that will be applied against the patient's pleural space. **B,** Schematic drawing of a modern manufactured three-chamber drainage system. (From Shapiro BA, Kacmarek RM, Cane RD et al: *Clinical application of respiratory care,* ed 4, St. Louis, 1991, Mosby–Year Book. Used by permission.)

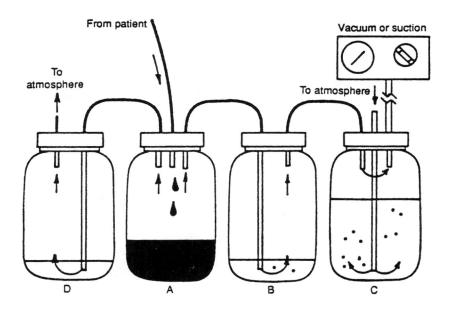

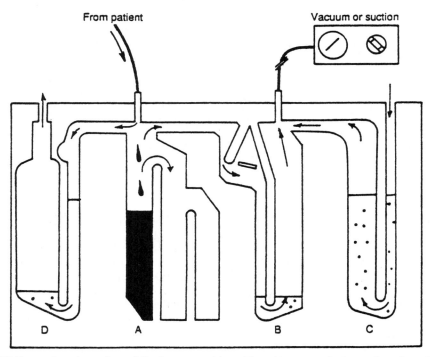

Fig. 17-7 Four-chamber pleural drainage systems. **Top,** Homemade four-chamber drainage system. The depth that the suction column tube in chamber C is placed under water determines the level of vacuum that will be applied against the patient's pleural space. **Bottom,** Schematic drawing of a modern manufactured four-chamber drainage system. The fourth chamber acts to vent high pressure air if the vacuum should be turned off or malfunction. (From Pilbeam SP, Deshpande VM: Chest tubes and pleural drainage, *Current Review in Respiratory Therapy* 5:151, 1983. Used by permission.)

Table 17-4. Troubleshooting Problems with Chest Drainage Systems

Problem	Corrective Action
Drainage system is cracked open or drainage tubing is permanently disconnected from the drainage system	If the patient has a leaking pneumothorax: Leave the tube open to room air so the pleural air will be vented out
	As quickly as possible, place the distal end of tubing into a glass of water to create a water seal.
	If the patient does not have a leaking pneumothorax, clamp the distal end of the tube to prevent room air from being drawn into the pleural space.
	In either case attach the tube to a new drainage system as soon as possible.
No bubbling through the suction control chamber	Increase the vacuum pressure.
	Correct any leak in the system.
Water is spouting out of the suction control chamber (3-bottle system)	Turn on the vacuum.
	Remove obstruction inside tubing between vacuum and drainage system.
Air leak through the water seal chamber	Check the patient for a pneumothorax; report a new air leak to the physician.
	Check for a leaking seal between the drainage tube and the patient's chest.
	Check for a hole in the drainage tube, a loose connection between the tube and the drainage system, or if a fenestration in the tubing has pulled out of the chest wall.
Fluid has filled a dependent loop in the tubing	Drape the tubing so that there are no loops or kinks.
No change in drainage	Check for loops or kinks in tube.
	Milk the tube to remove any clots.
	No action if drainage has ceased.
Full drainage collection chamber	Prepare another unit, clamp the tube while making the exchange, unclamp the tube after the new unit is functioning.

d.   Assist with the thoracentesis procedure. (IIIE1b) [R, Ap]

Thoracentesis is the surgical puncture and drainage of the thoracic cavity. The respiratory therapist will probably only assist with a thoracentesis of the pleural space. Thoracentesis is performed to aid in the diagnosis of inflammatory or neoplastic diseases of the pleura or lung. It is also performed as a therapeutic procedure to remove air or fluid that has accumulated in the pleural space.

The respiratory therapist may be responsible for preparing the patient, disinfecting the puncture site, setting up the sterile field around it, and preparing the equipment and supplies. Each hospital or physician may have a prescribed way of doing this. The general steps are listed here:

1. Inform the patient of the procedure and have him or her sign the medical release form.
2. Have a sedative or pain relieving agent administered if needed.
3. Position the patient properly. Usually this means sitting on the side of the bed and leaning on the overbed table as shown in Fig. 17-9. Or the

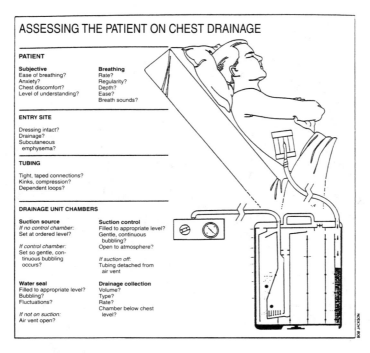

Fig. 17-8 Assessing the patient on chest drainage. (From Erickson RA: Chest drainage, II, *Nursing89,* 19(6):47-49, 1989. Used by permission.)

patient may straddle a chair and rest his or her arms and head on the back of the chair. The patient who cannot sit up is positioned on his or her side with the unaffected lung down on the bed.

4. If necessary, shave the insertion site clear of body hair.
5. Put on a sterile mask, cap, gown, and gloves according to protocol.
6. Disinfect the insertion site with a Betadine (iodine) soaked sterile 4 × 4-inch gauze pad. Place the pad at the center of the insertion site and move in a widening spiral away from the center. This step should be repeated with a second gauze pad. Let the Betadine dry.
7. Protect around the insertion site with a sterile fenestrated surgical drape.
8. Prepare the sterile field with these supplies:

    a. Have a local anesthestic such as 1% Xylocaine available in a 5-ml syringe with a 25-gauge × $\frac{5}{8}$-inch needle. The physician will inject some of the Xylocaine into the skin and deeper tissues (see Fig. 17-10, **A** and **B**).

    b. Have the following needles available: 1) 21-gauge × $1\frac{1}{2}$-inch for injecting Xylocaine into the periosteum of the rib. 2) 16-gauge × $3\frac{1}{2}$-inch for withdrawing the sample from the pleural space.

    c. 50-ml syringe for collecting the sample.

    d. Two-way valve or three-way stopcock to place between the 16-gauge needle and the 50-ml syringe.

    e. Rubber drainage tube to carry the sample from the valve/stopcock to the specimen tubes.

    f. Three 10-ml specimen tubes with caps.

    g. Adhesive bandage.

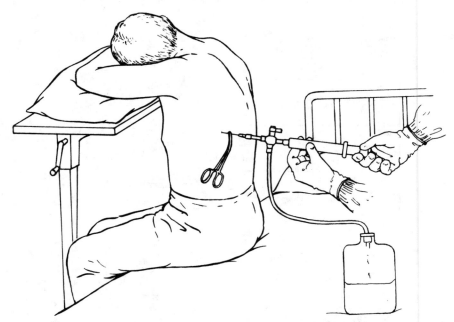

Fig. 17-9 Technique for thoracentesis. The patient sits up leaning on the overbed table. The pleural fluid is withdrawn through the needle by the syringe and then directed into the collection jar by turning the three-way stopcock. (From Anderson HL, Bartlett RH: Respiratory care of the surgical patient. In Burton GG, Hodgkin JE, Ward JJ, editors: *Respiratory care: a guide to clinical practice,* ed 3, Philadelphia, 1991, JB Lippincott. Used by permission.)

Note: A Curity Thoracentesis Tray or other prepackaged tray will contain the supplies that will most commonly be used.

9. Assist the physician into his or her sterile mask, cap, gown, and gloves.
10. Assist the physician with the procedure as needed.
11. Make any adjustments in the patient's respiratory care equipment as needed.
12. Dispose of any used supplies and so forth after the procedure is completed.
13. Tend to the patient's comfort.

Removal of Pleural Fluid

General steps in the procedure:

1. Check the patient's chest x-ray for the location of the pleural fluid or tissue for biopsy and its relationship to the ribs and other tissues.
2. Prepare the patient as described previously.
3. The physician will anesthetize the thoracentesis site as shown in Fig. 17-10, **A** and **B.**
4. The physician will insert the 16-gauge needle (with attached 50-ml syringe) into the pleural fluid (see Fig. 17-10, **C**) or the suspicious tissue.

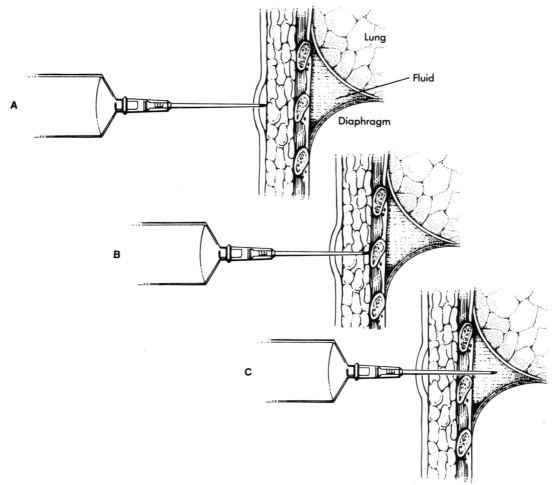

Fig. 17-10 Anesthetizing the needle insertion site and performing a thoracentesis. **A,** A 25-gauge needle is used to inject Xylocaine into the thoracentesis puncture site until the skin is raised. **B,** A 22-gauge needle is used to inject Xylocaine into the periosteum of the rib and surrounding tissues. The properly anesthetized patient should feel no pain during the thoracentesis. **C,** A 22- or larger-gauge aspirating needle is pushed through the numbed tissues, over the top edge of the rib, and into the pleural space. The fluid sample can now be aspirated. (From Martin L: *Pulmonary physiology in clinical practice: the essentials for patient care and evaluation,* St. Louis, 1987, Mosby–Year Book. Used by permission.)

5. The sample is then aspirated. If there is more than 50 ml of pleural fluid, the two-way valve or three-way stopcock, rubber hose, and collection tube are assembled to remove the fluid (see Fig. 17-9).
6. The needle is removed and a bandage is placed over the puncture site.
7. Place the patient with the unaffected side down on the bed.
8. Observe the patient for dizziness, cyanosis, and changes in heart rate and/or respiratory rate. (See Table 17-5 for the commonly seen complications.)
9. Send the collected sample to the laboratory for analysis.

Table 17-5. Common Complications of
a Thoracentesis

Infection
Hemothorax
Subcutaneous emphysema
Air embolism
Pneumothorax
Sudden mediastinal shift from removal of a large
  amount of pleural fluid (usually greater than
  1500 ml in an adult)
Unstable vital signs from the sudden mediastinal
  shift
Pulmonary edema from the sudden reexpansion
  of the lung and mediastinal shift

Insertion of a Pleural Chest Tube

It is unlikely that a respiratory therapist will be called on to assist with the insertion of a chest tube into the mediastinum or pericardial space. These are usually placed into the patient in the operating room as part of an open heart surgery procedure. However, if called on to help, the therapist's duties would be about the same as those described next for the insertion of a pleural tube.

The respiratory therapist may be responsible for preparing the patient, disinfecting the puncture site, setting up the sterile field around it, and preparing the equipment and supplies. Each hospital or physician may have a prescribed way of doing this. The general steps are listed here:

1. Inform the patient of the procedure and have him or her sign the medical release form if time permits.
2. Have a sedative or pain relieving agent administered if needed.
3. Position the patient properly. Usually this means the patient will lie on his or her back or with the unaffected lung down on the bed.
4. If necessary, shave the insertion site clear of body hair.
5. Put on a sterile mask, cap, gown, and gloves according to protocol.
6. Disinfect the insertion site with a Betadine (iodine) soaked sterile 4 × 4-inch gauze pad. Place the pad at the center of the insertion site and move in a widening spiral away from the center. This step should be repeated with a second gauze pad. Let the Betadine dry.
7. Protect around the insertion site with a sterile fenestrated surgical drape.
8. Prepare the sterile field with these supplies:

    a. Have a local anesthetic such as 1% Xylocaine available in a 5-ml syrine with a 25-gauge × $\frac{5}{8}$-inch needle. The physician will inject some of the Xylocaine into the skin (see Fig. 17-10, **A**).
    b. Have a 21-gauge × $1\frac{1}{2}$-inch needle available for attaching to the 5-ml syringe for injecting Xylocaine into the periosteum of the rib (see Fig. 17-10, **B**).
    c. 50-ml syringe for collecting a fluid sample if needed.
    d. Scalpels, hemostats, scissors, and Trocars as dictated by the hospital's policy or the physician's preference.

e. A length of sterile rubber drainage tube to be inserted into the patient to carry the air and/or fluid to the drainage system; it must have several fenestrations (openings) in the patient end so it will not become clogged with clotted blood.
   f. Argyle, Pleurovac, or other brand of drainage system.
   g. Suture needles and threads, sterile 4 × 4-inch gauze pads, and adhesive bandage.
   Note: A Curity Thoracentesis Tray or other prepackaged tray will contain the supplies that will most commonly be used.

9. Assist the physician into his or her sterile mask, cap, gown, and gloves.
10. Assist the physician with the procedure as needed.
11. Make any adjustments in the patient's respiratory care equipment as needed.
12. Dispose of any used supplies and so forth after the procedure is completed.
13. Tend to the patient's comfort.

General steps in inserting a pleural chest tube:

1. Check the patient's chest x-ray for the location of the air or fluid in the pleural space and its relationship to the ribs and other tissues.
2. Prepare the patient as described in the previous list.
3. The physician will anesthetize the tube insertion site as shown in Fig. 17-10, **A** and **B**.
4. The physician will create an opening into the patient's chest wall to place the chest tube (see Fig. 17-4). A tube to remove *air* will be placed over the top edge of a rib into the second to fourth intercostal space. The insertion site will be aligned with either the mid-clavicular line or mid-axillary line (preferred site). The tube is then advanced toward the apex of the lung. A tube to remove *fluid* will be placed over the top edge of the rib into the sixth to eighth intercostal space. It will be inserted at the mid-axillary line and advanced toward the posterior base of the lung.

   Mediastinal or pericardial tubes will be placed via an opening below the xiphoid process and placed posterior to the heart. This is most commonly done after open heart surgery.
5. The tube will be secured by sutures and/or a 4 × 4-inch gauze pad and bandage.
6. The other end of the tube is connected to the drainage system (discussed earlier).
7. Place the patient with his or her back against the bed or with the unaffected side down on the bed. The physician may want the head of the bed elevated or flat.
8. Observe the patient for dizziness, cyanosis, and changes in heart rate and/or respiratory rate. (See Table 17-5 for the most commonly seen complications.)

It is important to note that in the case of an emergency when the patient has a tension pneumothorax and rapidly worsening vital signs, the physician may choose to rapidly remove the air from the chest. This is done by placing a large bore needle (16-gauge or larger) through the second or third intercostal space in the midclavicular line. The intrapleural air will leave the chest allowing the lung to expand. A chest tube will then be inserted for a long-term solution to the problem.

4.   Intubation. (IIIE1i) [R, Ap]

The procedure for a therapist performing oral endotracheal intubation was discussed in Section 11. The following discussion is limited to assisting a physician who is performing a nasal endotracheal intubation. This procedure is usually only performed by an anesthesiologist or physician who has been trained in the procedure. Most commonly, the respiratory therapist is the assistant. See Table 17-6 for indications and contraindications and Table 17-7 for complications of nasal endotracheal intubation. There are two different procedures for passing an endotracheal tube by the nasal route: blind nasotracheal intubation and direct vision nasotracheal intubation.

Blind Nasotracheal Intubation

Be prepared to assist in blind nasotracheal intubation by positioning the patient properly, providing supplemental oxygen or manual ventilation to the patient, and getting and preparing the endotracheal tube or other equipment. A stylet is usually not indicated. Often the physician will order the patient to be prepared by having 1% phenylephrine sprayed into the nares. This medication vasoconstricts the blood vessels. This dilates the nasal passages making intubation easier and also reduces the risk of bleeding. Often 4% Lidocaine is sprayed into the nares for its local anesthetic effect. The distal end of the endotracheal tube is usually also covered with sterile Lidocaine ointment.

This procedure is done without the aid of a laryngoscope to visualize the patient's anatomy and expose the trachea. The general procedure is to place the patient in the sniffer's position, advance the tube to the oropharynx, and then advance it only on inspiration. The physician puts his or her ear near the proximal end of the tube to feel any air movement and listen for a change in sound as signs that the trachea has been intubated. Different head positions, pressure over the larynx, or pulling on the tongue may be needed to help guide the tube into the

---

Table 17-6. Indications and Contraindications for Nasal Endotracheal Intubation

General Indications for Endotracheal Intubation
Provide a secure, patent airway.
Provide a route for mechanical ventilation.
Prevent aspiration of stomach or mouth contents.
Provide a route for suctioning the lungs.
General anesthesia.

Indications for Nasal Intubation
Patient has a cervical spine abnormality or injury.
Use of muscle relaxants may cause a complete
    loss of the airway.
Limited movement of the cervical spine or
    mandible.
Lower facial injury or surgery.

Contraindications for Nasal Intubation
Basilar skull fracture
Nasal tumors
Deviated nasal septum
Severe coagulation disorder

Table 17-7. Complications of Nasal
Endotracheal Intubation

General Complications
Reflex laryngospasm
Perforation of the esophagus or pharynx
Esophageal intubation
Bronchial intubation
Reflex bradycardia
Tachycardia or other arrhythmias from hypoxemia
Hypotension
Bronchospasm
Aspiration of tooth, blood, gastric contents,
   laryngoscope bulb
Laceration of pharynx or larynx
Nosocomial infection
Vocal cord injury
Laryngeal or tracheal injury from the tube or the
   excessive cuff pressure

Mucosal bleeding
Trauma to the larynx during an attempted blind
   intubation
Sinusitis

Complications After Extubation
Reflex laryngospasm
Aspiration of stomach contents or oral secretions
Sore throat
Hoarseness
Laryngeal edema (postintubation croup)

trachea. In addition, there are several different devices that can aid in this intubation. The physician may choose to place a so-called *"trigger" tube* into the patient. This special endotracheal tube has a wire placed into it along the inside curve to the tip (see Fig. 11-15 in Section 11). The wire is pulled when the tube is near the larynx to bend the tip more anterior to aim it into the trachea. A *lighted stylet* can be passed through the tube so that the light source is at the distal tip. The light will shine through the skin over the larynx. When this is seen, the tube is advanced and the stylet is removed. A *fiberoptic bronchoscope* can be placed through the tube and guided into the patient's trachea. The tube is then advanced and the bronchoscope removed. Another choice is the *intubation guide*. This is a stylet with a flexible tip that can be bent by the physician through a proximal handle (see Fig. 17-11). The intubation guide is passed through and beyond the distal end of the endotracheal tube. When the guide is in the oropharynx the tip can be bent in an anterior direction and directed into the trachea. The tube is then advanced over the guide and into the trachea. The guide is then removed.

Direct Vision Nasotracheal Intubation

The respiratory therapist will assist with direct vision nasotracheal intubation and prepare the patient and endotracheal tube as with blind endotracheal intubation. This procedure is different from the previous procedure in that intubation equipment is used to visualize the patient's anatomy and see the glottis. Prepare

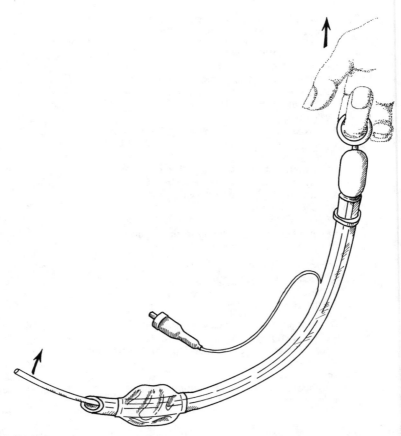

Fig. 17-11 An intubation guide stylet. The flexible tip can be guided by pulling or pushing on a ring attached to a wire running to the distal end. Once the end of the guide is directed into the trachea the endotracheal tube is slipped over it. After the intubation the guide is withdrawn. (Modified from Heffner JE: Managing difficult intubations in critically ill patients, *Respir Management* 19(3), 1989.)

a laryngoscope handle, the physician's choice of either a straight or curved blade, and a Magill forceps.

The lubricated tube is advanced to the oropharynx. The laryngoscope blade is then placed into the mouth and used to expose the glottis. The Magill forceps is then placed into the mouth. It is used to grasp the endotracheal tube and guide it into the trachea (see Fig. 17-12). Care must be taken not to place the pinchers over the cuff to avoid tearing it.

With either method, the tube must be properly positioned so that the cuff is in the trachea beyond the vocal cords (see Fig. 17-13). The cuff is then inflated, its pressure adjusted to a safe level, and the tube secured in place by tape.

5. Tracheostomy. (IIIE1d) [R, Ap]

A *tracheostomy* is a surgical opening in the anterior tracheal wall. The opening is usually placed below the cricoid cartilage and through the second, third, or fourth ring of tracheal cartilage (see Fig. 17-14, **A**). The term *tracheotomy* is used to describe the surgical procedure itself (the two terms are often used interchangeably).

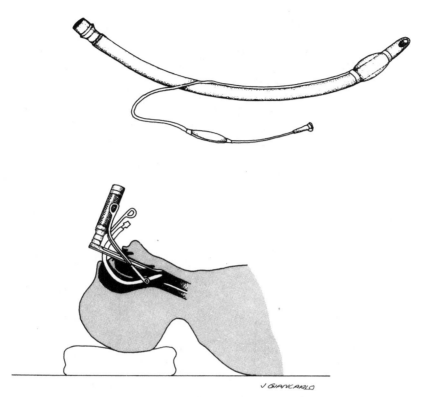

Fig. 17-12 Direct vision nasotracheal intubation. Note that the Magill forceps and laryngoscope and blade are both used. The Magill forceps is used to grasp the tip of the endotracheal tube and pull it anterior into the trachea. (From Shapiro BA, Harrison RA, Cane RD: *Clinical application of respiratory care,* ed 4, St. Louis, 1991, Mosby–Year Book. Used by permission.)

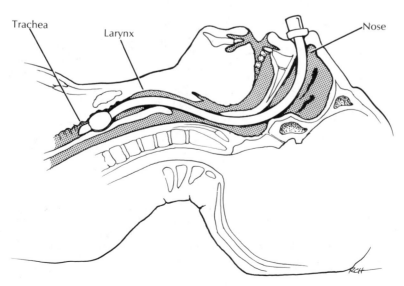

Fig. 17-13 A properly placed nasotracheal tube. (From Shapiro BA, Harrison RA, Cane RD: *Clinical application of respiratory care,* ed 4, St. Louis, 1991, Mosby–Year Book. Used by permission.)

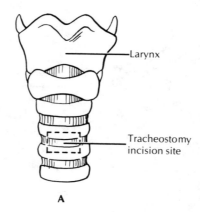

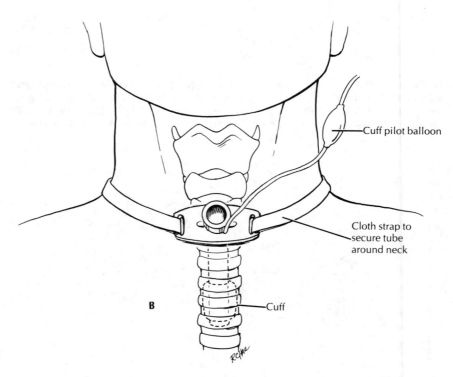

Fig. 17-14 Anatomy of the larynx and insertion of a tracheostomy tube. **A,** Close-up of the larynx and the tracheostomy incision site. **B,** Anterior cut-away view of the tracheostomy tube after its insertion. **C,** Lateral cut-away view of the tracheostomy tube after its insertion. (From Eubanks DH, Bone RC: *Comprehensive respiratory care: a learning system,* ed 2, St. Louis, 1990, Mosby–Year Book. Used by permission.)

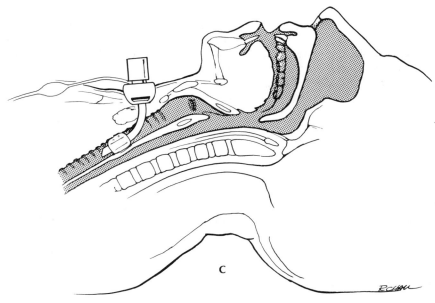

Fig. 17-14 (*cont.*)

Commonly the tracheostomy is created in the operating room under sterile conditions. When the respiratory therapist is called to assist, it is usually because of a patient emergency. The situation commonly involves an upper airway obstruction such as facial trauma or surgery where an endotracheal tube cannot be placed by either the oral or nasal route. Because of time contraints, the full sterile technique may be skipped over in favor of a clean technique. The physician's preference and the situation itself will dictate how the procedure will be performed. The respiratory therapist may also be called to assist in the procedure when the patient is already intubated. Usually this involves an unstable patient who requires long-term mechanical ventilation. Because of the patient's critical condition, the physician makes the decision to perform the tracheostomy at the bedside rather than in the operating room. The respiratory therapist may be responsible for preparing the patient, disinfecting the tracheostomy site, setting up the sterile field around it, and setting up the equipment and supplies. Each hospital or physician may have a prescribed way that this is done. The general steps are listed here:

1. Inform the patient of the procedure and have him or her sign the medical release form if time permits.
2. Have a sedative or pain relieving agent administered if needed.
3. If necessary, shave the insertion site clear of body hair.
4. Put on a sterile mask, cap, gown, and gloves according to protocol.
5. Disinfect the insertion site with a Betadine (iodine) soaked sterile 4 × 4-inch gauze pad. Place the pad at the center of the insertion site and move in a widening spiral away from the center. This step should be repeated with a second gauze pad. Let the Betadine dry.
6. Protect around the insertion site with a sterile fenestrated surgical drape.
7. Prepare the sterile field where the tracheostomy tube, scalpel, supplies, and so forth. Have a local anesthestic such as Xylocaine available in a syringe with needle. The physician will inject this into the insertion site.

8. Assist the physician into his or her sterile mask, cap, gown, and gloves.
9. Get the properly sized tracheostomy tube (see Table 11-3 in Section 11).
10. Assist the physician with the procedure as needed. If the patient is already intubated, withdraw the endotracheal tube after the tracheostomy has been created and the physician is ready to place the tracheostomy tube into the opening.
11. Make any adjustments in the patient's respiratory care equipment as needed.
12. Dispose of any used supplies and so forth after the procedure is completed.
13. Tend to the patient's comfort.

See Section 11 for further discussion on the indications for the various airway routes and when to routinely change a tracheostomy tube. Table 17-8 lists the common complications of a tracheostomy.

6.   Transtracheal aspiration. (IIIE1c) [R, Ap]

Transtracheal aspiration is a procedure where a large bore needle is inserted through the cricothyroid membrane. A catheter is then passed through the needle and advanced into the trachea where a sputum sample is aspirated (see Figs. 17-14 and 17-15). The purpose of this procedure is to obtain a sputum sample that is uncontaminated by oral flora. Samples gotten by the patient coughing up sputum or through nasotracheal suctioning or bronchoscopy are usually contaminated by upper airway organisms. Transtracheal aspiration is quite safe but does have possible complications of infection, bleeding, and subcutaneous emphysema.

The respiratory therapist may be responsible for preparing the patient, disinfecting the puncture site, setting up the sterile field around it, and preparing the equipment and supplies. Each hospital or physician may have a prescribed way of doing this. The general steps are listed here:

1. Inform the patient of the procedure and have him or her sign the medical release form.
2. Have a sedative or pain relieving agent administered if needed.
3. Position the patient properly. Usually this means the patient will lie on his or her back with the neck hyperextended into the sniff position.
4. If necessary, shave the insertion site clear of body hair.
5. Put on a sterile mask, cap, gown, and gloves according to protocol.

Table 17-8. Common Complications of a Tracheostomy

Complication	Approximate Time of Onset
Bleeding	During and after surgery for up to 24 hours; if possible do not replace the first tube for 2 to 3 days
Pneumothorax	During the procedure
Infection of the stoma or lungs	Usually seen after second day
Subcutaneous or mediastinal emphysema	May be seen during the procedure or at any later time

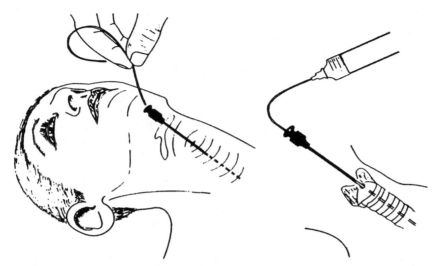

Fig. 17-15 Procedure for transtracheal aspiration. (From Couperus JJ, Elder HA: Infectious disease aspects of respiratory therapy. In Burton GG, Hodgkin JE, editors: *Respiratory care: a guide to clinical practice,* ed 2, Philadelphia, 1984, JB Lippincott. Used by permission.)

6. Disinfect the insertion site with a Betadine (iodine) soaked sterile 4 × 4-inch gauze pad. Place the pad at the center of the insertion site and move in a widening spiral away from the center. This step should be repeated with a second gauze pad. Let the Betadine dry.
7. Protect around the insertion site with a sterile fenestrated surgical drape.
8. Prepare the sterile field with these supplies:

   a. Local anesthestic such as 1% Xylocaine available in a 5-ml syringe with a 25-gauge × ⅝-inch needle. The physician will inject some of the Xylocaine into the skin.
   b. 14-gauge × 3-inch needle available for inserting through the cricothyroid membrane into the larynx.
   c. Catheter small enough to pass through the 14-gauge needle for removing the mucus sample.
   d. 10-ml syringe for collecting the mucus sample.
   e. 10-ml syringe with sterile, preservative-free saline for instillation into the trachea if needed.
   f. Sterile 2 × 2-inch gauze pads and adhesive bandage.
   g. Assist the physician into his or her sterile mask, cap, gown, and gloves.

10. Assist the physician with the procedure as needed.
11. Make any adjustments in the patient's respiratory care equipment as needed.

12. Dispose of any used supplies and so forth after the procedure is completed.
13. Tend to the patient's comfort.

General steps in the transtracheal aspiration procedure:

1. Check the patient's upper airway and/or chest x-ray as indicated.
2. Prepare the patient as described earlier.
3. The physician will anesthetize the needle insertion site.
4. The physician will insert the needle in alignment with the trachea.
5. Insert the catheter through the needle into the trachea. If possible, do not allow the patient to cough.
6. Attach the syringe to the catheter and apply vacuum to obtain a sample of mucus. If the secretions are too viscous to be aspirated, a 2 to 5 ml bolus of sterile, preservative-free saline may be instilled into the trachea through the catheter. This should make the aspiration easier.
7. Withdraw the catheter and needle.
8. Apply the gauze pad and/or bandage to the insertion site.
9. Observe the patient for bleeding, subcutaneous emphysema, cyanosis, and changes in heart rate and/or respiratory rate.
10. Send the collected sample to the laboratory for analysis.

7.   Transtracheal oxygen catheter placement.
   a.   Put the transtracheal catheter together, make sure that it works properly, and identify any problems with it. (IIB1a) [R, Ap]

See Section 5 for the discussion and Figure 5-3, **A** for an illustration of the catheter and stylet.

   b.   Fix any problems with the equipment. (IIB2a5) [R, Ap, An]

See Section 5 for the discussion.

   c.   Assist with the procedure. (IIIE1f) [R, Ap]

The respiratory therapist may be responsible for preparing the patient, disinfecting the puncture site, setting up the sterile field around it, and preparing the equipment and supplies. Each hospital or physician may have a prescribed way of doing this. The following procedure is based on recommendations by the manufacturer of the SCOOP Transtracheal Catheter (Transtracheal Systems of Denver, Colo).
General steps in the transtracheal procedure:

1. Inform the patient of the procedure and have him or her sign the medical release form.
2. (Optional) One hour before the procedure have a nurse give 4.5 mg of oxycodone for cough suppression, 500 mg of acetaminophen for pain relief, and 500 mg of cephalexin for infection prophylaxis.
3. Position the patient properly. Usually this means the patient will sit in a comfortable reclining chair with head rest with the neck hyperextended into the sniff position.
4. The patient should have his or her supplemental oxygen given by nasal

cannula throughout the procedure. Place a pulse oximeter on the patient's finger or ear to monitor his or her saturation.

5. If necessary, shave the insertion site clear of body hair.
6. Mark with a surgical pen the following anatomical landmarks: notch of the thyroid cartilage, cricothyroid membrane, and notch of the manubrium.
7. Premeasure around the patient's lower neck the bead-chain that will be used to hold the catheter in place. Two fingers should fit under the chain. The puncture site is where the chain crosses the trachea.
8. Remove the chain and disinfect the site with an alcohol swab.
9. Prepare the sterile field with these supplies:

   a. 5-ml syringe of 2% Xylocaine mixed with epinephrine (1 : 100,000) with a 27-gauge × 2-inch needle
   b. 21-gauge × 2-inch needle
   c. 18-gauge × 4-inch needle and 5-ml syringe (Draw 2 ml sterile normal saline into the syringe.)
   d. # 15 scalpel
   e. Two 3-0 nylon sutures with needle holder
   f. Sterile wire guide, 10 French dilator, and 9 French tubular stent (From Transtracheal Systems, Denver, Colo)
   g. Sterile lubricating jelly
   h. Several 4 × 4-inch sterile gauze pads

10. The physician will anesthetize the skin with the 27-gauge needle and syringe (about 2 ml are used).
11. The physician will anesthetize the deeper tissues through to the trachea with the 21-gauge needle and syringe (about 1 ml is used).
12. Air is aspirated back into the syringe to ensure that the needle is within the air column of the trachea. (Air will freely bubble through the saline.)
13. The remainder of the Xylocaine and epinephrine is squirted into the trachea and the needle is quickly withdrawn because the patient will probably cough.
14. Sterile gloves are put on. A sterile mask, cap, and gown may be put on according to protocol.
15. Disinfect the insertion site with a Betadine (iodine) soaked sterile 4 × 4-inch gauze pad. Place the pad at the center of the insertion site and move in a widening spiral away from the center. This step should be repeated with a second gauze pad. Let the Betadine dry.
16. Protect around the insertion site with a sterile surgical drape.
17. The scalpel is used to make a 1-cm vertical incision through the dermis and fat at the puncture site.
18. The 18-gauge × 4-inch needle attached to the 5-ml syringe with 2 ml of saline is pushed through the incision at a cartilage interspace.
19. Aspirate air from the trachea. The syringe is removed and the needle is angled down toward the carina.
20. The blunt end of the wire guide is inserted through the needle into the trachea. Advance it 10 cm to the black mark.
21. The needle is withdrawn over the wire guide and a 10 French dilator (Transtracheal Systems) is advanced over the guide wire into the trachea. Do not advance it beyond the 8 cm mark.
22. The dilator is removed over the wire guide. The tip of a nonfunctional 9 French stent is coated with lubricant and passed over the guide wire into the trachea all the way to the hub.

23. The wire guide is removed.
24. The stent is sewn to the skin with the two sutures.
25. A sterile 4 × 4-inch gauze dressing is taped over the stent.
26. Dispose of any used supplies and so forth after the procedure is completed.
27. A chest and neck x-ray is taken to confirm the position of the stent within the trachea and the absence of subcutaneous emphysema or pneumothorax.
28. (Optional) 250 mg of Cephalexin is prescribed four times per day for 7 days.
29. The patient can be sent home after the procedure unless there is a complication.

General steps in the 1-week postinsertion procedure:

1. The wire guide is inserted through the stent, which is then removed.
2. A functional 9 French transtracheal catheter with a single distal port is inserted over the wire guide and 11 cm into the trachea (Transtracheal Systems). The catheter flange will be next to the patient's neck. It is secured with the bead-chain (see Fig. 5-3 in Section 5).
3. About 9 cm of catheter is left outside of the patient's body. This is attached to regular oxygen tubing.
4. Pulse oximetry is used to titrate the proper level of inspired oxygen at rest and while walking. An SpO_2 of 90% to 91% is the usual goal. Normally the patient will be able to maintain this level at a lower inspired oxygen level; often as low as 0.25 L/min. Arterial blood gases may also be drawn to check all respiratory values.
5. Teach the patient to clean the catheter with 3 ml of instilled normal saline and a cleaning rod. This should be done twice a day.
6. Contact the home care company about the patient's new oxygen requirements.
7. One week later the patient is scheduled to come back and have the respiratory therapist remove the original catheter for cleaning and replacement.
8. Answer any of the patient's questions and reinstruct if necessary.

General steps in the 6-8 weeks postinsertion procedure:

1. Between 6 and 8 weeks later the 9 French catheter is removed. The catheter tract should be inspected for lack of infection.
2. An 8 French transtracheal catheter with multiple side ports is inserted (Transtracheal Systems). No guide wire should be needed because the tract should be mature and not close off. If the 8 French catheter cannot be easily inserted, it is removed. The guide wire is inserted into the stoma and the 9 French catheter is inserted over it again. This catheter is left in place for another two weeks to make sure that the tract is mature and lined with epithelial cells. The patient is instructed to come back once a week for a catheter cleaning.
3. After the tract is found to be mature the patient is taught to remove the 8 French catheter, clean it to prevent the accumulation of mucus on it (mucus balls), and reinsert the catheter. This should be done twice a day.
4. Answer any questions. Educate the patient as needed. Schedule the patient to come back in one week for catheter and tract inspection and redemonstration of the patient's skills at catheter care.

5. The patient is scheduled to come back every 3 months for routine catheter and tract inspection and further evaluation.

8. Stress testing.
a. Review the patient's chart for information on any previous pulmonary stress testing. (IA1j) [R]

Before starting a stress test the patient's chart should be reviewed for information on previous stress testing. It is important to know the type of testing that was performed, how the patient tolerated it, and what caused the patient to stop the test. Review the physician's evaluation of the test results and the patient's diagnosis.

b. Recommend pulmonary stress testing to get additional information on the patient's condition. (IA2k) [R, Ap, An]

Stress testing is performed to determine a patient's limits to exercise. The limiting factor(s) to exercise tell much about a patient's medical condition. Table 17-9 lists the indications for stress testing.

c. Assist with the procedure. (IIIE1e) [R, Ap]

Stress testing is the intentional exercising of the patient to the point of exhaustion or physiologic deterioration when the test must be stopped because the patient cannot continue. Because of this, the procedure is inherently risky to the patient. It is imperative that the patient be carefully evaluated before, during, and after the procedure. An informed consent statement must be signed by the patient before

---

Table 17-9. Indications for Exercise Testing

Evaluation of nonspecific dyspnea on exertion

Evaluation of the patient's ventilatory response to increased work

Evaluation of the patient's need for supplemental oxygen

Serial testing of the patient to help in evaluating the response to therapy, medication, smoking cessation, or a rehabilitation program

To determine the presence and/or nature of ventilatory limits to exercise, such as decreased flows, increased or decreased lung volumes, and/or decreased diffusing capacity

To determine the presence and/or nature of cardiovascular limits to exercise, such as heart rate, cardiac output, arrhythmias, blood pressure, and/or angina pectoris

To determine the presence and/or nature of muscular limits to exercise such as general deconditioning or decreased local perfusion

Preoperative assessment for a lung resection or transplantation

Assessment for the degree of impairment for disability evaluation

Assess an apparently healthy adult more than 40 years old before starting a vigorous exercise program

---

Table 17-10. Patient Evaluation
Before Testing

History of acute or chronic illness leading to the
   need for stress testing
General physical exam
Resting 12-lead electrocardiogram to exclude
   unexpected cardiac disease
Chest x-ray
Laboratory studies for complete blood count and
   serum electrolytes
Spirometry with measurement of flows, all lung
   volumes and capacities, and maximum
   voluntary ventilation
Carbon monoxide diffusing capacity
Pulse oximetry or arterial blood gases for PaO_2
Before and after bronchodilator spirometry
   studies if the patient is using an inhaled B_2
   medication or has a history of exercise-induced
   asthma

beginning. A physician should be present during the test along with the therapist and possibly a nurse.

Despite the risks involved in the procedure, it is an important diagnostic or clinical evaluation tool for many patients. Table 17-10 lists the steps in the patient workup before testing can be safely performed. Table 17-11 lists the contraindications to exercise testing. Patients with any of these problems are too ill to be jeoparized by the procedure.

Commonly Measured Patient Parameters Specific to Exercise Testing

Metabolic Equivalent of Basal Metabolic Rate

A person who is sleeping or totally relaxed is consuming the minimum number of calories and least amount of oxygen to stay alive. The minimum amount of carbon dioxide is being produced as a waste product of metabolism. He or she is said to be at basal metabolic rate (BMR). At BMR a person consumes about 3.5 ml of oxygen/kilogram of body weight/minute. Multiplying this value by the person's body weight produces the metabolic equivalent of basal metabolic rate for oxygen, or MET as it is abbreviated. The average adult at BMR consumes about 250 ml of oxygen/minute and produces about 200 ml of carbon dioxide/minute. Obviously, the more active a person is the more calories and oxygen are consumed and the more carbon dioxide is produced. Often a person's exercise limit is quantified in terms of how many METs he or she can perform. For example, light household cleaning might be 2 METs of exercise while competetive swimming might be 10 METs of exercise.

Respiratory Quotient and Respiratory Exchange Ratio

Respiratory quotient (RQ) is the ratio, at the cellular level, of the amount of carbon dioxide produced in 1 minute to the amount of oxygen consumed in 1 minute. Using the numbers discussed earlier, the RQ of a resting adult would be calculated as:

Table 17-11. Contraindications to
Exercise Testing

Arterial blood gases:
  PaO_2 less than 50 mm Hg when breathing room
    air
  SpO_2 less than 85% when breathing room air
Pulmonary:
  Severe pulmonary hypertension
  Recent pulmonary embolism
  Untreated or unstable asthma
  $FEV_{1.0}$ less than 30% of predicted
Cardiovascular:
  Myocardial infarction within the last 4 weeks
  Dissecting thoracic or abdominal aortic
    aneurysm
  Dissecting ventricular aneurysm
  Thrombophlebitis
  Systemic embolism
  Uncontrolled hypertension
  Unstable angina pectoris
  Second-degree or third-degree heart block
  Atrial arrhythmias with a rapid ventricular
    response
  Frequent premature ventricular contractions or
    other life-threatening ventricular arrythmias
  Congestive heart failure with pulmonary edema
  Severe aortic stenosis
  Acute pericarditis
  Resting diastolic blood pressure greater than
    110 torr or resting systolic blood pressure
    greater than 200 torr
Neuromuscular disorders that prevent or limit the
  testing
Orthopedic disorders that prevent or limit the
  testing

$$RQ = \frac{\dot{V}CO_2}{\dot{V}O_2} = \frac{200 \, ml \, CO_2}{250 \, ml \, O_2} = .8$$

The RQ of .8 remains quite steady during light to moderate exercise. A normal person can quite easily increase the amount of oxygen consumed and eliminate the extra carbon dioxide produced during exercise. This is what is seen during aerobic metabolism when all body systems are functioning smoothly. It is only during heavy exercise that the body has difficulty coping and must eventually stop. It must be readily apparent that it is impossible to directly measure the RQ because it looks at cellular metabolism; however, the same gases can be easily measured in the lungs.

Respiratory exchange ratio (R or RER) is the ratio, at the alveolar level, of the amount of carbon dioxide produced in 1 minute to the amount of oxygen consumed in 1 minute. Using the earlier numbers and equation, the RER of a resting adult would be calculated as .8 (the same as the RQ).

Maximum Oxygen Consumption and Maximum Carbon Dioxide Production

The maximum oxygen consumption ($\dot{V}O_{2\,max}$) is the highest oxygen consumption attainable by a person. Men have a greater capacity for oxygen consumption than women, and both sexes have a natural decline with age. The oxygen consumption at less than a maximum level is recorded as the volume in milliliters of oxygen used in a minute and abbreviated as $\dot{V}O_2$. The maximum carbon dioxide production ($\dot{V}CO_{2\,max}$) is the highest carbon dioxide production attainable by a person. The carbon dioxide production at less than a maximum level is recorded as the volume in milliliters of CO_2 produced in 1 minute and abbreviated as $\dot{V}CO_2$.

Anaerobic Threshold

Anaerobic threshold (AT) is the highest oxygen consumption during exercise, above which a sustained lactic acidosis occurs. The anaerobic threshold is confirmed as a respiratory quotient of 1.0. This value is reached during heavy exercise at about 50% to 60% of the $\dot{V}O_{2\,max}$. At this exercise level insufficient oxygen reaches the muscles resulting in the formation of lactic acid. This then converts to additional carbon dioxide until the level of CO_2 production equals the level of oxygen consumption. Elderly persons or patients with cardiopulmonary disease are rarely intentionally stressed to the anaerobic threshold.

Maximum Heart Rate

The maximum heart rate (HR_{max}) is the highest heart rate that a person should be able to achieve. Either of the following prediction equations for maximum heart rate in beats per minute can be used (the standard deviation for these formulas is ± 10 to 15 beats per minute):

$$HR_{max} \text{ for males and females} = 210 - (0.65 \times \text{age in years})$$

$$HR_{max} \text{ for males and females} = 220 - (\text{age in years})$$

Because it is obviously hazardous to exercise anyone to their maximum heart rate for a prolonged time, a lower target heart rate is usually calculated. Initially, a target heart rate of 60% to 70% of maximum is often used. Later, as the patient becomes better conditioned, the target heart rate may be raised.

There are many other concepts and formulas that may be studied by the student who wishes to learn more and become more skilled in performing and interpreting stress tests.

Exercise Equipment

Whether the patient is exercising on a treadmill or a bicycle, it is necessary to analyze the exhaled gas for oxygen and carbon dioxide. There are two different types of systems for this. One utilizes a mixing chamber from which the patient's gases are periodically analyzed. The other is a breath-by-breath system that samples and analyzes each exhaled breath (see Fig. 17-16). The measured patient parameters in both systems usually include: a) fraction of exhaled oxygen (F_EO_2), b) fraction of exhaled carbon dioxide (F_ECO_2), c) respiratory rate, d) exhaled gas temperature, e) exhaled volume, and f) time from the start of the test.

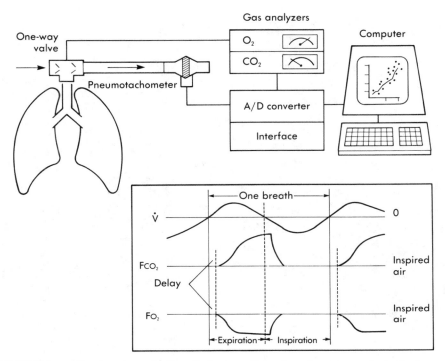

Fig. 17-16 Schematic drawing of a breath-by-breath system for gas analysis during exercise testing. Gas is taken continuously from the sampling port. The gas sample in combination with the pneumotachometer information are integrated by the computer to yield data on average mixes of exhaled oxygen (F_EO_2) and carbon dioxide (F_ECO_2), respiratory rate, tidal volume, minute volume, VO_2, VCO_2, and respiratory quotient. The insert shows a single breath. During inspiration, the oxygen percentage increases and carbon dioxide percentage decreases. During expiration, the oxygen percentage decreases and carbon dioxide percentage increases. There is an unavoidable delay as the gas flows to the analyzer to determine the gas concentrations and send the data to the computer for display. The information that is displayed will still be on a breath-by-breath basis but not synchronized with the patient's real time breathing efforts. (From Ruppel G: *Manual of pulmonary function testing*, ed 5, St. Louis, 1991, Mosby–Year Book. Used by permission.)

Treadmill

The treadmill is a motorized continuously looped belt combined with a ramp. The belt's speed may be adjusted from the stopped position to 1.5 to 10 miles per hour (great enough to exhaust a trained runner). The ramp may be adjusted from flat (0% grade) to sloped (30% grade) (great enough to require the patient to run to keep from falling off the back). There is a railing for the patient to hold if necessary. Commonly there is also an emergency button that the patient can hit to stop the unit. Adjunct equipment is nearby for monitoring the electrocardiogram, exhaled gases, and so forth (see Figure 17-17). The treadmill has an advantage over the bicycle ergometer in that it trains the patient's muscles that are needed for walking. This is an important practical consideration for most patients. However, it is more difficult to quantitate the exercise test results from a treadmill compared to a bicycle because the patient's stride and mechanics of walking vary as the speed increases.

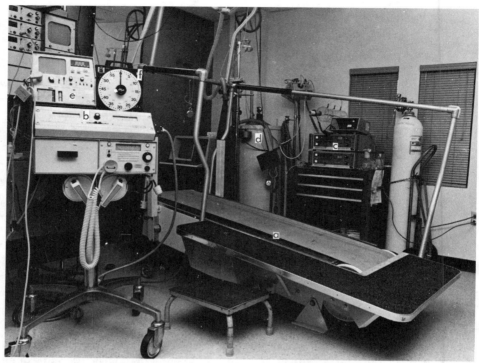

Fig. 17-17 A, A typical treadmill set up for an exercise test. Additional equipment includes: **B,** treadmill controls for speed and slope; **C,** rapid analyzers for oxygen and carbon dioxide (metabolic cart); **D,** Tissot spirometer for measuring the exhaled volume during the test; **E,** electrocardiogram monitor with recorder; **F,** electric timer for the test. (From Ruppel G: *Manual of pulmonary function testing,* ed 5, St. Louis, 1991, Mosby–Year Book. Used by permission.)

Bicycle Ergometer

The bicycle ergometer is a stationary cycle with seat, handle bars, and electronics for calculating distance, effort, and so forth. The electromechanical units as shown in Fig. 17-18 have electronic brakes to increase the patient's workload. Although less practical in training muscles for everyday tasks such as walking, the ergometer allows for easier workload adjustments and calculation of the exercise test results. Other exercise methods such as an arm ergometer or a rowing machine are rarely performed on patients.

Exercise Protocols

There are a number of exercise protocols that may be followed. Basically they fall into one of the two following test catagories and may be performed on either a treadmill or a bicycle ergometer.

Progressive Multistage Test

This test is designed to examine the effects of rapidly increasing work loads on the cardiopulmonary system. A steady state may or may not be reached because the goals are to trend the measured exercise parameters and find the maximum

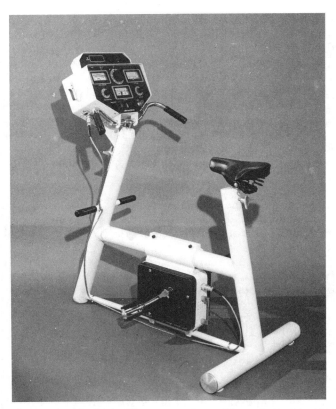

Fig. 17-18 An electromechanical bicycle ergometer with controls for electronic braking, pedaling resistance, test timer, meters for pedaling frequency in revolutions per minute (RPM), and external work load in watts. (From Warren E. Collings, Braintree, Mass. Used by permission.)

work load. The following parameters are measured: maximum oxygen consumption, maximum carbon dioxide production, maximum minute ventilation, and maximum heart rate. This is a less exhausting test than the steady state and may be repeated if necessary. This test may be used for its own purposes or to establish maximum work loads before having the patient perform the steady state test.

Steady State Test

This test is designed to measure cardiopulmonary parameters under steady metabolic conditions. Commonly these levels are 50% and 75% of the predicted maximum oxygen consumption. The following parameters are measured: oxygen consumption, carbon dioxide production, minute ventilation, and heart rate. This is a more exhausting test than the progressive multistage test because it takes longer. It usually is not repeated the same day.

General Steps in the Procedure

1. Explain the procedure to the patient. Answer any questions. Show the patient how to stop the test in case of an emergency. Develop a hand

signal system so that the patient can approve an increase in work load (thumb up) or warn you of the need to stop the test (thumb down).
2. Set up the following monitoring equipment on the patient:

    a. Electrocardiogram with chest leads placed as usual and limb leads moved to the shoulder areas and lower abdominal areas
    b. Pulse oximetry monitor for SpO_2 or (rarely) arterial line for monitoring PaO_2, other blood gas values, and continuous blood pressure
    c. Arm cuff and sphygmomanometer for automatic or manual blood pressure monitoring if an arterial line is not inserted
    d. Mouthpiece with one-way valves or head hood to gather exhaled gases for analysis

3. Have the patient breathe normally through the system and take a set of baseline parameters. Tell the patient to warm up on the equipment by exercising at a low level (approximately 25% of $\dot{V}O_{2\,max}$). Take a set of parameters.
    Note: Steps 4, 5, and 6 are for the steady state test. With the progressive multistage test, the patient will exercise at a given level for only a few minutes before moving to a higher work level.
4. Begin the test by having the patient exercise at a predetermined moderate level (approximately 50% of $\dot{V}O_{2\,max}$) for 5 to 8 minutes. Take a set of parameters in the last 1 to 2 minutes.
5. Increase the work load (approximately 75% of $\dot{V}O_{2\,max}$) and have the patient exercise at it for 5 to 8 minutes. Take a set of parameters in the last 1 to 2 minutes. Alternatively, the patient may be given a short rest period or low exercise period between the steps of increased work load.
6. Repeat step 5, if necessary, at a higher work load until the patient is exhausted or cannot continue because of one of the conditions listed in Table 17-12. The rate of increased work load should be rapid enough that the patient has to stop within 6 to 10 minutes.
7. Have the patient exercise at a low level for several minutes during a cool down/recovery period. It is important to monitor the patient during the recovery period because a sudden drop in blood pressure and fainting are known to occur if exercise should stop too quickly. Note how long it takes for the patient to return to baseline conditions.

Interpret the Results from the Procedure
Normal physiologic changes:

a. Tidal volume, respiratory rate, and minute volume: All patients will find the combination of tidal volume and respiratory rate that allows the most efficient ventilation. Patients with normal lungs will increase their tidal volume to about 60% of their vital capacity. They will then increase the respiratory rate to produce the $\dot{V}_{E\,max}$. Patients with obstructive airways disease are flow limited and cannot increase their respiratory rate adequately. They attempt to raise their tidal volume to increase minute volume but must stop exercising earlier than predicted. Patients with restrictive lung disease cannot increase their tidal volume as expected. Instead, they increase their respiratory rate to raise their minute volume. They too must stop exercising earlier than predicted.
b. Heart rate, stroke volume, and cardiac output: At low and moderate work loads the stroke volume increases from about 80 ml to 110 ml in healthy adults. Increases in heart rate account for the rest of the increase in cardiac output from low to heavy exercise. The heart rate increases are almost parallel with the increases

in $\dot{V}O_2$ (see Fig. 17-19). Patients with diseased left ventricles or heart block are unable to increase cardiac output sufficiently when exercising and must stop earlier than predicted.

c. Oxygen consumption, carbon dioxide production, and respiratory quotient: Both the oxygen consumption and carbon dioxide production will increase linearly with low and moderate exercise. The respiratory quotient will remain about 0.8 or increase slightly. As the subject exercises at levels closer and closer to the $\dot{V}O_{2\,max}$, the muscles are progressively starved for oxygen. This results in local anaerobic metabolism with lactic acid production. Lactic acid in turn converts to carbon dioxide. Because of this added CO_2, the respiratory center is stimulated to increase ventilation even more than expected. Eventually this fails to keep up with the increased production and the CO_2 level increases. The anaerobic threshold is reached when oxygen consumption equals carbon dioxide production and the respiratory quotient reaches 1.0.

d. Blood gases and pH: PaO_2, $PaCO_2$, and pH will remain stable in the normal ranges during low and moderate exercise. The cardiopulmonary system is able to

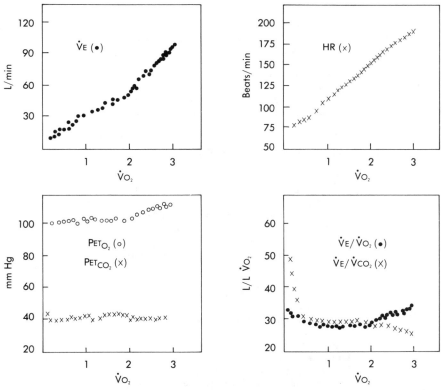

Fig. 17-19 Exercise data showing 30-second averages from a normal adult subject. Heart rate increases linearly as work load is increased and is not the limiting factor in this exercise test. The other three graphic displays show that the anaerobic threshold (AT) occurs at 2 L/min of VO_2. The following key points should be noted: a) minute volume ($\dot{V}_E$) increases sharply at AT; b) end-tidal carbon dioxide ($P_{ET}CO_2$) and the ventilatory equivalent for carbon dioxide (V_E/VCO_2) both decrease at the AT, which shows a disproportionate increase in CO_2 production secondary to lactic acid formation; and c) end-tidal oxygen ($P_{ET}O_2$) and the ventilatory equivalent for oxygen (V_E/VO_2) both increase at the AT. (From Ruppel G: *Manual of pulmonary function testing*, ed 5, St. Louis, 1991, Mosby–Year Book. Used by permission.)

deliver adequate oxygen to the tissues and remove sufficient carbon dioxide to keep the body functioning properly. However, at high levels of work, a lactic acid buildup occurs and a progressive metabolic acidosis is seen. This forces the patient to decrease the exercise level. Some may need to stop. Patients with cardiopulmonary disease will not be able to exercise heavily because they can provide only very limited increases of oxygen to the muscles or eliminate the extra carbon dioxide produced during even moderate exercise. Fig. 17-19 shows the parameter changes seen as a healthy individual exercises from a low to a maximal level.

Limitations Due to Abnormal Physiology

Patients who are forced to stop exercising at a lower than predicted work load will probably fall into one of the following three broad catagories. Table 17-12 lists conditions that would require that the stress test be stopped. Table 17-13 lists parameters that will help in differentiating between deconditioned muscles, pulmonary limitations, or cardiac limitations as the reason that exercise had to be stopped.

Table 17-12. Indications for Stopping an Exercise Test

Arterial blood gases
   PaO_2 decreasing to less than 55 mm Hg
   Acidosis with or without a rise in the $PaCO_2$
   SpO_2 less than 83% or 10% less than the
      baseline value
Pulmonary
   Exercise-induced bronchospasm
   Severe dyspnea
Cardiovascular
   20 torr fall in systolic blood pressure below the
      baseline value
   Systolic blood pressure greater than 250 mm Hg
   Diastolic blood pressure greater than 120 mm Hg
   Onset of angina pectoris
   Frequent premature ventricular contractions
      (PVCs)
   Ventricular tachycardia
   ST segment depression or elevation of more
      than 1 mm
   Onset of second-degree or third-degree heart
      block
   Onset of left or right bundle branch block
Equipment
   Monitoring equipment failure
   Unavailability of CPR equipment and defibrillator
Miscellaneous
   Request by patient, lightheadedness, mental
      confusion, or headache
   Muscle cramping
   Nausea or vomiting
   Sweating and pallor
   Cyanosis

Table 17-13. Exercise Intolerance: Differentiating Between Heart Disease, Lung Disease, and Deconditioned Muscles

Parameter	Heart Disease	Lung Disease	Deconditioned Muscles
$VO_{2\,max}$	D	D	D
Heart rate reserve	D	I	I
Breathing reserve	N	D	N
Exercise PaO_2 or SpO_2	N	D	N
VO_2 at anaerobic threshold	D	N	D
VO_2/heart rate	D	N	N
Exercise A-aDO_2	N	I	N
Exercise V_D/V_T	N	I	N
Exercise electrocardiogram	Abnormal	Normal	Normal
Common chief complaint	Chest pain	Dyspnea Bronchospasm	Leg fatigue or cramps

D, decreased; I, increased; N, normal.
(Based on a table in Sue D: Exercise testing and the patient with cardiopulmonary disease. In Goldman AL, editor: *Problems in pulmonary disease*, 2(1), 1986.)

Deconditioned Muscles

Normal, healthy people are quite commonly seen in this catagory. They are deconditioned from lack of exercise. These people are able to do quite well in a training program if there are no underlying cardiopulmonary limitations.

Pulmonary Limitations

As discussed earlier, patients with obstructive airways disease or restrictive lung disease have limited ventilatory reserve. This limits their exercise tolerance even if they have a normal cardiovascular system. If the limitation is due to bronchospasm, this may be treated by inhaling a bronchodilator before exercising. These patients may also be able to increase their exercise tolerance if given supplemental oxygen to prevent desaturation.

Cardiovascular Limitations

Patients with a damaged or diseased left ventricle, heart block, exercise-induced angina because of coronary artery disease, hypertension, and so forth are unable to exercise to expected levels. Medical or surgical intervention may enable them to increase their work level.

9. Sleep apnea studies.
    a. Review the patient's chart for information on any previous sleep studies. (IA1i1) [R]

It is important to review the results of any previous sleep study. Determine what physiologic parameters were measured and how the patient's parameters varied during the sleep study. Be sure to review the physician's interpretation of the sleep study results.

b. Assist with a sleep apnea study. (IIIE1g) [R, Ap]

A sleep apnea study is performed to determine if the patient has sleep disordered breathing. Furthermore, it can help to determine the type of disorder and follow the patient's response to treatment. See Table 17-14 for the indications for a cardiopulmonary sleep study. As a point of understanding, a cardiopulmonary sleep study means that the physician is primarily interested in the patient's cardiac and pulmonary variables found during sleep. A polysomnography sleep study has a broader meaning and refers to a method of identifying and evaluating the patient's sleep-state and a number of physiologic variables during sleep. The following physiologic parameters are usually measured during a cardiopulmonary sleep study:

a. Sleep stages through an electroencephalogram (EEG) recording of brain wave activity and electrooculogram (EOG) recording of eye movements
b. Inspiratory and expiratory airflow by nasal thermistor, pneumotachograph, or end-tidal carbon dioxide analyzer
c. Inspiratory and expiratory effort by esophageal pressure measurement or respiratory inductive plethysmography
d. Oxygen saturation by ear or bridge of nose oximetry; finger oximetry is not recommended because of patient movement
e. Body position related to normal and abnormal breathing patterns
f. Periodic arm and leg movements
g. Electrocardiogram for monitoring purposes

The respiratory therapist may be responsible for preparing the patient and setting up the equipment and supplies. Each hospital or physician may have a prescribed way of doing this. The general steps are listed here:

1. Inform the patient of the procedure and have him or her sign the medical release form.
2. Attach the monitoring leads and equipment to the patient.
3. Calibrate the equipment and make sure that it is working properly.
4. Assist the physician with the procedure as needed. Record the patient's parameters during the course of a 6-hour or longer sleep period. The patient may also be video and audio recorded during the sleep period.
5. Make any adjustments in the patient's respiratory care equipment as needed.

Table 17-14. Indications for a Cardiopulmonary Sleep Study

Patient with COPD whose awake PaO_2 is greater than 55 mm Hg but who has pulmonary hypertension, right heart failure (cor pulmonale), or polycythemia.
Patient whose awake PaO_2 is less than 55 mm Hg without continuous supplemental oxygen and who needs to have the proper oxygen flow rate set for sleeping at night. Overnight sleep ear oximetry should be performed.
Patient with restrictive ventilatory impairment secondary to chest wall or neuromuscular disturbances who also has chronic hypoventilation, polycythemia, pulmonary hypertension, disturbed sleep, morning headaches, or daytime somnolence and fatigue.
Patient with awake $PaCO_2$ greater than 45 mm Hg who also has polycythemia, pulmonary hypertension, disturbed sleep, morning headaches, or daytime somnolence and fatigue.
Patient with snoring, obesity, and other symptoms indicating disturbed sleep pattern.
Patient with excessive daytime sleepiness or sleep maintenance insomnia.
Patient with nocturnal cyclic bradytachyarrhythmias, atrioventricular conduction abnormalities while asleep, or increased abnormal ventricular beats compared to when awake.

6. Dispose of any used supplies and so forth after the procedure is completed.
7. Tend to the patient's comfort.

The cardiopulmonary sleep study is important but only as part of the patient's work-up for a diagnosis. The following steps are usually also performed:

History of the problem from both the patient's and the bed partner's viewpoint
Physical examination including neck, upper airway, blood pressure, heart rate, and respiratory rate and pattern
Arterial blood gases
Hemoglobin
Thyroid function
Chest and upper airway x-rays; may include a computed axial tomographic scan of the upper airway if obstructive sleep apnea is suspected
Electrocardiogram

c. Interpret the results of a sleep study. (IB9o and IC1g) [R, Ap, An]

Apnea is the cessation of breathing for 10 seconds or longer. For a diagnosis of sleep apnea to be given to a patient, he or she must experience at least 30 apneic periods during 6 hours of sleep. The EEG tracing should confirm that the apnea periods occur during both of the major sleep stages. The first stage is called *nonrapid eye movement* (non-REM) sleep and starts soon after the person loses consciousness. The second stage is called *rapid eye movement* (REM) sleep and follows after the non-REM stage. Normally people cycle through both stages about every 1 to 1½ hours during the night. This normal cycle of sleep is important for both mental and physical health. People with disturbed sleep do not dream as they should and are not physically rested when they rise for the day.

Obstructive Sleep Apnea

Obstructive sleep apnea results when the patient's upper airway is obstructed despite continued breathing efforts (see Figs. 17-20 and 17-21). Patients with this problem often exhibit the following symptoms: loud snoring (reported by the bed partner), morning headache, excessive daytime sleepiness, depression or other personality changes, decreased intellectual ability, sexual dysfunction, bed wetting (nocturnal enuresis), and/or abnormal limb movements during sleep.

Obstructive sleep apnea is associated with the following: middle age males, obesity, short neck, hypothyroidism, testosterone administration, myotonic dystrophy, temporomandibular joint disease (TMJ disease), narrowed upper airway from excessive pharyngeal tissue, enlarged tongue (macroglossia), enlarged tonsils or adenoids, deviated nasal septum, recessed jaw (micrognathia), goiter, laryngeal stenosis or web, or pharyngeal neoplasm. Management of patients with obstructive sleep apnea may include any of the following:

Weight reduction
Sleeping on either side or the abdomen; do not sleep in the supine position
Continuous positive airway pressure (CPAP) mask or BiPAP mask
Surgery to open the airway: mandibular advancement, palatopharyngoplasty, or tracheostomy

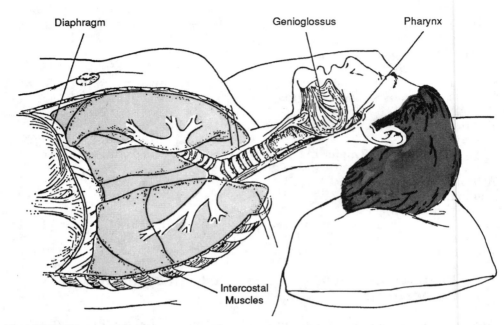

Fig. 17-20 Obstructive sleep apnea. These patients often obstruct when lying supine and the genioglossus muscle of the tongue fails to oppose the negative force on the airway during an inspiration. (From Des Jardins TL: *Clinical manifestations of respiratory disease*, ed 2, St. Louis, 1990, Year Book Medical. Used by permission.)

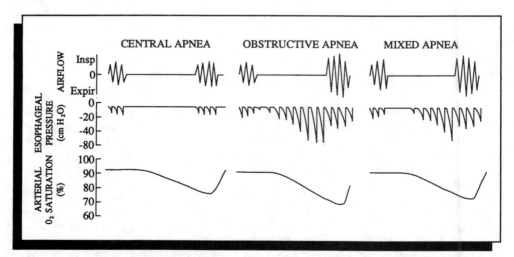

Fig. 17-21 Typical patterns of airflow, esophageal pressure showing respiratory effort, and arterial oxygen saturation produced by central, obstructive, and mixed sleep apnea. Central apnea shows a lack of respiratory effort resulting in no airflow. Obstructive apnea shows a continued respiratory effort but no airflow due to the airway obstruction. Mixed apnea starts out with an initial lack of respiratory effort (central apnea). Later, breathing efforts are made but there is no airflow due to the airway obstruction (obstructive apnea). Arterial desaturation results from all three types of apnea. When the desaturation becomes great enough and the carbon dioxide level high enough, the patient (hopefully) awakens enough to breathe again. (From Des Jardins TL: *Clinical manifestations of respiratory disease*, ed 2, St. Louis, 1989, Mosby–Year Book. Used by permission.)

The medication protriptyline (Triptil, Vivactil) to decrease REM sleep when
most obstructive episodes occur

Have the patient wear a tongue-retaining device to prevent it from
obstructing the pharynx

Have the patient wear a neck collar to keep the head and neck aligned with
the body

Central Sleep Apnea

Central sleep apnea is diagnosed when the respiratory center of the medulla
fails to signal the respiratory muscles for breathing to occur. The patient makes no
respiratory effort and there is no air movement (see Fig. 17-21). Patients with
this problem often exhibit these symptoms or traits: normal weight; mild snoring;
insomnia; and lesser levels of daytime sleepiness, depression, or sexual dysfunction
than the obstructive sleep apnea patient.

Central sleep apnea is associated with the following: primary alveolar (idio-
pathic) hypoventilation (Ondine's curse), muscular dystrophy, bilateral cervical
cordotomy, bulbar poliomyelitis, encephalitis, brain stem infarction or neoplasm,
spinal surgery, and hypothyroidism. Management of patients with central sleep
apnea may include the following:

Negative pressure ventilation for sleeping

Intubation or trachesotomy and positive pressure ventilation if the patient
has acute ventilatory failure

Phrenic nerve pacemaker

Mixed Sleep Apnea

Mixed sleep apnea is diagnosed when the patient shows evidence of both
central and obstructive apnea. It is usually found that the patient first stops all
breathing efforts (central apnea). After a period of time, the patient makes attempts
to breathe but cannot because the upper airway is blocked (obstructive apnea) (see
Fig. 17-21). Patients with mixed sleep apnea may show a variety of symptoms
and traits from those listed earlier. Clinical management may include any of the
treatments mentioned that prove to be effective.

Whatever the cause of the sleep apnea, it must be treated. If left to continue
its pathological course, the patient may develop a number of problems such as
pulmonary hypertension, cor pulmonale, polycythemia, cardiac arrhythmias, and
even unexplained nocturnal death. Minimally, the patient's personal, family, and
social life will suffer.

This ends the general discussion on special procedures that the respiratory
therapist is expected to be able to perform. They may be tested on both of the
registry exams.

Module C.   Patient assessment.

1.   Examine all the data to determine the patient's pathophysiological condition. (IC3a) [R, Ap, An]

Some discussion on pathophysiology was presented in the earlier discussions.
It is recommended that further study of cardiopulmonary and related disease states
and conditions be undertaken if necessary.

2. Take part in the development of the respiratory care plan. (IC3b) [An]

Be prepared to work with other members of the health care team to determine the patient's care plan. Based on the patient's progress or failure to meet the plan's objectives, be prepared to make recommendations on how the care plan should be modified.

Module D. Perform respiratory care quality assurance procedures. (IC3b) [R, Ap, An]

The broad concept of quality assurance can be viewed as a personal and department philosophy that ensures constant improvement in production and service. There are a number of ways to approach the subject. A key to quality assurance is understanding what the respiratory care department is there to do for the patients, the physicians, the nurses, and other allied health professionals, as well as the hospital. Once these are determined the quality assurance program can be instituted. Minimally, the following can be done:

1. Make sure that all respiratory care equipment is working properly or, if malfunctioning, is repaired.
2. Audit the patient's medical records to find out if all ordered services were performed. If not, find out why.
3. Communicate with patients during their hospitalization and after discharge to find out their impressions of the care they received.
4. Communicate with the physicians, nurses, and so forth to find out if their needs are being met for optimizing patient care.
5. Work with the hospital administration to find ways to contain unnecessary costs, expand into new areas as opportunities arise, and so forth.

Module E. Monitor the effectiveness of equipment sterilization procedures. (IIA2) [Ap]

Surveillance is the term used to describe the monitoring of equipment to be sure that the disinfection or sterilization process was successful and that in-use equipment is not a source of patient contamination. Processing indicators are used to ensure that disinfection or sterilization was done correctly. Examples include special tapes used to hold wrapping around packages of equipment being autoclaved or placed into ethylene oxide. These tapes turn color when the autoclave has reached the proper temperature or the correct concentration of ethylene oxide has been reached. Besides showing the user that the package was processed correctly, it identifies sterile from unsterile wrapped packages.

Another example is a biological indicator placed into the wrapped package before it is sterilized. These biological indicators are bacterial spores that are only killed if the required conditions are met. After the equipment and spores have been sent through the sterilization process, the spores are placed into conditions favorable for growth. If no growth occurs, they are dead. It can then be concluded that no other living organisms survived.

Equipment that is held in storage or being used in patient care is also randomly sampled for contamination. There are three ways that a sample is taken for culturing of possible organisms. The first involves a sterile swab being wiped onto an equipment surface. It is then rubbed over a plate of growth medium or placed into a tube of liquid broth. The second is used to check inside lengths of tubing. It requires a liquid broth to be poured through the tube and into a sterile container. The third involves sampling the aerosol that a nebulizer produces. Usually, a hose is attached to the outlet of the nebulizer. The other end of the hose is connected to a funnel that is attached to a culture plate where the droplets impact. In all three examples, the growth of any organisms in the growth medium indicates a form of contamination. The laboratory then determines if the organism is pathogenic. If it is, measures will need to be taken to improve the disinfection or sterilization process.

BIBLIOGRAPHY

AARC Clinical Practice Guideline: Exercise testing for evaluation of hypoxemia and/or desaturation, *Respir Care* 37(8):907-912, 1992.

Anderson HL, Bartlett RH: Respiratory care of the surgical patient. In Burton GG, Hodgkin JE, Ward JJ, editors: *Respiratory care: a guide to clinical practice*, ed 3, Philadelphia, 1991, JB Lippincott.

Bloom BS, Daniel JM, Wiseman M et al: Transtracheal oxygen delivery and patients with chronic obstructive pulmonary disease, *Respir Med* 83:281-288, 1989.

Brutinel WM, Cortese DA: Bronchoscopy. In Burton GG, Hodgkin JE, Ward JJ, editors: *Respiratory care: a guide to clinical practice*, ed 3, Philadelphia, 1991, JB Lippincott.

Chadha TS, Schneider AW, Tobin MJ et al: Noninvasive monitoring of breathing patterns during wakefulness and sleep, *Respir Ther* 27-40, May/June 1985.

Chavis AD, Grum CM: Fiberoptic bronchoscopy with mechanical ventilation, *Choices in Respiratory Management* 21(1):4-9, 1991.

Chavis AD, Grum CM: Pulmonary procedures during mechanical ventilation, *Choices in Respiratory Management* 21(2):29-33, 1991.

Christopher KL, Spofford BT, Petrun MD et al: A program for transtracheal oxygen delivery, *Ann Intern Med* 107:802-980, 1987.

Cofer JI, Greeley HP: *Quality improvement techniques for respiratory care*, Marblehead, Mass, 1994, Opus Communications.

Coppolo DP, Brienza LT, Pratt DS et al: A role for the respiratory therapist in flexible fiberoptic bronchoscopy, *Respir Care* 30(5):323-327, 1985.

Couperus JJ, Elder HA: Infectious disease aspects of respiratory therapy. In Burton GG, Hodgkin JE, editors: *Respiratory care: a guide to clinical practice*, ed 2, Philadelphia, 1984, JB Lippincott.

Curity thoracentesis tray package insert, Kendall Hospital Products, Boston, Mass.

Decker MJ, Smith BL, Strohl KP: Center-based vs. patient-based diagnosis and therapy of sleep-related respiratory disorders and role of the respiratory care practitioner, *Respir Care* 39(4):390-400, 1994.

Deshpande VM, Pilbeam SP, Dixon RJ: *A comprehensive review in respiratory care*, East Norwalk, Conn, 1988, Appleton & Lange.

Des Jardins TL: *Clinical manifestations of respiratory disease*, ed 2, St. Louis, 1990, Year Book Medical.

Erickson RA: Chest drainage. I, *Nursing89* 19(5):37-43, 1989.

Erickson RA: Chest drainage. II, *Nursing89* 19(6):47-49, 1989.

Eubanks DH, Bone RC: *Comprehensive respiratory care: a learning system*, ed 2, St. Louis, 1990, Mosby–Year Book.

Garay SM: Therapeutic options for obstructive sleep apnea, *Respir Management* 17(4):11-17, 1987.

Guidelines for fiberoptic bronchoscopy, *ATS News* 12(2):14-15, 1986.

Howard TP: Foreign body extraction by means of combined rigid and flexible bronchoscopy: a case report, *Respir Care* 33(9):786-789, 1988.

Indications and standards for cardiopulmonary sleep studies, *Am Rev Respir Dis* 139:559-568, 1989.

Kaplan J: Diagnosis and therapy of sleep-disordered breathing. In Burton GG, Hodgkin JE, Ward JJ, editors: *Respiratory care: a guide to clinical practice*, ed 3, Philadelphia, 1991, JB Lippincott.

Lough MD: Transportation of the high-risk infant. In Lough MD, Williams TJ, Rawson JE, editors: *Newborn respiratory care*, Chicago, 1979, Year Book Medical.

Manufacturer's literature, Transtracheal Oxygen Systems, Denver, Colo.

Mathewson HS: Drug therapy for obstructive sleep apnea, *Respir Care* 31(8):717-719, 1986.

Mims BC: You *can* manage chest tubes confidently, *RN* 39-44, Jan 1985.

Mishoe SC: The diagnosis and treatment of sleep apnea syndrome, *Respir Care* 32(3):183-201, 1987.

Peters RM: Chest trauma. In Moser KM, Spragg RG, editors: *Respiratory emergencies*, ed 2, St. Louis, 1982, Mosby–Year Book.

Phillipson EA: Breathing disorders during sleep, *Basics Respir Dis* 7(3):1-6, 1979.

Plevak DJ, Ward JJ: Airway management. In Burton GG, Hodgkin JE, Ward JJ, editors: *Respiratory care: a guide to clinical practice*, ed 3, Philadelphia, 1991, JB Lippincott.

Podnos SD, Chappell TR: Hemoptysis: a clinical update, *Respir Care* 30(11):977-985, 1985.

Rapaport DM: Techniques for administering nasal CPAP, *Respir Management* 17(4):17-21, 1987.

Scanlan CL, Gupta TL: Synopsis of cardiopulmonary diseases. In Scanlan CL, Spearman CB, Sheldon RL, editors: *Egan's fundamentals of respiratory care*, ed 5, St. Louis, 1990, Mosby–Year Book.

Shapiro BA, Kacmarek RM, Cane RD et al: *Clinical application of respiratory care*, ed 4, St. Louis, 1991, Mosby–Year Book.

Sills, JR: *Respiratory care certification guide—the complete review resource for the entry level exam*, ed 2, St. Louis, 1994, Mosby–Year Book.

Simmons KF: Airway care. In Scanlan CL, Spearman CB, Sheldon RL, editors: *Egan's fundamentals of respiratory care*, ed 5, St. Louis, 1990, Mosby–Year Book.

Van Hooser DT: The role of the RCP in transtracheal oxygen therapy: looking beyond the nasal cannula, *NBRC Horizons* 18(5):1-3, 1992.

Williams SF, Thompson JM: Respiratory disorders, St. Louis, 1990, Mosby–Year Book.

SELF-STUDY QUESTIONS

1. Your patient is being mechanically ventilated when the nurse calls you to evaluate her condition. You discover that the patient's breath sounds are absent over the left lung field, the left-sided percussion note is hyperresonant, and the peak airway pressures have increased from 40 to 65 cm water. What would you recommend?
   A. Place a pleural chest tube into the right side.
   B. Increase the tidal volume to better inflate the atelectatic left lung.
   C. Change the mode to SIMV from assist/control.
   D. Place a pleural chest tube into the left side.
   E. Decrease the respiratory rate to allow a longer expiratory time to minimize air trapping.

2. You notice that air is bubbling through the water seal of the patient's pleural drainage system when she coughs. This tells you that:
   A. The vacuum has to be increased.
   B. There is still air leaking through a tear in the lung.
   C. The proper level of vacuum has been set.
   D. There is a leak in the system.
   E. The patient should not be allowed to cough.

3. The best way to obtain a sample of mucus that will contain only those organisms from the lower respiratory tract would be:
   A. Bronchoscopy
   B. Have the patient cough into an open container for transport to the lab.
   C. Nasotracheal suctioning
   D. Transtracheal aspiration
   E. Oropharyngeal suctioning

4. After a sleep study has been performed, your patient is given a diagnosis of obstructive sleep apnea. His physician asks for your advice on the best method of management. You would recommend:
   A. The patient should use nasal CPAP when sleeping.
   B. The patient should sleep with an oropharyngeal airway to keep the tongue forward in the mouth.
   C. Have the patient always sleep on his back.
   D. The patient should have a home negative pressure ventilator for sleeping.
   E. A tracheostomy should be performed and he should be placed on a volume cycled ventilator to sleep.

5. You are assisting a physician with a tracheostomy procedure on a patient with an oral endotracheal tube. When should you withdraw the endotracheal tube?
   A. After the tracheostomy tube has been inserted.
   B. After the cuff of the tracheostomy tube has been inflated.
   C. As the tracheostomy tube is placed into the stoma.
   D. Before the stoma is made.
   E. As the trachea is surgically entered.

6. Your mechanically ventilated patient is going to have a flexible fiberoptic bronchoscopy performed. What kinds of considerations must you be aware of?
   I. The tidal volume must be monitored for a leak.
   II. The inspiratory flow resistance will increase.
   III. The inspiratory pressure will decrease.
   IV. The inspiratory pressure will increase.
   A. I
   B. II
   C. III
   D. II, III
   E. I, II, IV

7. During the transportation of your patient the chest tube drainage system is pulled off of the drainage tubing and cracked open. Your best response is to:
   A. Call the physician for instructions.
   B. Clamp the tube near the patient's chest at once.
   C. Hold the distal end of the tubing a few centimeters below the surface of a bottle of sterile water or saline.
   D. Leave the tube open to the atmosphere.

E.   Have the patient perform the Valsalva maneuver until a new system can be set up.

8.   All the following should be done when preparing to helicopter transport an adult patient EXCEPT:
   A.   Select a heated humidification system with the smallest internal compressible volume.
   B.   Calculate the duration of the oxygen cylinder that will be used.
   C.   Select a ventilator that uses a demand valve IMV system rather than one with an external reservoir IMV system.
   D.   Select a lightweight and portable ventilator.

9.   A subject was found to have a $\dot{V}O_2$ of 2000 ml and a $\dot{V}CO_2$ of 1700 ml during an exercise test. Calculate her respiratory exchange ratio (RER).
   A.   .85
   B.   1.18
   C.   3700
   D.   2000
   E.   1700

10.   Your patient is performing an exercise test and has the following signs and symptoms: systolic blood pressure of 260 mm Hg, cyanosis, headache, and dizziness. Which of the following would you recommend?
   A.   Continue the test until the anaerobic threshold is reached.
   B.   Continue the test until the patient's RQ hits 1.1.
   C.   Stop the test.
   D.   Continue the test until the patient complains of shortness of breath.
   E.   Continue the test at a lower work level.

11.   When preparing to assist the physician with the cardioversion of a patient it is important to check the following:
   I.   A strong R wave should be seen on the ECG monitor.
   II.   The charge level should be set as ordered.
   III. The electrode paddles should be kept clean so that there is the best possible conduction.
   IV.   Make sure the ECG electrodes are attached properly.
   A.   I, III
   B.   I, II, IV
   C.   III, IV
   D.   I, II, III, IV
   E.   I, III, IV

12.   The respiratory quotient (RQ) found at the anaerobic threshold is:
   A.   .7
   B.   .8
   C.   .9
   D.   1.0
   E.   1.1

13.   Calculate the maximum heart rate for a 55-year-old woman who is about to undergo a stress test.
   A.   55/minute
   B.   175/minute
   C.   275/minute

D.   265/minute
E.   110/minute

14.   You are going to assist in the thoracentesis of a mechanically ventilated patient. She cannot sit up on the edge of the bed because of weakness. You would recommend the following position for the procedure:
A.   Lying with the abnormal side down on the bed
B.   Lying supine on the bed
C.   Lying face down on the bed
D.   Supine on the bed with the head down 30°
E.   Lying with the normal side down on the bed

15.   Which of the following statements is true of ventilation during low to moderate exercise?
A.   It decreases as VO_2 increases.
B.   It decreases as V_D/V_D increases.
C.   It varies unpredictably in normal adult subjects.
D.   It increases as workload levels increase.
E.   It remains constant in normal subjects as workload levels increase.

16.   After assisting with a thoracentesis where 1400 ml of straw yellow fluid was removed, the patient complains of shortness of breath and has an increased heart and respiratory rate. What would you recommend to further evaluate the patient's reaction to the procedure?
I.   Pulse oximetry
II.   Chest x-ray
III.   Send the fluid to the laboratory for analysis
IV.   Remove additional fluid
A.   I
B.   I, II
C.   III
D.   III, IV
E.   II, IV

17.   All the following are tasks that would be performed by a respiratory therapist in a transtracheal catheter placement EXCEPT:
A.   Inserting the catheter into the patient's trachea.
B.   Informing the patient about the procedure.
C.   Preparing the necessary supplies.
D.   Monitoring the patient's pulse oximetry value and vital signs.
E.   Adjusting the patient's inspired oxygen flow.

Answer Key

1. D; 2. B; 3. D; 4. A; 5. C; 6. E; 7. C; 8. A; 9. A; 10. C; 11. B; 12. D; 13. B;
14. E; 15. D; 16. B; 17. A.

Appendix 1
Posttest: Practice Written
Registry Examination

Instructions

Select the best answer to each question. No calculators or notes may be used. The test must be finished within 2 hours. See the answer key and explanations at the end of the test to evaluate your performance.

Note: This examination is modeled on actual retired Written Registry Examinations given by the NBRC. The same styles of questions are used. It is made up of the same mix of questions that have historically been seen on the actual Written Registry Examinations. (See "Relative Weights of the Various Tested Areas on the Written Registry Exam" in the frontmatter.) However, no claim is made that the actual NBRC exam will match this practice exam.

1. The pulmonary capillary wedge pressure (PCWP) best represents:
   A. Right ventricular pressure
   B. Left atrial pressure
   C. Right atrial pressure
   D. Pulmonary artery pressure

2. Based on the following lung volume results, what is this patient's TLC?

   VC = 3500 ml
   FRC = 4000 ml
   ERV = 1200 ml

   A. 4700 ml
   B. 2800 ml
   C. 6300 ml
   D. 5200 ml

3. Your patient has adult respiratory distress syndrome (ARDS) and is being managed on a volume ventilator. What is the best way to reduce the patient's intrapulmonary shunting?
   A. Increase the level of therapeutic PEEP.
   B. Increase the sigh volume.
   C. Decrease the expiratory time.
   D. Add inflation hold.

4. A patient with an upper airway obstruction is receiving helium-oxygen therapy by a non-rebreathing mask. The respiratory therapist notices that the reservoir bag is completely collapsing on inspiration. What is the cause of the problem?

    A.   The mask is loose on the patient's face.
    B.   The one-way valves on the mask are on backwards.
    C.   The flow of helium and oxygen to the reservoir bag is too low.
    D.   The helium and oxygen mixture is too dense.

5.   The presence of subcutaneous emphysema would be identified on a chest x-ray by:
    A.   A dark area without lung markings
    B.   Increased lucency in soft tissues of the axilla or neck areas
    C.   Mediastinal shift
    D.   Increased opacification of the lungs

6.   A 50-year-old polio victim with a permanent tracheostomy is recovering from pneumonia. He is only placed on the ventilator at night to rest. The respiratory therapist should suggest that the patient's usual tracheostomy tube be changed to the following during the day:
    A.   A metal tube without a cuff
    B.   A transtracheal oxygen catheter
    C.   An endotracheal tube that has been cut shorter
    D.   A fenestrated tube with a low pressure cuff

7.   In which of the following situations should the respiratory therapist make the recommendation to minimize the aerosol output of a nebulizer?
    I.   An adult patient with dried, retained secretions complains of increased dyspnea.
    II.   An adult patient has chronic bronchitis.
    III.   An infant has pulmonary edema.
    A.   II
    B.   III
    C.   II, III
    D.   I, III

8.   Which of the following would be a normally observed respiratory rate for a newborn?
    A.   14 to 19/minute
    B.   20 to 24/minute
    C.   25 to 30/minute
    D.   30 or more/minute

9.   A patient entering a pulmonary rehabilitation program should be told to expect to realize long-term benefits in all the following areas EXCEPT:
    A.   His or her disease will be reversed.
    B.   Increased energy for activities of daily living.
    C.   Better tolerance of dyspnea.
    D.   Fewer hospitalizations.

10.   You are helping in a resuscitation attempt of a 200 pound man who is in ventricular fibrillation. The physician has just attempted defibrillation with 200 joules (watt-seconds) of power. Because the ECG monitor shows the patient to still be in ventricular fibrillation, what should you recommend?
    A.   Reattempt defibrillation at 200 joules.
    B.   Increase the power to 300 joules and reattempt defibrillation.
    C.   Instill racemic epinephrine (Vaponephrine) down the endotracheal tube.
    D.   Increase the power to 400 joules and reattempt defibrillation.

11. To calculate a dead space to tidal volume ratio (V_D/V_T), which of the following must be known?
    I. PaO_2
    II. PvO_2
    III. $PaCO_2$
    IV. P_ECO_2
    A. I, II
    B. III, IV
    C. II, IV
    D. II, III, IV

12. Bilevel positive pressure ventilation with a nasal mask and the BiPAP device is indicated in patients with all the following EXCEPT:
    A. Patient with upper airway obstruction and sleep apnea.
    B. Patient with chronic ventilatory muscle dysfunction as an aid to sleeping.
    C. Patient in ventilatory failure refuses intubation.
    D. Patient with variable airway resistance and lung compliance.

13. Your patient with moderate emphysema is about to be discharged. He is going to need 1 liter per minute of oxygen on a continuous basis. He wants to be able to walk his pet dog around the block. Which of the following would you, as his home care therapist, get for him?
    I. A Linde Walker unit
    II. An oxygen concentrator
    III. A bank of H cylinders of oxygen
    IV. An E cylinder of oxygen
    A. I
    B. II
    C. II, IV
    D. I, II

14. The respiratory therapist must perform a calibration check on a water seal spirometer. Which of the following should be performed?
    I. Check the accuracy of the timer, recorder, and kymograph.
    II. Make sure that there are no air leaks in the circuit, valves, and gas sampling devices.
    III. Check the accuracy of the thermometer.
    IV. Use a super syringe to confirm the volume accuracy of the unit.
    A. I, II
    B. I, II, III, IV
    C. II, IV
    D. I, II, III

15. Your patient is being mechanically ventilated and requires PEEP to keep an acceptable PaO_2. Despite 30 mm Hg pressure in the cuff, there is still a significant tidal volume leak. Which of the following should be done?
    A. Insert a larger diameter endotracheal tube with a high volume, low pressure cuff.
    B. Leave the cuff inflated to 30 mm Hg.
    C. Deflate the cuff to less than 20 mm Hg and increase the delivered tidal volume to compensate for the leak.
    D. Deflate the cuff to less than 20 mm Hg and increase the respiratory rate to compensate for the leak.

16. A thermodilution flow-directed pulmonary artery (Swan-Ganz) catheter has been placed into a patient. The following data have been obtained:

    Pulmonary capillary wedge pressure (PCWP) = 9 mm Hg
    Pulmonary artery pressure (PAP) = 45/25 mm Hg
    Cardiac output (CO) = 5.5 L/min

    The patient most likely has:
    A. Heart failure
    B. Hypovolemic shock
    C. Mitral valve stenosis
    D. Pulmonary hypertension

17. A worried parent has brought her 18-month-old child into the emergency room. The child has a history of suddenly developing inspiratory stridor while eating. Which of the following would be the most important in helping to determine the cause of the child's respiratory distress?
    A. Arterial blood gases
    B. Anteroposterior chest x-ray
    C. Upper airway x-ray
    D. Maximum inspiratory force test done at the bedside

18. A patient is receiving postural drainage therapy to drain the right posterior basal segment. The patient begins to cough vigorously. What would you do?
    A. Give the patient a tissue to cough into.
    B. Turn the patient onto the right side.
    C. Nebulize Xylocaine into the patient's airway to stop the coughing.
    D. Have the patient sit up to cough.

19. The respiratory therapist is asked by the physician to prepare a tray for an oral intubation of an 19-year-old patient. All the following would be needed EXCEPT:
    A. An intubation handle
    B. A straight (Miller) laryngoscope blade
    C. A curved (MacIntosh) laryngoscope blade
    D. Magill forceps

20. You are called to participate in the helicopter transportation of an adult patient with multiple trauma. It is important to do all the following in preparation for the flight EXCEPT:
    A. Calculate how long the oxygen cylinder will last at the expected flow rate.
    B. Select a heated humidifier for an adult.
    C. Choose a transport ventilator that is small and lightweight.
    D. Select a transport ventilator that uses a demand valve for IMV rather than a reservoir system.

21. When initiating positive expiratory pressure (PEP) therapy it is important that the patient:
    I. Have an I : E ratio of about 1 : 3.
    II. Generate a positive expiratory pressure of between 5 and 10 cm water.
    III. Inhale a deeper than normal tidal volume.
    IV. Have an I : E ratio of about 1 : 1.
    V. Generate a positive expiratory pressure of between 10 and 20 cm water.
    A. II, IV
    B. III, IV, V

C.   I, III, V
D.   II, III, IV

22.   A tracheostomy button is indicated to:
A.   Stabilize a transtracheal oxygen catheter
B.   Allow for positive pressure ventilation without a high pressure cuff
C.   Keep a patent tracheostomy stoma
D.   Allow a patient who had his or her larynx removed to vocalize

23.   A pneumothorax would be identified on a chest x-ray as:
A.   A white butterfly or bat-wing–shaped pattern
B.   A dark area that contains lung markings
C.   A white area with air bronchograms
D.   A dark area that does not contain any lung markings

24.   For which of the following can a flow-directed pulmonary artery (Swan-Ganz) catheter be used?
I.   To obtain a sample of mixed venous blood
II.   To measure pulmonary artery pressure
III.   To measure pulmonary capillary wedge pressure
IV.   To estimate the left ventricular end-diastolic pressure
A.   III, IV
B.   I, II
C.   II, III, IV
D.   I, II, III, IV

25.   A neonate is being mechanically ventilated on the IMV mode. During the last 2 hours the patient's PaO_2 has decreased from 60 to 45 mm Hg. The physician orders an increase in the mean airway pressure. Which of the following would you recommend to accomplish this?
I.   Increase expiratory time.
II.   Increase the pressure limit if it is being reached during the IMV breaths.
III.   Increase inspiratory time.
A.   I
B.   III
C.   I, II
D.   II, III

26.   A 42-year-old female patient has Guillain-Barré syndrome. Which of the following bedside spirometry tests is most important to follow to determine her need for mechanical ventilation?
A.   Decreased expiratory reserve volume
B.   Decreased peak flow
C.   When her vital capacity equals her tidal volume
D.   Increased residual volume

27.   Two days after surgery to remove her spleen, a 52-year-old patient is able to reach her incentive spirometry goal of 1.5 liters. The respiratory therapist should recommend the following to encourage the patient to increase her performance.
A.   Change to IPPB with a tidal volume of 2 liters.
B.   See if morphine and Valium can be given to decrease the patient's anxiety.
C.   The patient's goal should be increased to 2 liters.
D.   Change the patient to a hand-held nebulizer treatment with normal saline.

28. A patient is being managed on a volume ventilator with the following settings:

   Tidal volume = 850 ml
   Rate = 10/minute
   Minute volume = 8.8 liters
   Oxygen = 35%

   The following arterial blood gas results are found on these settings:

   PaO_2 = 51 torr
   $PaCO_2$ = 53 torr
   pH = 7.30
   Bicarbonate = 24 mEq/L
   SaO_2 = 85%

   Based on this information, what should the respiratory therapist do?
   A. Decrease the tidal volume, increase the respiratory rate, and keep the same oxygen percentage.
   B. Increase the inspired oxygen percentage and add mechanical dead space.
   C. Increase the oxygen percentage and increase either minute volume or tidal volume.
   D. Increase the inspired oxygen, increase the rate, and decrease the tidal volume to keep the same minute volume.

29. A patient in the intensive care unit complains of sudden, crushing substernal chest pain. Which of the following should you do first?
   A. Perform electrocardiogram monitoring on the patient.
   B. Analyze the patient's arterial blood gases.
   C. Recommend that a chest x-ray be taken.
   D. Defibrillate the patient.

30. A 70 kg (154 lb) patient with advance emphysema is being cared for on a volume ventilator. The following settings and blood gases have been recorded:

	10:00 AM	*11:00AM*
Tidal volume	600 ml	600 ml
Rate	10/minute	13/minute
Oxygen	35%	35%
PaO_2	71 torr	64 torr
$PaCO_2$	64 torr	71 torr
pH	7.31	7.28
HCO_3^-	36 mEq/L	36 mEq/L

   Based on this information, which of the following would you recommend to correct the blood gases?
   A. Increase the inspired oxygen to 45%.
   B. Add 5 cm water of PEEP.
   C. Add inflation hold.
   D. Make an increase in the tidal volume.

31. All the following are assessed to determine the Apgar score EXCEPT:
   A. Skin color
   B. Temperature

    C.   Reflex irritability
    D.   Muscle tone

32.   A 35-year-old, 300-pound patient with obstructive sleep apnea is being managed with a bilevel ventilator delivered through a nasal mask. His arterial blood gases show a $PaCO_2$ of 50 mm Hg. When sleeping he still has episodes of obstructive apnea. Ventilator settings are:

        Mode = SIMV
        Tidal volume = approximately 850 ml
        Rate = 10
        Oxygen = 30%
        High pressure setting = 30 cm water
        Low pressure setting = 5 cm water

    All the following ventilator adjustments would be appropriate EXCEPT:
    A.   Raise the high pressure setting.
    B.   Reduce the low pressure setting.
    C.   Increase the ventilator delivered rate.
    D.   Raise the low pressure setting.

33.   When a patient performs a maximum voluntary ventilation (MVV) test, all of the following are important for testing accuracy EXCEPT:
    A.   The patient's volume should be less than a vital capacity but more than a tidal volume.
    B.   The patient must give a maximal effort.
    C.   The patient should perform the test for 15 seconds.
    D.   The patient should breathe at a rate between 70 and 120 per minute.

34.   Which of the following cardiac arrhythmias should the respiratory therapist recommend be treated with defibrillation without delay?
    A.   Atrial fibrillation
    B.   Premature ventricular contraction
    C.   Ventricular fibrillation
    D.   Paroxysmal supraventricular tachycardia

35.   You have placed an unconscious 80 kg (176 lb) postoperative thoracotomy patient on the ventilator with these settings:

        Mode = SIMV
        Rate = 12/minute
        Oxygen = 40%
        Tidal volume = 1100 ml

    Arterial blood gases after 20 minutes show:

        PaO_2 = 93 torr
        $PaCO_2$ = 29 torr
        pH = 7.52
        HCO_3^- = 25 mEq/L

    Based on this information, what would you recommend?
    A.   Reduce the SIMV rate.
    B.   Decrease the oxygen to 35%.

C.   Add 50 ml of mechanical dead space.

D.   Change to assist/control mode at a rate of 12/minute.

36. A patient was in a car accident and broke several ribs. A pleural effusion is found on the chest x-ray. The fluid that will be drained out is most likely to be:

A.   Purulent

B.   Serous

C.   Milky

D.   Serosanguinous

37. You are working with a patient with status asthmaticus who was placed on a ventilator 2 hours ago. In checking the patient's dynamic compliance you determine that it is worse now than it was initially. What would you recommend to the physician to most rapidly improve the patient's dynamic compliance value?

A.   Nebulize isoproterenol (Isuprel).

B.   Give the patient diazepam (Valium) for sedation.

C.   Nebulize isoetharine (Bronkosol).

D.   Nebulize cromolyn sodium (Intal).

38. A premature newborn with bilateral atelectasis is breathing spontaneously. The patient is being given 60% oxygen inside an oxyhood. Blood gases were drawn from the umbilical artery catheter with these results:

$$PaO_2 = 45 \text{ torr}$$
$$PaCO_2 = 35 \text{ torr}$$
$$pH = 7.39$$
$$Bicarbonate = 23 \text{ mEq/L}$$

What would the respiratory therapist recommend to improve the newborn's oxygenation?

A.   Place the neonate inside an Isolette (incubator).

B.   Initiate mechanical ventilation.

C.   Place the neonate inside an oxygen tent.

D.   Start nasal CPAP.

39. The following pulmonary function testing results were obtained from a patient:

	Predicted	Observed	Percent of Predicted
FVC (L)	4.5	3.1	69
FEV_1/FVC (%)	70	20	29
$FEF_{25\%-75\%}$ (L/sec)	4.3	1.8	42
RV (L)	1.1	1.6	145
TLC (L)	6.8	8.9	131

Based on these results, what is the most likely conclusion?

A.   Severe obstructive lung disease

B.   Within normal limits

C.   Mild restrictive lung disease

D.   Mild obstructive lung disease

40. A physician asks you what the usual dose of metaproterenol sulfate (Alupent) would be for an adult by hand-held nebulizer. You would answer:

A.   0.15 ml

    B.   0.20 ml
    C.   0.30 ml
    D.   0.60 ml

41.   If a patient is being mechanically ventilated and needs an increase in alveolar ventilation, what is the best way to accomplish this?
    A.   Adding therapeutic PEEP.
    B.   Increasing the tidal volume.
    C.   Increasing the rate.
    D.   Giving a respiratory stimulant to the patient.

42.   Your patient had his TLC measured in a body plethysmograph and by the helium dilution method. It is noticed that the TLC in the body plethysmograph was larger. This difference represents:
    A.   Closing volume
    B.   Alveolar dead space
    C.   Helium leakage through a ruptured tympanic membrane
    D.   Nonventilated lung volume (blebs)

43.   An unconscious, hypoventilating patient is brought into the emergency room. He is a known heroin user and is suspected of having overdosed. What medication would you recommend be given to him as a respiratory stimulant?
    A.   Theophylline ethylenediamine (Aminophylline)
    B.   Doxapram (Dopram)
    C.   Naloxone (Narcan)
    D.   Nallorphine (Nalline)

44.   Which of the following is best treated with pressure control ventilation (PCV)?
    A.   Asthma
    B.   Adult respiratory distress syndrome with a pulmonary air leak
    C.   Lobar pneumonia
    D.   Carbon monoxide poisoning

45.   During the palpation of a patient's chest, it is noticed that the left side rises while the right side falls. Which of the following would be the most likely to cause this?
    A.   Left pneumothorax
    B.   Polio leading to paralysis of both hemidiaphragms
    C.   Flail chest
    D.   Pneumonia in both lungs

46.   After a patient has been extubated, racemic epinephrine (Vaponephrine) should be nebulized to treat laryngeal edema rather than isoproterenol (Isuprel) because:
    A.   It causes decongestion by stimulating alpha receptors.
    B.   It has less beta-1 stimulation while still being an effective bronchodilator.
    C.   It is less expensive because it is a naturally occuring hormone.
    D.   It causes decongestion by blocking alpha receptors.

47.   An adult patient has been weaned from the assist/control mode on a volume ventilator to a T-piece (Briggs' adapter) with heated aerosol. After 30 minutes the patient is agitated and using accessory muscles during inspiration. The following blood gases are obtained on 40% oxygen:

        PaO_2 = 59 torr
        $PaCO_2$ = 36 torr

pH = 7.42
BE = − 1

What would you recommend, based on this information?
A.   Place the patient on the ventilator in the pressure support mode.
B.   Give the patient a tranquilizer such as diazepam (Valium).
C.   Give the patient a nebulized bronchodilator.
D.   Switch to a cool aerosol.

48.   Two days after surgery to remove her gall bladder, a patient is confused and diapho-
retic. She is breathing 28 times per minute, has a pulse of 130 per minute, a blood
pressure of 135/90, and says that she cannot catch her breath. What is the *initial*
thing that you would recommend to evaluate the patient?
A.   Urinalysis
B.   Arterial blood gases
C.   Sputum culture and sensitivity
D.   Bedside spirometry

49.   Which of the following represents a pulmonary capillary wedge pressure (PCWP)
that is within normal limits?
A.   0 to 2 mm Hg
B.   4 to 10 mm Hg
C.   12 to 20 mm Hg
D.   22 to 28 mm Hg

50.   Inserting an endotracheal tube too far will most likely result in its entering the:
A.   Esophagus
B.   Right mainstem bronchus
C.   Right middle lobe bronchus
D.   Left mainstem bronchus

51.   It is most important to make sure that the following electrolyte value is within normal
limits:
A.   Sodium
B.   Bicarbonate
C.   Potassium
D.   Calcium

52.   A mechanically ventilated adult patient is being cared for in the intensive care unit.
The following data have been reported:

Urine output = 10 ml/hour
Central venous pressure = 3 cm water
Pulmonary capillary wedge pressure (PCWP) = 3 mm Hg
Mean pulmonary artery pressure = 10 mm Hg
Cardiac output (CO) = 4.5 L/min
PvO_2 = 46 mm Hg

Based on this information, what would you recommend?
A.   Give a diuretic such as Lasix.
B.   Increase the inspired oxygen.
C.   Measure static and dynamic compliances to determine how much airway resis-
tance the patient has.
D.   Increase the rate of giving fluids by the intravenous route.

53. An apneic 55-kg (120-lb) patient is being ventilated with a volume ventilator on the assist/control mode. Her ventilator settings are as shown:

    Tidal volume = 550 ml
    Rate = 12
    Oxygen = 60%
    Mechanical dead space = 75 ml

    Her arterial blood gases show:

    PaO_2 = 56 torr
    $PaCO_2$ = 52 torr
    pH = 7.32
    Base excess = +3

    Considering this information, all these individual ventilator adjustments would improve her arterial blood gas values EXCEPT:
    A.   Increase the respiratory rate to 14/minute.
    B.   Increase the tidal volume to 650 ml.
    C.   Change to an IMV mode with a rate of 12/minute.
    D.   Remove the mechanical dead space.

54. While working in the ICU you look up at a patient's ECG monitor. It shows ventricular tachycardia. You go to the patient and find him to be without a pulse. What is the best treatment in this situation?
    A.   Give the patient intracardiac epinephrine.
    B.   Defibrillate the patient.
    C.   Insert a cardiac pacemaker.
    D.   Give the patient intravenous sodium bicarbonate.

55. Which of the following tests should the respiratory therapist recommend to evaluate a patient who is suspected of having an upper airway obstruction?
    A.   Maximal expiratory flow volume loop (MEFV)
    B. FEV_1
    C.   Nitrogen washout
    D. $FEF_{25\%-75\%}$

56. You are working with a mechanically ventilated patient who is confused and disoriented. He is supposed to receive a tidal volume of 900 ml, 60% oxygen, and 10 cm PEEP. Due to his struggling, he has pulled the ventilator circuit off of the endotracheal tube several times. This results in hypoxemia and arrhythmias. What would you now recommend?
    A.   Increase the oxygen to 70%.
    B.   Decrease the tidal volume to 700 ml.
    C.   Sedate the patient.
    D.   Remove the ventilator and attach a Brigg's adapter with 70% oxygen to the endotracheal tube.

57. Your patient is recovering from Guillain-Barré syndrome and wishes to begin breathing again on her own. Unfortunately, her tidal volume and vital capacity values are too low to place her safely onto a Brigg's adapter. Currently she is being ventilated in the assist/control mode. What mode of ventilation would you recommend for her?
    A.   Mandatory minute ventilation (MMV)
    B.   Continuous positive airway pressure (CPAP)

    C. Pressure control inverse ratio ventilation (PCIRV)
    D. Assist/control (A/C)

58. A patient has been smoking a pack of cigarettes a day for 10 years. To determine if he has early small airways disease, which of the following tests would you recommend?
    A. $FEF_{200-1200}$
    B. RV/TLC%
    C. FEV_1
    D. $FEF_{25\%-75\%}$

59. Your intensive care unit patient has pulmonary edema. There is a question about whether it is of a pulmonary or cardiac origin. Which of the following would help you to differentiate the problem?
    A. Pulmonary capillary wedge pressure
    B. Systemic blood pressure
    C. Central venous pressure
    D. Pulmonary artery pressure

60. A patient you are helping to care for is on a volume ventilator and is about to undergo a flexible fiberoptic bronchoscopy. As part of your duties as the assistant, it is important that the ventilator be monitored for:
    I. An increase in the peak pressure
    II. An increase in the resistance to air flow
    III. Variable tidal volume
    A. I
    B. I, II
    C. II, III
    D. I, II, III

61. When calibrated on room air, which of the following devices would have a calibration point of zero mm Hg?
    A. Hygrometer
    B. Clark electrode
    C. Nitrogen analyzer
    D. Capnography device

62. An intubated intensive care unit patient is receiving 35% oxygen with aerosol through a T-adapter (Briggs' adapter). You notice that each time the patient inhales, the mist disappears from the end of the T-adapter. Corrective action would include all of the following:
    I. Adjust the nebulizer to increase the inspired oxygen percentage.
    II. Increase the oxygen flow to the nebulizer.
    III. Add 100 ml of reservoir tubing to the T-adapter.
    A. II
    B. II, III
    C. I
    D. III

63. The respiratory therapist has just finished assisting in a flexible fiberoptic bronchoscopy and transbronchial lung biopsy of a patient on a volume ventilator. When checking the ventilator settings, it is noticed that the peak pressure has increased markedly. What could have caused this to happen?
    I. Pneumothorax
    II. Laryngeal edema

    III.   Bronchospasm
    IV.   Hemorrhage from the biopsy site
    A.   I, III, IV
    B.   II, III
    C.   I, IV
    D.   I, II, III, IV

64.   Which of the following patient conditions is best monitored by a diffusing capacity ($D_{L\,CO}$) test?
    A.   Emphysema
    B.   Asthma
    C.   Laryngeal edema
    D.   Myasthenia gravis

65.   Your patient is on a mechanical ventilator and being monitored by capnography. All of the following would affect the accuracy of the readings EXCEPT:
    A.   The inspired oxygen percentage is decreased.
    B.   The exhalation valve of the circuit is not sealing completely.
    C.   The water trap is loose on the capnograph.
    D.   The gas sampling line is plugged.

66.   You discover that a muscular dystrophy patient being ventilated with a chest cuirass has a chest shell piece that does not fit properly. Which of the following will be observed?
    A.   The flow will increase.
    B.   The tidal volume will vary.
    C.   The respiratory rate will change.
    D.   The low minute volume alarm will sound.

67.   The respiratory therapist is checking a flow-directed pulmonary artery (Swan-Ganz) catheter. It is noticed that the infusion tubing contains only fluid. There is a slow upstroke on the pulmonary artery pressure wave and it lacks a dicrotic notch. What should be done initially?
    A.   Aspirate back 2 to 4 ml of blood, then fast-flush the catheter.
    B.   Increase the pressure on the infusion bag.
    C.   Advance the catheter and recheck the pressure waveform.
    D.   Make sure that the transducer is set at the proper level.

68.   When doing equipment rounds, the respiratory therapist notices that a mist tent does not have as much aerosol in it as it did before. All the following could be the cause EXCEPT:
    A.   The nebulizer water reservoir jar is filled to just over the "refill" line.
    B.   The gas flow into the nebulizer jet has been decreased.
    C.   The water reservoir jar is partially unscrewed from the base of the nebulizer.
    D.   The capillary tube is partially obstructed with debris.

69.   When assembling an independent high frequency jet ventilator system, all the following are needed EXCEPT:
    A.   Humidification system
    B.   High pressure oxygen source
    C.   Injector line or adapter
    D.   Spirometer for measuring exhaled volume

70. When calibrating a thermal conductivity helium analyzer with room air, it should read:
    A. 100%
    B. The partial pressure of atmospheric helium
    C. 20.95%
    D. Zero

71. An automobile accident victim has suffered multiple injuries including several broken ribs and a pulmonary contusion. The decision has been made to intubate the patient and institute mechanical ventilation. Due to extreme pain and agitation the patient will be medicated. What would you recommend for the control of pain and to ensure that the patient does not fight against the ventilator?
    A. Diazepam (Valium)
    B. Succinylcholine chloride (Anectine)
    C. Morhpine sulfate (morphine)
    D. Neostigmine bromide (Prostigmin)

72. A 55-year-old patient with emphysema is receiving IPPB for the delivery of an aerosol-ized bronchodilator. His I : E ratio is 1 : 2 and expiratory wheezing can be heard. Which of the following is indicated?
    A. Add inflation hold until the wheezing is minimized.
    B. Add a mucolytic acetylcysteine (Mucomyst).
    C. Add expiratory retard until the wheezing is minimized.
    D. Increase the tidal volume by increasing the set pressure.

73. What would be the most likely cause of bilateral fluffy infiltrates seen on a chest x-ray?
    A. Hemothorax
    B. Pulmonary edema
    C. Neoplasm
    D. Emphysema

74. All the following would be needed to prepare for a transtracheal oxygen catheter insertion EXCEPT:
    A. Nasal catheter
    B. Chain-link necklace
    C. Wire guide
    D. Oxygen tubing

75. You are assisting the physician with the synchronous cardioversion of a conscious, sedated patient. After the first attempt, it is noticed that the unit did not discharge. What should you check?
    I. Make sure that the electrocardiogram monitor shows an R wave.
    II. Make sure that the defibrillator is properly charged.
    III. Check that the chest leads are on properly.
    IV. Make sure that the electrocardiogram monitor shows a T wave.
    A. I
    B. II
    C. III, IV
    D. I, II, III

76. The following are observed when evaluating a patient breathing spontaneously through the natural airway: tachypnea, tracheal deviation to the left, decreased breath

sounds on the right, and hyperresonant percussion note on the right. Which is the most likely etiology to cause this?

A. Tension pneumothorax
B. Bronchiectasis
C. Pneumomediastinum
D. Status asthamaticus

77. A 17-year-old asthmatic patient has had a reoccurance of bronchospasm. The physician wants to increase the dose of bronchodilator. She asks you to calculate how much 1 : 100 isoproterenol (Isuprel) it would take to deliver 4 mg of active ingredient by hand-held nebulizer.

A. 40 ml
B. 0.4 ml
C. 4 ml
D. 0.2 ml

78. Your patient is being maintained on a Siemens Servo 900 C ventilator with the following settings:

    Rate = 10/minute
    Minute volume = 8 liters
    Oxygen = 40%
    Inspiratory time = 25%
    Pause time = 0%

To improve the patient's oxygenation the physician wants to begin pressure control inverse ratio ventilation. The most appropriate thing to do in this situation is:

A. Add 10% pause time
B. Increase the inspiratory time percentage.
C. Decrease the respiratory rate
D. Increase the minute volume by 10%

79. You are working with a patient who was rescued from a house fire. A pulse oximetry probe attached to his finger shows an SpO_2 reading of 99%. An arterial blood gas drawn with the patient wearing a non-rebreather mask has been analyzed through a CO oximeter. The results show a PaO_2 of 130 mm Hg, $PaCO_2$ of 30 mm Hg, and SaO_2 of 75%. What would best explain the differences in saturation?

A. The CO oximeter is out of calibration.
B. The patient has a higher than normal level of carboxyhemoglobin (COHb).
C. The measuring cuvette has been incorrectly placed.
D. The patient's skin is darkly pigmented.

80. Your mechanically ventilated patient has a central venous pressure (CVP) catheter in place. When would be the most appropriate time to make a CVP reading?

A. During the plateau pressure
B. At the end of exhalation
C. At the beginning of inspiration
D. At the peak airway pressure

81. When making a home care visit, the patient tells the respiratory therapist that she cannot feel any oxygen coming out of the nasal cannula. In addition, the oxygen concentrator is seen to have an alarm light on and to be making cycling noises. The respiratory therapist checks the cannula and finds that no gas is coming through the

prongs. Based on this information, the respiratory therapist should do all the following EXCEPT:
  A.   Add water to the humidifier bottle.
  B.   Put the patient on her back-up system of an oxygen tank.
  C.   Check the cannula tubing to look for a kink or knot.
  D.   Feel if any gas is leaving the oxygen concentrator.

82.   A patient has a -15 cm water pressure maximum inspiratory pressure (MIP) during a bedside test. What can you conclude from this result?
  I.   The patient has weak inspiratory muscles.
  II.   The patient has restrictive lung disease.
  III. The patient has obstructive airways disease.
  A.   I
  B.   II
  C.   I, II
  D.   I, III

83.   It is important to follow the sequence of pressures seen during the insertion of a flow-directed pulmonary artery (Swan-Ganz) catheter. Which of the following would indicate that the tip of the catheter has entered the pulmonary artery?
  A.   120/80 mm Hg
  B.   25/8 mm Hg
  C.   10 mm Hg
  D.   25/0 mm Hg

84.   You are assisting during a CPR attempt. The physician asks you to recommend the type of airway to place into the patient because she will be put on a mechanical ventilator. Based on this information, you would recommend:
  A.   Performing a tracheotomy to place a tracheostomy tube
  B.   Placing an oral endotracheal tube
  C.   Inserting an oral airway and strapping a resuscitation mask onto the patient
  D.   Placing a nasotracheal tube

85.   Four days after abdominal surgery a 65-year-old patient has a fever and a white blood cell count of 21,000/mm³. Her chest x-ray shows patchy infiltrates in both lung fields with air bronchograms. What is the most likely diagnosis of her condition?
  A.   Atelectasis
  B.   Pulmonary edema
  C.   Pleural effusion
  D.   Pneumonia

86.   You are assisting with CPR on an intubated patient with asystole. Neither the nurse nor physician is able to start an intravenous line. What would you now suggest to help with the resuscitation attempt?
  A.   Give the patient intracardiac epinephrine.
  B.   Call a surgeon to start an intravenous line in the subclavian vein.
  C.   Give the patient sodium bicarbonate by instilling it down the endotracheal tube.
  D.   Give the patient epinephrine by instilling it down the endotracheal tube.

87.   A patient should be extubated at peak inspiration to:
  A.   Ensure carbon dioxide removal
  B.   Provide a large enough volume for an effective cough to remove secretions
  C.   Not injure the vocal cords
  D.   Ensure that the lungs are full of supplemental oxygen

88. The respiratory therapist is working with a neonate with infant respiratory distress syndrome (IRDS) and an occasional patent ductus arteriosus. The physician wants transcutaneous oxygen monitoring used on the patient. Where would you recommend an electrode be placed?
    I. Abdomen
    II. Upper part of the right chest
    III. Right thigh
    IV. Left thigh
    V. Upper part of the left chest
    A. II
    B. II, V
    C. III, IV
    D. I, V

89. Calculate the dead space volume given the following:

    PaO_2 = 85 mm Hg
    PvO_2 = 39 mm Hg
    $PaCO_2$ = 45 mm Hg
    P_ECO_2 = 25 mm Hg
    Tidal volume = 700 ml

    A. 444 ml
    B. 252 ml
    C. 380 ml
    D. 310 ml

90. A 28-year-old patient is brought into the emergency room. He has a cervical spine injury from a diving accident and is wearing a neck brace. The patient is unconscious and inspiratory stridor can be heard. Arterial blood gases on 40% oxygen show: PaO_2 57, $PaCO_2$ 56, and pH 7.30. The physician has decided to establish a secure airway. What device would you recommend be used:
    A. 7 mm nasotracheal tube
    B. Berman oral airway
    C. 6 mm nasopharyngeal airway
    D. 9 mm nasotracheal tube

91. A lecithin/sphingomyelin (L/S) ratio of 1 : 1 is found during an amniocentesis before a neonate is delivered by cesarean section. Based on this, the neonate will probably show:
    A. Expiratory grunting
    B. Bradycardia
    C. Kussmaul's breathing
    D. Strong reflex irritability

92. Which of the following conditions can cause an increase in the V_D/V_T ratio?
    A. Pleural effusion
    B. Tracheostomy
    C. Pulmonary embolism
    D. Laryngotracheobronchitis

93. When selecting a suction catheter to be placed through an endotracheal tube, it is important that:
    A. The catheter is no more than one fourth the internal diameter of the endotracheal tube.

B.   The catheter is no more than three fourths the internal diameter of the endotracheal tube.
C.   The catheter is no more than one half the internal diameter of the endotracheal tube.
D.   It should be as close to the internal diameter of the endotracheal tube as possible.

94.   You are working in the intensive care unit with a patient on a mechanical ventilator. She has a flow-directed pulmonary artery (Swan-Ganz) catheter that can give continuous data on SvO_2. The nurse calls you over to help in interpreting the most recent mixed venous blood gas values: PvO_2 of 27 mm Hg and SvO_2 of 54%. How would you interpret these values?
A.   The peak pressure on the ventilator is artifically lowering the patient's values.
B.   The patient is adequately oxygenated.
C.   They cannot be interpreted because there are no venous pH and $PvCO_2$ values or arterial blood gas values for a comparison.
D.   The patient is hypoxemic.

95.   The respiratory therapist is performing quality control procedures on regulators and flowmeters. If a flowmeter is backpressure compensated, which of the following will be seen?
A.   The float will move up if a resistance is placed at the outlet.
B.   The gas density inside the tube will decrease as the resistance is increased.
C.   The float will move down if a resistance is placed at the outlet.
D.   A needle valve is placed between the gas inlet and the flow tube.
E.   The float will not move if a resistance is placed at the outlet.

96.   All the following parameters indicate that your patient can be successfully extubated EXCEPT:
A.   The alveolar-arterial difference in oxygen $P(A - a)O_2$ on 100% oxygen is 85 mm Hg.
B.   There are few tracheal secretions.
C.   The patient has a vital capacity of 17 ml/kg of body weight.
D.   The patient is in a coma.

97.   A 45-year-old patient has a high resistance to inspiratory flow because of a tracheal tumor. Despite being managed on a volume ventilator, gas distribution is unequal throughout the lungs. What should the respiratory therapist recommend to correct this problem?
A.   Increase the inspiratory flow.
B.   Decrease the tidal volume.
C.   Add an inspiratory plateau.
D.   Increase the tidal volume.

98.   The respiratory therapist is assisting the physician during a tracheostomy procedure on a patient with a nasal endotracheal tube. When should the endotracheal tube be withdrawn?
A.   As the cartilage of the trachea is being removed.
B.   Before the trachea is entered to form the tracheostomy opening.
C.   As the tracheostomy tube is being inserted.
D.   Before the skin is cut.

99.   The differential diagnosis of central versus obstructive sleep apnea requires the following information:
I.   EEG

II. Nasal air flow
III. ECG
IV. Chest wall and abdominal wall impedence (movement)
A. II
B. III, IV
C. I, II, III
D. II, IV

100. All of the following are indications to stop an exercise test EXCEPT:
A. Angina pectoris is felt.
B. The patient is nauseated.
C. The patient's blood pressure is 265/135.
D. The patient's SpO_2 is 91%.

⟨END OF EXAMINATION⟩

Answer Key

1. B;	26. C;	51. C;	76. A;
2. C;	27. C;	52. D;	77. B;
3. A;	28. C;	53. C;	78. B;
4. C;	29. A;	54. B;	79. B;
5. B;	30. D;	55. A;	80. B;
6. D;	31. B;	56. C;	81. A;
7. D;	32. B;	57. A;	82. A;
8. D;	33. C;	58. D;	83. B;
9. A;	34. C;	59. A;	84. B;
10. B;	35. A;	60. D;	85. D;
11. B;	36. D;	61. D;	86. D;
12. D;	37. C;	62. B;	87. B;
13. D;	38. D;	63. A;	88. B;
14. B;	39. A;	64. A;	89. D;
15. A;	40. C;	65. A;	90. A;
16. D;	41. B;	66. B;	91. A;
17. C;	42. D;	67. A;	92. C;
18. D;	43. C;	68. A;	93. C;
19. D;	44. B;	69. D;	94. D;
20. B;	45. C;	70. D;	95. C;
21. C;	46. A;	71. C;	96. D;
22. C;	47. A;	72. C;	97. C;
23. D;	48. B;	73. B;	98. C;
24. D;	49. B;	74. A;	99. D;
25. D;	50. B;	75. D;	100. D.

Explanations for the Practice Written Registry Examination

Code: c = Correct
      a = Acceptable but not best
      u = Unsatisfactory
      h = Potentially harmful

Interpretation of the Final Score

The National Board for Respiratory Care (NBRC) has set a minimum pass level of 70% for the Written Registry Exam. However, a raw score of 70 correct out of 100 questions may not be the minimum passing score. This is because each question is individually weighted based on its difficulty. For example, Recall questions are less valuable than Analysis questions. A multiplier for the exam is determined based on the total mix of questions. Historically, this has resulted in the examinee needing a raw score only in the mid to upper 60% range to pass the exam.

It is not possible to develop a multiplier for this practice exam. Use 70 correct answers for the minimum pass level. The student or examinee who takes this practice exam should not feel too encouraged or discouraged by either passing or failing it. Instead, it should be used to identify areas that may need improvement. Continue to study so that you are better prepared to pass the actual NBRC examination.

1.
u A. Right ventricular pressure is only seen as the catheter passes through the chamber.
c B. With the balloon inflated, the pulmonary capillary wedge pressure reflects pressure changes in the left atrium.
u C. Right atrial pressure is only seen as the catheter passes through the chamber.
u D. This pressure is seen when the balloon is left deflated.

2.
u A. See C.
u B. See C.
c C. The following two equations are used to derive the answer:

TLC (total lung capacity) = VC (vital capacity) + RV (residual volume)

$$TLC = 3500 + 2800$$
$$TLC = 6300\,ml$$

RV = FRC (functional residual capacity) − ERV (expiratory reserve volume)

$$RV = 4000 - 1200$$
$$RV = 2800$$

u D. See C.

3.
c A. This should increase the patient's functional residual capacity and decrease the shunt percentage.
u B. This will not affect the shunt percentage.
u C. Same as B.
u D. Same as B.

4.
u   A.   If this were true, the bag would not collapse.
u   B.   If this were true, the bag would overinflate.
c   C.   Raising the flow of gas should result in the bag refilling.
u   D.   This gas mix is less dense than room air or oxygen.

5.
u   A.   This is seen in a pneumothorax.
c   B.   Air in the tissues makes them more lucent; they will be darker on the chest x-ray.
u   C.   This is seen in a tension pneumothorax.
u   D.   This is seen with infiltrates or a neoplasm.

6.
u   A.   This would have to be replaced with a standard tracheostomy tube if mechanical ventilation had to be quickly started.
u   B.   This will not maintain a patent airway.
u   C.   This should not be used unless a tracheostomy tube is unavailable.
c   D.   This will allow the patient to speak. Inserting the inner cannula will quickly allow the patient to be placed on mechanical ventilation if needed.

7.
u   A.   This is an indication for aerosol.
a   B.   True, but not the only reason.
u   C.   See B and C.
c   D.   Both are indications to decrease aerosol output.

8.
u   A.   This may be seen in an alert adult.
u   B.   Mild tachypnea in an adult.
u   C.   Moderate tachypnea in an adult; normal for an infant.
c   D.   Normal rate in a newborn.

9.
c   A.   There is no evidence that the patient's underlying disease improves.
u   B.   This should be expected.
u   C.   This should be expected.
u   D.   This should be expected.

10.
h   A.   This will probably not be successful a second time; more power is needed. Any delay lessens the patient's chance of recovery.
c   B.   This is an appropriate increase in power for the second attempt at defibrillation.
u   C.   This medication is not indicated is this situation. While probably not harmful, it does delay the appropriate action.
h   D.   This is too great of an increase in power for only the second attempt at defibrillation. Too much power can injure the patient.

11.
u   A.   See B.
c   B.   Arterial carbon dioxide and average exhaled carbon dioxide are needed to calculate the dead space to tidal volume ratio.
u   C.   See B.
u   D.   See B.

12.
u   A.   This is an indication.
u   B.   This is an indication.
u   C.   This is an indication.
c   D.   Patients with variable airway resistance and lung compliance should be intubated and placed on a volume cycled ventilator.

13.
u   A.   A Linde Walker is ideal for mobility but is too expensive to use as a primary oxygen source in the home.
u   B.   An oxygen concentrator is ideal for use as a primary oxygen source in the home but does not offer any mobility for outside.
a   C.   An E cylinder is acceptable for mobility but not as good as a Linde Walker.
c   D.   The combination of an oxygen concentrator and Linde Walker is best for providing oxygen both in the home and outside.

14.
u   A.   See B.
c   B.   All are necessary to ensure the accuracy of the unit.
u   C.   See B.
u   D.   See B.

15.
c   A.   This is the only way to seal the trachea at a safe cuff pressure and maintain the tidal volume and PEEP.
h   B.   The cuff pressure is high enough to damage the tracheal mucosa.
u   C.   Increasing the delivered tidal volume will only result in a larger gas leak.
u   D.   Increasing the respiratory rate will only result in a more frequent gas leak.

16.
u   A.   The cardiac output is normal.
u   B.   The pulmonary capillary wedge pressure (PCWP) is normal.
u   C.   Same as B.
c   D.   The pulmonary vascular resistance (PVR) is increased. It is found by subtracting the PCWP from the diastolic PAP:

$$PVR = (\text{diastolic PAP} - \text{PCWP})$$
$$= (25 - 9)$$
$$= 16 \text{ mm Hg (The normal PVR is 2 to 5 mm Hg.)}$$

17.
u   A.   This will not tell you the cause of the distress.
u   B.   This should be done after finding that the upper airway x-ray is negative. It could help to locate a thoracic foreign body.
c   C.   The history and symptoms point to an upper airway obstruction. This x-ray should confirm or deny it.
h   D.   This should not be done. The negative force could pull a foreign body deeper into the airway.

18.
h   A.   It is potentially harmful to have the patient cough in a head-down position.
h   B.   Same as A.
h   C.   Same as A. Also, no medication can be given without an order.
c   D.   Have the patient sit up to cough to reduce the intracranial pressure.

19.
u A. This is always needed.
u B. The physician may prefer this style of blade.
u C. The physician may prefer this style of blade.
c D. The Magill forceps is only used during a nasal intubation.

20.
u A. This is important.
c B. This is not important because a heat moisture exchanger could be used for the short time the patient may have to be transported on a mechanical ventilator.
u C. This is important.
u D. This is important.

21.
u A. See C for best answer.
u B. See C for best answer.
c C. Ideally, the patient will have an I : E ratio of about 1 : 3, inhale a deeper than normal tidal volume, and generate between 10 and 20 cm water positive expiratory pressure.
u D. See C for best answer.

22.
u A. The transtracheal oxygen catheter is placed through an opening only large enough to accomodate it.
u B. A cuffed endotracheal or tracheostomy tube is needed for positive pressure ventilation.
c C. The tracheostomy button maintains the stoma until it is determined that it can safely be allowed to heal over.
u D. The tracheostomy button is not a substitute larynx.

23.
u A. This is seen with congestive heart failure and pulmonary edema.
u B. This may be seen with hyperinflation.
u C. This is seen with consolidation.
c D. The lung is collapsed with a pneumothorax so no markings will be seen.

24.
a A. True, but not the only purpose.
a B. Same as A.
a C. Same as A.
c D. All of these can be performed with a pulmonary artery catheter.

25.
u A. This will lower the mean airway pressure and result in a drop in the PaO_2.
a B. This will increase the mean airway pressure. See D.
u C. Only option II will increase the mean airway pressure.
c D. Both of these will increase the mean airway pressure.

26.
u A. This will decrease as the vital capacity decreases.
u B. This will decrease as the vital capacity decreases.
c C. Intubation and mechanical ventilation should be initiated because the patient will be unable to cough out her secretions or protect her airway.
u D. This cannot be measured at the bedside and will decrease with this disease.

27.
u   A.   IPPB is an unnecessarily expensive way to increase the volume goal.
u   B.   These medications will probably result in excessive sedation so that the patient will be unable to perform incentive spirometry.
c   C.   This is a reasonable increase in the volume goal.
u   D.   No mention was made of the patient having a secretion problem.

28.
u   A.   See C.
u   B.   See C.
c   C.   Increasing the oxygen percentage should help to increase the patient's PaO_2. Increasing the minute volume or tidal volume should help to both decrease the $PaCO_2$ and increase the PaO_2.
u   D.   See C.

29.
c   A.   Electrocardiogram monitoring is needed to know if the patient is having cardiac arrhythmias.
u   B.   This would require you to be away from the patient for an extended period of time.
u   C.   This might be a helpful procedure; however, it is time consuming when the patient is experiencing a problem that requires emergency action.
u   D.   Defibrillation is not called for without first knowing if the patient has a life-threatening arrhythmia. See A.

30.
u   A.   This will not correct the respiratory acidosis and may blunt the patient's hypoxic drive to breathe.
h   B.   PEEP is contraindicated in patients with emphysema because of the increased risk of barotrauma.
u   C.   This will have no effect on the respiratory acidosis.
c   D.   This will decrease the carbon dioxide level and result in an increase in the pH.

31.
u   A.   This is part of the score. Normally a child will not be cyanotic.
c   B.   This value is not scored.
u   C.   This is part of the score. Normally a child will grimace or sneeze if a catheter is placed into a nostril.
u   D.   This is part of the score. Normally a child will have good muscle tone.

32.
u   A.   Raising the high pressure setting will decrease the $PaCO_2$.
c   B.   Reducing the low pressure setting will result in more airway obstruction.
u   C.   Increasing the respiratory rate will decrease the $PaCO_2$.
u   D.   Raising the low pressure setting should help to prevent airway obstruction.

33.
u   A.   This would be an appropriate MVV volume.
u   B.   The patient has to perform maximally for this test.
c   C.   The test does not need to be performed for more than 12 seconds.
u   D.   This would be an appropriate MVV rate.

34.
h   A.   See C.

h	B.	See C.
c	C.	Of the arrhythmias shown, ventricular fibrillation is the only one that is immediately life threatening and treated with defibrillation. All the others are treated by medications.
h	D.	See C.

35.
c	A.	This will result in a lower minute volume and correct the respiratory alkalosis.
u	B.	This will have no affect on the respiratory alkalosis.
u	C.	While helpful, this is not enough mechanical dead space to correct the respiratory alkalosis.
u	D.	This will result in the same minute volume.

36.
u	A.	This would be seen if there were an infection.
u	B.	This would be seen if there were pulmonary edema.
u	C.	This would be seen with a chylothorax.
c	D.	This is a mixture of blood and plasma.

37.
a	A.	While this is a powerful bronchodilator, it also causes tachycardia.
u	B.	Sedation will have no affect on bronchospasm.
c	C.	Bronkosol is a fast-acting, effective, safe bronchodilator.
h	D.	Intal is only useful in preventing an asthma attack. It can worsen an existing asthma attack because it will irritate the airway.

38.
u	A.	This will not improve the neonate's oxygenation.
u	B.	This step is not necessary at this time because the $PaCO_2$ is normal.
u	C.	This will not improve the neonate's oxygenation and will make it difficult to work with the patient.
c	D.	Nasal CPAP should help to increase the functional residual capacity, which will increase the PaO_2.

39.
c	A.	The combination of low flows and increased RV and TLC are seen only with obstructive lung disease. These results indicate severe disease.
u	B.	See B.
u	C.	See B.
u	D.	See B.

40.
u	A.	See C.
u	B.	See C.
c	C.	The manufacturer's recommended dose is 0.30 ml.
u	D.	See C.

41.
u	A.	This will increase the functional residual capacity but not increase alveolar ventilation.
c	B.	This will directly increase alveolar ventilation.
u	C.	This does not affect alveolar ventilation.
u	D.	The patient may breathe more frequently but this does not affect the alveolar ventilation.

42.

u A. This is a test of early small airways disease.

u B. Neither of these tests can measure alveolar dead space.

a C. Possible, but unlikely to show a significant difference.

c D. The body plethysmograph can measure nonventilated lung volume that the helium dilution method cannot.

43.

u A. This will not be helpful with a narcotic overdose.

u B. This will not be helpful with a narcotic overdose.

c C. Narcan is the antagonist of choice in a narcotic overdose.

a D. Nalline will act as an antagonist in a case of narcotic overdose but Narcan is the medication of choice.

44.

u A. Asthma is characterized by increased airway resistance, not low lung compliance.

c B. Pressure control ventilation is indicated for patients with bilateral low compliance conditions. If a pulmonary air leak is present, PCV should help to minimize the leak.

u C. A patient with lobar pneumonia would not present with low compliance in both lungs.

u D. The ideal treatment for carbon monoxide poisoning is 100% oxygen by whatever means is necessary. PCV offers no advantage.

45.

u A. This would make the right side rise.

u B. Both sides would be affected equally.

c C. This would cause the asymmetrical movement.

u D. Both sides would be affected equally.

46.

c A. Alpha receptor stimulation should reduce congestion in the larynx and trachea.

u B. This is true but the patient does not need a bronchodilator.

u C. This is irrelevant.

u D. This is false. See A.

47.

c A. The pressure support mode will enable the patient to have greater control over his or her breathing while overcoming the airway resistance caused by the endotracheal tube.

h B. Do not sedate a patient who is failing a weaning trial.

u C. This will probably not help the patient.

48.

u A. This will delay identifying the seriousness of the patient's problem.

c B. This will identify if the patient is hypoxemic.

a C. If the patient has pneumonia, this would be needed later to identify the pathogen and best antibiotic to treat it.

u D. This will delay identifying the seriousness of the patient's problem.

49.

u A. This pressure is abnormally low.

c B. 4 to 10 mm Hg is the normal range for the pulmonary capillary wedge pressure.

u C. This pressure is above normal.

u D. This pressure is dangerously above normal.

50.

u A. See B.

c B. Due to the relatively small angle of the right mainstem bronchus off of the trachea, the endotracheal tube is most likely to enter it.

u C. See B.

u D. See B.

51.

u A. An abnormal sodium level is unlikely to be life threatening.

u B. The kidneys retain or excrete bicarbonate to compensate for a respiratory acidosis or alkalosis and correct the pH.

c C. Either an elevated or decreased potassium level can lead to serious cardiac rhythm disturbances and even cardiac arrest.

u D. An abnormal calcium level is unlikely to be life threatening.

52.

h A. Because the patient is dehydrated, giving a diuretic can be harmful.

u B. This will have no effect on the problem.

u C. This will have no effect on the problem.

c D. This will help to correct the patient's dehydration.

53.

u A. This will help to remove carbon dioxide and the PaO_2 may also increase.

u B. This will decrease the $PaCO_2$ and raise the PaO_2.

c C. This will not change the minute volume, so the blood gases will remain the same.

u D. This will help to lower the $PaCO_2$.

54.

h A. This is not called for yet. Serious complications can result from this procedure.

c B. Pulseless ventricular tachycardia is one of the indications for defibrillation.

h C. This time-consuming procedure will delay immediate care for the patient.

h D. This medication is not called for at this time.

55.

c A. This test could confirm or deny an upper airway obstruction.

u B. This test is useful in determining significant small airways disease.

u C. This test is used for determining functional residual capacity.

u D. This test is used to look for early small airways disease.

56.

u A. The patient will still fight against the ventilator.

u B. Same as A.

c C. Sedating the patient will keep him from fighting against the ventilator.

h D. The loss of PEEP will probably result in hypoxemia.

57.

c A. MMV will ensure that she does not hypoventilate while she breathes on her own.

h B. CPAP offers no support to her breathing if she should become tired or apneic.

h C. PCIRV is not indicated because her lung compliance is normal. In fact, PCIRV may result in barotrauma or decreased cardiac output.

u D. She is currently on the A/C mode and does not care for it. She cannot do any spontaneous breathing on this mode.

58.

u A. This will only be decreased if there is significant obstruction to expiration.

u B. This will be normal in early obstructive airways disease.

u C. This will only be decreased if there is significant obstruction to expiration.

c D. This test is fairly sensitive to obstructed exhalation through medium to small airways.

59.

c A. A high wedge pressure is usually found with a cardiac problem; a normal wedge pressure is usually found with a pulmonary problem.

u B. See A.

u C. See A.

u D. See A.

60.

a A. This is important but not the only thing to check.

a B. These are important but not the only things to check.

a C. These are important but not the only things to check.

c D. All three are important to check.

61.

u A. This would show the amount of water vapor in the air.

u B. There is about 21% oxygen in the air.

u C. There is about 78% nitrogen in the air.

c D. Because there is only a trace of carbon dioxide in the atmosphere, the analyzer is set at zero mm Hg.

62.

a A. True, but not the only solution.

c B. Increasing oxygen flow will increase the total flow. The reservoir will result in less or no room air being inspired.

u C. This will result in less flow to the T-adapter.

u D. True, but not the only solution.

63.

c A. Pneumothorax, bronchospasm, and hemorrhage could all result from the biopsy.

u B. See A. Laryngeal edema cannot be a problem because the patient is intubated.

u C. See A.

u D. See A.

64.

c A. Because emphysema results in loss of both alveoli and pulmonary capillaries, the diffusing capacity test is an important way to monitor these patients' lung function.

u B. Diffusing capacity is not indicated in asthma. Between attacks these patients have normal lung function.

u C. These patients have normal lung function. Their problem is upper airway obstruction.

u D. These patients suffer from muscular weakness. Their lung function is fundamentally normal.

65.
c   A.   Changing the oxygen percentage will have no affect on exhaled carbon dioxide.
u   B.   A leaking exhalation valve will allow some tidal volume to pass through the circuit during inspiration.
u   C.   A loose water trap will allow exhaled gas to escape and not be analyzed.
u   D.   A plugged gas sampling line will not allow any gas to enter the analyzer.

66.
u   A.   An inappropriate chest shell piece will not affect the flow.
c   B.   A chest shell that is either too large or too small will not fit properly and the tidal volume will vary.
u   C.   A chest shell that is either too large or too small will not affect the rate.
u   D.   There is no low minute volume alarm on these ventilators.

67.
c   A.   This will remove any clot that has formed at the catheter tip.
u   B.   This will have no affect on the problem.
h   C.   Advancing a properly positioned catheter can be dangerous.
u   D.   This will have no affect on the problem.

68.
c   A.   This will not affect the aerosol output.
u   B.   This will decrease the aerosol output.
u   C.   Same as B.
u   D.   Same as B.

69.
u   A.   This is a required component.
u   B.   This is a required component.
u   C.   This is a required component.
c   D.   Exhaled volume is not measurable.

70.
u   A.   The atmosphere contains less than 1% helium.
a   B.   Because there is less than 1% helium in the atmosphere, the analyzer is calibrated at zero.
u   C.   The percentage of oxygen is not being analyzed.
c   D.   Because there is less than 1% helium in the atmosphere, the analyzer is calibrated for zero.

71.
u   A.   This is a sedative that will not control pain.
u   B.   This will paralyze the patient but not control pain.
c   C.   Morphine will control pain and sedate the patient.
u   D.   Prostigmin is used to antagonize nondepolarizing neuromuscular blocking agents.

72.
u   A.   Inflation hold is only used with volume ventilation.
u   B.   Mucomyst will have no affect on expiratory flow. A medication cannot be added without a physician's order.
c   C.   Expiratory retard is similar to pursed lips breathing. It applies backpressure on the airways so that they are less prone to collapse. Exhalation will be prolonged and wheezing should be decreased.
u   D.   Increasing the tidal volume will probably worsen the air trapping.

73.
u   A.   The sign does not fit this condition. It should be reviewed.
c   B.   The infiltrates are fluid that has leaked out of the pulmonary capillary bed.
u   C.   The sign does not fit this condition. It should be reviewed.
u   D.   The sign does not fit this condition. It should be reviewed.

74.
c   A.   A nasal catheter is sometimes used to deliver oxygen through the upper airway. A transtracheal catheter is inserted through the anterior of the trachea.
u   B.   The chain-link necklace is used to hold the catheter in place.
u   C.   The wire guide is used to help guide the catheter into the trachea.
u   D.   Oxygen tubing is used to connect the catheter to the oxygen source.

75.
a   A.   This is necessary but not enough by itself.
a   B.   This is necessary but not enough by itself.
u   C.   The chest leads must be on properly. It is not necessary to see a T wave on ECG.
c   D.   All of these are necessary.

76.
c   A.   All the signs fit this condition.
u   B.   The signs do not fit this condition. It should be reviewed.
u   C.   The signs do not fit this condition. It should be reviewed.
u   D.   The signs do not fit this condition. It should be reviewed.

77.
u   A.   See B.
c   B.   A 1 : 100 drug concentration means that there is 1 part of active ingredient in 100 parts of the solution. Or there would be 1 ml or g of active ingredient in 100 ml or g of the solution. This converts to 1000 mg/100 ml. Set up the following proportion:

$$\frac{1000 \text{ mg active ingredient}}{100 \text{ ml total solution}} = \frac{4 \text{ mg}}{X \text{ ml needed}} \quad \text{(Cross multiply.)}$$

400 ml = 1000 X   (Divide both sides of the equation by 1000.)

X = 0.4 ml of Isuprel should be given.

u   C.   See B.
u   D.   See B.

78.
u   A.   This will hold the patient's breath in for a longer time but is not PCIRV.
c   B.   Increasing the inspiratory time percentage is appropriate. Also, the pressure limit will have to be set at a desired level.
u   C.   This will not affect the initial PCIRV settings.
u   D.   PCIRV does not usually deliver a consistent tidal volume or minute volume.

79.
a   A.   Possible but unlikely given the patient's history.
c   B.   Pulse oximeters read COHb as functional hemoglobin. Also, a high PaO_2 and low SaO_2 is usually seen with carbon monoxide poisoning.
a   C.   Possible but unlikely given the patient's history.

u D. This could result in a lowered pulse oximetry reading but have no effect on the CO oximetry reading.

80.
u A. See B.
c B. The intrathoracic pressure will be lowest at the end of exhalation; therefore the CVP will be the most accurate.
u C. See B.
u D. See B.

81.
c A. The water level in the humidifier bottle should have an effect on gas flowing through the system.
u B. The patient will need to be placed on her back-up system while the primary oxygen system is being evaluated.
u C. This should be checked.
u D. This should be checked.

82.
c A. The negative inspiratory force (NIF) is a test of inspiratory muscle strength.
u B. The NIF test is not diagnostic of restrictive lung disease.
u C. The NIF test is not diagnostic of restrictive lung disease.
u D. The NIF test is not diagnostic of obstructive airways disease.

83.
u A. This is normal systolic pressure.
c B. This is a normal pulmonary artery pressure.
u C. This is a normal pulmonary artery wedge pressure.
u D. This is a normal right ventricular pressure.

84.
h A. This surgical procedure is not indicated at this time.
c B. This is a relatively safe and easy procedure.
u C. This is only done in the operating room as indicated.
u D. This time-consuming procedure requires an anesthesiologist and special equipment.

85.
u A. The sign does not fit this condition. It should be reviewed.
u B. The sign does not fit this condition. It should be reviewed.
u C. The sign does not fit this condition. It should be reviewed.
c D. All these signs are seen with pneumonia.

86.
h A. This method of giving epinephrine is unnecessary because of the endotracheal tube route. It is also potentially dangerous—heart and lung damage can result from a misplaced needle.
u B. This wastes time.
h C. Sodium bicarbonate should not be given by the pulmonary route.
c D. Studies have shown that giving epinephrine by the pulmonary route is as effective as giving it by the intravenous route.

87.
u A. Ongoing carbon dioxide removal is dependent on normal ventilation.

c   B.   There are usually secretions pooled in the oropharynx that must be coughed out to prevent them from being aspirated.

u   C.   This is dependent on the size of the tube and how long it was in place.

u   D.   Most patients are given an aerosol mask with supplemental oxygen after extubation.

88.

a   A.   See B.

c   B.   The key to detecting a patent ductus arteriosus is to measure a difference in preductal and postductal oxygenation. To do this, a monitor must be placed in the right upper chest to measure preductal oxygen tension. Another monitor must be placed downstream from the ductus arteriosus to measure postductal oxygen tension. This second monitor may be placed on the left upper chest, abdomen, or either thigh. Measuring only preductal or only postductal blood gives only half of the needed information.

a   C.   See B.

a   D.   See B.

89.

u   A.   See D.

u   B.   See D.

u   C.   See D.

c   D.   Dead space volume $= \dfrac{PaCO_2 - P_ECO_2}{PaCO_2} \times$ tidal volume

$$= \frac{45 - 25}{45} \times 700$$

$$= \frac{20}{45} \times 700$$

$$= .444 \times 700$$

$$= 310\,ml$$

90.

c   A.   This is an appropriate size nasotracheal tube for an adult.

u   B.   Although this will keep the tongue forward, it does not provide a secure airway.

u   C.   Although this will keep the tongue forward, it does not provide a secure airway.

u   D.   This is probably too large of a nasotracheal tube.

91.

c   A.   The L/S ratio indicates infant respiratory distress syndrome (IRDS). Expiratory grunting is performed to prevent alveolar collapse.

u   B.   Tachycardia is likely to be seen with IRDS.

u   C.   This is seen during diabetic ketoacidosis.

u   D.   This Apgar sign is likely to be weak rather than strong.

92.

u   A.   This will compress lung tissue.

u   B.   This will decrease the dead space to tidal volume ratio.

c   C.   A pulmonary embolism reduces blood flow without affecting tidal volume; therefore dead space is increased.

u   D.   This may decrease the dead space.

93.

u   A.   This catheter is too small. Extra passes will be needed to remove all of the secretions.

u   B.   This catheter is too large. The patient will not be able to breathe around it and too much air will be removed from the lungs.

c   C.   This is an appropriate size.

u   D.   This catheter is too large. The patient will not be able to breathe around it and too much air will be removed from the lungs.

94.

u   A.   The peak pressure on the ventilator should have no effect on mixed venous blood gas values. A high peak pressure may artificially increase the pulmonary capillary wedge pressure.

h   B.   The patient is not adequately oxygenated. The patient could be harmed by not taking action to raise the oxygen level.

u   C.   It is not necessary to have other venous or arterial blood gas values to interpret the PvO_2 and SvO_2.

c   D.   Both PvO_2 below 30 mm Hg and SvO_2 below 56% indicate tissue hypoxemia.

95.

u   A.   See C.

u   B.   Gas density will increase as pressure is applied against it.

c   C.   Backpressure-compensated flowmeters will accurately show the flow through them in the face of resistance.

u   D.   This is seen in non-backpressure compensated flowmeters.

u   E.   See C.

96.

u   A.   This is within normal limits.

u   B.   This is normal.

u   C.   This is acceptable.

c   D.   Being in a coma places a patient at risk for aspiration, atelectasis, and possibly other complications.

97.

h   A.   This will make the problem worse.

u   B.   This will have no affect on the problem.

c   C.   An inspiratory plateau will hold the gas in the lungs for the set period of time so that it can be more evenly distributed.

u   D.   This may either have no affect or make the problem worse.

98.

u   A.   This would leave the patient without a secure, patent airway.

u   B.   Same as A.

c   C.   This would result in a simultaneous changing of the breathing tubes.

u   D.   Same as A.

99.

a   A.   Nasal air flow is necessary but not enough by itself.

u   B.   ECG is important to monitor but does not give information that relates to the type of sleep apnea. Chest and abdominal movement are necessary to follow.

u   C.   See A and B.

c   D.   Both nasal air flow and chest and abdominal movements are necessary to follow.

100.

u   A.   This type of pain indicates that the heart is hypoxemic.

u   B.   The patient might vomit.

u   C.   The patient is hypertensive.

c   D.   This is a safe oxygenation level.

Appendix 2
Practice Clinical Simulation
Examination Problems

The two problems in this appendix are modeled after the format of the actual clinical simulation problems. They should be helpful in understanding how the actual problems are designed. Use the special felt-tip marker to reveal the latent image answers. Gently rub the marker in the bracketed area until the double asterisks (**) are found at the end of the answer. Make your selections and turn to the indicated pages for the answers and analysis. Allow yourself 20 minutes to complete each problem. When finished, turn to the answer keys for scoring the problems.

Fred Smith

You are a staff therapist in a 400-bed metropolitan hospital working the evening shift. By way of pager you are called to come to the emergency room (E.R.) because an automobile accident victim is being transported by ambulance. The patient should arrive in about 5 minutes; it is now 9:00 PM. Radio communication from the accident tells you and the rest of the E.R. team that the patient is a 47-year-old male who was involved in a two-car accident. He is conscious and stable but has a chest injury and facial lacerations. He is reported to have hit the steering wheel because he was not wearing a seat belt.

When the patient arrives, the E.R. physician asks you to do an assessment of the patient and make any recommendations. Select AS MANY of the following as you think are indicated at this time:

Fred Smith, Section 1

Options	Answers
1. Heart rate	[ ]
2. Respiratory rate	[ ]
3. Blood pressure	[ ]
4. Sensorium	[ ]
5. Breath sounds	[ ]

Options	*Answers*
6. Chest symmetry	[
	]
7. Tracheal position	[ ]
8. Arterial blood gases	[ ]
9. Pulse oximetry	[
	]
10. Peripheral reflexes	[ ]
11. Pulmonary artery pressure	[ ]
12. Pulmonary wedge pressure	[ ]
13. Cardiac output	[ ]
14. Bedside spirometry: tidal volume, vital capacity, maximum inspiratory pressure	[
	]
15. Chest x-ray	[ ]
16. Neck x-ray	[ ]
17. General appearance	[
	]
18. Respiratory pattern	[
	]
19. Urine output and color	[
	]
20. Ventilation/perfusion scan	[ ]
21. Sputum culture and sensitivity	[ ]
22. Complete blood count	[ ]
23. Urinalysis	[ ]

WHEN FINISHED WITH THIS LIST, TURN TO SECTION 2.

Fred Smith, Section 2

Based on what you have just learned, which of the following would you recommend to the physician? Make ONLY ONE SELECTION in this section unless directed to do otherwise.

Options	*Answers*
1. Place a 4 L/min nasal cannula on the patient	[
	]
2. Place a non-rebreather mask at 8 L/min on the patient.	[
	]

3. Institute mechanical ventilation in   [
    the IMV mode.

                                                                         ]

4. Place a 35% venturi mask at   [
    6 L/min on the patient.
                                                                         ]
5. Intubate the patient and place a   [
    T-piece (Briggs' adapter) with
    35% oxygen and heated aerosol.
                                                                         ]
6. Institute mechanical ventilation in   [
    the assist/control mode.

                                                                         ]

Fred Smith, Section 3

Twenty minutes after starting supplemental oxygen on the patient, he is stabilized and sent to the radiology department for chest x-rays. He has had an upright
posteroanterior and upright lateral x-ray taken. When he is laid on his right side
for a supine x-ray he complains of a sudden pain in his right anterior chest. He
demands to sit up and says he is having a hard time breathing. You quickly assess
him and notice that his breath sounds are absent over the right upper lobe and his
trachea has shifted to the left. Based on this and previous information, what would
you recommend to the physician?

Make ONLY ONE SELECTION in this section unless directed to do otherwise.

Options   *Answers*

1. Place a pleural chest tube into the   [
    6th interspace in the mid-axillary
    line on the left side.
                                                                         ]
2. Have a coaxial tomography study   [
    done of the patient's chest since
    you are already in the radiology
    department. It should reveal the   ]
    problem.
3. Place a pleural chest tube into the   [
    6th interspace in the mid-axillary
    line on the right side.   ]
4. Place a pleural chest tube into the   [
    3rd interspace in the mid-
    clavicular line on the right side.   ]
5. Institute mask CPAP at 5 cm water   [
    to correct the hypoxemia.

                                                                         ]

Fred Smith, Section 4

After the chest tube has been placed, the previously drawn arterial blood gas results arrive from the laboratory. They show: PaO_2 53 torr, $PaCO_2$ 33 torr, pH 7.43, SaO_2 87%, and base excess +1. The physician decides to have another chest x-ray taken with the chest tube in place. After viewing the before and after chest x-rays, the physician determines that the patient has a right pneumothorax; a flail segment with ribs 4, 5, and 6 on the right side broken in two places; and a pulmonary contusion of the right upper and middle lobes. The physician makes the decision to intubate the patient and place him on a ventilator. The nurses's notes indicate that he is 5 feet 11 inches tall and weighs 180 pounds. What would you recommend in this situation?

Make ONLY ONE SELECTION in this section unless directed to do otherwise.

Options		*Answers*	
1.	Place the patient on a BEAR II ventilator with the following parameters: Assist/control mode, tidal volume 900 ml., rate 14, 40% oxygen, sigh volume 1300 ml every 6 minutes, 3 cm water of PEEP. Sedate the patient with Valium and relieve his pain with morphine.	[	]
2.	Place the patient on a Bennett 7200 ventilator with the following parameters: Pressure support mode, pressure level 20 cm water, 40% oxygen.	[	]
3.	Place the patient on a Servo 900 C Ventilator with the following parameters: SIMV mode, tidal volume 900 ml, rate 10, 35% oxygen. Sedate the patient with Valium and relieve his pain with morphine.	[	]
4.	Place the patient on Bird Mark 7 ventilator with the following parameters: pressure level sufficient to get a tidal volume of at least 850 ml, rate 10, 40% oxygen.	[	]

Fred Smith, Section 5

Based on your decision, what would you like to know to evaluate your patient's response? Select AS MANY of the following as you think are indicated at this time:

Options   *Answers*

  1. Heart rate   [   ]
  2. Respiratory rate   [   ]
  3. Blood pressure   [   ]
  4. Sensorium   [   ]
  5. Breath sounds   [   ]
  6. Chest symmetry   [   ]
  7. Tracheal position   [   ]
  8. Arterial blood gases   [

                                                                                  ]
  9. Venous blood gases   [   ]
10. Peripheral reflexes   [

                                                                                  ]
11. Pulmonary artery pressure   [   ]
12. Pulmonary wedge pressure   [   ]
13. Cardiac output   [   ]
14. Bedside spirometry: tidal volume, [
      vital capacity, maximum
      inspiratory pressure   ]
15. Chest x-ray   [

                                                                                  ]
16. General appearance   [
                                                                                  ]
17. Respiratory pattern   [
                                                                                  ]
18. Urine output and color   [
                                                                                  ]
19. Ventilation/perfusion scan   [   ]
20. Sputum culture and sensitivity   [   ]
21. Complete blood count   [
                                                                                  ]

WHEN FINISHED WITH THIS LIST, TURN TO SECTION 7.

Fred Smith, Section 6

Based on your decision, what would you like to know to evaluate your patient's response? Select AS MANY of the following as you think are indicated at this time:

Options	*Answers*	
1. Heart rate	[	]
2. Respiratory rate	[	]
3. Blood pressure	[	]
4. Sensorium	[	]
5. Breath sounds	[	]
6. Chest symmetry	[	]
7. Tracheal position	[	]
8. Arterial blood gases	[	
		]
9. Venous blood gases	[	]
10. Peripheral reflexes	[	
		]
11. Pulmonary artery pressure	[	]
12. Pulmonary wedge pressure	[	]
13. Cardiac output	[	]
14. Bedside spirometry: tidal volume, vital capacity, negative inspiratory pressure	[	
		]
15. Chest x-ray	[	
		]
16. General appearance	[	
		]
17. Respiratory pattern	[	
		]
18. Urine output and color	[	
		]
19. Ventilation/perfusion scan	[	]
20. Sputum culture and sensitivity	[	]
21. Complete blood count	[	
		]

WHEN FINISHED WITH THIS LIST, TURN TO SECTION 8.

Fred Smith, Section 7

Based on this information, what would you recommend at this time? Make ONLY ONE SELECTION in this section unless directed to do otherwise.

Options	*Answers*
1. Leave the settings as they are.	[ ]
2. Decrease the rate of 12 per minute and and decrease the inspired oxygen to 35%.	[ ]
3. Decrease the tidal volume of 750 ml and decrease the inspired oxygen to 35%.	[ ]
4. Increase the tidal volume to 1000 ml and decrease the rate to 12 per minute.	[ ]
5. Remove the PEEP.	[ ]

END OF PROBLEM. See the answer key to calculate your score.

Fred Smith, Section 8

Based on this information, what would you recommend at this time? Make ONLY ONE SELECTION in this section unless directed to do otherwise.

Options	*Answers*
1. Leave the settings as they are.	[ ]
2. Decrease the tidal volume to 750 ml, increase the rate to 12 per minute, and increase the inspired oxygen to 45%.	[ ]
3. Increase the rate to 12 and increase the inspired oxygen to 40%.	[ ]
4. Increase the tidal volume to 1300 ml and increase the inspired oxygen to 45%.	[ ]
5. Add 5 cm water PEEP.	[ ]

END OF PROBLEM. See the answer key to calculate your score.

Answer Key for Fred Smith

Each item available in the information-gathering and decision-making sections is scored for its relative value. The reasoning behind the score is given in parentheses. The minimum passing scores for both information gathering and decision making are provided at the end of this answer key. Also, the best pathway and an acceptable pathway through the decision-making sections are provided at the end of this answer key.

Try to avoid getting too excited at passing or too upset at failing this sample problem. Rather, use what you have learned to help you prepare for the real examination process.

Fred Smith, Section 1

Options	*Answers*	*Score*
1. Heart rate	120/minute (Vital signs are fast and easy to measure and give important information.)	+2
2. Respiratory rate	20/minute (Same reasons as heart rate.)	+2
3. Blood pressure	110/70 (Same reasons as heart rate.)	+1
4. Sensorium	Alert and complaining of pain. (It is helpful to know if the patient can cooperate.)	+1
5. Breath sounds	Bilateral but diminished on right. (Fast and easy to evaluate and important in a patient with a chest injury.)	+3
6. Chest symmetry	Right anterior is not symmetrical with left anterior. (Fast and easy to evaluate and important in a patient with a chest injury.)	+3
7. Tracheal position	Midline (Same reasons as chest symmetry.)	+2
8. Arterial blood gases	Drawn, results pending. (Invasive; does give important information on the patient's oxygenation. Other values are less important.)	+2
9. Pulse oximetry	88% saturation on room air. (Noninvasive; gives important information on the patient's oxygenation.)	+3
10. Peripheral reflexes	Intact and normal. (Neither helpful nor harmful in this case.)	0

Options	*Answers*	
11. Pulmonary artery pressure	Physician disagrees. (Placing a pulmonary artery catheter is an invasive, time-consuming, and potentially harmful procedure. Not indicated in this case.)	−2
12. Pulmonary wedge pressure	Physician disagrees. (Same reasons as pulmonary artery pressure.)	−2
13. Cardiac output	Physician disagrees. (Same reasons as pulmonary artery pressure.)	−2
14. Bedside spirometry: tidal volume, vital capacity, maximum inspiratory pressure	Tidal volume 540 ml, vital capacity 2500 ml, MIP refused due to pain. (Somewhat valuable information.)	+1
15. Chest x-ray	Ordered. (Very important in a patient with a chest injury.)	+3
16. Neck x-ray	Physician disagrees. (Not necessary because there is no neck injury.)	−1
17. General appearance	Anxious, sweating, slightly cyanotic. (Fast and easy to evaluate and gives helpful information.)	+2
18. Respiratory pattern	Irregular, grimaces at end of inspiration. (Fast and easy to evaluate and gives helpful information.)	+2
19. Urine output and color	Voided 75 ml of pale yellow. (Neither helpful nor harmful in this case.)	0
20. Ventilation/perfusion scan	Physician disagrees. (Expensive, time consuming, and not indicated in this case.)	−2
21. Sputum culture and sensitivity	Physician disagrees. (Expensive, time consuming, and not indicated in this case.)	−1
22. Complete blood count	Drawn, results pending. (It is important to know if the patient has lost an excessive amount of blood.)	+1
23. Urinalysis	Physician disagrees. (Neither helpful nor harmful in this case.)	0

WHEN FINISHED WITH THIS LIST, TURN TO SECTION 2.

Fred Smith, Section 2

Options	*Answers*	*Score*
1. Place a 4 L/min nasal cannula on the patient.	Physician agrees. Turn to Section 3. (Supplemental oxygen is justified based on cyanosis and low saturation on pulse oximetry.)	+2
2. Place a non-rebreather mask at 8 L/min on the patient.	Physician disagrees. Make another selection in this section. (While supplemental oxygen is justified, the patient does not need to receive 100%.)	−1
3. Institute mechanical ventilation in the IMV mode.	Physician disagrees. Make another selection in this section. (Mechanical ventilation is not justified at this time.)	−3
4. Place a 35% venturi mask at 6 L/min on the patient.	Physician agrees. Turn to Section 3. (Supplemental oxygen is justified based on cyanosis and low saturation on pulse oximetry. It is best to give a known percentage.)	+3
5. Intubate the patient and place a T-piece (Briggs' adapter) with 35% oxygen and heated aerosol.	Physician disagrees. Make another selection in this section. (Intubation is not justified at this time.)	−2
6. Institute mechanical ventilation in the assist/control mode.	Physician disagrees. Make another selection in this section. (Mechanical ventilation is not justified at this time.)	−3

WHEN FINISHED WITH THIS LIST, TURN TO SECTION 3.

Fred Smith, Section 3

Options	*Answers*	*Score*
1. Place a pleural chest tube into the 6th interspace in the mid-axillary line on the left side.	Physician disagrees. Make another selection in this section. (This would place the chest tube into the wrong side.)	−3

Options	*Answers*	
2. Have a coaxial tomography study done of the patient's chest since you are already in the radiology department. It should reveal the problem.	Physician disagrees. Make another selection in this section. (This delays taking care of the patient's pneumothorax.)	−2
3. Place a pleural chest tube into the 6th interspace in the mid-axillary line on the right side.	Physician agrees. Turn to Section 4. (This is the ideal location to place the pleural chest tube.)	+3
4. Place a pleural chest tube into the 3rd interspace in the mid-clavicular line on the right side.	Physician agrees. Turn to Section 4. (This is an acceptable location to place the pleural chest tube; however, it is being placed through the injured part of the chest wall and will leave a visible scar.)	+2
5. Institute mask CPAP at 5 cm water to correct the hypoxemia.	Physician disagrees. Make another selection in this section. (This delays taking care of the patient's pneumothorax. Also, the positive pressure may make the air leak worse.)	−2

WHEN FINISHED WITH THIS LIST, TURN TO SECTION 4.

Fred Smith, Section 4

Options	*Answers*	*Score*
1. Place the patient on a BEAR II ventilator with the following parameters: Assist/control mode, tidal volume 900 ml, rate 14, 40% oxygen, sigh volume 1300 ml every 6 minutes, 3 cm water of PEEP. Sedate the patient with Valium and relieve his pain with morphine.	Physician agrees. Turn to Section 5. (Volume ventilation with relatively large volumes and a small amount of PEEP is justified to help stabilize the chest wall and prevent atelectasis. Sedation and relief of pain will keep the patient from fighting the ventilator.)	+3
2. Place the patient on a Bennett 7200 ventilator with the following parameters: Pressure support mode, pressure level 20 cm water, 40% oxygen.	Physician disagrees. Make another selection in this section. (Pressure support requires the patient to trigger each breath, which will prevent the chest wall from stabilizing. Also, tidal volumes will vary considerably.)	−1

Options	*Answers*	
3. Place the patient on a Servo 900 C ventilator with the following parameters: SIMV mode, tidal volume 900 ml, rate 10, 35% oxygen. Sedate the patient with Valium and relieve his pain with morphine.	Physician agrees. Turn to Section 6. (Volume ventilation with SIMV is acceptable; however, if the patient should take any spontaneous breaths, the chest wall will move asynchronously over the flail segment. A sigh would help to prevent atelectasis.)	+2
4. Place the patient on Bird Mark 7 ventilator with the following parameters: Pressure level sufficient to get a tidal volume of at least 850 ml, rate 10, 40% oxygen.	Physician disagrees. Make another selection in this section. (This unit will give quite variable tidal volumes. Alarm systems must be added on and are rather limited in function.)	−2

Fred Smith, Section 5

Options	*Answers*	*Score*
1. Heart rate	105/minute (Vital signs are easy to measure and give helpful information.)	+1
2. Respiratory rate	14/minute (Same reasons as heart rate.)	+1
3. Blood pressure	120/80 (Same reasons as heart rate.)	+1
4. Sensorium	Sedated. (Sensorium cannot be measured in a sedated patient.)	0
5. Breath sounds	Equal bilaterally. (This is fast, easy, and gives important information about this situation.)	+3
6. Chest symmetry	Equal movement. (This is fast, easy, and gives important information about this situation.)	+2
7. Tracheal position	Midline. (Same reasons as chest symmetry.)	+1
8. Arterial blood gases	PaO_2 120 torr, SaO_2 99%, $PaCO_2$ 30 torr, pH 7.49, BE −1 (Arterial blood gases must be drawn after mechanical ventilation is instituted.)	+3

Options	*Answers*	
9. Venous blood gases	Physician disagrees. (This will not give useful information about the patient's ventilatory status.)	−1
10. Peripheral reflexes	Patient sedated; cannot evaluate. (This is wasteful of time and effort.)	−1
11. Pulmonary artery pressure	Physician disagrees. (This requires the placement of a pulmonary artery catheter. It is a time-consuming, expensive, and potentially dangerous procedure that is not indicated in this case.)	−2
12. Pulmonary wedge pressure	Physician disagrees. (Same reasons as pulmonary artery pressure.)	−2
13. Cardiac output	Physician disagrees. (Same reasons as pulmonary artery pressure.)	−2
14. Bedside spirometry: tidal volume, vital capacity, maximum inspiratory effort	Patient sedated; cannot evaluate. (This is a waste of time and effort.)	−1
15. Chest x-ray	Endotracheal tube in mid-trachea, pleural tube in right side, both lungs expanded. (This is very important information.)	+2
16. General appearance	Normal coloration; not diaphoretic. (Easy and fast to evaluate and gives important information.)	+1
17. Respiratory pattern	Regular with a rate of 14 from the ventilator. (Easy and fast to evaluate and gives important information.)	+1
18. Urine output and color	50 ml per hour, light yellow. (Neither helpful nor harmful in this case.)	0
19. Ventilation/perfusion scan	Physician disagrees. (Expensive, time consuming, and not needed in this case.)	−1
20. Sputum culture and sensitivity	Physician disagrees. (Not needed because there is no sign of infection.)	0
21. Complete blood count	Normal RBC and WBC values. (It is helpful to know if the patient has lost an excessive	+1

Options	*Answers*
	amount of blood or if an infection is developing.)

WHEN FINISHED WITH THIS LIST, TURN TO SECTION 7.

Fred Smith, Section 6

Options	*Answers*	*Score*
1. Heart rate	105/minute (Vital signs are easy to measure and give helpful information.)	+1
2. Respiratory rate	10/minute (Same reasons as heart rate.)	+1
3. Blood pressure	120/80 Same reasons as heart rate.)	+1
4. Sensorium	Sedated. (Sensorium cannot be measured in a sedated patient.)	0
5. Breath sounds	Equal bilaterally. (This is fast, easy, and gives important information about this situation.)	+3
6. Chest symmetry	Equal movement. (This is fast, easy, and gives important information about this situation.)	+2
7. Tracheal position	Midline. (Same reasons as chest symmetry.)	+1
8. Arterial blood gases	PaO_2 61 torr, SaO_2 90%, $PaCO_2$ 48 torr, pH 7.36, BE +3 (Arterial blood gases must be drawn after mechanical ventilation is instituted.)	+3
9. Venous blood gases	Physician disagrees. (This will not give useful information about the patient's ventilatory status.)	−1
10. Peripheral reflexes	Patient sedated; cannot evaluate. (This is wasteful of time and effort.)	−1
11. Pulmonary artery pressure	Physician disagrees. (This requires the placement of a pulmonary artery catheter. It is a time-consuming, expensive, and potentially dangerous procedure that is not indicated in this case.)	−2

Options	Answers	
12. Pulmonary wedge pressure	Physician disagrees. (Same reason as pulmonary artery pressure.)	−2
13. Cardiac output	Physician disagrees. (Same reason as pulmonary artery pressure.)	−2
14. Bedside spirometry: tidal volume, vital capacity, maximum inspiratory effort	Patient sedated; cannot evaluate. (This is a waste of time and effort.)	−1
15. Chest x-ray	Endotracheal tube in midtrachea, pleural tube in right side, both lungs expanded. (This is very important information.)	+2
16. General appearance	Normal coloration; not diaphoretic. (Easy and fast to evaluate and gives important information.)	+1
17. Respiratory pattern	Regular with a rate of 10 by the ventilator. (Easy and fast to evaluate and gives important information.)	+1
18. Urine output and color	50 ml per hour, light yellow. (Neither helpful nor harmful in this case.)	0
19. Ventilation/perfusion scan	Physician disagrees. (Expensive, time consuming, and not needed in this case.)	−1
20. Sputum culture and sensitivity	Physician disagrees. (Not needed because there is no sign of infection.)	0
21. Complete blood count	Normal RBC and WBC values. (It is helpful to know if the patient has lost an excessive amount of blood or if an infection is developing.)	+1

WHEN FINISHED WITH THIS LIST, TURN TO SECTION 8.

Fred Smith, Section 7

Options	Answers	Score
1. Leave the settings as they are.	Physician disagrees. Make another selection in this section. (Arterial blood gases show that the carbon dioxide level should be raised and the oxygen level lowered.)	−1

Options	*Answers*	
2. Decrease the rate to 12 per minute and decrease the inspired oxygen to 35%.	Physician agrees. End of problem. (This should correct the excessively high PaO_2 and low $PaCO_2$.)	+3
3. Decrease the tidal volume to 750 ml and decrease the inspired oxygen to 35%.	Physician disagrees. Make another selection in this section. (This tidal volume will deliver less than 10 ml/kg of body weight and could result in atelectasis. Decreasing the inspired oxygen is appropriate.)	−2
4. Increase the tidal volume to 1000 ml and decrease the rate to 12 per minute.	Physician disagrees. Make another selection in this section. (The increased tidal volume will result in further hyperventilation and respiratory alkalosis.)	−2
5. Remove the PEEP.	Physician disagrees. Make another selection in this section. (Removing the PEEP will result in a drop in the PaO_2, but at the expense of losing some of the functional residual capacity. Removing the PEEP will have no effect on the $PaCO_2$.)	−1

END OF PROBLEM. See the answer key to calculate your score.

Fred Smith, Section 8

Options	*Answers*	*Score*
1. Leave the settings as they are.	Physician disagrees. Make another selection in this section. (The patient's PaO_2 is too low and the $PaCO_2$ is too high.)	−2
2. Decrease the tidal volume to 750 ml, increase the rate to 12 per minute, and increase the inspired oxygen to 45%.	Physician disagrees. Make another selection in this section. (This tidal volume and rate combination will give the same minute volume as the previous settings. The $PaCO_2$ will not be changed. It is appropriate to increase the inspired oxygen.)	−2

Options	*Answers*	
3. Increase the rate to 12 and increase the inspired oxygen to 40%.	Physician agrees. End of problem. (This should correct the hypoventilation and hypoxemia.)	+3
4. Increase the tidal volume to 1300 ml and increase the inspired oxygen to 45%.	Physician disagrees. Make another selection in this section. (This tidal volume will deliver more than 15 ml/kg of body weight to the patient. Hyperventilation and possibly barotrauma could result. It is appropriate to increase the inspired oxygen.)	−2
5. Add 5 cm water PEEP.	Physician disagrees. Make another selection in this section. (Adding PEEP should help to correct the hypoxemia. It will not have any effect on the high $PaCO_2$.)	+1

END OF PROBLEM. See the answer key to calculate your score.

Scoring

The maximum passing score for the information-gathering sections is: 45
The minimum passing score for the information-gathering sections is: 31

The maximum passing score for the decision-making sections is: 12
The minimum passing score for the decision-making sections is: 7

The ideal pathway and an acceptable pathway through the decision-making sections is shown as follows:

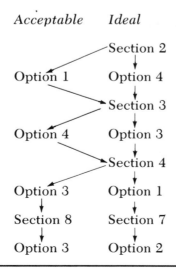

Acceptable   *Ideal*

Section 2
↓
Option 1   Option 4
↓
Section 3
↓
Option 4   Option 3
↓
Section 4
↓
Option 3   Option 1
↓   ↓
Section 8   Section 7
↓   ↓
Option 3   Option 2

Baby Wanda

You are a staff therapist working the night shift at a 300-bed community hospital. You receive a call from the nursery to come up and assist in a delivery. When you arrive, Dr. Roberts, an anesthesiologist, asks you to assist. She has put in a call for the mother's obstetric physician to come to the hospital. Because it will be at least half an hour for the obstetrician to arrive, Dr. Roberts asks you to help her in what appears to be an imminent delivery for the 42-year-old patient. She asks if there is anything else that you would like to know or if you have any suggestions. Select AS MANY of the following as you think are indicated at this time:

Baby Wanda, Section 1

Options	*Answers*
1. Fetal heart rate	[ ]
2. Fetal respiratory rate	[ ]
3. Mother's blood pressure	[ ]
4. Sensorium	[ ]
5. Transillumination of the chest	[ ]
6. Dubowitz score	[ ]
7. Mother's pulse oximetry value	[ ]
8. Amniocentesis	[ ]
9. Silverman Score	[ ]
10. Bedside spirometry: tidal volume, vital capacity, maximum inspiratory pressure	[ ]
11. Mother's chest x-ray	[ ]
12. Mother's pelvic x-ray	[ ]
13. Mother's general appearance	[ ]
14. Mother's respiratory pattern	[ ]
15. Urine output and color	[ ]
16. Fetal ultrasound	[ ]

Options   *Answers*

17. Maternal history   [

                                                                                    ]

18. Complete blood count   [
                                                                                    ]
19. Urinalysis   [   ]

WHEN FINISHED WITH THIS LIST, TURN TO SECTION 2.

Baby Wanda, Section 2

The mother, Mrs. Jackson, has been prepared for the birth and moved to the delivery room. As you are placing a simple oxygen mask on her at 4 L/min, she tells you that the baby has been predetermined to be a girl. She will be named Wanda.

Dr. Roberts calls for you as the baby's head crowns in the birth canal. It is covered in meconium. With Mrs. Jackson's next push the head is delivered. Based on what you have just learned, which of the following would you recommend to the physician? Make ONLY ONE SELECTION in this section unless directed to do otherwise.

Options   *Answers*

1. Tell the mother to push Wanda   [
   out. Place a 2 L/min neonatal
   nasal-cannula on the infant.   ]
2. Intubate the infant while telling   [
   the mother to stop pushing. Apply
   suction directly to the endotra-   ]
   cheal tube until as much
   meconium as possible has been
   removed from the trachea and
   upper airway.
3. As soon as Wanda is born and   [
   wiped off, place her into an
   incubator at 5 L/min of oxygen.   ]

Options	*Answers*
4. Use a suction bulb and suction catheter to remove as much meconium as possible from the upper airway.	[ ]
5. Have the mother stop pushing and stop the delivery until her obstetrician arrives.	[ ]

Baby Wanda, Section 3

After Baby Wanda has been stabilized, Dr. Roberts wants you to evaluate her. Select AS MANY of the following as you think are needed at this time:

Options	*Answers*
1. Neonatal heart rate	[ ]
2. Neonatal respiratory rate	[ ]
3. Neonatal blood pressure	[ ]
4. Transillumination of the chest	[ ]
5. Dubowitz score	[ ]
6. Neonatal pulse oximetry	[ ]
7. Weight	[ ]
8. Silverman score	[ ]
9. Bedside spirometry: tidal volume, vital capacity, maximum inspiratory pressure	[ ]
10. Neonatal chest x-ray	[ ]
11. Apgar score	[ ]
12. Urine output and color	[ ]
13. Lecithin/sphingomyelin ratio	[ ]
14. Arterial blood gases	[ ]
15. Complete blood count	[ ]
16. Urinalysis	[ ]

WHEN FINISHED WITH THIS LIST, TURN TO SECTION 4.

Baby Wanda, Section 4

Wanda has been moved from the delivery room to the nursery. She has been given a diagnosis of meconium aspiration syndrome (MAS). Based on what you have just learned, which of the following would you recommend to the physician? Make ONLY ONE SELECTION in this section unless directed to do otherwise.

Options   *Answers*

1. Institute nasal CPAP at 3 cm   [
   water and 40% oxygen.

                                                                                    ]

2. Intubate the infant and place her   [
   on a BEAR Cub ventilator with
   the following settings: Frequency   ]
   20/min by SIMV, 50% oxygen,
   pressure limit 15 cm water, I : E
   ratio 1 : 4, gas flow at 5 L/min.

3. Intubate Baby Wanda and place   [
   her on a Secrist ventilator with the
   following settings: Frequency   ]
   25/min by SIMV, 70% oxygen,
   pressure limit 15 cm water, I : E
   ratio 1 : 3, gas flow at 6 L/min.

4. Put Wanda into an incubator with   [
   oxygen hood delivering 30%
   oxygen. Call the nearest hospital   ]
   that can transfer her to their
   neonatal intensive care unit.

5. Place her into an incubator with 6   [
   L/min of oxygen running into it.
   Put her on a high frequency   ]
   ventilator once it arrives from a
   local rental company.

Baby Wanda, Section 5

After Baby Wanda has been stabilized on the ventilator, Dr. Roberts wants you to evaluate her again. Select AS MANY of the following as you think are needed at this time:

Options   *Answers*

1. Neonatal heart rate   [   ]
2. Neonatal respiratory rate   [

                                                                                    ]

Options	*Answers*	
3. Neonatal blood pressure	[	]
4. Transillumination of the chest	[	
		]
5. Dubowitz score	[	
		]
6. Neonatal pulse oximetry	[	]
7. Weight	[	]
8. Silverman score	[	
		]
9. Bedside spirometry: tidal volume, vital capacity, maximum inspiratory pressure	[	
		]
10. Neonatal chest x-ray	[	
		]
11. Apgar score	[	
		]
12. Urine output and color	[	]
13. Lecithin/sphingomyelin ratio	[	]
14. Arterial blood gases	[	
		]
15. Complete blood count	[	]
16. Urinalysis	[	
		]

WHEN FINISHED WITH THIS LIST, TURN TO SECTION 6.

Baby Wanda, Section 6

Based on what you have just learned, which of the following would you recommend to the physician? Make AS MANY selections in this section as you believe are indicated for proper patient care.

Options	*Answers*	
1. Decrease the amount of inspired oxygen by 10% and redraw an arterial blood gas in 20 minutes.	[	]
2. Place an umbilical artery catheter.	[	]
3. Decrease the amount of inspired oxygen by 20% and redraw an arterial blood gas in 20 minutes.	[	]

Options	*Answers*	
4. Instill exogenous surfactant to improve the lungs' compliance.	[	]
5. Begin postural drainage therapy and suction the endotracheal tube as often as needed.	[	]

END OF PROBLEM. See the answer key to calculate your score.

Answer Key for Baby Wanda

Each item available in the information-gathering and decision-making sections is scored for its relative value. The reasoning behind the score is given in parentheses. The minimum passing score for both information gathering and decision making is provided at the end of the answer key. Also, the best pathway and an acceptable pathway through the decision-making sections are provided at the end of the answer key.

Try to avoid getting too excited at passing or too upset at failing this sample problem. Rather, use what you have learned to help you prepare for the real examination process.

Baby Wanda, Section 1

Options	*Answers*	*Score*
1. Fetal heart rate	Range is between 105 to 130/minute; shows variable deceleration pattern. (Very important because it indicates if the fetus is doing well during labor.)	+3
2. Fetal respiratory rate	This cannot be measured. (Asking this wastes time and indicates to the physician that you may not be competent in neonatal care.)	−1
3. Mother's blood pressure	130/90 (Easy to perform. Indicates how the mother is tolerating the labor.)	+2
4. Sensorium	The mother is awake and alert. (Easy to evaluate.)	+1
5. Transillumination of the chest	Cannot be performed on a fetus. (Asking this wastes time and indicates to the physician that you may not be competent in neonatal care.)	−1
6. Dubowitz score	Cannot be performed on a fetus. (Asking this wastes time and indicates to the physician that you may not be competent in neonatal care.)	−1

Options	*Answers*	
7. Mother's pulse oximetry value	95% saturation. (Easy to evaluate. If the mother is hypoxic, so is the fetus.)	+1
8. Amniocentesis	Should not be performed during labor. (This would be a dangerous procedure. Suggesting it indicates to the physician that you may not be competent in neonatal care.)	−3
9. Silverman score	Cannot be performed on a fetus. (Asking this wastes time and indicates to the physician that you may not be competent in neonatal care.)	−1
10. Bedside spirometry: tidal volume, vital capacity, maximum inspiratory pressure	Mother cannot perform while doing coached breathing during labor. (Attempting to do this is a waste of your time and the mother's energy. It is probably of no clinical value.)	−2
11. Mother's chest x-ray	Physician disagrees. (There is no indication of the mother having pulmonary or cardiac disease.)	−1
12. Mother's pelvic x-ray	Physician does not think this is indicated at this time. (This would be indicated only if later the mother's birth canal seemed too narrow to allow for natural childbirth.)	0
13. Mother's general appearance	Sweating from labor; no cyanosis. (Easy to observe.)	+1
14. Mother's respiratory pattern	Normal except during Lamaze breathing (Easy to observe.)	+1
15. Urine output and color	Volume not measured when last voided. (Not pertinent. A waste of time and money.)	−1
16. Fetal ultrasound	Normal 1 month ago. (Helpful to know if there was a history of fetal complications.)	+2
17. Maternal history	This is the 42-year-old mother's first child. The baby is 7 days past term. A large amount of amniotic fluid leaked through the birth canal an hour ago and was stained with meconium. (Critical information to know because it relates to fetal distress.)	+3

Options	*Answers*	
18. Complete blood count	Not performed on admission. (Worth asking about if only to know that the mother is normal.)	+1
19. Urinalysis	Physician disagrees. (Not pertinent. A waste of time and money.)	−1

WHEN FINISHED WITH THIS LIST, TURN TO SECTION 2.

Baby Wanda, Section 2

Options	*Answers*	*Score*
1. Tell the mother to push Wanda out. Place a 2 L/min neonatal nasal cannula on the infant.	Physician disagrees. Make another selection in this section. (This is dangerous because Baby Wanda will aspirate the meconium deeply into her lungs. The supplemental oxygen will be of little value.)	−3
2. Intubate the infant while telling the mother to stop pushing. Apply suction directly to the endotracheal tube until as much meconium as possible has been removed from the trachea and upper airway.	Physician agrees. Done. Turn to Section 3. (This is probably the most effective way to remove the meconium from the lungs and upper airway. Later care will be made much easier and effective.)	+3
3. As soon as Wanda is born and wiped off, place her into an incubator at 5 L/min of oxygen.	Physician disagrees. Make another selection in this section. (This is dangerous because Baby Wanda will aspirate the meconium deeply into her lungs. The supplemental oxygen will be of little value.)	−3
4. Use a suction bulb and suction catheter to remove as much meconium as possible from the upper airway.	Physician agrees. Done. Turn to Section 3. (This is probably an effective way to remove the meconium from the upper airway. It is doubtful if meconium in the trachea will be removed. Later care will be made easier.)	+2
5. Have the mother stop pushing and stop the delivery until her obstetrician arrives.	Physician disagrees. Make another selection to this section. (This is not practical. It is also	−3

Options	Answers
	likely to be harmful to the fetus and mother.)

WHEN FINISHED WITH THIS LIST, TURN TO SECTION 3.

Baby Wanda, Section 3

Options	Answers	Score
1. Neonatal heart rate	170/minute (Very important because it shows how the infant is tolerating breathing on her own.)	+3
2. Neonatal respiratory rate	65/minute (Very important because it shows how the infant is tolerating breathing on her own.)	+3
3. Neonatal blood pressure	60/30 mm Hg (Very important because it shows how the infant is tolerating breathing on her own.)	+3
4. Transillumination of the chest	Physician disagrees. (There is no clinical sign of the baby having a pneumothorax.)	−2
5. Dubowitz score	48 (This shows the neurological and physical maturity of the newborn.)	+2
6. Neonatal pulse oximetry	83% (Easy to perform and indicates Wanda's saturation level.)	+2
7. Weight	3800 grams (Lets you know if Wanda is an appropriate weight for her age.)	+1
8. Silverman score	8 (The most complete assessment of how she is ventilating. A score of 8 indicates she is having serious difficulty.)	+3
9. Bedside spirometry: tidal volume, vital capacity, negative inspiratory force	Cannot be performed. (Attempting this is a serious waste of your time.)	−2
10. Neonatal chest x-ray	Shows patchy infiltrates in both lung fields. (This will show you if she has a serious cardiopulmonary problem.)	+2

Options	*Answers*	
11. Apgar score	1-minute score is 8. 5-minute score is 3. (Most widely accepted initial assessment of how an infant has tolerated being born.)	+3
12. Urine output and color	Output not measured; color light yellow. (An insignificant test considering the serious breathing problem that Wanda is showing.)	−1
13. Lecithin/sphingomyelin ratio	Cannot be performed. (This can only be performed on amniotic fluid. None was saved.)	−1
14. Arterial blood gases	PaO_2 47 mm Hg, $PaCO_2$ 49 mm Hg, pH 7.33, Saturation 82%; drawn on room air. (Critical information to let you know how Baby Wanda is tolerating breathing on her own.)	+3
15. Complete blood count	Within normal limits. (This is helpful to know only if it shows everything to be normal.)	+1
16. Urinalysis	Physician disagrees. (An insignificant test considering the serious breathing problem that Wanda is showing.)	−1

WHEN FINISHED WITH THIS LIST, TURN TO SECTION 4.

Baby Wanda, Section 4

Options	*Answers*	*Score*
1. Institute nasal CPAP at 3 cm water and 40% oxygen.	Physician disagrees. Make another selection in this Section. (CPAP may help to increase her oxygenation but will not correct her hypercapnea.)	−2
2. Intubate the infant and place her on a BEAR Cub ventilator with the following settings: Frequency 20/min by SIMV, 50% oxygen, pressure limit 15 cm water, I : E ratio 1 : 4, gas flow at 5 L/min	Physician agrees. Done. Go to Section 5. (These initial ventilator settings are appropriate.)	+3

Options	Answers	
3. Intubate Baby Wanda and place her on a Secrist ventilator with the following settings: Frequency 25/min by SIMV, 70% oxygen, pressure limit 15 cm water, I : E ratio 1 : 3, gas flow at 6 L/min	Physician agrees. Done. Go to Section 5. (These initial ventilator settings are acceptable; 70% oxygen is probably excessive.)	+2
4. Put Wanda into an incubator with oxygen hood delivering 30% oxygen. Call the nearest hospital that can transfer her to their neonatal intensive care unit.	Physician disagrees. Make another selection in this section. (30% oxygen will probably not correct her hypoxemia. Without the support of a mechanical ventilator she will probably tire out and stop breathing.)	−3
5. Place her into an incubator with 6 L/min of oxygen running into it. Put her on a high frequency ventilator once it arrives from a local rental company.	Physician disagrees. Make another selection in this section. (There is no way to predict what percentage of oxygen will be delivered to Wanda. It will probably not correct her hypoxemia. Without the support of a mechanical ventilator she will probably tire out and stop breathing.)	−3

WHEN FINISHED WITH THIS LIST, TURN TO SECTION 5.

Baby Wanda, Section 5

Options	Answers	Score
1. Neonatal heart rate	130/minute (This will help you to evaluate how well Wanda is tolerating being on the ventilator.)	+3
2. Neonatal respiratory rate	SIMV rate plus 5 spontaneous breaths. (This will help you to evaluate how well Wanda is tolerating being on the ventilator.)	+3
3. Neonatal blood pressure	62/42 mm Hg (This will help you to evaluate how well Wanda is tolerating being on the ventilator.)	+3
4. Transillumination of the chest	Physician disagrees as unnecessary. (There is no clinical sign of a pneumothorax.)	−1

Options	*Answers*	
5. Dubowitz score	Physician disagrees as unnecessary.	−1
	(This score would not change this quickly.)	
6. Neonatal pulse oximetry	99%	+2
	(This is important because it lets you know that Wanda is not hypoxemic.)	
7. Weight	Unchanged	−2
	(This value would not change this quickly. It could be dangerous to move Wanda.)	
8. Silverman score	Cannot evaluate on the ventilator.	−1
	(A waste of time to try.)	
9. Bedside spirometry: tidal volume, vital capacity, maximum inspiratory pressure	Cannot evaluate on the ventilator.	−2
	(A waste of time to try.)	
10. Neonatal chest x-ray	Endotracheal tube in mid-trachea. No change in infiltrates.	+2
	(It is always necessary to get a chest x-ray after intubation.)	
11. Apgar score	Physician disagrees as unnecessary.	−1
	(This is only done soon after birth.)	
12. Urine output and color	Patient has not voided.	−1
	(A waste of time.)	
13. Lecithin/sphingomyelin ratio	Cannot perform.	−1
	(No amniotic fluid was saved.)	
14. Arterial blood gases	PaO_2 125 mm Hg, $PaCO_2$ 38 mm Hg, pH 7.41, Saturation 99% on ordered oxygen percentage	+3
	(This is critical to determining if the ventilator settings are appropriate or if changes need to be made.)	
15. Complete blood count	Within normal limits.	−2
	(This is an unnecessary test because Baby Wanda's values were normal just a short time ago.)	
16. Urinalysis	Physician disagrees as unnecessary.	−1
	(Not necessary at this time because there is no indication of renal disease.)	

WHEN FINISHED WITH THIS LIST, TURN TO SECTION 6.

Baby Wanda, Section 6

Options	Answers	Score
1. Decrease the amount of inspired oxygen by 10% and redraw an arterial blood gas in 20 minutes.	Physician agrees. Done. (This will help to correct Wanda's hyperoxia. Always get another arterial blood gas value after making a change in oxygen percentage.)	+3
2. Place an umbilical artery catheter.	Physician agrees. Done. (This will make getting samples for arterial blood gases and other laboratory studies much easier. Wanda will not need to have painful venipunctures performed with the catheter in place.)	+2
3. Decrease the amount of inspired oxygen by 20% and redraw an arterial blood gas in 20 minutes.	Physician disagrees. (While helping to correct Wanda's hyperoxia, this is too great of a decrease in the inspired oxygen for a patient who is still unstable. Always get another arterial blood gas value after making a change in oxygen percentage.)	−1
4. Instill exogenous surfactant to improve the lungs' compliance.	Physician disagrees. (Exogenous surfactant is only indicated in neonates with Infant Respiratory Distress Syndrome.)	−2
5. Begin postural drainage therapy and suction the endotracheal tube as often as needed.	Physician agrees. Done. (These procedures should help in clearing the meconium out of the airways.)	+2

END OF PROBLEM. See the answer key to calculate your score.

Scoring

The maximum passing score for the information-gathering sections is: 57
The minimum passing score for the information-gathering sections is: 35

The maximum passing score for the decision-making sections is: 13
The minimum passing score for the decision-making sections is: 7

The ideal pathway and an acceptable pathway through the decision-making sections is shown as follows:

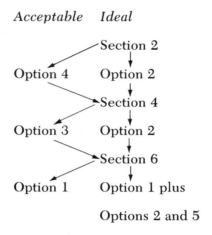

INDEX